WITHDRAWN

Advanced Information and Knowledge Processing

Also in this series

Gregoris Mentzas, Dimitris Apostolou, Andreas Abecker and Ron Young
Knowledge Asset Management
1-85233-583-1

Michalis Vazirgiannis, Maria Halkidi and Dimitrios Gunopulos
Uncertainty Handling and Quality Assessment in Data Mining
1-85233-655-2

Asunción Gómez-Pérez, Mariano Fernández-López, Oscar Corcho
Ontological Engineering
1-85233-551-3

Arno Scharl (Ed.)
Environmental Online Communication
1-85233-783-4

Shichao Zhang, Chengqi Zhang and Xindong Wu
Knowledge Discovery in Multiple Databases
1-85233-703-6

Jason T.L. Wang, Mohammed J. Zaki, Hannu T.T. Toivonen and Dennis Shasha (Eds)
Data Mining in Bioinformatics
1-85233-671-4

C.C. Ko, Ben M. Chen and Jianping Chen
Creating Web-based Laboratories
1-85233-837-7

K.C. Tan, E.F. Khor and T.H. Lee
Multiobjective Evolutionary Algorithms and Applications
1-85233-836-9

Manuel Graña, Richard Duro, Alicia d'Anjou and Paul P. Wang (Eds)
Information Processing with Evolutionary Algorithms
1-85233-886-0

Dirk Husmeier, Richard Dybowski and
Stephen Roberts (Eds)

Probabilistic Modeling in Bioinformatics and Medical Informatics

With 218 Figures

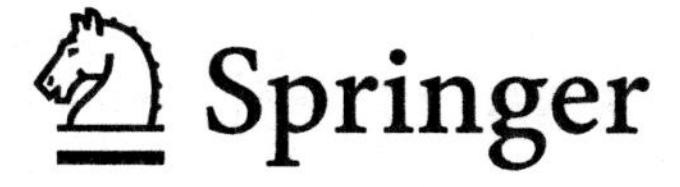

Dirk Husmeier DiplPhys, MSc, PhD
Biomathematics and Statistics-BioSS, UK

Richard Dybowski BSc, MSc, PhD
InferSpace, UK

Stephen Roberts MA, DPhil, MIEEE, MIoP, CPhys
Oxford University, UK

Series Editors
Xindong Wu
Lakhmi Jain

British Library Cataloguing in Publication Data
Probabilistic modeling in bioinformatics and medical
informatics. — (Advanced information and knowledge
processing)
1. Bioinformatics — Statistical methods 2. Medical
informatics — Statistical methods
I. Husmeier, Dirk, 1964- II. Dybowski, Richard III. Roberts,
Stephen
570.2′85
ISBN 1852337788

Library of Congress Cataloging-in-Publication Data
Probabilistic modeling in bioinformatics and medical informatics / Dirk Husmeier,
Richard Dybowski, and Stephen Roberts (eds.).
p. cm. — (Advanced information and knowledge processing)
Includes bibliographical references and index.
ISBN 1-85233-778-8 (alk. paper)
1. Bioinformatics—Methodology. 2. Medical informatics—Methodology. 3. Bayesian
statistical decision theory. I. Husmeier, Dirk, 1964- II. Dybowski, Richard, 1951- III.
Roberts, Stephen, 1965- IV. Series.
QH324.2.P76 2004
572.8′0285—dc22 2004051826

AI&KP ISSN 1610-3947
ISBN 1-85233-778-8 Springer-Verlag London Berlin Heidelberg
Springer Science+Business Media
springeronline.com

Printed and bound in the United States of America

Typesetting: Electronic text files prepared by authors
34/3830-543210 Printed on acid-free paper SPIN 10961308

Preface

> We are drowning in information,
> but starved of knowledge.
> – John Naisbitt, *Megatrends*

The turn of the millennium has been described as the dawn of a new scientific revolution, which will have as great an impact on society as the industrial and computer revolutions before. This revolution was heralded by a large-scale DNA sequencing effort in July 1995, when the entire 1.8 million base pairs of the genome of the bacterium *Haemophilus influenzae* was published – the first of a free-living organism. Since then, the amount of DNA sequence data in publicly accessible data bases has been growing exponentially, including a working draft of the complete 3.3 billion base-pair DNA sequence of the entire human genome, as pre-released by an international consortium of 16 institutes on June 26, 2000.

Besides genomic sequences, new experimental technologies in molecular biology, like microarrays, have resulted in a rich abundance of further data, related to the transcriptome, the spliceosome, the proteome, and the metabolome. This explosion of the "omes" has led to a paradigm shift in molecular biology. While pre-genomic biology followed a hypothesis-driven reductionist approach, applying mainly qualitative methods to small, isolated systems, modern post-genomic molecular biology takes a holistic, systems-based approach, which is data-driven and increasingly relies on quantitative methods. Consequently, in the last decade, the new scientific discipline of *bioinformatics* has emerged in an attempt to interpret the increasing amount of molecular biological data. The problems faced are essentially statistical, due to the inherent complexity and stochasticity of biological systems, the random processes intrinsic to evolution, and the unavoidable error-proneness and variability of measurements in large-scale experimental procedures.

Since we lack a comprehensive theory of life's organization at the molecular level, our task is to learn the theory by induction, that is, to extract patterns from large amounts of noisy data through a process of statistical inference based on model fitting and learning from examples.

Medical informatics is the study, development, and implementation of algorithms and systems to improve communication, understanding, and management of medical knowledge and data. It is a multi-disciplinary science at the junction of medicine, mathematics, logic, and information technology, which exists to improve the quality of health care.

In the 1970s, only a few computer-based systems were integrated with hospital information. Today, computerized medical-record systems are the norm within the developed countries. These systems enable fast retrieval of patient data; however, for many years, there has been interest in providing additional decision support through the introduction of knowledge-based systems and statistical systems.

A problem with most of the early clinically-oriented knowledge-based systems was the adoption of ad hoc rules of inference, such as the use of certainty factors by MYCIN. Another problem was the so-called knowledge-acquisition bottleneck, which referred to the time-consuming process of eliciting knowledge from domain experts. The renaissance in neural computation in the 1980s provided a purely data-based approach to probabilistic decision support, which circumvented the need for knowledge acquisition and augmented the repertoire of traditional statistical techniques for creating probabilistic models.

The 1990s saw the maturity of Bayesian networks. These networks provide a sound probabilistic framework for the development of medical decision-support systems from knowledge, from data, or from a combination of the two; consequently, they have become the focal point for many research groups concerned with medical informatics.

As far as the methodology is concerned, the focus in this book is on probabilistic graphical models and Bayesian networks. Many of the earlier methods of data analysis, both in bioinformatics and in medical informatics, were quite ad hoc. In recent years, however, substantial progress has been made in our understanding of and experience with probabilistic modelling. Inference, decision making, and hypothesis testing can all be achieved if we have access to conditional probabilities. In real-world scenarios, however, it may not be clear what the conditional relationships are between variables that are connected in some way. Bayesian networks are a mixture of graph theory and probability theory and offer an elegant formalism in which problems can be portrayed and conditional relationships evaluated. Graph theory provides a framework to represent complex structures of highly-interacting sets of variables. Probability theory provides a method to infer these structures from observations or measurements in the presence of noise and uncertainty. This method allows a system of interacting quantities to be visualized as being composed of simpler subsystems, which improves model transparency and facilitates system interpretation and comprehension.

Many problems in computational molecular biology, bioinformatics, and medical informatics can be treated as particular instances of the general problem of learning Bayesian networks from data, including such diverse problems as DNA sequence alignment, phylogenetic analysis, reverse engineering of genetic networks, respiration analysis, Brain-Computer Interfacing and human sleep-stage classification as well as drug discovery.

Organization of This Book

The first part of this book provides a brief yet self-contained introduction to the methodology of Bayesian networks. The following parts demonstrate how these methods are applied in bioinformatics and medical informatics.

This book is by no means comprehensive. All three fields – the methodology of probabilistic modeling, bioinformatics, and medical informatics – are evolving very quickly. The text should therefore be seen as an introduction, offering both elementary tutorials as well as more advanced applications and case studies.

The first part introduces the methodology of statistical inference and probabilistic modelling. Chapter 1 compares the two principle paradigms of statistical inference: the frequentist versus the Bayesian approach. Chapter 2 provides a brief introduction to learning Bayesian networks from data. Chapter 3 interprets the methodology of feed-forward neural networks in a probabilistic framework.

The second part describes how probabilistic modelling is applied to bioinformatics. Chapter 4 provides a self-contained introduction to molecular phylogenetic analysis, based on DNA sequence alignments, and it discusses the advantages of a probabilistic approach over earlier algorithmic methods. Chapter 5 describes how the probabilistic phylogenetic methods of Chapter 4 can be applied to detect interspecific recombination between bacteria and viruses from DNA sequence alignments. Chapter 6 generalizes and extends the standard phylogenetic methods for DNA so as to apply them to RNA sequence alignments. Chapter 7 introduces the reader to microarrays and gene expression data and provides an overview of standard statistical pre-processing procedures for image processing and data normalization. Chapters 8 and 9 address the challenging task of reverse-engineering genetic networks from microarray gene expression data using dynamical Bayesian networks and state-space models.

The third part provides examples of how probabilistic models are applied in medical informatics.

Chapter 10 illustrates the wide range of techniques that can be used to develop probabilistic models for medical informatics, which include logistic regression, neural networks, Bayesian networks, and class-probability trees.

The examples are supported with relevant theory, and the chapter emphasizes the Bayesian approach to probabilistic modeling.

Chapter 11 discusses Bayesian models of groups of individuals who may have taken several drug doses at various times throughout the course of a clinical trial. The Bayesian approach helps the derivation of predictive distributions that contribute to the optimization of treatments for different target populations.

Variable selection is a common problem in regression, including neural-network development. Chapter 12 demonstrates how Automatic Relevance Determination, a Bayesian technique, successfully dealt with this problem for the diagnosis of heart arrhythmia and the prognosis of lupus.

The development of a classifier is usually preceded by some form of data preprocessing. In the Bayesian framework, the preprocessing stage and the classifier-development stage are handled separately; however, Chapter 13 introduces an approach that combines the two in a Bayesian setting. The approach is applied to the classification of electroencephalogram data.

There is growing interest in the application of the variational method to model development, and Chapter 14 discusses the application of this emerging technique to the development of hidden Markov models for biosignal analysis.

Chapter 15 describes the Treat decision-support system for the selection of appropriate antibiotic therapy, a common problem in clinical microbiology. Bayesian networks proved to be particularly effective at modelling this problem task.

The medical-informatics part of the book ends with Chapter 16, a description of several software packages for model development. The chapter includes example codes to illustrate how some of these packages can be used.

Finally, an appendix explains the conventions and notation used throughout the book.

Intended Audience

The book has been written for researchers and students in statistics, machine learning, and the biological sciences. While the chapters in Parts II and III describe applications at the level of current cutting-edge research, the chapters in Part I provide a more general introduction to the methodology for the benefit of students and researchers from the biological sciences.

Chapters 1, 2, 4, 5, and 8 are based on a series of lectures given at the Statistics Department of Dortmund University (Germany) between 2001 and 2003, at Indiana University School of Medicine (USA) in July 2002, and at the "International School on Computational Biology", in Le Havre (France) in October 2002.

Website

The website

http://robots.ox.ac.uk/~parg/pmbmi.html

complements this book. The site contains links to relevant software, data, discussion groups, and other useful sites. It also contains colored versions of some of the figures within this book.

Acknowledgments

This book was put together with the generous support of many people.

Stephen Roberts would like to thank Peter Sykacek, Iead Rezek and Richard Everson for their help towards this book. Particular thanks, with much love, go to Clare Waterstone.

Richard Dybowski expresses his thanks to his parents, Victoria and Henry, for their unfailing support of his endeavors, and to Wray Buntine, Paulo Lisboa, Ian Nabney, and Peter Weller for critical feedback on Chapters 3, 10, and 16.

Dirk Husmeier is most grateful to David Allcroft, Lynn Broadfoot, Thorsten Forster, Vivek Gowri-Shankar, Isabelle Grimmenstein, Marco Grzegorczyk, Anja von Heydebreck, Florian Markowetz, Jochen Maydt, Magnus Rattray, Jill Sales, Philip Smith, Wolfgang Urfer, and Joanna Wood for critical feedback on and proofreading of Chapters 1, 2, 4, 5, and 8. He would also like to express his gratitude to his parents, Gerhild and Dieter; if it had not been for their support in earlier years, this book would never have been written. His special thanks, with love, go to Ulli for her support and tolerance of the extra workload involved with the preparation of this book.

Edinburgh, London, Oxford
UK
July 2003

Dirk Husmeier
Richard Dybowski
Stephen Roberts

Contents

Part I Probabilistic Modeling

1 A Leisurely Look at Statistical Inference
Dirk Husmeier 3
1.1 Preliminaries 3
1.2 The Classical or Frequentist Approach 5
1.3 The Bayesian Approach 10
1.4 Comparison 12
References 15

2 Introduction to Learning Bayesian Networks from Data
Dirk Husmeier 17
2.1 Introduction to Bayesian Networks 17
2.1.1 The Structure of a Bayesian Network 17
2.1.2 The Parameters of a Bayesian Network 25
2.2 Learning Bayesian Networks from Complete Data 25
2.2.1 The Basic Learning Paradigm 25
2.2.2 Markov Chain Monte Carlo (MCMC) 28
2.2.3 Equivalence Classes 35
2.2.4 Causality 38
2.3 Learning Bayesian Networks from Incomplete Data 41
2.3.1 Introduction 41
2.3.2 Evidence Approximation and Bayesian Information Criterion 41
2.3.3 The EM Algorithm 43
2.3.4 Hidden Markov Models 44
2.3.5 Application of the EM Algorithm to HMMs 49
2.3.6 Applying the EM Algorithm to More Complex Bayesian Networks with Hidden States 52
2.3.7 Reversible Jump MCMC 54
2.4 Summary 55

References 55

3 A Casual View of Multi-Layer Perceptrons as Probability Models
Richard Dybowski 59
3.1 A Brief History 59
3.1.1 The McCulloch-Pitts Neuron 59
3.1.2 The Single-Layer Perceptron 60
3.1.3 Enter the Multi-Layer Perceptron 62
3.1.4 A Statistical Perspective 63
3.2 Regression 63
3.2.1 Maximum Likelihood Estimation 65
3.3 From Regression to Probabilistic Classification 65
3.3.1 Multi-Layer Perceptrons 67
3.4 Training a Multi-Layer Perceptron 69
3.4.1 The Error Back-Propagation Algorithm 70
3.4.2 Alternative Training Strategies 73
3.5 Some Practical Considerations 73
3.5.1 Over-Fitting 74
3.5.2 Local Minima 75
3.5.3 Number of Hidden Nodes 77
3.5.4 Preprocessing Techniques 77
3.5.5 Training Sets 78
3.6 Further Reading 78
References 79

Part II Bioinformatics

4 Introduction to Statistical Phylogenetics
Dirk Husmeier 83
4.1 Motivation and Background on Phylogenetic Trees 84
4.2 Distance and Clustering Methods 90
4.2.1 Evolutionary Distances 90
4.2.2 A Naive Clustering Algorithm: UPGMA 93
4.2.3 An Improved Clustering Algorithm: Neighbour Joining .. 96
4.2.4 Shortcomings of Distance and Clustering Methods 98
4.3 Parsimony 100
4.3.1 Introduction 100
4.3.2 Objection to Parsimony 104
4.4 Likelihood Methods 104
4.4.1 A Mathematical Model of Nucleotide Substitution 104
4.4.2 Details of the Mathematical Model of Nucleotide Substitution 106
4.4.3 Likelihood of a Phylogenetic Tree 111
4.4.4 A Comparison with Parsimony 118

4.4.5 Maximum Likelihood 120
4.4.6 Bootstrapping 127
4.4.7 Bayesian Inference 130
4.4.8 Gaps 135
4.4.9 Rate Heterogeneity 136
4.4.10 Protein and RNA Sequences 138
4.4.11 A Non-homogeneous and Non-stationary Markov Model of Nucleotide Substitution 139
4.5 Summary 141
References 142

5 Detecting Recombination in DNA Sequence Alignments
Dirk Husmeier, Frank Wright 147
5.1 Introduction 147
5.2 Recombination in Bacteria and Viruses 148
5.3 Phylogenetic Networks 148
5.4 Maximum Chi-squared 152
5.5 PLATO 156
5.6 TOPAL 159
5.7 Probabilistic Divergence Method (PDM) 162
5.8 Empirical Comparison I 167
5.9 RECPARS 170
5.10 Combining Phylogenetic Trees with HMMs 171
5.10.1 Introduction 171
5.10.2 Maximum Likelihood 175
5.10.3 Bayesian Approach 176
5.10.4 Shortcomings of the HMM Approach 180
5.11 Empirical Comparison II 181
5.11.1 Simulated Recombination 181
5.11.2 Gene Conversion in Maize 184
5.11.3 Recombination in *Neisseria* 184
5.12 Conclusion 187
5.13 Software 188
References 188

6 RNA-Based Phylogenetic Methods
Magnus Rattray, Paul G. Higgs 191
6.1 Introduction 191
6.2 RNA Structure 193
6.3 Substitution Processes in RNA Helices 196
6.4 An Application: Mammalian Phylogeny 201
6.5 Conclusion 207
References 208

7 Statistical Methods in Microarray Gene Expression Data Analysis
Claus-Dieter Mayer, Chris A. Glasbey ... 211
7.1 Introduction ... 211
7.1.1 Gene Expression in a Nutshell ... 211
7.1.2 Microarray Technologies ... 212
7.2 Image Analysis ... 214
7.2.1 Image Enhancement ... 215
7.2.2 Gridding ... 216
7.2.3 Estimators of Intensities ... 216
7.3 Transformation ... 218
7.4 Normalization ... 222
7.4.1 Explorative Analysis and Flagging of Data Points ... 222
7.4.2 Linear Models and Experimental Design ... 225
7.4.3 Non-linear Methods ... 227
7.4.4 Normalization of One-channel Data ... 228
7.5 Differential Expression ... 228
7.5.1 One-slide Approaches ... 228
7.5.2 Using Replicated Experiments ... 229
7.5.3 Multiple Testing ... 232
7.6 Further Reading ... 234
References ... 235

8 Inferring Genetic Regulatory Networks from Microarray Experiments with Bayesian Networks
Dirk Husmeier ... 239
8.1 Introduction ... 240
8.2 A Brief Revision of Bayesian Networks ... 241
8.3 Learning Local Structures and Subnetworks ... 244
8.4 Application to the Yeast Cell Cycle ... 247
8.4.1 Biological Findings ... 248
8.5 Shortcomings of Static Bayesian Networks ... 251
8.6 Dynamic Bayesian Networks ... 252
8.7 Accuracy of Inference ... 252
8.8 Evaluation on Synthetic Data ... 253
8.9 Evaluation on Realistic Data ... 257
8.10 Discussion ... 263
References ... 265

9 Modeling Genetic Regulatory Networks using Gene Expression Profiling and State-Space Models
Claudia Rangel, John Angus, Zoubin Ghahramani, David L. Wild ... 269
9.1 Introduction ... 269
9.2 State-Space Models (Linear Dynamical Systems) ... 272
9.2.1 State-Space Model with Inputs ... 272

9.2.2 EM Applied to SSM with Inputs 274
9.2.3 Kalman Smoothing 275
9.3 The SSM Model for Gene Expression 277
9.3.1 Structural Properties of the Model 277
9.3.2 Identifiability and Stability Issues 278
9.4 Model Selection by Bootstrapping 281
9.4.1 Objectives 281
9.4.2 The Bootstrap Procedure 281
9.5 Experiments with Simulated Data 283
9.5.1 Model Definition 283
9.5.2 Reconstructing the Original Network 283
9.5.3 Results 283
9.6 Results from Experimental Data 288
9.7 Conclusions 289
References 291

Part III Medical Informatics

10 An Anthology of Probabilistic Models for Medical Informatics
Richard Dybowski, Stephen Roberts 297
10.1 Probabilities in Medicine 297
10.2 Desiderata for Probability Models 297
10.3 Bayesian Statistics 298
10.3.1 Parameter Averaging and Model Averaging 299
10.3.2 Computations 300
10.4 Logistic Regression 301
10.5 Bayesian Logistic Regression 302
10.5.1 Gibbs Sampling and GLIB 304
10.5.2 Hierarchical Models 306
10.6 Neural Networks 307
10.6.1 Multi-Layer Perceptrons 307
10.6.2 Radial-Basis-Function Neural Networks 308
10.6.3 "Probabilistic Neural Networks" 309
10.6.4 Missing Data 310
10.7 Bayesian Neural Techniques 311
10.7.1 Moderated Output 311
10.7.2 Hyperparameters 312
10.7.3 Committees 313
10.7.4 Full Bayesian Models 314
10.8 The Naïve Bayes Model 316
10.9 Bayesian Networks 317
10.9.1 Probabilistic Inference over BNs 318
10.9.2 Sigmoidal Belief Networks 321

10.9.3 Construction of BNs: Probabilities 321
10.9.4 Construction of BNs: Structures 322
10.9.5 Missing Data 322
10.10 Class-Probability Trees 323
10.10.1 Missing Data 324
10.10.2 Bayesian Tree Induction 325
10.11 Probabilistic Models for Detection 326
10.11.1 Data Conditioning 327
10.11.2 Detection, Segmentation and Decisions 330
10.11.3 Cluster Analysis 331
10.11.4 Hidden Markov Models 335
10.11.5 Novelty Detection 338
References 338

11 Bayesian Analysis of Population Pharmacokinetic/Pharmacodynamic Models
David J. Lunn 351
11.1 Introduction 351
11.2 Deterministic Models 352
11.2.1 Pharmacokinetics 352
11.2.2 Pharmacodynamics 359
11.3 Stochastic Model 360
11.3.1 Structure 360
11.3.2 Priors 363
11.3.3 Parameterization Issues 364
11.3.4 Analysis 365
11.3.5 Prediction 366
11.4 Implementation 367
11.4.1 PKBugs 367
11.4.2 WinBUGS Differential Interface 368
References 369

12 Assessing the Effectiveness of Bayesian Feature Selection
Ian T. Nabney, David J. Evans, Yann Brulé, Caroline Gordon 371
12.1 Introduction 371
12.2 Bayesian Feature Selection 372
12.2.1 Bayesian Techniques for Neural Networks 372
12.2.2 Automatic Relevance Determination 374
12.3 ARD in Arrhythmia Classification 375
12.3.1 Clinical Context 375
12.3.2 Benchmarking Classification Models 376
12.3.3 Variable Selection 379
12.3.4 Conclusions 380
12.4 ARD in Lupus Diagnosis 381
12.4.1 Clinical Context 381

12.4.2 Linear Methods for Variable Selection ... 383
12.4.3 Prognosis with Non-linear Models ... 383
12.4.4 Bayesian Variable Selection ... 385
12.4.5 Conclusions ... 386
12.5 Conclusions ... 387
References ... 388

13 Bayes Consistent Classification of EEG Data by Approximate Marginalization
Peter Sykacek, Iead Rezek, and Stephen Roberts ... 391
13.1 Introduction ... 391
13.2 Bayesian Lattice Filter ... 393
13.3 Spatial Fusion ... 396
13.4 Spatio-temporal Fusion ... 400
13.4.1 A Simple DAG Structure ... 401
13.4.2 A Likelihood Function for Sequence Models ... 402
13.4.3 An Augmented DAG for MCMC Sampling ... 403
13.4.4 Specifying Priors ... 404
13.4.5 MCMC Updates of Coefficients and Latent Variables ... 405
13.4.6 Gibbs Updates for Hidden States and Class Labels ... 407
13.4.7 Approximate Updates of the Latent Feature Space ... 408
13.4.8 Algorithms ... 409
13.5 Experiments ... 411
13.5.1 Data ... 412
13.5.2 Classification Results ... 413
13.6 Conclusion ... 415
References ... 416

14 Ensemble Hidden Markov Models with Extended Observation Densities for Biosignal Analysis
Iead Rezek, Stephen Roberts ... 419
14.1 Introduction ... 419
14.2 Principles of Variational Learning ... 421
14.3 Variational Learning of Hidden Markov Models ... 423
14.3.1 Learning the HMM Hidden State Sequence ... 425
14.3.2 Learning HMM Parameters ... 426
14.3.3 HMM Observation Models ... 427
14.3.4 Estimation ... 431
14.4 Experiments ... 435
14.4.1 Sleep EEG with Arousal ... 435
14.4.2 Whole-Night Sleep EEG ... 435
14.4.3 Periodic Respiration ... 436
14.4.4 Heartbeat Intervals ... 437
14.4.5 Segmentation of Cognitive Tasks ... 439
14.5 Conclusion ... 440

A Model Free Update Equations 442
B Derivation of the Baum-Welch Recursions 443
C Complete KL Divergences 445
C.1 Negative Entropy 446
C.2 KL Divergences 446
C.3 Gaussian Observation HMM 447
C.4 Poisson Observation HMM 448
C.5 Linear Observation Model HMM 448
References 449

15 A Probabilistic Network for Fusion of Data and Knowledge in Clinical Microbiology
Steen Andreassen, Leonard Leibovici, Mical Paul, Anders D. Nielsen, Alina Zalounina, Leif E. Kristensen, Karsten Falborg, Brian Kristensen, Uwe Frank, Henrik C. Schønheyder 451
15.1 Introduction 451
15.2 Institution of Antibiotic Therapy 453
15.3 Calculation of Probabilities for Severity of Sepsis, Site of Infection, and Pathogens 454
15.3.1 Patient Example (Part 1) 454
15.3.2 Fusion of Data and Knowledge for Calculation of Probabilities for Sepsis and Pathogens 456
15.4 Calculation of Coverage and Treatment Advice 461
15.4.1 Patient Example (Part 2) 461
15.4.2 Fusion of Data and Knowledge for Calculation of Coverage and Treatment Advice 466
15.5 Calibration Databases 467
15.6 Clinical Testing of Decision-support Systems 468
15.7 Test Results 468
15.8 Discussion 469
References 470

16 Software for Probability Models in Medical Informatics
Richard Dybowski 473
16.1 Introduction 473
16.2 Open-source Software 474
16.3 Logistic Regression Models 474
16.3.1 S-Plus and R 475
16.3.2 BUGS 476
16.4 Neural Networks 477
16.4.1 Netlab 477
16.4.2 The Stuttgart Neural Network Simulator 478
16.5 Bayesian Networks 478
16.5.1 Hugin and Netica 481
16.5.2 The Bayes Net Toolbox 481

16.5.3 The OpenBayes Initiative 483
16.5.4 The Probabilistic Networks Library 483
16.5.5 The gR Project 484
16.5.6 The VIBES Project 484
16.6 Class-probability trees 484
16.7 Hidden Markov Models 485
16.7.1 Hidden Markov Model Toolbox for Matlab 486
References 487

A Appendix: Conventions and Notation
.... 491

Index 495

Part I

Probabilistic Modeling

1

A Leisurely Look at Statistical Inference

Dirk Husmeier

Biomathematics and Statistics Scotland (BioSS)
JCMB, The King's Buildings, Edinburgh EH9 3JZ, UK
dirk@bioss.ac.uk

Summary. Statistical inference is the basic toolkit used throughout the whole book. This chapter is intended to offer a short, rather informal introduction to this topic and to compare its two principled paradigms: the frequentist and the Bayesian approach. Mathematical rigour is abandoned in favour of a verbal, more illustrative exposition of this subject, and throughout this chapter the focus will be on concepts rather than details, omitting all proofs and regularity conditions. The main target audience is students and researchers in biology and computer science, who aim to obtain a basic understanding of statistical inference without having to digest rigorous mathematical theory.

1.1 Preliminaries

This section will briefly revise Bayes' rule and the concept of conditional probabilities. For a rigorous mathematical treatment, consult a textbook on probability theory.

Consider the Venn diagram of Figure 1.1, where, for example, G represents the event that a hypothetical oncogene (a gene implicated in the formation of cancer) is over-expressed, while C represents the event that a person suffers from a tumour.

The conditional probabilities are defined as

$$P(G|C) = \frac{P(G,C)}{P(C)} \tag{1.1}$$

$$P(C|G) = \frac{P(G,C)}{P(G)} \tag{1.2}$$

where $P(G, C)$ is the joint probability that a person suffers from cancer *and* shows an over-expression of the indicator gene, while $P(G)$ and $P(C)$ are the marginal probabilities of contracting cancer or showing an over-expression of the indicator gene, respectively.

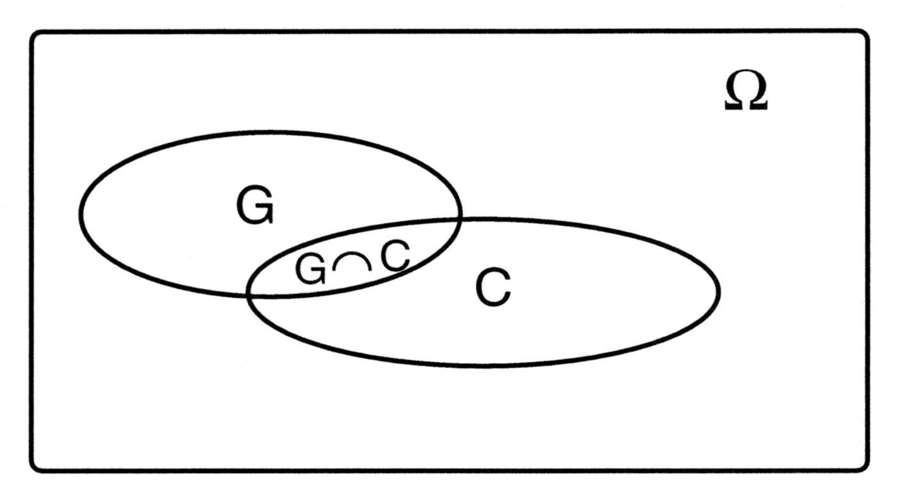

Fig. 1.1. Illustration of Bayes' rule. See text for details.

The first conditional probability, $P(G|C)$, is the probability that the oncogene of interest is over-expressed given that its carrier suffers from cancer. The estimation of this probability is, in principle, straightforward: just determine the fraction of cancer patients whose indicator gene is over-expressed, and approximate the probability by the relative frequency, by the law of large numbers (see, for instance, [9]).

For diagnostic purposes more interesting is the second conditional probability, $P(C|G)$, which predicts the probability that a person will contract cancer given that their indicator oncogene is over-expressed. A direct determination of this probability might be difficult. However, solving for $P(G,C)$ in (1.1) and (1.2),

$$P(G,C) = P(G|C)P(C) = P(C|G)P(G) \tag{1.3}$$

and then solving for $P(C|G)$ gives:

$$P(C|G) = \frac{P(G|C)P(C)}{P(G)} \tag{1.4}$$

Equation (1.4) is known as *Bayes' rule*, which allows expressing a conditional probability of interest in terms of the complementary conditional probability and two marginal probabilities. Note that, in our example, the latter are easily available from global statistics. Consequently, the diagnostic conditional probability $P(C|G)$ can be computed without having to be determined explicitly.

Now, the objective of *inference* is to learn or *infer* these probabilities from a set of training data, $\mathcal{D}$, where the training data result from a series of observations or measurements. Suppose you toss a coin or a thumbnail. There

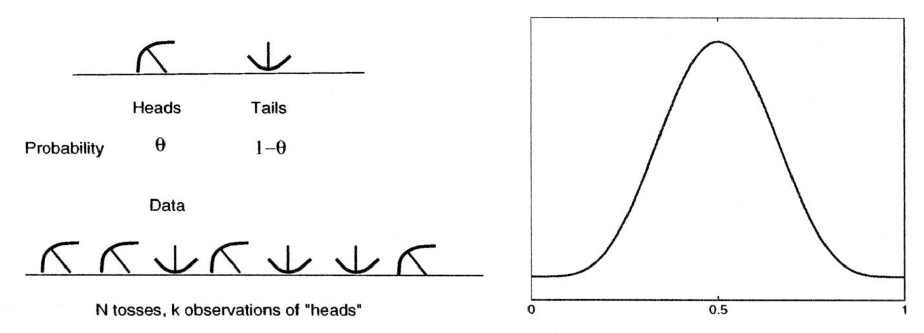

Fig. 1.2. Thumbnail example. *Left:* To estimate the parameter θ, the probability of a thumbnail showing heads, an experiment is carried out, which consists of a series of thumbnail tosses. *Right:* The graph shows the likelihood for the thumbnail problem, given by (1.5), as a function of θ, for a true value of $\theta = 0.5$. Note that the function has its maximum at the true value. Adapted from [6], by permission of Cambridge University Press.

are two possible outcomes: heads (1) or tails (0). Let θ be the probability of the coin or thumbnail to show heads. We would like to infer this parameter from an experiment, which consists of a series of thumbnail (or coin) tosses, as shown in Figure 1.2. We also would like to estimate the uncertainty of our estimate. In what follows, I will use this example to briefly recapitulate the two different paradigms of statistical inference.

1.2 The Classical or Frequentist Approach

Let $\mathcal{D} = \{y_1, \ldots, y_N\}$ denote the training data, which is a set of observations or measurements obtained from our experiment. In our example, $y_t \in \{0, 1\}$, and $\mathcal{D} = \{1, 1, 0, 1, 0, 0, 1\}$, where $y_t = 0$ represents the outcome *tails*, $y_t = 1$ represents the outcome *heads*, and $t = 1, \ldots, N = 7$. The probability of observing the data $\mathcal{D}$ in the experiment, $P(\mathcal{D}|\theta)$, is called the *likelihood* and is given by

$$P(\mathcal{D}|\theta) = \binom{N}{k} \theta^k (1 - \theta)^{N-k} \tag{1.5}$$

where k is the number of heads observed, and $\binom{N}{k} = \frac{N!}{(N-k)!k!}$. A plot of this function is shown in Figure 1.2 for a true value of $\theta = 0.5$. Since the true value is usually unknown, we would like to infer θ from the experiment, that is, we would like to find the "best" estimate $\hat{\theta}(\mathcal{D})$ most supported by the data. A standard approach is to choose the value of θ that maximizes the likelihood (1.5). This so-called *maximum likelihood* (ML) estimate satisfies several optimality criteria: it is consistent and asymptotically unbiased with minimum estimation uncertainty; see, for instance, [1] and [5]. Note, however, that the unbiasedness of the ML estimate is an asymptotic result, which is occasionally

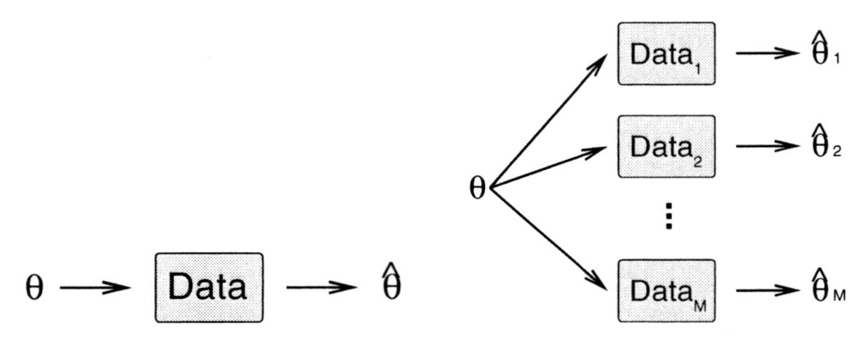

Fig. 1.3. The frequentist paradigm. *Left:* Data are generated by some process with true, but unknown parameters θ. The parameters are estimated from the data with maximum likelihood, leading to the estimate $\hat{\theta}$. This estimate is a function of the data, which themselves are subject to random variation. *Right:* When the data-generating process is repeated M times, we obtain an ensemble of M identically and independently distributed data sets. Repeating the estimation on each of these data sets gives an ensemble of estimates $\hat{\theta}_1, \ldots, \hat{\theta}_M$, from which the intrinsic estimation uncertainty can be determined.

severely violated for small sample sizes. Figure 1.2, right, shows that for the thumbnail problem, the likelihood has its maximum at the true value of θ. To obtain the ML estimate analytically, we take a log transformation, which simplifies the mathematical derivations considerably and does not, due to its strict monotonicity, affect the location of the maximum. Define $C = \log \binom{N}{k}$, which is a constant independent of the parameter θ. Setting the derivative of the *log likelihood* to zero gives:

$$\log P(D|\theta) = k \log \theta + (N - k) \log(1 - \theta) + C \tag{1.6}$$

$$\frac{d}{d\theta} \log P(D|\theta) = \frac{k}{\theta} - \frac{N - k}{1 - \theta} = 0 \tag{1.7}$$

which results in the following intuitively plausible maximum likelihood estimate:

$$\hat{\theta} = \frac{k}{N} \tag{1.8}$$

Hence the maximum likelihood estimate for θ, the probability of observing heads, is given by the relative frequency of the occurrence of heads.

Now, the number of observed heads, k, is a random variable, which is susceptible to statistical fluctuations. These fluctuations imply that the maximum likelihood estimate itself is subject to statistical fluctuations, and our next objective is to estimate the ensuing estimation uncertainty. Figure 1.3 illustrates the philosophical concept on which the classical or frequentist approach to this problem is based. The data, $\mathcal{D}$, are generated by some unknown process of interest. From these data, we want to estimate the parameters θ of a model for the data-generating process. Since the data $\mathcal{D}$ are usually subject

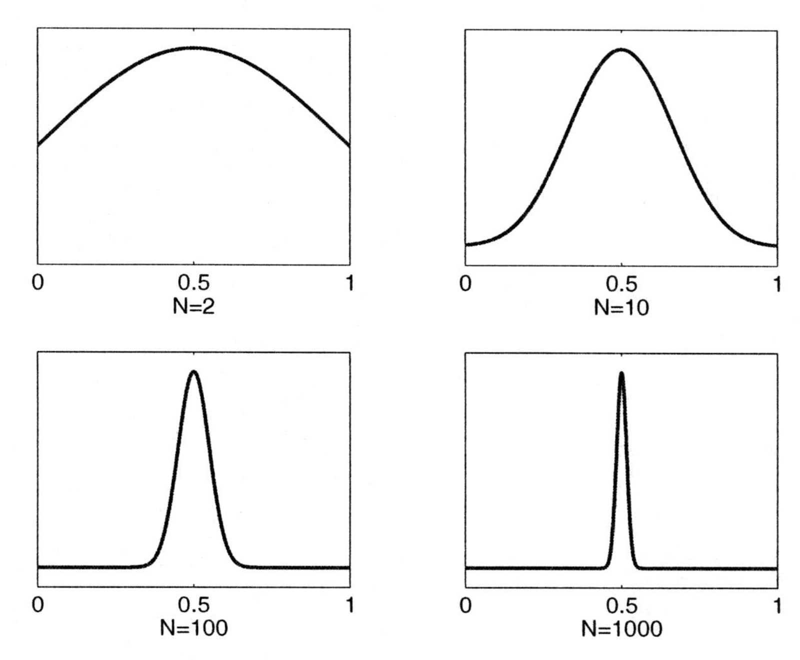

Fig. 1.4. Distribution of the parameter estimate. The figures show, for various sample sizes N, the distribution of the parameter estimate $\hat{\theta}$. In all samples, the numbers of heads and tails were the same. Consequently, all distributions have their maximum at $\hat{\theta} = 0.5$. Note, however, how the estimation uncertainty decreases with increasing sample size.

to random fluctuations and intrinsic uncertainty, repeating the whole process of data collection and parameter estimation under identical conditions will most likely lead to slightly different results. Thus, if we are able to repeat the data-generating processes several times, we will get a distribution of parameter estimates $\hat{\theta}$, from which we can infer the intrinsic uncertainty of the estimation process.

Unfortunately, repeating the data-generating process is usually impossible. For instance, the diversity of contemporary life on Earth is the consequence of the intrinsically stochastic process of evolution. Methods of phylogenetic inference, to be discussed later in Chapter 4, have to take this stochasticity into account and estimate the intrinsic estimation uncertainty. Obviously, we cannot set back the clock by 4.5 billion years and restart the course of evolution, starting from the first living cell in the primordial ocean. Consequently, the frequentist approach of Figure 1.3 has to be interpreted in terms of hypothetical parallel universes, and the estimation of the estimation uncertainty is based on hypothetical data that could have been generated by the underlying data-generating process, but, in fact, happened not to be.

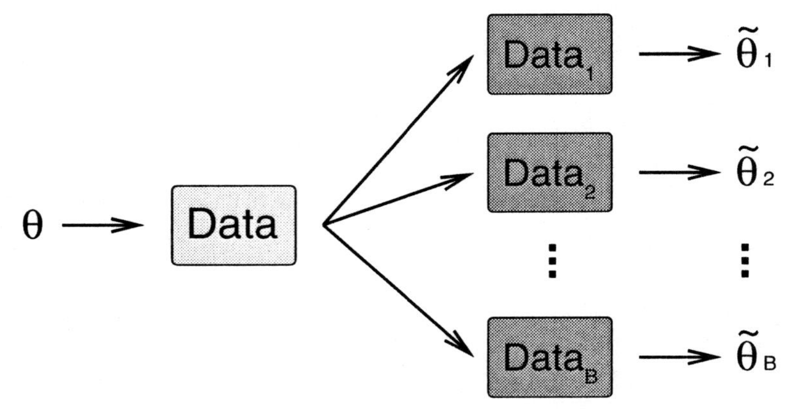

Fig. 1.5. Bootstrapping. From the observed data set of size N, B bootstrap replicas are generated by drawing N data points with replacement from the original data. The parameter estimation is repeated on each bootstrap replica, which leads to an ensemble of bootstrap parameters $\tilde{\theta}_i$, $i = \{1, \ldots, B\}$. If N and B are sufficiently large, the distribution of the bootstrap parameters $\tilde{\theta}_i$ is a good approximation to the distribution that would result from the conceptual, but practically intractable process of Figure 1.3.

Now, in a simple situation like the thumbnail example, this limitation does not pose any problems. Here, we can easily compute the distribution of the parameter estimate $\hat{\theta}$ without actually having to repeat the experiment (where an experiment is a batch of N thumbnail tosses). To see this, note that the probability of k observations of heads in a sample of size N is given by

$$P(k) \;=\; \theta^k \,(1-\theta)^{N-k} \binom{N}{k} \tag{1.9}$$

Substituting $k = N\hat{\theta}$, by equation (1.8), leads to

$$P(\hat{\theta}) \;=\; \theta^{N\hat{\theta}} \,(1-\theta)^{N(1-\hat{\theta})} \binom{N}{N\hat{\theta}} C \tag{1.10}$$

where the constant C results from the transformation of the discrete distribution $P(k)$ into the continuous distribution $P(\hat{\theta})$ (see [2], Section 8.4). The distribution (1.10) is plotted, for various sample sizes N, in Figure 1.4, and the graphs reflect the obvious fact that the intrinsic uncertainty decreases with increasing sample size N.

In more complicated situations, analytic solutions, like (1.10), are usually not available. In this case, one either has to make simplifying approximations, which are often not particularly satisfactory, or resort to the computational procedure of *bootstrapping* [3], which is illustrated in Figure 1.5. In fact, bootstrapping tries to approximate the conceptual, but usually unrealizable scenario of Figure 1.3 by drawing samples with replacement from the original

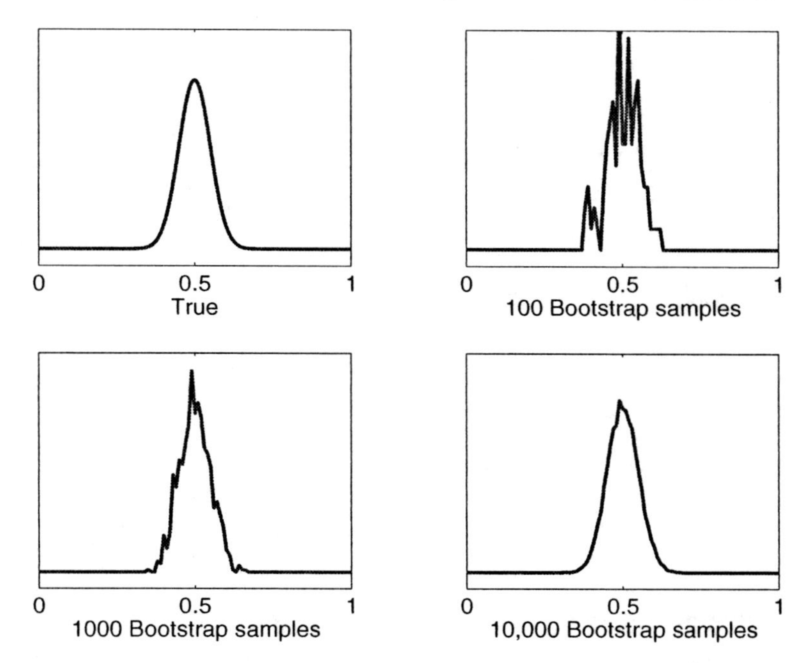

Fig. 1.6. Bootstrap example: thumbnail. The figures show the true distribution of the parameter estimate $\hat{\theta}$ (top, left), and three distributions obtained with bootstrapping, using different bootstrap sample sizes. Top right: 100, bottom left: 1000, bottom right: 10,000. The graphs were obtained with a Gaussian kernel estimator.

data. This procedure generates a synthetic set of replicated data sets, which are used as surrogates for the data sets that would be obtained if the data-generating process was repeated. An estimation of the parameters from each bootstrap replica gives a distribution of parameter estimates, which for sufficiently large data size N and bootstrap sample size B is a good approximation to the true distribution, that is, the distribution one would obtain from the hypothetical process of Figure 1.3. As an illustration, Figure 1.6 shows the distribution $P(\hat{\theta})$ obtained for the thumbnail example, $N = 100$, for three different bootstrap sample sizes: $B = 100$, 1000 and 10,000. Even for a relatively small bootstrap sample size of $B = 100$ the resulting distribution is qualitatively correct. Increasing the bootstrap sample size to $B = 10{,}000$, the difference between the true and the bootstrap distribution becomes negligible. More details and a good introduction to the bootstrap method can be found in [4]. Applications of bootstrapping can be found in Section 4.4.6, and in Chapter 9, especially Section 9.4.

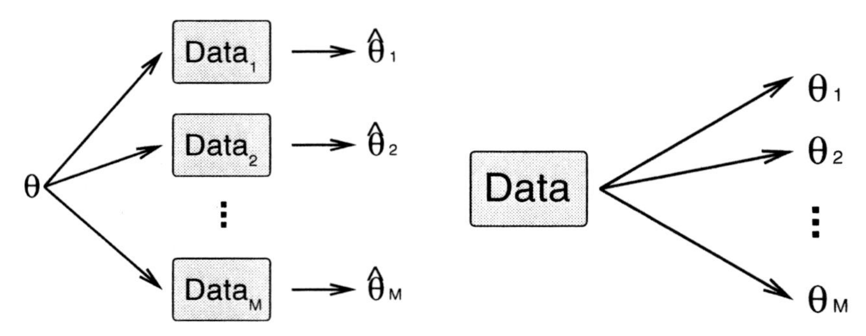

Fig. 1.7. Comparison between the frequentist and Bayesian paradigms. *Left:* In the frequentist approach, the entity of interest, θ, is a parameter and *not* a random variable. The estimation of the estimation uncertainty is based on the concept of hypothetical parallel statistical universes, that is, on data sets that could have been observed, but happened not to be. *Right:* In the Bayesian approach, the entity of interest, θ, is treated as a random variable. This implies that the estimation of the estimation uncertainty can be based on a single data set: the one observed in the experiment.

1.3 The Bayesian Approach

In the frequentist approach, probabilities are interpreted in terms of repeatable experiments. More precisely, a probability is defined as the limiting case of an experimentally observed frequency, which is justified by the law of large numbers (see, for instance, [9]). This definition implies that the entities of interest, like θ in the thumbnail example, are *parameters* rather than *random variables*. For estimating the uncertainty of estimation, the frequentist approach is based on hypothetical parallel statistical universes, as discussed above. The Bayesian approach overcomes this rather cumbersome concept by interpreting all entities of interest as random variables. This interpretation is impossible within the frequentist framework. Assume that, in the previous example, you were given an oddly deshaped thumbnail. Then θ is associated with the physical properties of this particular thumbnail under investigation, whose properties – given its odd shape – are fixed and unique. In phylogenetics, discussed in Chapter 4, θ is related to a sequence of mutation and speciation events during evolution. Obviously, this process is also unique and non-repeatable. In both examples, θ can *not* be treated as a random variable within the frequentist paradigm because no probability can be obtained for it. Consequently, the Bayesian approach needs to extend the frequentist probability concept and introduce a generalized definition that applies to unique entities and non-repeatable events. This extended probability concept encompasses the notion of *subjective uncertainty*, which represents a person's prior belief about an event. Once this definition has been accepted, the mathematical procedure is straightforward in that the uncertainty of the entity of interest θ, given the data $\mathcal{D}$, can immediately be obtained from Bayes' rule:

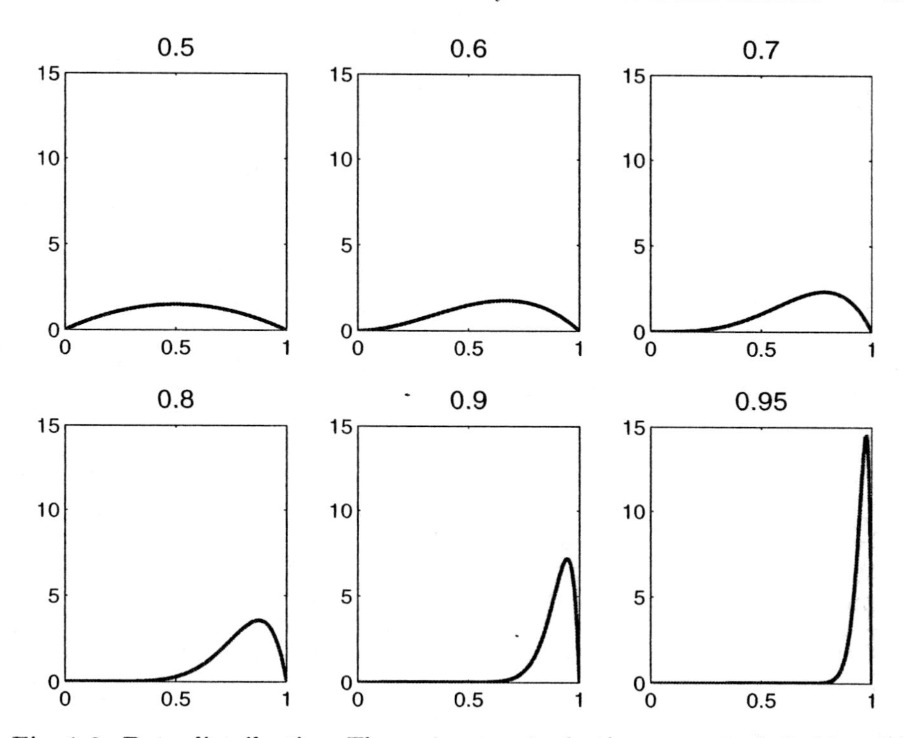

Fig. 1.8. Beta distribution. The conjugate prior for the parameter θ of a binomial distribution is a beta distribution, which depends on two hyperparameters, α and β. The mean of the distribution is $\mu = \frac{\alpha}{\alpha+\beta}$. The subfigures show plots of the distribution for different values of μ, indicated at the top of each subfigure, when $\beta = 2$ is fixed.

$$P(\theta|\mathcal{D}) \propto P(\mathcal{D}|\theta)P(\theta) \tag{1.11}$$

where $P(\mathcal{D}|\theta)$ is the likelihood, and $P(\theta)$ is the prior probability of θ before any data have been observed. This latter term is related to the very notion of subjective uncertainty, which is an immediate consequence of the extended probability concept and inextricably entwined with the Bayesian framework. Now, equation (1.11) has the advantage that the estimation of uncertainty is solely based on the actually observed data $\mathcal{D}$ and no longer needs to resort to any unobserved, hypothetical data. An illustration is given in Figure 1.7.

To demonstrate the Bayesian approach on an example, let us revisit the thumbnail problem. We want to apply (1.11) to compute the *posterior* probability $P(\theta|\mathcal{D})$ from the *likelihood* $P(\mathcal{D}|\theta)$, given by (1.5), and the *prior* probability, $P(\theta)$. It is mathematically convenient to choose a functional form that is invariant with respect to the transformation implied by (1.11), that is, for which the *prior* and the *posterior* probability are in the same function family. Such a prior is called *conjugate* . The conjugate prior for the thumbnail example, that is, for the parameter $\theta \in [0,1]$ of a binomial distribution, is a beta distribution:

$$\mathcal{B}(\theta|\alpha,\beta) = \frac{\Gamma(\alpha+\beta)}{\Gamma(\alpha)\Gamma(\beta)}\theta^{\alpha-1}(1-\theta)^{\beta-1} \quad \text{if} \quad 0 \leq \theta \leq 1 \tag{1.12}$$

where

$$\Gamma(x) = \int_0^\infty \exp(-t)t^{x-1}dt \tag{1.13}$$

and the term with the $\Gamma(.)$ functions in (1.12) results from the normalization. For $\theta \notin [0,1]$, $\mathcal{B}(\theta|\alpha,\beta) = 0$. The conjugacy is easy to prove. Setting $P(\theta) = \mathcal{B}(\theta|\alpha,\beta)$ and inserting both this expression as well as the likelihood of (1.5) into (1.11) gives:

$$P(\theta|\mathcal{D}) \propto \theta^{k+\alpha-1}(1-\theta)^{N-k+\beta-1} \tag{1.14}$$

which, on normalization, leads to

$$P(\theta|\mathcal{D}) = \mathcal{B}(\theta|k+\alpha, N-k+\beta) \tag{1.15}$$

The beta distribution (1.12) depends on the so-called *hyperparameters* α and β. For $\alpha = \beta = 1$, the beta distribution is equal to the uniform distribution over the unit interval, that is, $\mathcal{B}(\theta|1,1) = 1$ for $\theta \in [0,1]$, and 0 otherwise. Some other forms of the beta distribution, for different settings of the hyperparameters, are shown in Figure 1.8.

Figure 1.9 shows several plots of the posterior probability $P(\theta|\mathcal{D})$ for a constant prior, $P(\theta) = \mathcal{B}(\theta|1,1)$, and for data sets of different size N. As in Figure 1.4, the uncertainty decreases with increasing sample size N, which reflects the obvious fact that our trust in the estimation increases as more training data become available. Since no prior information is used, the graphs in Figures 1.4 and 1.9 are similar. Note that a uniform prior is appropriate in the absence of any domain knowledge. If domain knowledge about the system of interest is available, for instance, about the physical properties of differently shaped thumbnails, it can and should be included in the inference process by choosing a more informative prior. We discuss this in more detail in the following section.

1.4 Comparison

An obvious difference between the frequentist and Bayesian approaches is the fact that the latter includes subjective prior knowledge in the form of a prior probability distribution on the parameters of interest. Recall from (1.11) that the posterior probability is the product of the prior and the likelihood. While the first term is independent of the sample size N, the second term increases

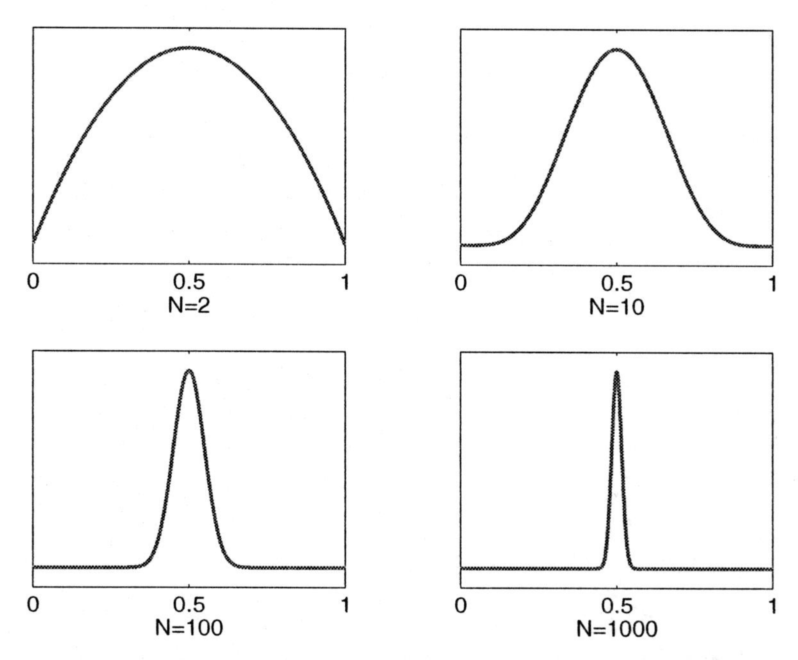

Fig. 1.9. Posterior probability of the thumbnail parameter. The subfigures show, for various values of the sample size N, the posterior distribution $P(\theta|\mathcal{D})$, assuming a constant prior on θ. In all data sets $\mathcal{D}$, the numbers of heads and tails are the same, which is reflected by the fact that the mode of the posterior distribution is always at $\theta = 0.5$. Note, however, how the uncertainty decreases with increasing sample size. Compare with Figure 1.4.

with N. Consequently, for a sufficiently large data set $\mathcal{D}$ and a reasonable prior (meaning a prior whose support covers the entire parameter domain), the weight of the likelihood term is considerably higher than that of the prior, and variations of the latter have only a marginal influence on the posterior probability. This implies that for $N \to \infty$, the *maximum a posteriori* (MAP) estimate,

$$\theta_{MAP} = \text{argmax}_\theta \{P(\theta|\mathcal{D})\} \tag{1.16}$$

and the *maximum likelihood* (ML) estimate

$$\theta_{ML} = \text{argmax}_\theta \{P(\mathcal{D}|\theta)\} \tag{1.17}$$

become identical. For small data sets, on the other hand, the prior can make a substantial difference. In this case, the weight of the likelihood term is relatively small, which comes with a concomitant uncertainty in the inference scheme, as illustrated in Figures 1.4 and 1.9. This inherent uncertainty suggests that including prior domain knowledge is a reasonable approach, as it may partially compensate for the lack of information in the data. Take, again, the thumbnail of the previous example, and suppose that you are only allowed to toss it a few times. You may, however, consult a theoretical physicist who can derive the torque acting on the falling thumbnail from its shape. Obviously, you would be foolish not to use this prior knowledge, since any inference based on your data alone is inherently unreliable. If, on the other hand, you are allowed to toss the thumbnail arbitrarily often, the data will "speak for itself", and including any prior knowledge no longer makes a difference to the prediction. Similar approaches can be found in ridge regression and neural networks. Here, our prior knowledge is that most real-world functions are relatively smooth. Expressing this mathematically in the form of a prior and applying (1.11) leads to a *penalty term*, by which the MAP estimate (1.16) differs from the ML estimate (1.17). For further details, see, for instance, [7].

The main difference between the frequentist and the Bayesian approach is the different interpretation of θ. Recall from the previous discussion that the frequentist statistician interprets θ as a parameter and aims to estimate it with a point estimate, typically adopting the maximum likelihood (1.17) approach. The Bayesian statistician, on the other hand, interprets θ as a random variable and tries to infer its whole posterior distribution, $P(\theta|\mathcal{D})$. In fact, computing the MAP estimate (1.16), although widely applied in machine learning, is not in the Bayesian spirit in that it only aims to obtain a point estimate rather than the entire posterior distribution. (As an aside, note that the MAP estimate, as opposed to the ML estimate, is not invariant with respect to non-linear coordinate transformations and therefore, in fact, not particularly meaningful as a summary of the distribution.) Although an exact derivation of $P(\theta|\mathcal{D})$ is usually impossible in complex inference problems, powerful computational approximations, based on Markov chain Monte Carlo, are available and will be discussed in Section 2.2.2.

Take, for instance, the problem of learning the weights in a neural network. By applying the standard *backpropagation* algorithm, discussed in Chapter 3, we get a point estimate in the high-dimensional space of weight vectors. This point estimate is usually an approximation to the proper maximum likelihood estimate or, more precisely, a *local maximum* of the likelihood surface. Now, it is well known that, for sparse data, the method of maximum likelihood is susceptible to over-fitting. This is because, for sparse data, there is substantial information in the curvature and (possibly) multimodality of the likelihood landscape, which is not captured by a point estimate of the parameters. The Bayesian approach, on the other hand, samples the network weights from the posterior probability distribution with MCMC and thereby captures much more information about this landscape. As demonstrated in [8], this leads to a considerable improvement in the generalization performance, and over-fitting is avoided even for over-complex network architectures.

The previous comparison is not entirely fair in that the frequentist approach has only been applied partially. Recall from Figure 1.3 that the point estimate of the parameters has to be followed up by an estimation of its distribution. Again, this estimation is usually analytically intractable, and the frequentist equivalent to MCMC is bootstrapping, illustrated in Figure 1.5. This approach requires running the parameter learning algorithm on hundreds of bootstrap replicas of the training data. Unfortunately, this procedure is usually prohibitively computationally expensive – much more expensive than MCMC – and it has therefore hardly been applied to complex inference problems. The upshot is that the full-blown frequentist approach is practically not viable in many machine-learning applications, whereas an incomplete frequentist approach without the bootstrapping step is inherently inferior to the Bayesian approach. We will revisit this important point later, in Section 4.4.7 and Figure 4.35.

Acknowledgments

I would like to thank Anja von Heydebreck, Wolfgang Urfer, David Allcroft and Thorsten Forster for critical feedback on a draft version of this chapter, as well as Philip Smith for proofreading it.

References

[1] G. Deco and D. Obradovic. *An Information-Theoretic Approach to Neural Computing.* Springer Verlag, New York, 1996.
[2] R. Durbin, S. R. Eddy, A. Krogh, and G. Mitchison. *Biological sequence analysis. Probabilistic models of proteins and nucleic acids.* Cambridge University Press, Cambridge, UK, 1998.
[3] B. Efron. Bootstrap methods: Another look at the jacknife. *Annals of Statistics*, 7:1–26, 1979.
[4] B. Efron and G. Gong. A leisurely look at the bootstrap, the jacknife, and cross-validation. *The American Statistician*, 37(1):36–47, 1983.
[5] P. G. Hoel. *Introduction to Mathematical Statistics.* John Wiley and Sons, Singapore, 1984.
[6] P. J. Krause. Learning probabilistic networks. *Knowledge Engineering Review*, 13:321–351, 1998.
[7] D. J. C. MacKay. Bayesian interpolation. *Neural Computation*, 4:415–447, 1992.
[8] R. M. Neal. *Bayesian Learning for Neural Networks*, volume 118 of *Lecture Notes in Statistics.* Springer, New York, 1996. ISBN 0-387-94724-8.
[9] A. Papoulis. *Probability, Random Variables, and Stochastic Processes.* McGraw-Hill, Singapore, 3rd edition, 1991.

2

Introduction to Learning Bayesian Networks from Data

Dirk Husmeier

Biomathematics and Statistics Scotland (BioSS)
JCMB, The King's Buildings, Edinburgh EH9 3JZ, UK
dirk@bioss.ac.uk

Summary. Bayesian networks are a combination of probability theory and graph theory. Graph theory provides a framework to represent complex structures of highly-interacting sets of variables. Probability theory provides a method to infer these structures from observations or measurements in the presence of noise and uncertainty. Many problems in computational molecular biology and bioinformatics, like sequence alignment, molecular evolution, and genetic networks, can be treated as particular instances of the general problem of learning Bayesian networks from data. This chapter provides a brief introduction, in preparation for later chapters of this book.

2.1 Introduction to Bayesian Networks

Bayesian networks (BNs) are interpretable and flexible models for representing probabilistic relationships between multiple interacting entities. At a *qualitative* level, the structure of a Bayesian network describes the relationships between these entities in the form of conditional independence relations. At a *quantitative level*, (local) relationships between the interacting entities are described by (conditional) probability distributions. Formally, a BN is defined by a graphical structure, $\mathcal{M}$, a family of (conditional) probability distributions, $\mathcal{F}$, and their parameters, $\mathbf{q}$, which together specify a joint distribution over a set of random variables of interest. These three components are discussed in the following two subsections.

2.1.1 The Structure of a Bayesian Network

The graphical structure $\mathcal{M}$ of a BN consists of a set of *nodes* or *vertices*, $\mathcal{V}$, and a set of *directed edges* or *arcs*, $\mathcal{E}$: $\mathcal{M} = (\mathcal{V}, \mathcal{E})$. The nodes represent random variables, while the edges indicate conditional dependence relations. If we have a directed edge from node A to node B, then A is called the *parent* of B, and B is called the *child* of A. Take, as an example, Figure 2.1, where

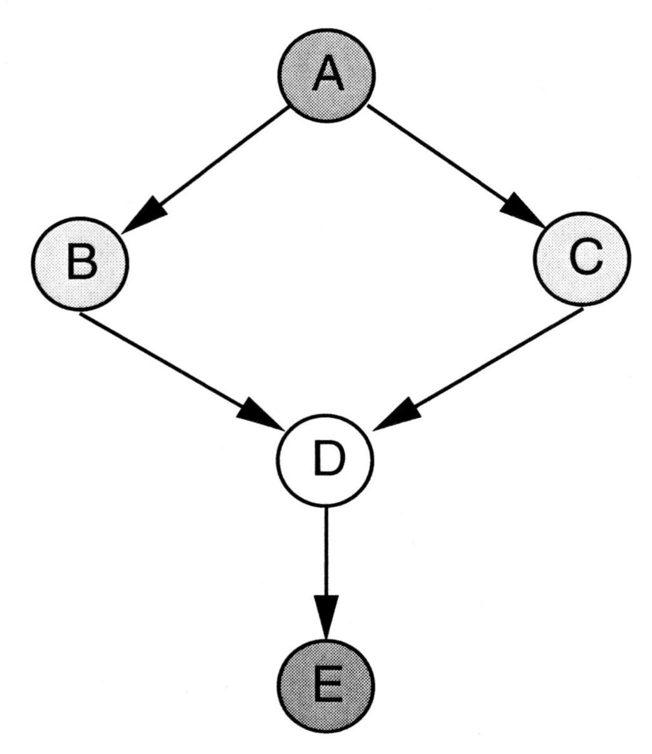

Fig. 2.1. Example of a Bayesian network. Nodes represent random variables, edges indicate conditional dependence relations. The joint probability $P(A, B, C, D, E)$ factorizes into the product $P(A)P(B|A)P(C|A)P(D|B, C)P(E|D)$. Reprinted from [23], by permission of Cambridge University Press.

we have the set of vertices $\mathcal{V} = \{A, B, C, D, E\}$, and the set of edges $\mathcal{E} = \{(A, B), (A, C), (B, D), (C, D), (D, E)\}$. Node A does not have any parents. Nodes B and C are the children of node A, and the parents of node D. Node D itself has one child: node E. The graphical structure has to take the form of a *directed acyclic graph* or DAG, which is characterized by the absence of directed cycles, that is, cycles where all the arcs point in the same direction. A BN is characterized by a simple and unique rule for expanding the joint probability in terms of simpler conditional probabilities. Let $X_1, X_2, \ldots, X_n$ be a set of random variables represented by the nodes $i \in \{1, \ldots, n\}$ in the graph, define $pa[i]$ to be the parents of node i, and let $\mathcal{X}_{pa[i]}$ represent the set of random variables associated with $pa[i]$. Then

$$P(X_1, X_2, \ldots, X_n) = \prod_{i=1}^{n} P(X_i|\mathcal{X}_{pa[i]}) \tag{2.1}$$

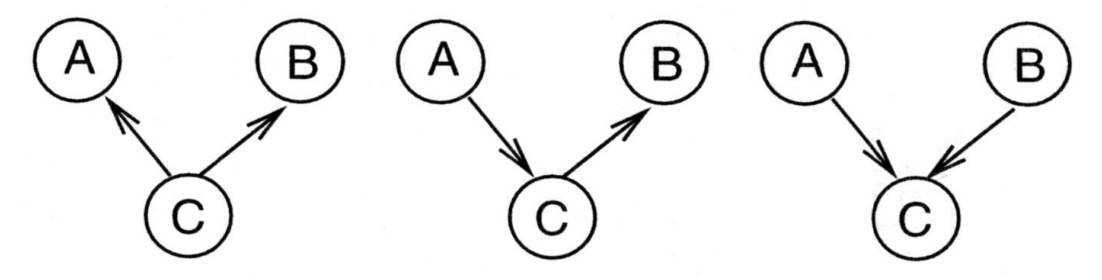

Fig. 2.2. Three elementary BNs. The BNs on the left and in the middle have equivalent structures: A and B are conditionally independent given C. The BN on the right belongs to a different equivalence class in that conditioning on C causes, in general, a dependence between A and B.

As an example, applying (2.1) to the BN of Figure 2.1, we obtain the factorization

$$P(A, B, C, D, E) = P(A)P(B|A)P(C|A)P(D|B, C)P(E|D) \quad (2.2)$$

An equivalent way of expressing these independence relations is based on the concept of the *Markov blanket*, which is the set of children, parents, and coparents (that is, other parents of the children) of a given node. This set shields the selected node from the remaining nodes in the graph. So, if $MB[i]$ is the Markov blanket of node i, and $\mathcal{X}_{MB[i]}$ is the set of random variables associated with $MB[i]$, then

$$P(X_k|X_1, \ldots, X_{k-1}, X_{k+1}, \ldots, X_n) = P(X_k|\mathcal{X}_{MB[i]}) \quad (2.3)$$

Applying (2.3) to Figure 2.1 gives:

$$P(A|B, C, D, E) = P(A|B, C) \quad (2.4)$$
$$P(B|A, C, D, E) = P(B|A, C, D) \quad (2.5)$$
$$P(C|A, B, D, E) = P(C|A, B, D) \quad (2.6)$$
$$P(D|A, B, C, E) = P(D|B, C, E) \quad (2.7)$$
$$P(E|A, B, C, D) = P(E|D) \quad (2.8)$$

To illustrate the equivalence of the factorization rule (2.1) and the notion of the Markov blanket (2.3), let us derive, for instance, (2.6) from (2.2):

$$\begin{aligned}
P(C|A, B, D, E) &= \frac{P(A, B, C, D, E)}{P(A, B, D, E)} \\
&= \frac{P(A)P(B|A)P(C|A)P(D|B, C)P(E|D)}{\sum_C P(A)P(B|A)P(C|A)P(D|B, C)P(E|D)} \\
&= \frac{P(A)P(E|D)P(B|A)P(C|A)P(D|B, C)}{P(A)P(E|D)P(B|A)\sum_C P(C|A)P(D|B, C)} \\
&= \frac{P(C|A)P(D|B, C)}{\sum_C P(C|A)P(D|B, C)}
\end{aligned}$$

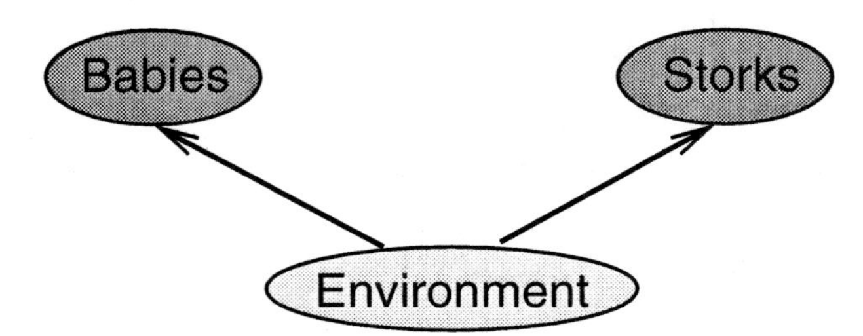

Fig. 2.3. Storks and babies. The numbers of stork sightings and new-born babies depend on common environmental factors. Without the knowledge of these environmental factors, the number of new-born babies seems to depend on the number of stork sightings, but conditional on the environmental factors, both events are independent.

where we have applied (2.2) for the factorization of the joint probability $P(A, B, C, D, E)$. Note that the last term does not depend on E, which proves (2.6) true. For a general proof of the equivalence of (2.1) and (2.3), see [24] and [34].

Consider the BN on the left of Figure 2.2. Expanding the joint probability according to (2.1) gives

$$P(A, B, C) = P(A|C)P(B|C)P(C) \tag{2.9}$$

For the conditional probability $P(A, B|C)$ we thus obtain:

$$P(A, B|C) = \frac{P(A, B, C)}{P(C)} = P(A|C)P(B|C) \tag{2.10}$$

Hence, A and B are *conditionally* independent given C. Note, however, that this independence does not carry over to the marginal probabilities, and that in general

$$P(A, B) \neq P(A)P(B) \tag{2.11}$$

As an example, consider the BN in Figure 2.3. The number of new-born babies has been found to depend on the number of stork sightings [39], which, in former times, even led to the erroneous conclusion that storks deliver babies. In fact, both events depend on several environmental factors. In an urban environment, families tend to be smaller as a consequence of changed living conditions, while storks are rarer due to the destruction of their natural habitat. The introduction of contraceptives has led to a decrease of the number of new-born babies, but their release into the environment also adversely affected the fecundity of storks. So while, without the knowledge of these environmental factors, the number of new-born babies depends on the number of stork sightings, conditionally on the environmental factors both events are independent.

The situation is similar for the BN in the middle of Figure 2.2. Expanding the joint probability by application of the factorization rule (2.1) gives:

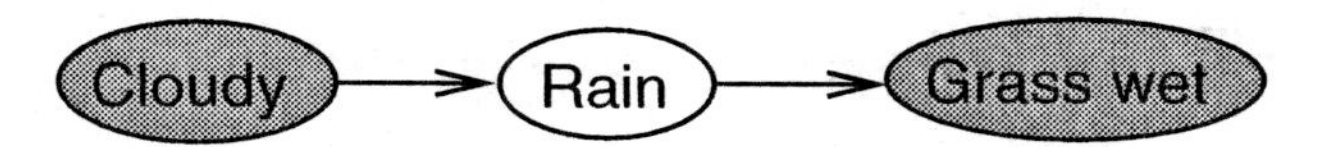

Fig. 2.4. Clouds and rain. When no information on the rain is available, the wetness of the grass depends on the clouds: the more clouds are in the sky, the more likely the grass is found to be wet. When information on the rain is available, information on the clouds is no longer relevant for predicting the state of wetness of the grass: conditional on the rain, the wetness of the grass is independent of the clouds.

$$P(A, B, C) = P(B|C)P(C|A)P(A) \tag{2.12}$$

For the conditional probability we thus obtain:

$$P(A, B|C) = \frac{P(A, B, C)}{P(C)} = P(B|C)\frac{P(C|A)P(A)}{P(C)} = P(B|C)P(A|C) \tag{2.13}$$

where we have used Bayes' rule, (1.4). So again we find that A and B are conditionally independent given C, while, in general, this does not hold for the marginal probabilities; see (2.11).

An example is shown in Figure 2.4. Clouds may cause rain, and rain makes grass wet. So if information on precipitation is unavailable, that is, if the node "rain" in Figure 2.4 is hidden, the state of wetness of the grass depends on the clouds: an increased cloudiness, obviously, increases the likelihood for the grass to be wet. However, if information on precipitation is available, meaning that the node "rain" in Figure 2.4 is observed, the wetness of the grass becomes independent of the clouds. If it rains, the grass gets wet no matter how cloudy it is. Conversely, if it does not rain, the grass stays dry irrespective of the state of cloudiness.

The situation is different for the BN on the right of Figure 2.2. Expanding the joint probability $P(A, B, C)$ according to (2.1) gives:

$$P(A, B, C) = P(C|A, B)P(A)P(B) \tag{2.14}$$

Marginalizing over C leads to

$$P(A, B) = \sum_C P(A, B, C) = P(A)P(B) \tag{2.15}$$

where we have used the fact that a probability function is normalized: $\sum_C P(C|A, B) = 1$. We thus see that, as opposed to the previous two examples, A and B are *marginally* independent. However, it can *not* be shown, in general, that the same holds for the conditional probabilities, that is, different from the previous examples we have

$$P(A, B|C) \neq P(A|C)P(B|C) \tag{2.16}$$

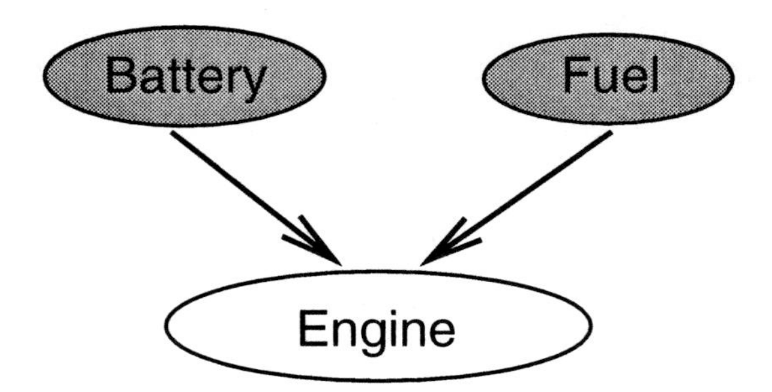

Fig. 2.5. Fuel and battery. Nationwide, the unfortunate events of having a flat car battery and running out of fuel are independent. This independence no longer holds when an engine failure is observed in a particular car, since establishing one event as the cause of this failure explains away the other alternative.

An illustration is given in Figure 2.5. Suppose you cannot start your car engine in the morning. Two possible reasons for this failure are: (1) a flat battery, B, or (2) an empty fuel tank, F. Nationwide, these two unfortunate events can be assumed to be independent: $P(B, F) = P(B)P(F)$. However, this independence no longer holds when you observe an engine failure, E, in your particular car: $P(B, F|E) \neq P(B|E)P(F|E)$. Obviously, on finding the fuel tank empty, there is little need to check the voltage of the battery: the empty tank already accounts for the engine failure and thus *explains away* any problems associated with the battery.

Figure 2.6 gives an overview of the independence relations we have encountered in the previous examples. The power of Bayesian networks is that we can deduce, in much more complicated situations, these independence relations between random variables from the network structure without having to resort to algebraic computations. This is based on the concept of *d-separation*, which is formally defined as follows (see [34], and references in [23]):

- Let A and B be two nodes, and let $\mathcal{Z}$ be a set of nodes.
- A *path* from A to B is *blocked* with respect to $\mathcal{Z}$
  - if there is a node $C \in \mathcal{Z}$ without converging edges, that is, which is *head-to-tail* or *tail-to-tail* with respect to the path, or
  - if two edges on the path converge on a node C, that is, the configuration of edges is *head-to-head*, and neither C nor any of its descendents are in $\mathcal{Z}$.
- A and B are *d-separated* by $\mathcal{Z}$ if and only if all possible paths between them are blocked.
- If A and B are d-separated by $\mathcal{Z}$, then A is conditionally independent of B given $\mathcal{Z}$, symbolically written as $A \perp B|\mathcal{Z}$.

An illustration is given in Figure 2.7. As a first example, consider the elementary BNs of Figure 2.8. Similar to the preceding examples, we want to decide whether A is independent of B conditional on those other nodes

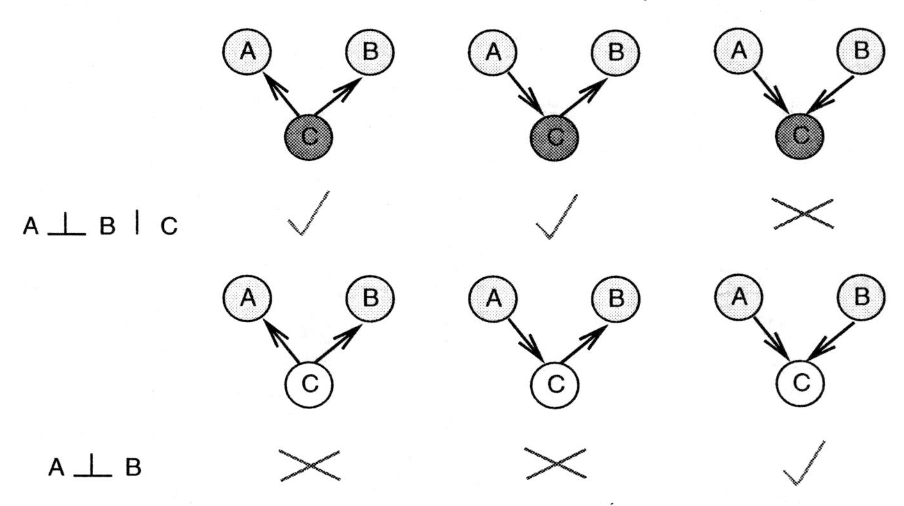

Fig. 2.6. Overview of elementary BN independence relations. $A \perp B$ means that A and B are marginally independent: $P(A, B) = P(A)P(B)$. $A \perp B|C$ means that A and B are conditionally independent: $P(A, B|C) = P(A|C)P(B|C)$. The figure summarizes the independence relations of Figures 2.3–2.5, which can easily be derived with the method of d-separation, illustrated in Figure 2.7. A tick indicates that an independence relation holds true, whereas a cross indicates that it is violated.

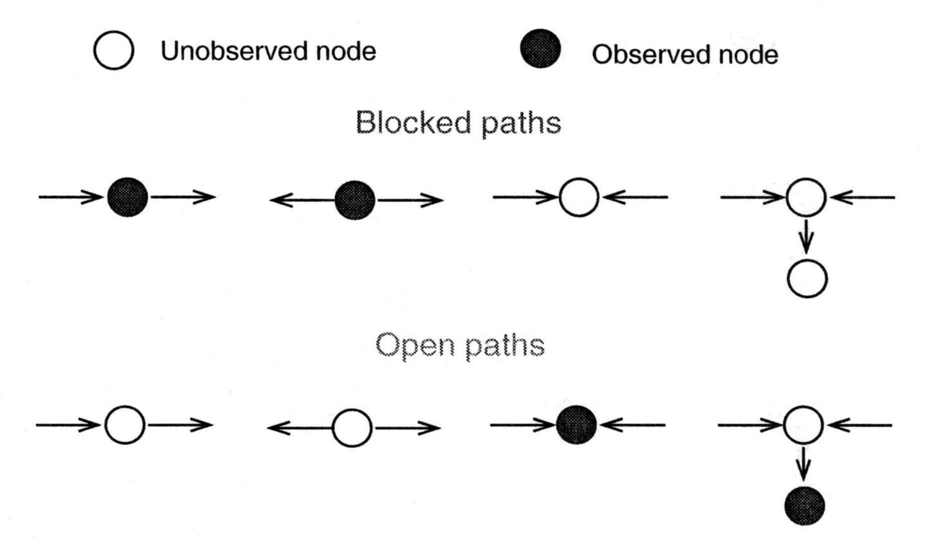

Fig. 2.7. Illustration of d-separation when the separating set $\mathcal{Z}$ is the set of observed nodes. Filled circles represent observed nodes, empty circles indicate hidden states (for which no data are available).

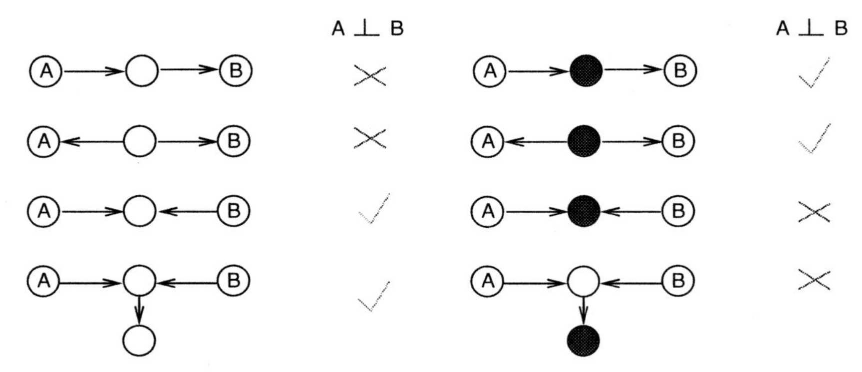

Fig. 2.8. Illustration of d-separation in elementary BN structures. Filled circles represent observed nodes, empty circles represent hidden nodes (for which no data are available). The column on the right of each subfigure indicates whether A and B are independent given $\mathcal{Z}$, where $\mathcal{Z}$ is the set of observed nodes. Compare with Figure 2.6.

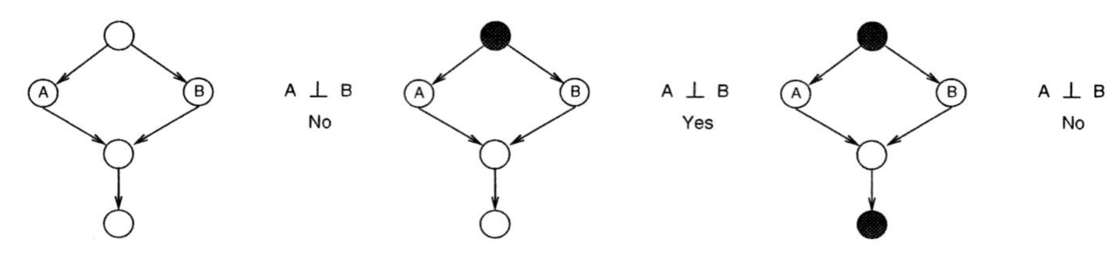

Fig. 2.9. Illustration of d-separation in a Bayesian network. Filled circles represent observed nodes, empty circles represent hidden nodes (for which no data are available). The legend on the right of each network indicates whether nodes A and B are independent given $\mathcal{Z}$, where $\mathcal{Z}$ is the set of observed nodes. Adapted from [23], by permission of Cambridge University Press.

in the graph that have been observed. It can easily be seen that testing for *d-separation* leads to the same results as before, but without having to go through the (albeit very simple) algebra of equations (2.10), (2.13), and (2.15). This is useful in more complex networks, where the algebra is more involved.

Take, as a second example, Figure 2.9. Again, we are interested in whether A is independent of B given the set of observed nodes, $\mathcal{Z}$. There are two paths connecting nodes A and B. If no other node is observed (Figure 2.9, left), the upper path is *not* blocked, because the edges do not converge and the separating node is not observed (that is, it is not in $\mathcal{Z}$). Consequently, A and B are *not* d-separated, and A and B are *not* conditionally independent given $\mathcal{Z}$, symbolically written as $A \not\perp B|\mathcal{Z}$. On observing the top node (Figure 2.9, middle), the upper path gets blocked. The lower path is also blocked, because the edges converge on the separating node, and neither the separating node itself nor its descendant is observed. Consequently, A and B are *d-separated*, and $A \perp B|\mathcal{Z}$. This changes when the descendant of the separating node is observed (Figure 2.9, right), which opens the lower path and thus destroys the d-separation between A and B, implying that $A \not\perp B | \mathcal{Z}$.

Here, we have used the observation of nodes as an obvious criterion for membership in the separating set $\mathcal{Z}$. However, other membership criteria can also be employed. For instance, when trying to infer genetic networks from microarray experiments, described in Chapters 8 and 9, we are particularly interested in the up- and down-regulation of gene expression levels. So rather than asking whether two genes A and B are independent given a set $\mathcal{Z}$ of measured mediating genes, we could ask whether A and B are independent conditional on a set $\mathcal{Z}'$ of up- or down-regulated genes. We will return to this issue later, in Chapter 8.

2.1.2 The Parameters of a Bayesian Network

Recall that a BN is defined by a graphical structure, $\mathcal{M}$, a family of (conditional) probability distributions, $\mathcal{F}$, and their parameters, $\mathbf{q}$. The structure $\mathcal{M}$ defines the independence relations between the interacting random variables, as discussed in the previous subsection and expressed in the factorization rule (2.1). The family $\mathcal{F}$ defines the functional form of the (conditional) probabilities in the expansion (2.1) and defines, for instance, whether these probabilities are Gaussian, multinomial, etc. To fully specify the conditional probabilities associated with the edges we need certain parameters, for instance, the mean and variance of a Gaussian, etc. In what follows, the function family $\mathcal{F}$ will be assumed to be fixed and known, chosen according to some criteria discussed in Section 8.2. Consequently, the probability distribution (2.1) is completely defined by the network structure, $\mathcal{M}$, henceforth also referred to as the *model*, and the vector of network *parameters*, $\mathbf{q}$. An illustration is given in Figure 2.10. Note that a parameter vector $\mathbf{q}$ is associated with its respective network structure $\mathcal{M}$, with structures of different degrees of connectivity having associated parameter vectors of different dimension. Consequently, it would be more accurate to write $\mathbf{q}_{\mathcal{M}}$ instead of $\mathbf{q}$. For the sake of simplicity of the notation, however, the subscript is dropped.

2.2 Learning Bayesian Networks from Complete Data

2.2.1 The Basic Learning Paradigm

Our next goal is to learn a Bayesian network from a set of training data, $\mathcal{D}$. These data are assumed to be complete, meaning that observations or measurements are available on *all nodes* in the network. The case of *incomplete data* will be treated later, in Section 2.3.

Recall from the discussion in Sections 1.2 and 1.3 that there are two principled inference paradigms in machine learning and statistics. *Bayesian networks* are not necessarily related to the concept of *Bayesian learning*, and

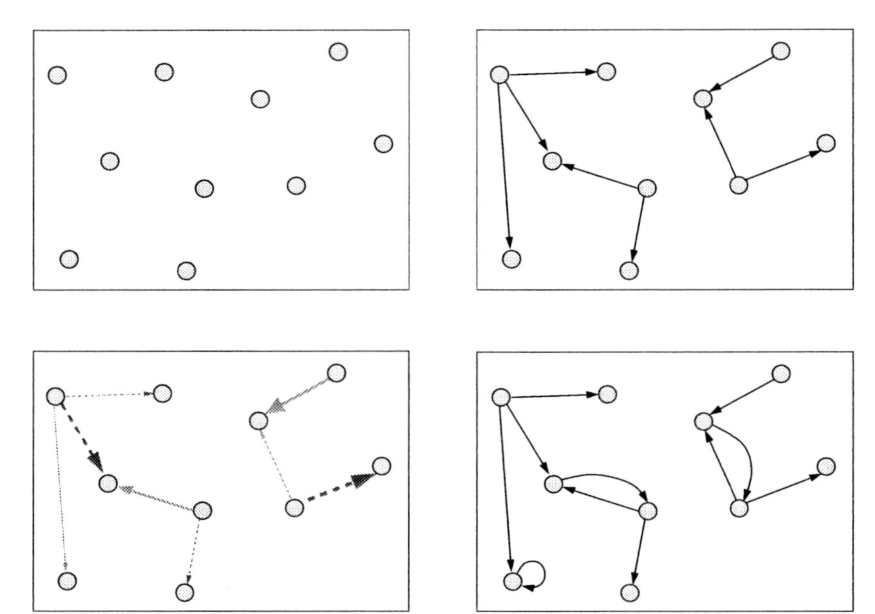

Fig. 2.10. Structure and parameters of a Bayesian network. *Top left:* A set of random variables for which we want to learn the Bayesian network, which is defined by its *structure* and its *parameters*. *Top right:* The structure $\mathcal{M}$ defines the set of edges between the nodes, which indicate the interactions between the entities of interest. *Bottom left:* The parameters $\mathbf{q}$ specify the functional form of the conditional probabilities associated with the edges, that is, they determine the nature of the interactions between the objects and indicate, for instance, whether an influence is strong (thick arrow) or weak (thin arrow) and whether an interaction is of an activating (solid line) or inhibitory (dashed line) nature. Note that the structure of the graph must satisfy the acyclicity constraint. A network with feedback loops, as shown in the *bottom right*, is *not* a Bayesian network.

learning Bayesian networks from data can, in fact, follow either of the two approaches discussed in Chapter 1. However, as pointed out in Section 1.3, and discussed in more detail in Section 4.4.7, a proper frequentist approach is often prohibitively computationally expensive. This chapter will therefore focus on the Bayesian approach.

Note from the discussion in the previous subsection that learning is a two-stage process, as illustrated in Figure 2.10. Given the data, we first want to find the posterior distribution of network *structures* $\mathcal{M}$ and, from this distribution, the structure $\mathcal{M}^*$ that is most supported by the data:

$$\mathcal{M}^* = \text{argmax}_{\mathcal{M}} \Big\{ P(\mathcal{M}|\mathcal{D}) \Big\} \tag{2.17}$$

Then, given the best structure $\mathcal{M}^*$ and the data, we want to find the posterior distribution of the parameters $\mathbf{q}$, and the best parameters:

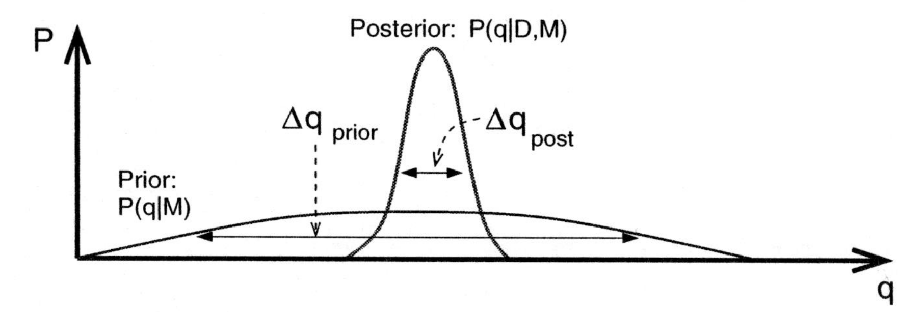

Fig. 2.11. Marginal likelihood and Occam factor. The figure shows a one-dimensional illustration of equation (2.20) to demonstrate the regularization effect of integrating out the network parameters. See text for details. Adapted from [3], by permission of Oxford University Press.

$$\mathbf{q}^* = \text{argmax}_{\mathbf{q}}\Big\{P(\mathbf{q}|\mathcal{M}^*, \mathcal{D})\Big\} \tag{2.18}$$

Applying Bayes' rule (1.4) to (2.17) gives:

$$P(\mathcal{M}|\mathcal{D}) \;\propto\; P(\mathcal{D}|\mathcal{M})P(\mathcal{M}) \tag{2.19}$$

where the marginal likelihood $P(\mathcal{D}|\mathcal{M})$ implies an integration over the whole parameter space:

$$P(\mathcal{D}|\mathcal{M}) \;=\; \int P(\mathcal{D}|\mathbf{q}, \mathcal{M})P(\mathbf{q}|\mathcal{M})d\mathbf{q} \tag{2.20}$$

Note that this marginal likelihood includes an inherent penalty for unnecessary complexity. To see this simply, consider the one-dimensional case of Figure 2.11. Assume that the posterior probability $P(\mathbf{q}|\mathcal{D}, \mathcal{M})$ is unimodal and peaked around its mode, $\hat{\mathbf{q}}$, with width $\triangle\mathbf{q}_{post}$. Also, assume that the prior can be approximated by a distribution that is uniform over some large interval $\triangle\mathbf{q}_{prior}$. With this approximation, (2.20) becomes:

$$P(\mathcal{D}|\mathcal{M}) \;=\; P(\mathcal{D}|\hat{\mathbf{q}}, \mathcal{M})\frac{\triangle\mathbf{q}_{post}}{\triangle\mathbf{q}_{prior}} \tag{2.21}$$

The first term on the right-hand side, $P(\mathcal{D}|\hat{\mathbf{q}}, \mathcal{M})$, is the likelihood, evaluated at the maximum likelihood parameters (note that for a uniform prior $P(\mathbf{q}|\mathcal{M})$, the MAP estimate $\hat{\mathbf{q}}$ is equal to the maximum likelihood estimate). Obviously, the likelihood is maximized for a complex structure with many edges, which is bound to over-fit to the observed data $\mathcal{D}$. The second term on the right-hand side, $\triangle\mathbf{q}_{post}/\triangle\,\mathbf{q}_{prior}$, referred to as the Occam factor in [3] and [26], measures the ratio of the posterior and prior accessible volumes in parameter space. For an over-complex model, this ratio will be small. The structure $\mathcal{M}$ with the largest marginal likelihood $P(\mathcal{D}|\mathcal{M})$ will be determined by the

Number of nodes	2	4	6	8	10
Number of topologies	3	543	3.7×10^6	7.8×10^{11}	4.2×10^{18}

Table 2.1. Number of Bayesian network topologies as a function of the number of nodes in the graph. From [32].

trade-off between having to fit the data well, so as to get a large likelihood $P(\mathcal{D}|\hat{\mathbf{q}}, \mathcal{M})$, and the need to do so with a low model complexity, so as to get a large Occam factor. Consequently, even for a flat prior $P(\mathcal{M})$, the posterior probability (2.19) includes a penalty for unnecessary complexity, which guards against over-fitting.

This chapter will not discuss the choice of prior. It is just noted that under certain regularity conditions, the parameter priors $P(\mathbf{q}|\mathcal{M})$ for all structures $\mathcal{M}$ can be specified using a single prior network, together with a "virtual" data count that describes the confidence in that prior [17].

Now, it can be shown that when certain regularity conditions for the prior $P(\mathbf{q}|\mathcal{M})$ and the likelihood $P(\mathcal{D}|\mathbf{q}, \mathcal{M})$ are satisfied and when the data are *complete*, then the integral in (2.20) becomes analytically tractable [16]. Unfortunately, this closed-form solution to (2.20) does not imply a straightforward solution to (2.17): the number of network structures increases super-exponentially with the number of nodes, as demonstrated in Table 2.1, and the optimization problem is known to be NP-hard [6]. We therefore have to resort to heuristic optimization methods, like hill-climbing or simulated annealing [22]. A heuristic acceleration of these procedures, which restricts the search in structure space to the most "relevant" regions, is discussed in [12].

2.2.2 Markov Chain Monte Carlo (MCMC)

In many situations, there is reason to question the appropriateness of the learning paradigm based on (2.17) altogether. For example, when inferring genetic network from microarray data, as discussed in Chapters 8 and 9, the data $\mathcal{D}$ are usually sparse, which implies that the posterior distribution over structures, $P(\mathcal{M}|\mathcal{D})$, is likely to be diffuse. Consequently, $P(\mathcal{M}|\mathcal{D})$ will not be adequately represented by a single structure $\mathcal{M}^*$, as illustrated in Figure 8.5 on page 245, and it is more appropriate to sample networks from the posterior probability

$$P(\mathcal{M}|\mathcal{D}) = \frac{P(\mathcal{D}|\mathcal{M})P(\mathcal{M})}{P(\mathcal{D})} = \frac{P(\mathcal{D}|\mathcal{M})P(\mathcal{M})}{\sum_{\mathcal{M}'} P(\mathcal{D}|\mathcal{M}')P(\mathcal{M}')} \tag{2.22}$$

so as to obtain a representative sample of high-scoring network structures, that is, structures that offer a good explanation of the data. Again, a direct approach is impossible due to the denominator in (2.22), which in itself is a sum over the whole model space and, consequently, intractable. A solution to this problem, proposed by Metropolis et al. [30] and Hastings [15], reviewed,

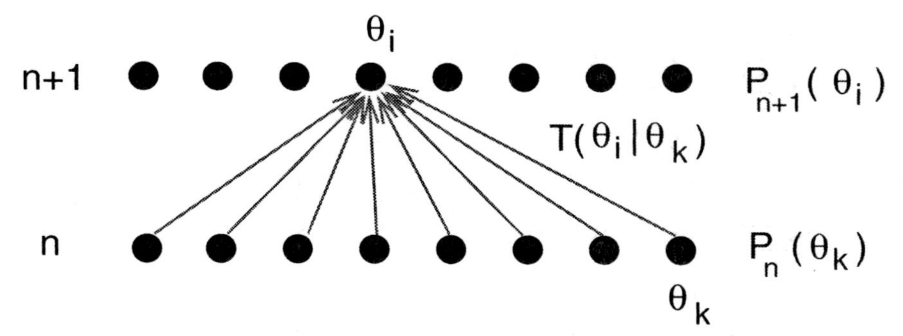

Fig. 2.12. Illustration of a Markov chain. $P_n(\theta_k)$ is the probability distribution in the nth step of the algorithm, where θ_k, in general, can be a structure, $\mathcal{M}_k$, a parameter vector, $\mathbf{q}_k$, or a combination of both, $(\mathcal{M}_k, \mathbf{q}_k)$. In the current application, we are only interested in the former, but applications of the other two cases will be discussed in later chapters of this book. The probability $P_n(\theta_k)$ evolves in time by application of the Markov transition matrix $\mathbf{T}$, which, in a single application, transforms $P_n(\theta_k)$ into $P_{n+1}(\theta_k)$. If the Markov chain is ergodic, $P_n(\theta_k)$ will converge to the equilibrium distribution $P_\infty(\theta_k)$, which is unique and independent of the initial conditions.

for instance, in [4], [13] and [28], and first applied to Bayesian networks by Madigan and York [29], is to devise a Markov chain

$$P_{n+1}(\mathcal{M}_i) = \sum_k T(\mathcal{M}_i|\mathcal{M}_k)P_n(\mathcal{M}_k) \tag{2.23}$$

that converges in distribution to the posterior probability $P(\mathcal{M}|\mathcal{D})$ of (2.22):

$$P_n(\mathcal{M}) \overset{n\to\infty}{\longrightarrow} P(\mathcal{M}|\mathcal{D}) \tag{2.24}$$

The Markov matrix $\mathbf{T}$ in (2.23) is a matrix of transition probabilities, with $T(\mathcal{M}_i|\mathcal{M}_k)$ denoting the probability of a transition from model $\mathcal{M}_k$ into model $\mathcal{M}_i$: $\mathcal{M}_k \to \mathcal{M}_i$. An illustration of (2.23) is given in Figure 2.12.

The important feature of a Markov chain is that, under the fairly weak condition of *ergodicity*,[1] the distribution $P_n(\mathcal{M}_k)$ converges to a *stationary distribution* $P_\infty(\mathcal{M}_k)$:

$$P_n(\mathcal{M}_k) \overset{n\to\infty}{\longrightarrow} P_\infty(\mathcal{M}_k) \tag{2.25}$$

This stationary distribution is independent of the initialization of the Markov chain and uniquely determined by the Markov transition matrix $\mathbf{T}$:

[1] A Markov chain is called *ergodic* if it is *aperiodic* and *irreducible*. An *irreducible* Markov chain is one in which all states are reachable from all other states. A sufficient test for *aperiodicity* is that each state has a "self-loop," meaning that the probability that the next state is the same as the current state is non-zero. In general it is difficult to prove that a Markov chain is ergodic. However, ergodicity can be assumed to hold in most real-world applications.

$$P_\infty(\mathcal{M}_i) = \sum_k T(\mathcal{M}_i|\mathcal{M}_k)P_\infty(\mathcal{M}_k) \tag{2.26}$$

The idea, therefore, is to construct the transition matrix $\mathbf{T}$ in such a way that the resulting Markov chain has the desired posterior probability $P(\mathcal{M}|\mathcal{D})$ of (2.22) as its stationary distribution: $P(\mathcal{M}|\mathcal{D}) = P_\infty(\mathcal{M})$. A sufficient condition for this to hold is the equation of *detailed balance*:

$$\frac{T(\mathcal{M}_k|\mathcal{M}_i)}{T(\mathcal{M}_i|\mathcal{M}_k)} = \frac{P(\mathcal{M}_k|\mathcal{D})}{P(\mathcal{M}_i|\mathcal{D})} = \frac{P(D|\mathcal{M}_k)P(\mathcal{M}_k)}{P(D|\mathcal{M}_i)P(\mathcal{M}_i)} \tag{2.27}$$

To prove that this holds true, we have to show that for a transition matrix $\mathbf{T}$ satisfying (2.27), the posterior probability $P(\mathcal{M}|\mathcal{D})$ of (2.22) is the stationary distribution and therefore obeys (2.26):

$$\sum_k T(\mathcal{M}_i|\mathcal{M}_k)P(\mathcal{M}_k|\mathcal{D}) = P(\mathcal{M}_i|\mathcal{D}) \tag{2.28}$$

Now, from (2.27) we have

$$T(\mathcal{M}_k|\mathcal{M}_i)P(\mathcal{M}_i|\mathcal{D}) = T(\mathcal{M}_i|\mathcal{M}_k)P(\mathcal{M}_k|\mathcal{D}) \tag{2.29}$$

and consequently

$$\begin{aligned}\sum_k T(\mathcal{M}_i|\mathcal{M}_k)P(\mathcal{M}_k|\mathcal{D}) &= \sum_k T(\mathcal{M}_k|\mathcal{M}_i)P(\mathcal{M}_i|\mathcal{D}) \\ &= P(\mathcal{M}_i|\mathcal{D})\sum_k T(\mathcal{M}_k|\mathcal{M}_i) \\ &= P(\mathcal{M}_i|\mathcal{D})\end{aligned} \tag{2.30}$$

which is identical to (2.28) and thus completes the proof. Note that the last step in (2.30) follows from the fact that $T(\mathcal{M}_k|\mathcal{M}_i)$ is a conditional probability, which is normalized.

In practically setting up a Markov chain, note that a transition into another structure, $\mathcal{M}_k \rightarrow \mathcal{M}_i$, consists of two parts. First, given $\mathcal{M}_k$, a new structure is proposed with a proposal probability $Q(\mathcal{M}_i|\mathcal{M}_k)$. In a second step, this new structure is then accepted with an acceptance probability $A(\mathcal{M}_i|\mathcal{M}_k)$. A transition probability is therefore given by the product of a proposal and an acceptance probability and can be written as

$$T(\mathcal{M}_k|\mathcal{M}_i) = Q(\mathcal{M}_k|\mathcal{M}_i)A(\mathcal{M}_k|\mathcal{M}_i) \tag{2.31}$$

The proposal probabilities $Q(\mathcal{M}_k|\mathcal{M}_i)$ are defined by the way we design our moves in the model space (see, for instance, Figure 2.15). From (2.27) and (2.31), we then obtain the following condition for the acceptance probabilities:

$$\frac{A(\mathcal{M}_k|\mathcal{M}_i)}{A(\mathcal{M}_i|\mathcal{M}_k)} = \frac{P(D|\mathcal{M}_k)P(\mathcal{M}_k)Q(\mathcal{M}_i|\mathcal{M}_k)}{P(D|\mathcal{M}_i)P(\mathcal{M}_i)Q(\mathcal{M}_k|\mathcal{M}_i)} \tag{2.32}$$

for which a sufficient condition is

$$A(\mathcal{M}_k|\mathcal{M}_i) = \min\left\{\frac{P(D|\mathcal{M}_k)P(\mathcal{M}_k)Q(\mathcal{M}_i|\mathcal{M}_k)}{P(D|\mathcal{M}_i)P(\mathcal{M}_i)Q(\mathcal{M}_k|\mathcal{M}_i)}, 1\right\} \tag{2.33}$$

To summarize: Accepting new configurations $\mathcal{M}_k$ with the probability (2.33) is a sufficient condition for satisfying the equation of detailed balance (2.27) which itself (assuming ergodicity) is a sufficient condition for the convergence of the Markov chain to the desired posterior distribution (2.22). While a direct computation of the posterior probability (2.22) is intractable due to the sum in the denominator, the equation of detailed balance (2.27) and the acceptance criterion (2.33) only depend on the ratio of the posterior probabilities. Consequently, the intractable denominator cancels out. The algorithm, thus, can be summarized as follows:

Metropolis–Hastings algorithm

- Start from an initial structure $\mathcal{M}^{(0)}$
- Iterate for $n = 1 \dots N$
  1. Obtain a new structure $\mathcal{M}^{(n)}$ from the proposal distribution $Q(\mathcal{M}^{(n)}|\mathcal{M}^{(n-1)})$
  2. Accept the new model with probability $A(\mathcal{M}^{(n)}|\mathcal{M}^{(n-1)})$, given by (2.33), otherwise leave the model unchanged: $\mathcal{M}^{(n)} = \mathcal{M}^{(n-1)}$
- Discard an initial equilibration or burn-in period to allow the Markov chain to reach stationarity. For example, discard $\mathcal{M}_1, \dots, \mathcal{M}_{N/2}$
- Compute expectation values from the MCMC sample $\{\mathcal{M}_{N/2+1}, \dots, \mathcal{M}_N\}$:

$$\langle f \rangle = \sum_{\mathcal{M}} f(\mathcal{M})P(\mathcal{M}|\mathcal{D}) \simeq \frac{2}{N} \sum_{n=N/2+1}^{N} f(\mathcal{M}_n)$$

An illustration is given in Figure 2.13. Note that this algorithm is not restricted to discrete (cardinal) entities, like topologies $\mathcal{M}$, but that it can equally be applied to continuous entities, like network parameters $\mathbf{q}$. In this case expectation values are typically given by integrals of the form $\langle f \rangle = \int f(\mathbf{q})P(\mathbf{q}|\mathcal{D})d\mathbf{q}$, which are approximated by discrete sums over the parameters $\{\mathbf{q}_1, \dots, \mathbf{q}_N\}$ sampled along the MCMC trajectory:

$$\langle f \rangle = \int f(\mathbf{q})P(\mathbf{q}|\mathcal{D})d\mathbf{q} \simeq \frac{2}{N} \sum_{n=N/2+1}^{N} f(\mathbf{q}_n)$$

The MCMC approximation is exact in the limit of an infinitely long Markov chain. In theory, the initialization of the Markov chain and the details of the proposal distribution are unimportant: if the condition of detailed balance (2.27) is satisfied, an ergodic Markov chain will converge to its stationary distribution (2.28) irrespective of these details. In practice, however, extreme starting values and unskillfully chosen proposal distributions may slow down

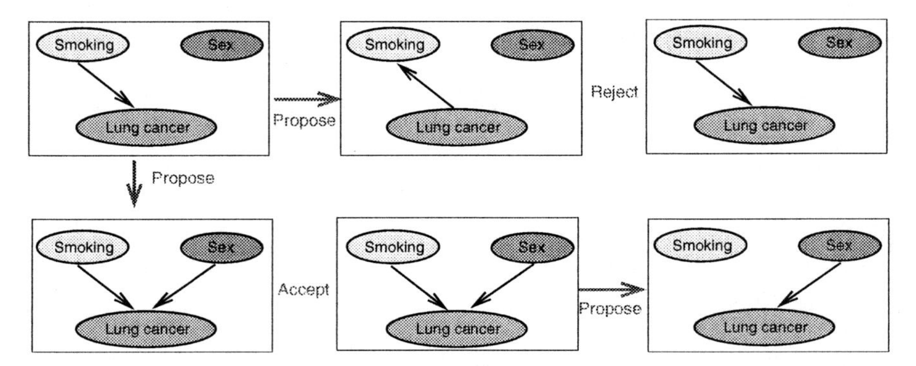

Fig. 2.13. Illustration of MCMC. Starting from the initial network shown in the top left, a new network is proposed (top middle) and accepted with a probability given by (2.33). In this example, the proposed network is rejected (top right). A new network is proposed (bottom left) and again accepted with a probability given by (2.33), which in this example leads to an acceptance of the proposed structure (bottom middle). This structure is now taken as the initial configuration, from which a new network is proposed in the next move (bottom right).

Step size λ	0.5	2.0	10.0
Relative error	79%	17%	58%

Table 2.2. Dependence of the relative prediction error on the steps size of the proposal scheme for the MCMC simulation of Figure 2.14.

the mixing and convergence of the chain and result in a very long burn-in, in which case the MCMC sampler may fail to converge towards the main support of the stationary distribution in the available simulation time. An example is given in Figure 2.14, where we want to infer the mean of a univariate Normal distribution from an MCMC sample of size 200, discarding a burn-in phase of the first 100 MCMC steps. (This is just an illustration. In practice we would not resort to an MCMC simulation to solve this simple problem.) Our entity of interest, in this case, is a single continuous random variable q, and we choose the proposal distribution $Q(q^{(n+1)}|q^{(n)})$ to be a uniform distribution over an interval of length λ (the *step size*), centred on the current value in the Markov chain, $q^{(n)}$. Figure 2.14 shows a trace plot of $q^{(n)}$ for three values of the step size λ. In the left subfigure, λ has been chosen too small, and the convergence of the Markov chain is slow. This is indicated by a high acceptance ratio of about 80% of the moves, which suggests that the step size should be increased. In the right subfigure, λ has been chosen too large, leading to a Markov chain that is too sticky and has a very low acceptance ratio of only 17%, wasting a lot of computer time by rejecting most of the moves. The subfigure in the middle shows an appropriate choice of λ, where the acceptance ratio is about 50%. This optimal choice results in the fastest convergence of the Markov chain and is reflected by the smallest prediction

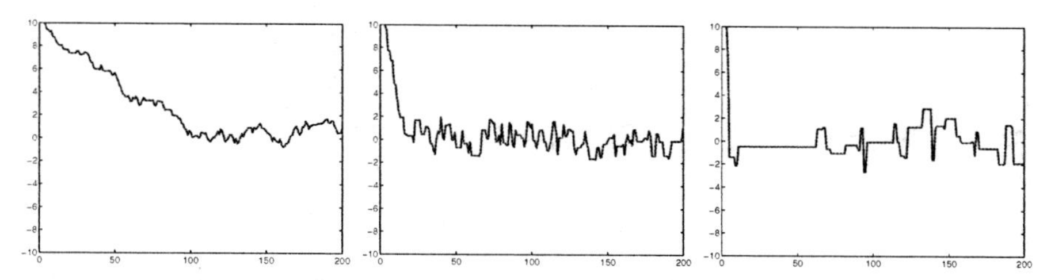

Fig. 2.14. Dependence of the MCMC convergence on the proposal distribution. The figures show MCMC trace plots of a univariate continuous random variable q with a (known) normal $N(0,1)$ distribution; hence the true mean is $\langle q \rangle = 0$. The proposal distribution $Q(q^{(n+1)}|q^{(n)})$ was chosen to be a uniform distribution over an interval of length λ, centred on the current value $q^{(n)}$. The figures were obtained for three different values of the step size λ. Left: $\lambda = 0.5$; middle: $\lambda = 2.0$; right: $\lambda = 10.0$.

error, as seen from Table 2.2. In this particular example, the choice of the proposal distribution (determined by λ) is not particularly critical because one can easily continue the MCMC simulation over about 10,000 or 100,000 steps, in which case all three alternatives give practically identical results. For more complex problems, however, where computer time is a critical issue, the optimization of the proposal distribution can become most important. The previous example suggests that, starting from a random choice of λ, one should adjust this parameter until an acceptance ratio of about 50% is reached. In general, the parameters of more complex proposal distributions should be tuned in a similar way. Note, however, that this tuning has to be restricted to the burn-in phase of the algorithm, and it must not be continued in the sampling phase. The reason is that optimizing the parameters of the proposal distribution on the basis of a history of past configurations violates the condition of detailed balance (2.27) and may therefore lead to a biased distribution that may not be representative of the true stationary distribution (2.28).

When the proposal distribution is symmetric, $Q(\mathcal{M}_k|\mathcal{M}_i) = Q(\mathcal{M}_i|\mathcal{M}_k)$, it cancels out in (2.33), and the algorithm reduces to the *Metropolis algorithm* [30]. For asymmetric proposal distributions, the scheme is called the *Metropolis–Hastings* algorithm [15], and the ratio of the proposal probabilities is usually referred to as the *Hastings ratio*. While in some cases the asymmetry of the proposal distribution is introduced deliberately as a means of accelerating the convergence of the Markov chain, it is often inherent in the nature of the proposal mechanism and needs to be considered carefully by the user in order to avoid biased results. Take, for example, the proposal mechanism for generating new DAGs, as illustrated in Figure 2.15. One might, naively, assume that the proposal distribution is symmetric. After all, there are only three elementary operations – edge creation, edge reversal, and edge deletion – all of which can be chosen with the same probability for the forward and the

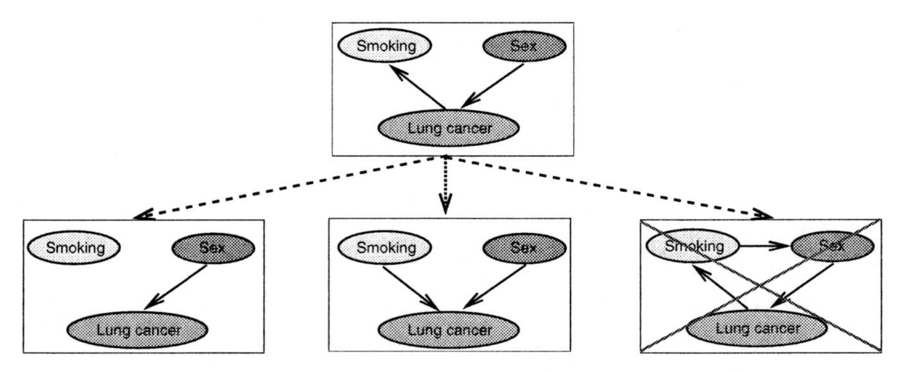

Fig. 2.15. Elementary MCMC moves for DAGs. The figure shows three typical elementary proposal moves: (1) deletion of an edge (left), (2) reversal of an edge (middle), and (3) creation of a new edge (right). Note that the last two operations may lead to graphs that violate the acyclicity constraint and therefore have to be discarded. An example is shown on the right.

backward move and, therefore, should cancel out when computing the Hastings ratio. A more careful consideration, however, reveals that this assumption is false. The reason for this fallacy is that, as a consequence of the acyclicity constraint, certain proposal moves will lead to invalid DAGs that have to be discarded (as illustrated in Figure 2.15). Figure 2.16 demonstrates how the Hastings ratio is computed properly. The figure shows the neighbourhoods of two DAGs, where the neighbourhood is the set of all valid DAGs that can be reached from the given DAG with one of the elementary operations of Figure 2.15. As a consequence of the acyclicity constraint, the neighbourhoods of two neighbouring DAGs are not necessarily of the same size. Consequently, the proposal probability of an MCMC move, which is given by the inverse of the neighborhood size, is not equal to that of the opposite move, leading to a Hastings ratio that is different from 1. For complex networks with large neighbourhoods, the computation of the Hastings ratio is therefore not trivial and requires the determination of the number of all valid (acyclic) graphs in the neighbourhoods of the two DAGs involved in the proposal move.

Recall that in theory an ergodic Markov chain converges to the true posterior distribution irrespective of the choice of the proposal distribution and the initialization. In practice, however, it is difficult to decide whether an MCMC simulation has sufficiently converged. A simple heuristic convergence test is shown in Figure 2.17. Note, however, that passing the indicated test is only a necessary rather than a sufficient condition for convergence as it may not distinguish between meta-stable disequilibrium and true equilibrium.

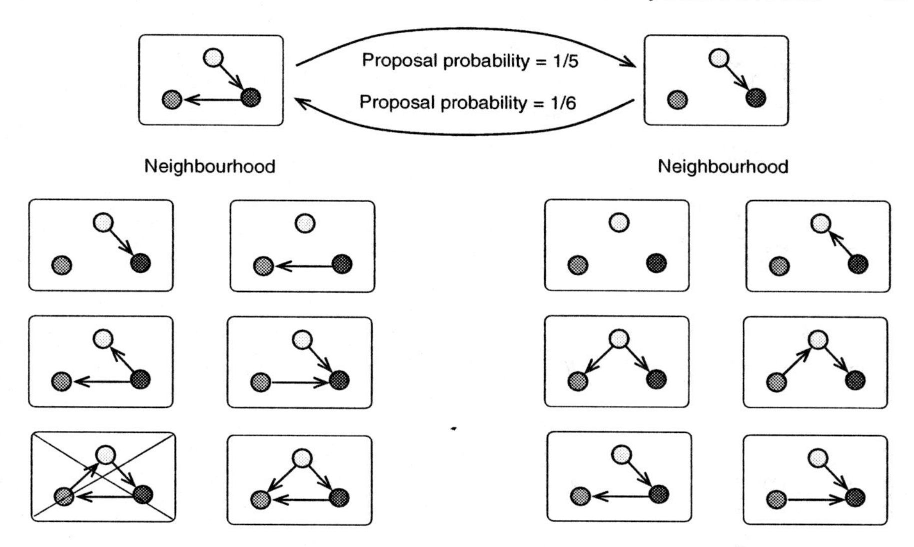

Fig. 2.16. DAG neighbourhoods and Hastings ratio. The figure shows the neighbourhoods of two DAGs, where the neighbourhood of a DAG is the set of all valid DAGs that can be reached from the specified DAG with one of the elementary operations of Figure 2.15. The neighbourhoods of two neighbouring DAGs are not necessarily of the same size: while the DAG on the right has six neighbours, the DAG on the left has only five because one of the graphs in its neighbourhood violates the acyclicity constraint. The Hastings ratio is given by the ratio of the neighbourhood sizes of the two networks involved in the proposal move. The Hastings ratio for an MCMC proposal move from the left to the right DAG is thus given by 5/6, while the Hastings ratio for the opposite move is 6/5.

2.2.3 Equivalence Classes

Figure 2.18 shows the four elementary Bayesian networks we have already encountered several times in this chapter. All networks have the same skeleton, which is the configuration of edges without their direction, but they differ with respect to the edge directions. However, expanding the joint probability $P(A, B, C)$ according to (2.1) gives the same factorization for three of the networks irrespective of the edge directions. These networks are therefore *equivalent*, that is, they show alternative ways of describing the same set of independence relations. In general, it can be shown that networks are equivalent if and only if they have the same skeleton and the same *v-structure*, where the latter denotes a configuration of two directed edges converging on the same node without an edge between the parents [5]. An equivalence class can be represented by a *partially directed acyclic graph* (PDAG), which is a graph that contains both directed and undirected edges. An example is given in the bottom of Figure 2.18, and in Figure 2.19, where the subfigure on the right shows the equivalence class that corresponds to the Bayesian network on

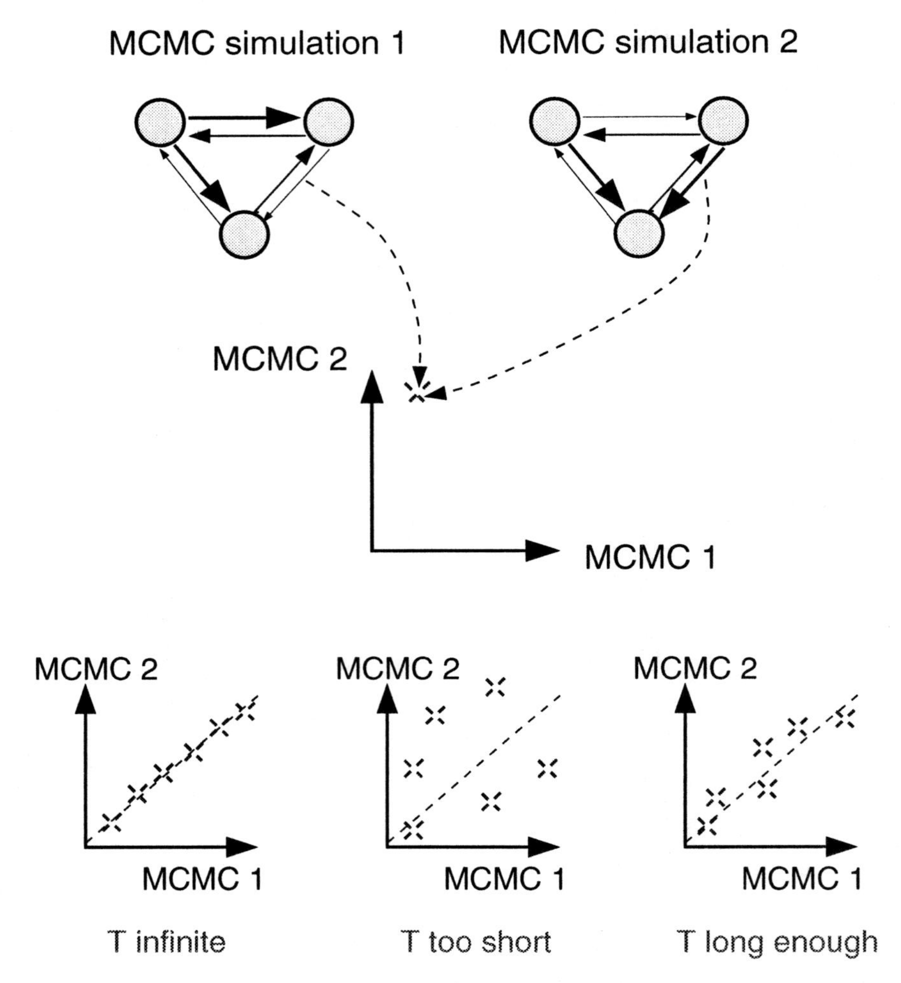

Fig. 2.17. Convergence test for MCMC simulations. *Top:* MCMC simulations are started from different initializations and/or different random number generator seeds. Corresponding posterior probabilities of the edges, obtained from different simulations, are plotted against each other. *Bottom left: Infinite simulation time T.* For an infinitely long simulation time, all MCMC simulations give the same results: the estimated posterior probabilities of the edges are equal to the true posterior probabilities irrespective of the initialization of the Markov chain, and the scatter plot has the form of a straight line. *Bottom middle: Simulation time T too short.* Insufficient convergence or mixing of the Markov chain is indicated by a scatter plot that strongly deviates from the straight line. This deviation indicates a strong dependence of the results on the initialization, resulting from insufficient convergence or mixing. *Bottom right: Simulation time T long enough.* A necessary condition for sufficient convergence and mixing is a scatter plot that does not deviate markedly from the diagonal line.

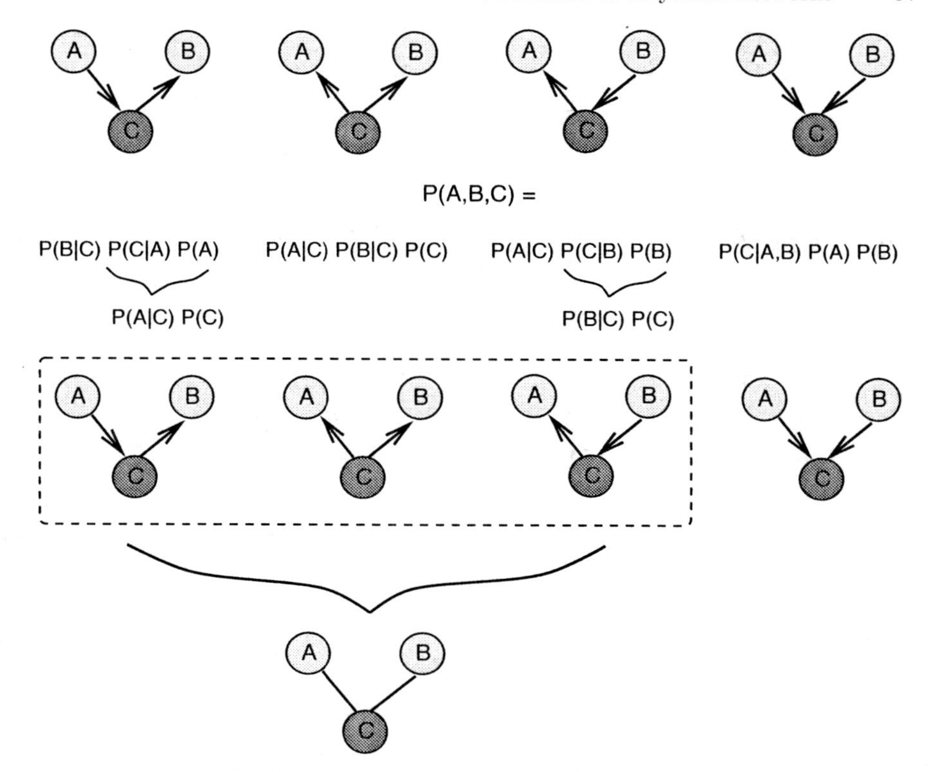

Fig. 2.18. Equivalent Bayesian networks. The top subfigure shows four BNs with their respective expansion of the joint probability distribution. The three BNs on the left are equivalent and lead to the same expansion. These BNs thus belong to the same equivalence class, which can be represented by the undirected graph at the bottom.

the left. Note that an undirected edge indicates that its direction is not unequivocal among the DAGs in the equivalence class represented by the PDAG. Conversely, a directed edge indicates that all DAGs in the equivalence class concur about its direction.

Under fairly general conditions, equivalent BNs have the same likelihood score [16].[2] Unless this symmetry is broken by the prior,[3] the posterior probabilities are the same, that is, equivalent BNs can *not* be distinguished on the basis of the data. This implies that, in general, we can only learn PDAGs

---

[2] Heckerman [16] distinguishes between *structure equivalence*, identical to the notion of equivalence used in the present chapter, and *distribution equivalence*. The latter equivalence concept is defined with respect to a distribution family $\mathcal{F}$ and implies invariance with respect to the likelihood.

[3] Heckerman et al. [17] discuss the choice of priors that do not break the symmetry of equivalence classes.

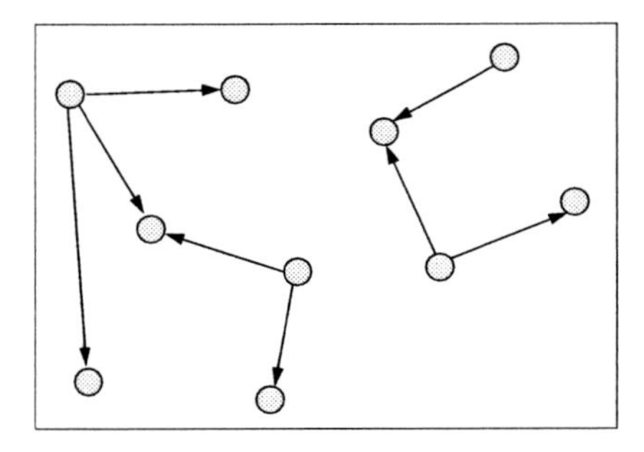

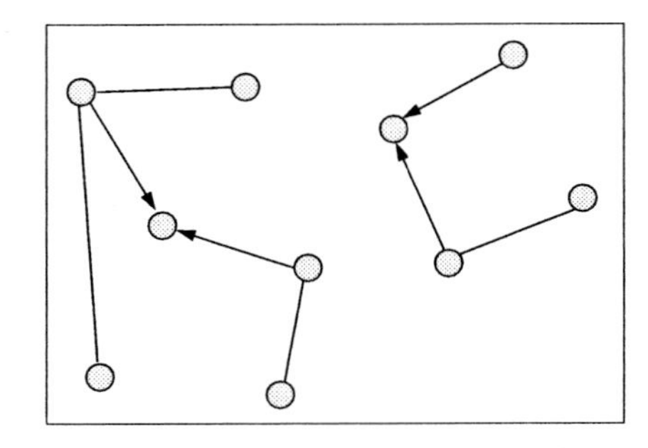

Fig. 2.19. DAG and PDAG. The left figure shows a DAG. The right figure shows the corresponding PDAG, which represents the equivalence class to which the DAG on the left belongs. Note that the skeleton and the v-structure, that is, the set of converging edge pairs, remain unchanged. Information about the directions of the remaining edges, however, gets lost.

rather than DAGs from the data. The consequence is that for a given network structure $\mathcal{M}$ learned from the data, or sampled from the posterior distribution $P(\mathcal{M}|\mathcal{D})$, one has to identify the whole equivalence class $\mathcal{C}(\mathcal{M})$ to which $\mathcal{M}$ belongs and then discard all those edge directions that are not unequivocal among all $\mathcal{M}' \in \mathcal{C}(\mathcal{M})$. For further details and references, see [5] and [16].

2.2.4 Causality

A Bayesian network conveys information about conditional dependence relations between interacting random variables: given its parents, a node is independent of its nondescendants. Ultimately, we might be more interested in the flow of causality and in finding a *causal network* as a model of the causal processes of the system of interest. In fact, we can interpret a DAG as a causal graph if we assign a stricter interpretation to the edges, whereby the parents of a variable are its immediate causes. Take, as an example, the DAG in Figure 2.4. Interpreting this DAG as a Bayesian network implies that given information about the rain the probability of finding the grass to be wet is independent of the clouds. Interpreted as a causal graph, the edges indicate that clouds are the immediate cause for rain, and that rain is the immediate cause for the wetness of the grass. Obviously, there is a relation between these two interpretations. Given information on the rain, the state of the wetness of the grass is completely determined and no longer depends on the clouds: if it rains, the grass gets wet irrespective of the cloud formation. This causal graph thus satisfies what is called the *causal Markov assumption:* given the values of a variable's immediate causes, this variable is independent of its earlier causes. When the causal Markov assumption holds, the causal network satisfies the Markov independence relations of the corresponding Bayesian network.

An important question is whether we can learn a causal network from the data. Obviously, a first difficulty in trying to achieve this objective is the exis-

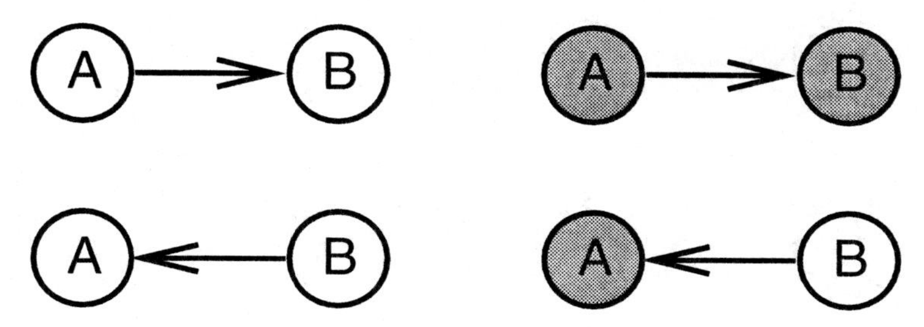

Fig. 2.20. Effect of intervention. The two DAGs on the left are in the same equivalence class, and the edge direction can *not* be inferred from observations alone. To infer the causal direction, the value for A has to be set externally. If A is a causal ancestor of B, this intervention is likely to lead to a changed value of B (top right). If, however, B is a causal ancestor of A, this intervention will have no effect on B (bottom right).

tence of equivalence classes. Recall from the discussion of the previous section that we can only learn equivalence classes of DAGs (represented by PDAGs) rather than DAGs themselves. This implies that effectively a lot of edge directions get lost, obstructing the inference of causality. In what follows we have to distinguish between *observations* and *interventions*. An *observation* is a passive measurement of variables in the domain of interest, for instance, the simultaneous measurement of gene expression levels in a standard microarray experiment.[4] In an *intervention*, the values of some variables are set from outside the system, for instance, by knocking out or over-expressing a particular gene. An example is given in Figure 2.20. More formally, recall that the likelihood scores of two BNs with equivalent DAGs, $\mathcal{M}$ and $\mathcal{M}'$, are the same, where the likelihood is computed from (2.1). When setting the value of node k externally to some value x_k^*, then $P(X_k = x_k^*|\mathcal{X}_{pa[k]}) = 1$. This is because setting a value by external force means that the respective node takes on this particular value with probability 1 irrespective of the values of the other nodes in the network. Consequently, the contributions of all those nodes that are subject to intervention effectively disappear from (2.1):

$$P(X_1, X_2, \ldots, X_n) = \prod_{i \notin I} P(X_i|\mathcal{X}_{pa[i]}) \tag{2.34}$$

where I is the set of intervened nodes. This modification can destroy the symmetry within an equivalence class, that is, the likelihood scores for $\mathcal{M}$ and $\mathcal{M}'$ might no longer be the same, which may resolve the ambiguity about certain edge directions.

A second and potentially more serious difficulty in trying to learn causal structures from data is the possible presence of hidden, unobserved variables. Figure 2.20, for instance, shows two possible DAG structures that explain

[4] See Chapter 7 for an introduction to microarray experiments.

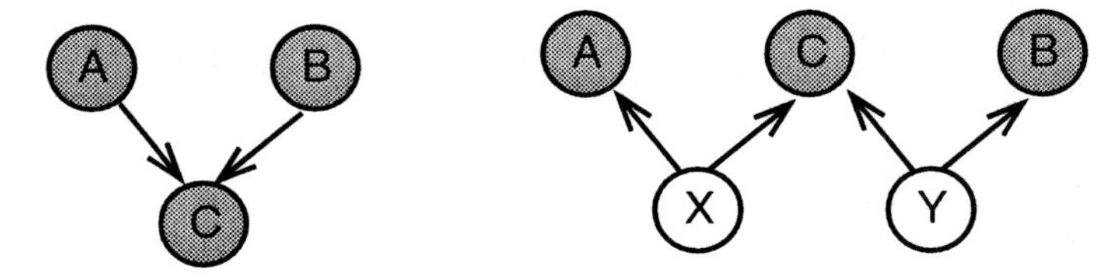

Fig. 2.21. Equivalence of networks with hidden variables. The network on the left without hidden variables is equivalent to the network on the right, which contains two additional hidden variables. Filled circles represent observed, empty circles represent hidden nodes.

a conditional dependence between two random variables. However, a third possibility is that both observed random variables depend on a third, hidden variable, as in Figure 2.3. Another example is given in Figure 2.21, where the network on the left, which only includes observed nodes, is equivalent to the network on the right, which contains two extra hidden nodes. This equivalence can easily be shown. Applying the factorization rule (2.1) to the graph on the right gives:

$$\begin{aligned} P(A, B, C, X, Y) &= P(A|X)P(X)P(C|X, Y)P(B|Y)P(Y) \\ &= P(X|A)P(A)P(C|X, Y)P(Y|B)P(B) \end{aligned}$$

where in the second step (1.3) has been used. Then, marginalizing over the unobserved variables X and Y yields

$$\begin{aligned} P(A, B, C) &= \sum_X \sum_Y P(A, B, C, X, Y) \\ &= P(A)P(B) \sum_X \sum_Y P(C|X, Y)P(X|A)P(Y|B) \\ &= P(A)P(B)P(C|A, B) \end{aligned}$$

This result is identical to the factorization one obtains from the structure on the left of Figure 2.21. Consequently, the two network structures in Figure 2.21 are equivalent, and we can *not* decide whether A and B are causal ancestors of C, or whether all three variables are controlled by some hidden causal ancestors. A more complex analysis [40] reveals that it is possible to characterize all networks with latent variables that can result in the same set of independence relations over the observed variables. However, it is not clear how to score such an equivalence class, which consists of many models with different numbers of latent variables, and this lack of a score defies any inference procedure.

2.3 Learning Bayesian Networks from Incomplete Data

2.3.1 Introduction

The previous section was based on the assumption that we can find a closed-form solution to the integral in (2.20). This is only possible if we have complete observation without any missing or *hidden* variables. In many applications this cannot be assumed, since observations may be missing either systematically or at random. Take, for example, a microarray experiment, where we measure the expression levels of hundreds or thousands of genes simultaneously. As described in Chapter 7, some genes get occasionally *flagged*, meaning that the data quality is so poor that these measurements are at best ignored. It is also known that certain interactions in genetic regulatory networks are mediated by transcription factors, whose activation is often undetectable at the level of gene expression. In phylogenetics, covered in Chapters 4–6, DNA or RNA sequences are only available for contemporary or extant species, while those for extinct species are systematically missing. Further examples will be given in later chapters of this book. In all these applications, the assumption of complete observation is violated, and the integration in (2.20) becomes intractable.

2.3.2 Evidence Approximation and Bayesian Information Criterion

A simple approximation to (2.20) is as follows. First, consider a focused model in which $P(\mathbf{q}|\mathcal{D},\mathcal{M})$ is assumed to be dominated by the likelihood, either because of assuming a uniform prior on the parameters, or by increasing the sample size. That is, we set (assuming prior parameter independence)

$$P(\mathbf{q}|\mathcal{M}) = \prod_{i=1}^{\nu} P(q_i|\mathcal{M}) = c^{\nu} \tag{2.35}$$

where $\nu = \dim(\mathbf{q})$ is the dimension of the parameter space, and c is a constant. Next, define

$$E(\mathbf{q}) = -\log P(\mathcal{D}|\mathbf{q},\mathcal{M}) \tag{2.36}$$

$$\hat{\mathbf{q}} = \text{argmin}_{\mathbf{q}} E(\mathbf{q}) = \text{argmax}_{\mathbf{q}} P(\mathcal{D}|\mathbf{q},\mathcal{M}) \tag{2.37}$$

$$\mathbf{H} = \Big[\nabla_{\mathbf{q}}\nabla_{\mathbf{q}}^{\dagger} E(\mathbf{q})\Big]_{\mathbf{q}=\hat{\mathbf{q}}} = -\nabla_{\mathbf{q}}\nabla_{\mathbf{q}}^{\dagger}\Big[\log P(\mathcal{D}|\mathbf{q},\mathcal{M})\Big]_{\mathbf{q}=\hat{\mathbf{q}}} \tag{2.38}$$

where $\hat{\mathbf{q}}$ is the vector of maximum likelihood parameters, and $\mathbf{H}$ is the Hessian or empirical *Fisher information matrix*. Inserting (2.36) and (2.35) into (2.20) gives

$$P(\mathcal{D}|\mathcal{M}) = \int P(\mathcal{D}|\mathbf{q},\mathcal{M})P(\mathbf{q}|\mathcal{M})d\mathbf{q} = c^{\nu}\int \exp\Big[-E(\mathbf{q})\Big]d\mathbf{q} \tag{2.39}$$

Approximating the negative log-likelihood by a second-order Taylor series expansion, the so-called *Laplace approximation*,

$$E(\mathbf{q}) \approx E(\hat{\mathbf{q}}) + \frac{1}{2}(\mathbf{q} - \hat{\mathbf{q}})^{\dagger}\mathbf{H}(\mathbf{q} - \hat{\mathbf{q}}) \tag{2.40}$$

where the superscript † denotes matrix transposition, and inserting (2.40) into (2.39), we get

$$P(\mathcal{D}|\mathcal{M}) \approx c^{\nu} \exp\Big[- E(\hat{\mathbf{q}})\Big] \int \exp\Big[- \frac{1}{2}(\mathbf{q} - \hat{\mathbf{q}})^{\dagger}\mathbf{H}(\mathbf{q} - \hat{\mathbf{q}})\Big] d\mathbf{q} \tag{2.41}$$

$$= P(\mathcal{D}|\hat{\mathbf{q}}, \mathcal{M}) c^{\nu} \sqrt{\frac{(2\pi)^{\nu}}{\det \mathbf{H}}} \tag{2.42}$$

Taking logs, this gives:

$$\log P(\mathcal{D}|\mathcal{M}) = \log P(\mathcal{D}|\hat{\mathbf{q}}, \mathcal{M}) - \frac{1}{2} \log \det \mathbf{H} + \frac{\nu}{2} \log(2\pi c^2) \tag{2.43}$$

Equation (2.43), which in the neural network literature is referred to as the *evidence approximation* [26], [27], decomposes $\log P(\mathcal{D}|\mathcal{M})$ into two terms: the maximum log likelihood score, $\log P(\mathcal{D}|\hat{\mathbf{q}}, \mathcal{M})$, and a *penalty* or *regularization* term that depends on the Hessian $\mathbf{H}$. The integration (2.20) is thus reduced to an optimization, to obtain $\log P(\mathcal{D}|\hat{\mathbf{q}}, \mathcal{M})$, and the computation of the Hessian. For complex models, this computation of the Hessian can be quite involved [18], [19]. Therefore, a further approximation is often applied. Note that the Hessian $\mathbf{H}$ is symmetric and positive semi-definite, as seen from (2.38), and it thus has ν real nonnegative eigenvalues, $\{\varepsilon_i\}$, $i = 1, \ldots, \nu$. The determinant of a matrix is given by the product of its eigenvalues, which allows (2.43) to be rewritten as follows:

$$\log P(\mathcal{D}|\mathcal{M}) = \log P(\mathcal{D}|\hat{\mathbf{q}}, \mathcal{M}) - \frac{1}{2} \sum_{i=1}^{\nu} \log \left(\frac{\varepsilon_i}{2\pi c^2}\right) \tag{2.44}$$

The eigenvalues ε_i determine the curvature of the log-likelihood surface along the eigendirections at the maximum likelihood parameters $\hat{\mathbf{q}}$. This curvature increases with the sample size N, so the eigenvalues can be assumed to be proportional to N: $\varepsilon_i \propto N$. Now, introducing the further approximation of isotropy, that is, assuming the same curvature along all eigendirections:

$$\varepsilon_i \approx 2\pi c^2 N \quad \forall i \tag{2.45}$$

we get (recall that $\nu = \dim(\mathbf{q})$):

$$\log P(\mathcal{D}|\mathcal{M}) \approx \log P(\mathcal{D}|\hat{\mathbf{q}}, \mathcal{M}) - \frac{\nu}{2} \log N \tag{2.46}$$

This simple formula, which is a variant of the *minimum description length* in information theory [37], is known as the BIC (Bayesian information criterion) approximation, introduced by Schwarz [38]. The first term is the maximum likelihood estimate for model $\mathcal{M}$. The second term is a regularization term, which penalizes model complexity and results from the integration; compare with the discussion in Section 2.2.1. However, for sparse data $\mathcal{D}$, neither the Laplace approximation nor the assumption of isotropy, (2.45), are reasonable. In particular, both approximations assume that the likelihood function is unimodal, which does not hold for many models. In fact, this deviation from unimodality becomes particularly noticeable for small data sets, which may render both the evidence and BIC approximations unreliable. A different, simulation-based approach that overcomes this shortcoming will be discussed in Section 2.3.7.

2.3.3 The EM Algorithm

The previous section has demonstrated that under certain approximations the integration (2.20) reduces to an optimization problem, namely, to find the maximum likelihood parameters $\hat{\mathbf{q}}$ for a given model $\mathcal{M}$. This optimization, however, may not be trivial due to the presence of hidden variables. Denote by $\mathcal{D}$ the data corresponding to observed nodes in the graph. Denote by $\mathcal{S} = \{S_1, \ldots, S_M\}$ the set of hidden nodes and their associated random variables. The log likelihood is given by

$$L(\mathbf{q}, \mathcal{M}) = \log P(\mathcal{D}|\mathbf{q}, \mathcal{M}) = \log \sum_{\mathcal{S}} P(\mathcal{D}, \mathcal{S}|\mathbf{q}, \mathcal{M}) \tag{2.47}$$

which involves a marginalization over all possible configurations of hidden states. If each hidden state S_i, $i = 1, \ldots, M$, has K discrete values, we have to sum over K^M different terms, which for large values of M becomes intractable. To proceed, let $Q(\mathcal{S})$ denote some arbitrary distribution over the set of hidden states, and define

$$F(\mathbf{q}, \mathcal{M}) = \sum_{\mathcal{S}} Q(\mathcal{S}) \log \frac{P(\mathcal{D}, \mathcal{S}|\mathbf{q}, \mathcal{M})}{Q(\mathcal{S})} \tag{2.48}$$

$$KL[Q, P] = \sum_{\mathcal{S}} Q(\mathcal{S}) \log \frac{Q(\mathcal{S})}{P(\mathcal{S}|\mathcal{D}, \mathbf{q}, \mathcal{M})} \tag{2.49}$$

KL in (2.49) is the Kullback–Leibler divergence between the distributions Q and P, which is always non-negative and zero if and only if $Q = P$. The proof is based on the concavity of the log function and the normalization condition for probabilities: $\sum_{\mathcal{S}} Q(\mathcal{S}) = 1$:

$$\log x \leq x - 1 \quad \Longrightarrow \quad \log \frac{P(\mathcal{S})}{Q(\mathcal{S})} \leq \frac{P(\mathcal{S})}{Q(\mathcal{S})} - 1$$

$$\Longrightarrow \; Q(\mathcal{S}) \log \frac{P(\mathcal{S})}{Q(\mathcal{S})} \leq P(\mathcal{S}) - Q(\mathcal{S}) \quad \Longrightarrow \quad \sum_{\mathcal{S}} Q(\mathcal{S}) \log \frac{P(\mathcal{S})}{Q(\mathcal{S})} \leq 0$$

$$\Longrightarrow \; KL[Q, P] \geq 0$$

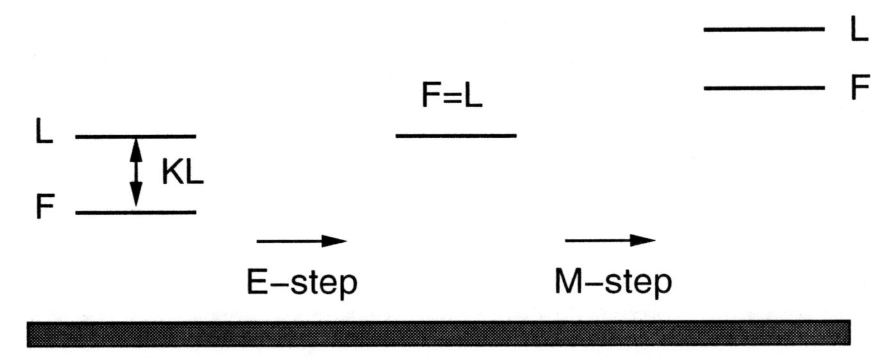

Fig. 2.22. Illustration of the EM algorithm. L, F, and KL are defined in equations (2.47)–(2.49). The algorithm is explained in the text.

From (2.47)–(2.49) we get:

$$L(\mathbf{q}, \mathcal{M}) \;=\; F(\mathbf{q}, \mathcal{M}) + KL[Q, P] \qquad (2.50)$$

This is the fundamental equation of the Expectation Maximization (EM) algorithm [8], [33]. An illustration is given in Figure 2.22. F is a lower bound on the log-likelihood L, with a difference given by KL. The E-step holds the parameters $\mathbf{q}$ fixed and sets $Q(\mathcal{S}) = P(\mathcal{S}|\mathcal{D}, \mathbf{q}, \mathcal{M})$; hence $KL(Q, P) = 0$ and $F = L$. The M-step holds the distribution $Q(\mathcal{S})$ fixed and computes the parameters $\mathbf{q}$ that maximize F. Since $F = L$ at the beginning of the M-step, and since the E-step does not affect the model parameters, each EM cycle is guaranteed to increase the likelihood unless the system has already converged to a (local) maximum (or, less likely, a saddle point). The power of the EM algorithm results from the fact that F is usually considerably easier to maximize with respect to the model parameters $\mathbf{q}$ than L. An example is given in Section 2.3.5.

2.3.4 Hidden Markov Models

A hidden Markov model (HMM) is a particular example of a Bayesian network with hidden nodes. In fact, the structure of an HMM is comparatively simple, which makes it an appropriate example for illustrating the concepts of the preceding subsection. Also, HMMs have been extensively applied in bioinformatics, and they will play an important role in later chapters of this book; see Section 5.10, Section 10.11.4, and Chapter 14. An illustrative example is given in Figure 2.23. Assume you are in a casino and take part in a gambling game that involves a die. You are playing against two croupiers: a fair croupier, who uses a fair die, and a corrupt croupier, who uses a loaded die. Unfortunately, the croupiers are hidden behind a wall, and all you observe is a sequence of die faces. The task is to predict which croupier is rolling the

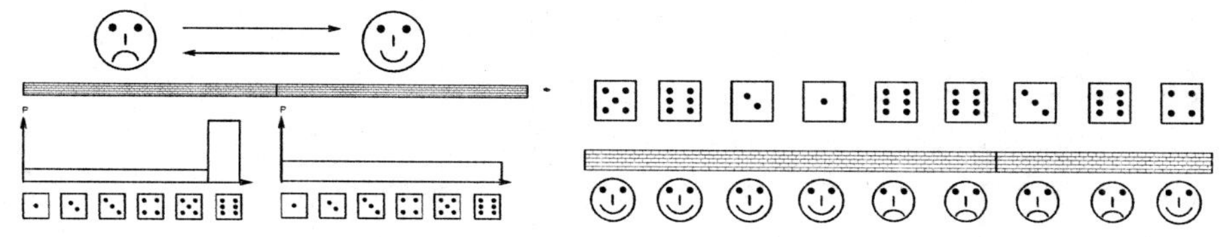

Fig. 2.23. The occasional corrupt casino. *Left:* Two croupiers are in a casino: a fair croupier, who uses a fair die, and a corrupt croupier, who uses a biased die. *Right:* The player only sees a sequence of die faces, but not the croupier, from whom he is separated by a wall. The task is to infer, from the sequence of observed die faces, which croupier has been rolling the die and to predict the breakpoint when the corrupt croupier is taking over. The idea for this illustration is taken from [9].

```
A C G T T A T A          A C G T T A T A
A G T C A T A      →     A – G T C A T A
```

Fig. 2.24. Pairwise DNA sequence alignment. The figure shows two hypothetical DNA sequences, each composed of the four nucleotides *adenine* (A), *cytosine* (C), *guanine* (G), and *thymine* (T). The sequences on the left are unaligned and seem to differ in all but one position. The sequences on the right have been aligned, and they differ only in two positions. Note that this alignment makes use of an extra symbol, the horizontal bar "–", which indicates an *indel* (an *insertion* or a *deletion*, depending on the reference sequence).

```
TGGAGACCAC CGTGAACGCC CATCA --- GG TCC T GCCCAA
TGGAGACCAC CGTGAACGCC CACCA --- AT TCT T GCCCAA
TGGAGACCAC CGTGAACGCC GCCCA TCT AT TCT T GCCCAA
TGGAGACCAC CGTGAACGCC CATCA --A AG TCT - GCCCAA
TGGAGACCAC CGTGAACGCC CACCA --- GG TCT T GCCCAA
```

Fig. 2.25. Multiple DNA sequence alignment. The figure shows a small section of a DNA sequence alignment of five strains of Hepatitis-B virus. Rows represent strains, and columns represent sequence positions. The letters represent the four nucleotides adenine (A), cytosine (C), guanine (G), and thymine (T), while the horizontal bars indicate gaps.

die at a given time and to predict the breakpoint where the corrupt croupier is taking over (in order to nab him).

As a second example, consider the problem of aligning DNA sequences. Recall that DNA is composed of an alphabet of four nucleotides: *adenine* (A), *cytosine* (C), *guanine* (G), and *thymine* (T). After obtaining the DNA sequences of the taxa of interest, we would like to compare homologous nucleotides, that is, nucleotides that have been acquired from the same common ancestor. The problem is complicated due to the possibility of *insertions* and *deletions* of nucleotides in the genome (referred to as *indels*). Take, for instance, Figure 2.24. A direct comparison of the two sequences on the left gives the erroneously small count of only a single site with identical nucleotides. This is due to the

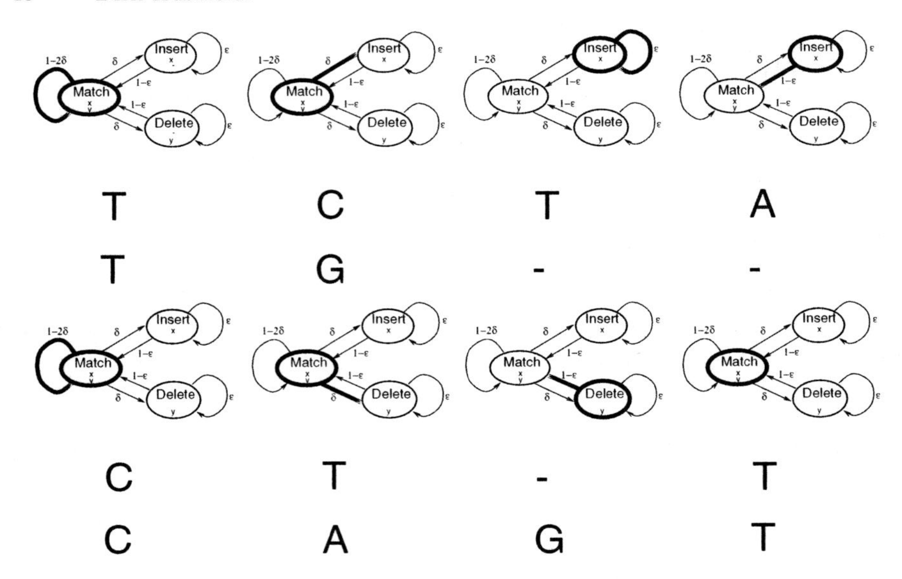

Fig. 2.26. Hidden states for pairwise DNA sequence alignment. The hidden states are represented by ellipses, and edges between these ellipses indicate possible transitions between the states. Active transitions are shown as thick lines. There are three different hidden states. (1) A *match* state emits a pair of nucleotides. (2) An *insert* state emits a nucleotide for the first sequence, and a gap for the second – so it "inserts" a nucleotide in the first sequence. (3) A *delete* state emits a nucleotide for the second sequence, and a gap for the first – hence it "deletes" a nucleotide in the first sequence.

insertion of a *C* in the second position of the first strand, or, equivalently, the deletion of a nucleotide at the second position of the second strand (the insertion of a so-called *gap*). A correct comparison leads to the alignment on the right of Figure 2.24, which suggests that the sequences differ in only two positions. The process of correcting for insertions and deletions is called DNA sequence alignment. Figure 2.25 shows a small subregion of a multiple DNA sequence alignment of five strains of Hepatitis-B virus.

The two examples given here have three important features in common. First, we can describe both processes in terms of a *hidden state* that has generated the observations. For the casino, this hidden state corresponds to the unknown croupier who is rolling the die. For the DNA sequence alignment, we can introduce conceptually a hidden state that indicates whether we have, at a given position, a nucleotide *match*, an *insertion*, or a *deletion*. An illustration is given in Figure 2.26. Second, the problem of finding the correct hidden states corresponding to a given sequence of observations is intrinsically stochastic. Observing, say, that the die face *six* occurs three times in a row gives some indication that the die may be biased. However, due to the inherent stochasticity of rolling a die this observation can also be obtained

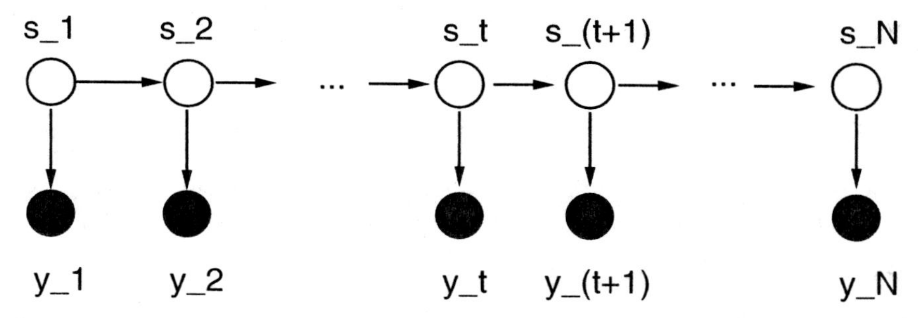

Fig. 2.27. Hidden Markov model. Black nodes represent observed random variables, white nodes represent hidden states, and arrows represent conditional dependencies. The joint probability factorizes into a product of *emission probabilities* (vertical arrows), *transition probabilities* (horizontal arrows), and the *initial probability*, that is, the probability of the initial state. The prediction task is to find the most likely sequence of hidden states given the observations.

from a fair die. Similarly, several mismatches between the nucleotides in corresponding DNA sequence positions may indicate that the sequences are misaligned. However, such mismatches can also occur in homologous sequences as a result of *mutations* during evolution. Consequently, we need probabilistic methods that allow robust inference in the presence of inherent stochasticity, and Bayesian networks are the ideal tools for this task. Third, and possibly most notably, both problems suffer from an explosion of the computational complexity. Given a sequence of observations – a sequence of die faces in the first example, or a sequence of nucleotide pairs in the second – we would like to find the *best* sequence of hidden states describing the observations. Given the intrinsic stochasticity mentioned above, *"best"* should be defined probabilistically as the mode of the posterior probability $P(\mathcal{S}|\mathcal{D})$, where $\mathcal{S}$ represents a sequence of hidden states, and $\mathcal{D}$ is the set of observations (the *"data"*). However, given K different hidden states ($K = 2$ for the casino, and $K = 3$ for the pairwise sequence alignment) and N sequence positions, there are K^N different hidden state sequences. Consequently, the number of hidden state sequences increases exponentially with the sequence length, which, in the most general scenario, prohibits an exhaustive search in sequence space.

To proceed, consider the Bayesian network in Figure 2.27, which contains two types of nodes. Filled circles represent observed random variables, $\mathbf{y}_t$ (which, in general, can be vectors). Empty circles represent hidden states, S_t. The index t can refer to time, as in the casino example, or to location, as in the alignment problem. Applying the expansion rule for Bayesian networks (2.1) to the network in Figure 2.27 gives:

$$P(\mathbf{y}_1, \ldots, \mathbf{y}_N, S_1, \ldots, S_N) = \prod_{t=1}^{N} P(\mathbf{y}_t|S_t) \prod_{t=2}^{N} P(S_t|S_{t-1})P(S_1) \qquad (2.51)$$

We refer to the set of $P(\mathbf{y}_t|S_t)$ as the *emission probabilities* (associated with the vertical edges), to $P(S_t|S_{t-1})$ as the *transition probabilities* (which are associated with the horizontal edges), and to $P(S_1)$ as the *initial probability*.

Since the dependence structure between the hidden states is obviously Markovian, the Bayesian network in Figure 2.27 is called a *hidden Markov model*. A consequence of this simplification is that the complexity of an exhaustive search in the space of hidden state sequences is no longer exponential in the sequence length. From (2.51) we obtain the recursion:

$$\begin{aligned}
\gamma_n(S_n) &= \max_{S_1,\ldots,S_{n-1}} \log P(\mathbf{y}_1,\ldots,\mathbf{y}_n,S_1,\ldots,S_n) \\
&= \max_{S_1,\ldots,S_{n-1}} \left[\sum_{t=1}^{n} \log P(\mathbf{y}_t|S_t) + \sum_{t=2}^{n} \log P(S_t|S_{t-1}) + \log P(S_1)\right] \\
&= \log P(\mathbf{y}_n|S_n) + \max_{S_{n-1}} \left[\log P(S_n|S_{n-1}) + \max_{S_1,\ldots,S_{n-2}} \left[\sum_{t=1}^{n-1} \log P(\mathbf{y}_t|S_t) \right.\right. \\
&\quad \left.\left. + \sum_{t=2}^{n-1} \log P(S_t|S_{t-1}) + \log P(S_1)\right]\right] \\
&= \log P(\mathbf{y}_n|S_n) + \max_{S_{n-1}} \left[\log P(S_n|S_{n-1}) + \gamma_{n-1}(S_{n-1})\right]
\end{aligned} \tag{2.52}$$

Obviously:

$$\begin{aligned}
\max_{S_1,\ldots,S_N} P(S_1,\ldots,S_N|\mathbf{y}_1,\ldots,\mathbf{y}_N) &= \max_{S_1,\ldots,S_N} \log P(\mathbf{y}_1,\ldots,\mathbf{y}_N,S_1,\ldots,S_N) \\
&= \max_{S_N} \gamma_N(S_N)
\end{aligned} \tag{2.53}$$

and the mode, $P(\hat{\mathcal{S}}|\mathcal{D}) = P(\hat{S}_1,\ldots,\hat{S}_N|\mathbf{y}_1,\ldots,\mathbf{y}_N)$, is obtained by recursive backtracking, starting from the initialization $\hat{S}_N = \text{argmax}_{S_N}\gamma_N(S_N)$, and continuing with the following iteration:

$$\hat{S}_{n-1} = \text{argmax}_{S_{n-1}} \left[\log P(\hat{S}_n|S_{n-1}) + \gamma_{n-1}(S_{n-1})\right] \tag{2.54}$$

This recursive iteration is called the *Viterbi algorithm* [36], which is a variant of *dynamic programming*. The computational complexity of a single step of the recursions (2.52) and (2.54) is $\mathcal{O}(K^2)$, that is, it only depends on the number of different states K, but is independent of the sequence length N. The total computational complexity of the algorithm is thus linear in N – rather than exponential in N – which enables us to carry out an exhaustive search even for long sequences. Note, again, that the hidden Markov assumption is at the heart of this reduction in computational complexity. This approximation corresponds to a casino where the decision about changing croupiers is made instantaneously, without considering earlier events in the past. In a pairwise DNA sequence alignment, the hidden Markov assumption restricts the explicit modelling of the dependence structure between nucleotides to interactions between neighbouring sites. Finally, note that the log transformation in the previous equations is not required for a derivation of the algorithm. It is, however, important in practical implementations in order to prevent a numerical underflow for long sequences.

2.3.5 Application of the EM Algorithm to HMMs

Recall from Section 2.1 that a Bayesian network is defined by a triplet $(\mathcal{M}, \mathcal{F}, \mathbf{q})$. $\mathcal{M}$ represents the network structure, given by Figure 2.27. $\mathcal{F}$ represents the family of transition, emission, and initial probabilities, which are assumed to be known and fixed. The probabilities are thus completely specified by the parameter vector $\mathbf{q} = (\mathbf{w}, \boldsymbol{\nu}, \boldsymbol{\pi})$, where $\mathbf{w}$ determines the emission probabilities, $P(\mathbf{y}_t|S_t, \mathbf{w})$, $\boldsymbol{\nu}$ determines the transition probabilities, $P(S_t|S_{t-1}, \boldsymbol{\nu})$, and $\boldsymbol{\pi}$ determines the initial probabilities, $P(S_1|\boldsymbol{\pi})$.[5] For a sequence of observations $\mathcal{D} = (\mathbf{y}_1, \ldots \mathbf{y}_N)$ and a state sequence $\mathcal{S} = (S_1, \ldots, S_N)$ we have the joint probability (from (2.51)):

$$\begin{aligned} P(\mathcal{D}, \mathcal{S}|\mathbf{q}) &= P(\mathbf{y}_1, \ldots, \mathbf{y}_N, S_1, \ldots, S_N|\mathbf{q}) \\ &= \prod_{t=1}^{N} P(\mathbf{y}_t|S_t, \mathbf{w}) \prod_{t=2}^{N} P(S_t|S_{t-1}, \boldsymbol{\nu}) P(S_1|\boldsymbol{\pi}) \end{aligned} \tag{2.55}$$

Assume we want to optimize the parameters in a maximum likelihood sense, that is, we want to maximize

$$L(\mathbf{q}) = \log P(\mathcal{D}|\mathbf{q}) = \log \sum_{\mathcal{S}} P(\mathcal{D}, \mathcal{S}|\mathbf{q}) \tag{2.56}$$

with respect to the parameter vector $\mathbf{q}$. The computation of L requires a summation over all hidden state sequences $\mathcal{S} = (S_1, \ldots, S_N)$, that is, over K^N terms. For all but very short sequence lengths N, this direct approach is intractable. A viable alternative, however, is given by the expectation maximization (EM) algorithm, discussed in Section 2.3.3. Let $Q(\mathcal{S})$ denote an arbitrary probability distribution over the hidden state sequences, and F the function defined in (2.48). Inserting (2.55) into (2.48) gives:

$$F(\mathbf{q}) = A(\mathbf{w}) + B(\boldsymbol{\nu}) + C(\boldsymbol{\pi}) + H \tag{2.57}$$

where $H = -\sum_{\mathcal{S}} Q(\mathcal{S}) \log Q(\mathcal{S})$ is a constant independent of the parameters $\mathbf{q}$, and

[5] Recall the convention that for different arguments, P denotes different functions. Also, note that the three probabilities stated here do not explicitly depend on t, that is, the Markov chain is assumed to be *homogeneous*. For example, if $S_t \in \{a_1, \ldots, a_K\}$, then $P(S_t = a_i|S_{t-1} = a_k) = P(S_{t'} = a_i|S_{t'-1} = a_k)\, \forall\, t, t'$.

$$A(\mathbf{w}) = \sum_{\mathcal{S}} \sum_{t=1}^{N} Q(\mathcal{S}) \log P(\mathbf{y}_t|S_t, \mathbf{w}) = \sum_{t=1}^{N} \sum_{S_t} Q(S_t) \log P(\mathbf{y}_t|S_t, \mathbf{w}) \quad (2.58)$$

$$B(\boldsymbol{\nu}) = \sum_{\mathcal{S}} \sum_{t=2}^{N} Q(\mathcal{S}) \log P(S_t|S_{t-1}, \boldsymbol{\nu})$$

$$= \sum_{t=2}^{N} \sum_{S_t} \sum_{S_{t-1}} Q(S_t, S_{t-1}) \log P(S_t|S_{t-1}, \boldsymbol{\nu}) \quad (2.59)$$

$$C(\boldsymbol{\pi}) = \sum_{\mathcal{S}} Q(\mathcal{S}) \log P(S_1|\boldsymbol{\pi}) = \sum_{S_1} Q(S_1) \log P(S_1|\boldsymbol{\pi}) \quad (2.60)$$

Note that these expressions depend only on the marginal univariate and bivariate distributions $Q(S_t)$ and $Q(S_t, S_{t-1})$, but no longer on the multivariate joint distribution $Q(\mathcal{S})$. This marginalization outside the argument of the log function is at the heart of the reduction in computational complexity inherent in the EM algorithm. Having derived an expression for the function F in (2.48), we are set for the application of the EM algorithm, as described in Section 2.3.3.

The probabilities $Q(S_t)$ and $Q(S_t, S_{t-1})$ are updated in the *E-step*, where we set:

$$Q(S_t) \longrightarrow P(S_t|\mathcal{D}, \mathbf{w}, \boldsymbol{\nu}, \boldsymbol{\pi}) \quad (2.61)$$

$$Q(S_t, S_{t-1}) \longrightarrow P(S_t, S_{t-1}|\mathcal{D}, \mathbf{w}, \boldsymbol{\nu}, \boldsymbol{\pi}) \quad (2.62)$$

These computations are carried out with the *forward–backward* algorithm for HMMs [36], which is a dynamic programming method that reduces the computational complexity from $O(K^N)$ to $O(NK^2)$, that is, from exponential to linear complexity in N. The underlying principle is similar to that of the Viterbi algorithm, discussed after equation (2.54), and is based on the sparseness of the connectivity in the HMM structure. Since the forward–backward algorithm has been discussed several times in the literature before, it will not be described in this chapter again. Details can be found in the tutorial article by Rabiner [36], or textbooks like [1] and [9], which also discuss implementation issues.

Now, all that remains to be done is to derive update equations for the parameters $\mathbf{q} = (\mathbf{w}, \boldsymbol{\nu}, \boldsymbol{\pi})$ so as to maximize the function F in the *M-step* of the algorithm. From (2.57) we see that this optimization problem breaks up into three separate optimization problems for $\mathbf{w}$, $\boldsymbol{\nu}$, and $\boldsymbol{\pi}$. As an example, consider the optimization of $C(\boldsymbol{\pi})$ in (2.60) with respect to $\boldsymbol{\pi}$. Assume the hidden state S_t is taken from a discrete letter alphabet, $S_t \in \{a_1, \ldots, a_K\}$. For the casino example, we have $K = 2$ "letters", corresponding to the two croupiers. For the pairwise sequence alignment, we have $K = \binom{6}{2} - 1 = 14$ letters, corresponding to all 2-element combinations from $\{A, C, G, T, -\}$ except for the concurrence of two gaps. Define $\boldsymbol{\pi} = (\Pi_1, \ldots, \Pi_K)$ and $P(S_1 = a_k|\boldsymbol{\pi}) = \Pi_k$ for positive, normalized scalars $\Pi_k \in [0, 1]$, that is, Π_k can be interpreted as a probability distribution over the alphabet $\{a_1, \ldots, a_K\}$. We can now rewrite (2.60) as follows:

$$C(\boldsymbol{\pi}) = \sum_{k=1}^{K} Q(k) \log \Pi_k = \sum_{k=1}^{K} Q(k) \log Q(k) - \sum_{k=1}^{K} Q(k) \log \frac{Q(k)}{\Pi_k}$$

The first term, $\sum_{k=1}^{K} Q(k) \log Q(k)$, does not depend on the parameters. The second term, $\sum_{k=1}^{K} Q(k) \log \frac{Q(k)}{\Pi_k}$, is the Kullback–Leibler divergence between the distributions $Q(k)$ and Π_k. In order to maximize $C(\boldsymbol{\pi})$, this term should be as small as possible. Now, recall from the discussion after equation (2.49) that the Kullback–Leibler divergence is always non-negative, and zero if and only if the two distributions are the same. Consequently, $C(\boldsymbol{\pi})$ is maximized for $\Pi_k = Q(S_1 = k)$.

The optimization of the other parameters, $\mathbf{w}$ and $\boldsymbol{\nu}$, is, in principle, similar. For multinomial distributions, complete update equations have been derived in [1], [9], and [36], and these derivations will not be repeated here. Instead, let us consider the maximization of $B(\boldsymbol{\nu})$ in (2.59) for a special case that will be needed later, in Section 5.10. Assume that we have only two different transition probabilities between the hidden states. Let $\nu \in [0, 1]$ denote the probability that a state will not change as we move from position $t - 1$ to position t. The probability for a state transition is given by the complement, $1 - \nu$. If a state transition occurs, we assume that all the transitions into the remaining $K - 1$ states are equally likely. An illustrative application is shown in Figure 5.20. We can then write the transition probabilities in the following form:

$$P(S_t|S_{t-1}, \nu) = \nu^{\delta_{S_t, S_{t-1}}} \left(\frac{1 - \nu}{K - 1} \right)^{1 - \delta_{S_t, S_{t-1}}} \tag{2.63}$$

where $\delta_{S_t, S_{t-1}}$ denotes the Kronecker delta symbol, which is 1 when $S_t = S_{t-1}$, and 0 otherwise. It is easily checked that (2.63) satisfies the normalization constraint $\sum_{S_t} P(S_t|S_{t-1}) = 1$. Note that the vector of transition parameters, $\boldsymbol{\nu}$, has been replaced by a scalar, ν. Now, define

$$\Psi = \sum_{t=2}^{N} \sum_{S_t} \sum_{S_{t-1}} Q(S_t, S_{t-1}) \delta_{S_t, S_{t-1}} = \sum_{t=2}^{N} \sum_{S_t} Q(S_t, S_{t-1} = S_t) \tag{2.64}$$

and note that

$$\sum_{t=2}^{N} \sum_{S_t} \sum_{S_{t-1}} Q(S_t, S_{t-1})[1 - \delta_{S_t, S_{t-1}}] = N - 1 - \Psi \tag{2.65}$$

Inserting (2.63) into (2.59) and making use of definitions (2.64) and (2.65) gives

$$B(\nu) = \Psi \log \nu + (N-1-\Psi) \log \left(\frac{1-\nu}{K-1} \right) \tag{2.66}$$

Setting the derivative of $B(\nu)$ with respect to ν to zero,

$$\frac{dB}{d\nu} = \frac{\Psi}{\nu} + \frac{N-1-\Psi}{\nu-1} = 0 \tag{2.67}$$

we obtain for the optimal parameter ν:

$$\nu = \frac{\Psi}{N-1} \tag{2.68}$$

This estimation is straightforward because, as seen from (2.64), Ψ depends only on $Q(S_{t-1}, S_t)$, which is obtained by application of the forward–backward algorithm in the E-step (see above). An example for optimizing $\mathbf{w}$ in (2.58) will be given in Section 5.10. Note that the three parameter optimizations for $\mathbf{w}$, $\boldsymbol{\pi}$, and $\boldsymbol{\nu}$ (or ν) constitute the M-step, which has to be applied repeatedly, in each loop of the EM algorithm.

2.3.6 Applying the EM Algorithm to More Complex Bayesian Networks with Hidden States

HMMs are a special class of Bayesian networks with hidden nodes. Their structure, $\mathcal{M}$, is particularly simple and known. The general scenario of learning arbitrary Bayesian networks with hidden states is more involved, but draws on the principles discussed in the previous sections. This section will provide a brief, not comprehensive, overview.

Let $\mathcal{D}$ denote the set of observations associated with the observable nodes, and denote by $\mathcal{S}$ the set of hidden states with their associated random variables. To optimize the network parameters $\mathbf{q}$ in a maximum likelihood sense, we would like to apply the EM algorithm of Section 2.3.3. The E-step requires us to compute the posterior probability of the hidden states, $P(\mathcal{S}|\mathcal{D}, \mathbf{q}, \mathcal{M})$. For HMMs, this computation is effected with the forward–backward algorithm, as discussed in Section 2.3.5. The update equations in the M-step depend only on the univariate and bivariate marginal posterior distributions, $P(S_t|\mathcal{D}, \mathbf{q}, \mathcal{M})$ and $P(S_t, S_{t-1}|\mathcal{D}, \mathbf{q}, \mathcal{M})$, as seen from (2.57)–(2.62), which leads to the considerable reduction in the computational complexity, from $O(K^N)$ to $O(NK^2)$.

Section 4.4.3 will describe the application of a similar algorithm, *Pearl's message-passing algorithm* [34], to tree-structured Bayesian networks. The most general algorithm for computing the posterior probability of the hidden states is the *junction-tree algorithm* [25], [7]. This algorithm is based on a transformation of the DAG structure into a certain type of undirected graph, the so-called junction tree. The computational complexity of the EM algorithm is exponential in the size of the largest clique in this graph [21]. Here, a *clique* denotes a maximal complete subgraph, where a *complete* graph is a graph with an edge between any pair of nodes, and a complete graph is *maximal* if it is not itself a proper subgraph of another complete graph. For HMMs, the size of the largest clique is two, hence we need to compute only univariate and bivariate posterior probabilities; see (2.61)–(2.62). The computational complexity is thus $O(K^2N)$, as stated before. If the size of the largest clique in the junction tree is m, the expressions in the M-step depend on m-variate posterior probabilities, and the computational complexity increases to $O(K^mN)$. For large values of m the computational costs thus become prohibitively large, which has motivated the exploration of faster, approximate techniques. Rather than set Q equal to the posterior probability $P(\mathcal{S}|\mathcal{D}, \mathbf{q}, \mathcal{M})$ in the E-step, which corresponds to an unrestricted free-form minimization of (2.49), one can define Q to be a member of a sufficiently simple function family, and then minimize (2.49) subject to this functional constraint. The simplest approach is to set Q equal to the product of its marginals, $Q(\mathcal{S}) = \prod_k Q(S_k)$, which corresponds to the *mean field approximation* in statistical physics (see, for instance, [2], Chapter 4). An application to inference in Bayesian network-like models can be found, for example, in [35]. An improved approach is to use a mixture of mean field approximators [20]. For a more comprehensive overview of these so-called *variational methods*, see [21]. Note, however, that by minimizing the Kullback–Leibler divergence in (2.49) – rather than setting it to zero – the likelihood is no longer guaranteed to increase after an EM step. In fact, this variational variant of the EM algorithm can only be shown to maximize a lower bound on the log-likelihood, rather than the log-likelihood itself [21].

Recall from the discussion in Sections 2.2.1 and 2.2.2 that the objective of inference is either to sample models from the posterior distribution $P(\mathcal{M}|\mathcal{D})$ or, if there is reason to assume that this distribution is peaked, to find the mode of $P(\mathcal{M}|\mathcal{D}) \propto P(\mathcal{D}|\mathcal{M})P(\mathcal{M})$, the *maximum a posteriori* (MAP) model (where due to the NP-hardness of the inference problem this mode, in practice, is usually a local maximum). Also, recall from Section 2.3.2 that under the BIC approximation, $\log P(\mathcal{D}|\mathcal{M}) = \log P(\mathcal{D}|\mathcal{M}, \mathbf{q}) - R(\mathbf{q})$, where $R(\mathbf{q}) = \frac{1}{2}\dim(\mathbf{q}) \log N$ is a regularization term; see (2.46). Now, it is straightforward to modify the EM algorithm such that it (locally) maximizes, for a given model $\mathcal{M}$, the penalized log-likelihood $\log P(\mathcal{D}|\mathcal{M}, \mathbf{q}) - R(\mathbf{q})$. Instead of maximizing F, defined in (2.48), in the M-step, we have to maximize the modified function $\tilde{F} = F - R(\mathbf{q})$. Then we repeat this procedure for different models $\mathcal{M}$, using heuristic hill-climbing techniques to find a high-scoring $\mathcal{M}$. However, each parameter optimization requires several EM cycles to be carried out. As discussed above, the E-step can be computationally expensive, and several E-steps are needed before a single change to the network structure $\mathcal{M}$ can be made. To overcome this shortcoming, Friedman suggested a variant of the EM algorithm, the *structural EM algorithm* [10], where both the parameters $\mathbf{q}$ *and* the model $\mathcal{M}$ are optimized simultaneously in the M-step. This modification reduces the total number of E-steps that have to be carried out, although at the price of increased computational costs for those

E-steps that are carried out. Friedman also suggested combining the EM algorithm with the integration (2.20) in what he called the *Bayesian structural EM algorithm* (BSEM) [11]. Formally, BSEM is based on a modification of equations (2.48)–(2.49), where the dependence on $\mathbf{q}$ is dropped so as to perform an optimization in model rather than parameter space. Recall that when certain regularity conditions are satisfied, the integral in (2.20) can be solved analytically. The idea in [11] is to carry out this integration within the E-step after imputing the missing values with their expectation values, where expectation values are taken with respect to the distribution obtained in the E-step. This approach is based on approximating the expectation value of a nonlinear function by the value of this function at the expectation value. Also, the expectation value has to be taken with respect to the posterior distribution $P(\mathcal{S}|\mathcal{D}, \mathcal{M})$ – as a result of the aforementioned modification of (2.48)–(2.49). Computing this expectation value is usually intractable. Hence, $P(\mathcal{S}|\mathcal{D}, \mathcal{M})$ is approximated by $P(\mathcal{S}|\mathcal{D}, \mathcal{M}, \hat{\mathbf{q}})$, where $\hat{\mathbf{q}}$ is the MAP parameter estimate for model $\mathcal{M}$; see [11] for details.

2.3.7 Reversible Jump MCMC

The EM algorithm, discussed in the previous subsections, is an optimization algorithm. Its application is motivated by the BIC score (2.46), according to which an integration over the parameters $\mathbf{q}$ can be replaced by an optimization. However, as discussed in Section 2.3.2, the BIC approximation becomes unreliable for sparse data. Also, for sparse data, the posterior distribution over structures, $P(\mathcal{M}|\mathcal{D})$, becomes diffuse and is not appropriately summarized by its mode, $\mathcal{M}^* = \text{argmax} P(\mathcal{M}|\mathcal{D})$. Consequently, the optimization approach should be replaced by a sampling approach when the training data are sparse.

Now, recall from page 31 that the MCMC scheme is not restricted to a space of cardinal entities (model structures), but can readily be extended to continuous entities (model parameters). So rather than perform the sampling in the structure space $\{\mathcal{M}\}$, which is impossible due to the intractability of (2.20), we can sample in the product space of structures and parameters, $\{\mathcal{M}, \mathbf{q}\}$, and then marginalize over the parameters $\mathbf{q}$. Examples for this will be given in Chapters 4–6. However, care has to be taken when the dimension of the model $\mathcal{M}$ changes. In modelling genetic networks, for instance, the model dimension may vary, changing every time we introduce or remove a hypothetical hidden agent (like a transcription factor[6]). In this case the probability distribution over the parameters $\mathbf{q}$ becomes singular when the model dimension increases, and this has to be taken care of in the formulation of the algorithm. A generalization of the classical Metropolis–Hastings algorithm that allows for these dimension changes has been given by Green [14] and is usually referred to as the *reversible jump MCMC* or *Metropolis–Hastings–Green* algorithm. The details are beyond the scope of this chapter.

---

[6] A transcription factor is a protein that initiates or modulates the transcription of a gene; see Figure 8.14.

2.4 Summary

This chapter has given a brief introduction to the problem of learning Bayesian networks from complete and incomplete data. The methods described here will reoccur several times in the remaining chapters of this book. For example, methods of phylogenetic inference from DNA or RNA sequence alignments, covered in Chapters 4 and 6, the detection of recombination between different strains of bacteria and viruses, discussed in Chapter 5, as well as the attempt to infer genetic regulatory interactions from microarray experiments, described in Chapters 8 and 9, are all based on the concepts and ideas outlined in the present chapter. The detailed procedures and methods for the particular applications will be discussed in the respective chapters.

Acknowledgments

Several ideas for this chapter have been taken from the tutorials by David Heckermann [16], Paul Krause [23], and Kevin Murphy [31], as well as a lecture given by Christopher Bishop at the 9th International Conference on Artificial Neural Networks in Edinburgh, 1999. I would like to thank Anja von Heydebreck, Marco Grzegorczyk, David Allcroft and Thorsten Forster for critical feedback on a first draft of this chapter, as well as Philip Smith for proofreading the final version.

References

[1] P. Baldi and P. Brunak. *Bioinformatics – The Machine Learning Approach.* MIT Press, Cambridge, MA, 1998.
[2] R. Balian. *From Microphysics to Macrophysics. Methods and Applications of Statistical Physics.*, volume 1. Springer-Verlag, 1982.
[3] C. M. Bishop. *Neural Networks for Pattern Recognition.* Oxford University Press, New York, 1995. ISBN 0-19-853864-2.
[4] S. Chib and E. Greenberg. Understanding the Metropolis-Hastings algorithm. *The American Statistician*, 49(4):327–335, 1995.
[5] D. M. Chickering. A transformational characterization of equivalent Bayesian network structures. *International Conference on Uncertainty in Artificial Intelligence (UAI)*, 11:87–98, 1995.
[6] D. M. Chickering. Learning Bayesian networks is NP-complete. In D. Fisher and H. J. Lenz, editors, *Learning from Data: Artificial Intelligence and Statistics*, volume 5, pages 121–130, New York, 1996. Springer.
[7] A. P. Dawid. Applications of general propagation algorithm for probabilistic expert systems. *Statistics and Computing*, 2:25–36, 1992.
[8] A. P. Dempster, N. M. Laird, and D. B. Rubin. Maximum likelihood from incomplete data via the EM algorithm. *Journal of the Royal Statistical Society*, B39(1):1–38, 1977.

[9] R. Durbin, S. R. Eddy, A. Krogh, and G. Mitchison. *Biological sequence analysis. Probabilistic models of proteins and nucleic acids.* Cambridge University Press, Cambridge, UK, 1998.

[10] N. Friedman. Learning belief networks in the presence of missing values and hidden variables. In D. H. Fisher, editor, *Proceedings of the Fourteenth International Conference on Machine Learning (ICML)*, pages 125–133, Nashville, TN, 1997. Morgan Kaufmann.

[11] N. Friedman. The Bayesian structural EM algorithm. In G. F. Cooper and S. Moral, editors, *Proceedings of the Fourteenth Conference on Uncertainty in Artificial Intelligence (UAI)*, pages 129–138, Madison, WI, 1998. Morgan Kaufmann.

[12] N. Friedman, I. Nachman, and D. Pe'er. Learning Bayesian network structure from massive datasets: The "sparse candidate" algorithm. In *Proceedings of the Fifteenth Annual Conference on Uncertainty in Artificial Intelligence*, pages 196–205, San Francisco, CA, 1999. Morgan Kaufmann Publishers.

[13] W. R. Gilks, S. Richardson, and D. J. Spiegelhalter. Introducing Markov chain Monte Carlo. In W. R. Gilks, S. Richardson, and D. J. Spieglehalter, editors, *Markov Chain Monte Carlo in Practice*, pages 1–19, Suffolk, 1996. Chapman & Hall. ISBN 0-412-05551-1.

[14] P. Green. Reversible jump Markov chain Monte Carlo computation and Bayesian model determination. *Biometrika*, 82:711–732, 1995.

[15] W. K. Hastings. Monte Carlo sampling methods using Markov chains and their applications. *Biometrika*, 57:97–109, 1970.

[16] D. Heckerman. A tutorial on learning with Bayesian networks. In M. I. Jordan, editor, *Learning in Graphical Models*, Adaptive Computation and Machine Learning, pages 301–354, The Netherlands, 1998. Kluwer Academic Publishers.

[17] D. Heckerman, D. Geiger, and D. M. Chickering. Learning Bayesian networks: The combination of knowledge and statistical data. *Machine Learning*, 20:245–274, 1995.

[18] D. Husmeier. *Neural Networks for Conditional Probability Estimation: Forecasting Beyond Point Predictions.* Perspectives in Neural Computing. Springer, London, 1999. ISBN 1-85233-095-3.

[19] D. Husmeier. The Bayesian evidence scheme for regularising probability-density estimating neural networks. *Neural Computation*, 12(11):2685–2717, 2000.

[20] T. S. Jaakola and M. I. Jordan. Improving the mean field approximation via the use of mixture distributions. In M. I. Jordan, editor, *Learning in Graphical Models*, Adaptive Computation and Machine Learning, pages 163–173, The Netherlands, 1998. Kluwer Academic Publishers.

[21] M. I. Jordan, Z. Ghahramani, T. S. Jaakola, and L. K. Saul. An introduction to variational methods for graphical models. In M. I. Jordan, editor, *Learning in Graphical Models*, pages 105–161, The Netherlands, 1998. Kluwer Academic Publishers.

[22] S. Kirkpatrick, C. D. Gelatt, and M. P. Vecchi. Optimization by simulated annealing. *Science*, 220:671–680, 1983.

[23] P. J. Krause. Learning probabilistic networks. *Knowledge Engineering Review*, 13:321–351, 1998.

[24] S. L. Lauritzen, A. P. Dawid, B. N. Larsen, and H. G. Leimer. Independence properties of directed Markov fields. *Networks*, 20:491–505, 1990.

[25] S. L. Lauritzen and D. J. Spiegelhalter. Local computations with probabilities on graphical structures and their applications to expert systems. *Journal of the Royal Statistical Society, Series B*, 50:157–224, 1988.

[26] D. J. C. MacKay. Bayesian interpolation. *Neural Computation*, 4:415–447, 1992.

[27] D. J. C. MacKay. A practical Bayesian framework for backpropagation networks. *Neural Computation*, 4:448–472, 1992.

[28] D. J. C. MacKay. Introduction to Monte Carlo methods. In M. I. Jordan, editor, *Learning in Graphical Models*, pages 301–354, The Netherlands, 1998. Kluwer Academic Publishers.

[29] D. Madigan and J. York. Bayesian graphical models for discrete data. *International Statistical Review*, 63:215–232, 1995.

[30] N. Metropolis, A. W. Rosenbluth, M. N. Rosenbluth, A. H. Teller, and E. Teller. Equation of state calculations by fast computing machines. *Journal of Chemical Physics*, 21:1087–1092, 1953.

[31] K. P. Murphy. An introduction to graphical models. Technical report, MIT Artificial Intelligence Laboratory, 2001. http://www.ai.mit.edu/~murphyk/Papers/intro_gm.pdf.

[32] K. P. Murphy. Bayes net toolbox. Technical report, MIT Artificial Intelligence Laboratory, 2002. http://www.ai.mit.edu/~murphyk/.

[33] R. M. Neal and G. E. Hinton. A view of the EM algorithm that justifies incremental, sparse, and other variants. In M. I. Jordan, editor, *Learning in Graphical Models*, pages 355–368, The Netherlands, 1998. Kluwer Academic Publishers.

[34] J. Pearl. *Probabilistic Reasoning in Intelligent Systems: Networks of Plausible Inference.* Morgan Kaufmann, San Francisco, CA, 1988.

[35] C. Petersen and J. R. Anderson. A mean field theory learning algorithm for neural networks. *Complex Systems*, 1:995–1019, 1987.

[36] L. Rabiner. A tutorial on hidden Markov models and selected applications in speech recognition. *Proceedings of the IEEE*, 77(2):257–286, 1989.

[37] J. J. Rissanen. Modeling by shortest data description. *Automatica*, 14:465–471, 1978.

[38] G. Schwarz. Estimating the dimension of a model. *Annals of Statistics*, 6:461–464, 1978.

[39] H. Sies. A new parameter for sex-education. *Nature*, 332:495, 1988.

[40] P. Spirtes, C. Meek, and T. Richardson. An algorithm for causal inference in the presence of latent variables and selection bias. In G. Cooper and C. Glymour, editors, *Computation, Causation, and Discovery*, pages 211–252. MIT Press, 1999.

3

A Casual View of Multi-Layer Perceptrons as Probability Models

Richard Dybowski

InferSpace, 143 Village Way, Pinner HA5 5AA, UK.
richard@inferspace.com

Summary. The purpose of this chapter is to introduce the reader to a type of artificial neural network called a multi-layer perceptron. The intention is not to present a detailed, comprehensive treatise on the subject; instead, we provide a brief, informal, tutorial in the spirit of Chapter 1.

We start with the historical background and then introduce the concept of regression. This concept holds for both continuous-valued and binary-valued response variables; however, when applied to the latter, probabilistic classification models are created.

In the context of medicine, probabilistic classification models are usually obtained using logistic regression analysis, but if logistic functions are nested to produce multi-layer perceptrons, the high flexibility of the resulting models enables them to handle complex classification tasks.

We discuss some important points that should be kept in mind when applying multi-layer perceptrons to classification problems. Finally, we end the tutorial with some recommended reading.

3.1 A Brief History

Artificial neural networks (ANNs) are a large class of mathematical models that possess a capacity to learn from examples. Some of these models are loosely based on the structures and functions of biological neural systems.

In this section, we summarize the historical development of the multi-layer perceptron via the McCulloch-Pitts neuron and the single-layer perceptron.

3.1.1 The McCulloch-Pitts Neuron

The original motivation for designing ANNs was the desire to model the cognitive processes of recognition and learning. In the 1920s, Nicolas Rashevsky began a research programme to model mathematically Pavlovian conditioning in terms of biological neural networks [20]. Rashevsky was joined by Warren McCulloch and Walter Pitts who, in 1943, published a simple model of the neuron called the *McCulloch-Pitts neuron* [16].

The McCulloch-Pitts neuron (Figure 3.1) consists of several "dendrites", each with an associated weight w_i. When w_i is positive, the associated "synapse" is excitatory; when w_i is negative, it is inhibitory. A set of values $x_1, \ldots, x_d$ received by the artificial neurone at its "synapsis" is converted to a weighted sum $w_1 x_1 + \cdots + w_n x_d$. If the sum exceeds a predefined threshold $-w_0$, the signal ξ produced by the artificial neurone equals 1; otherwise, it is 0. This process is analogous to the triggering of an impulse by the hillock zone of a real neurone when a membrane-potential threshold is exceeded.

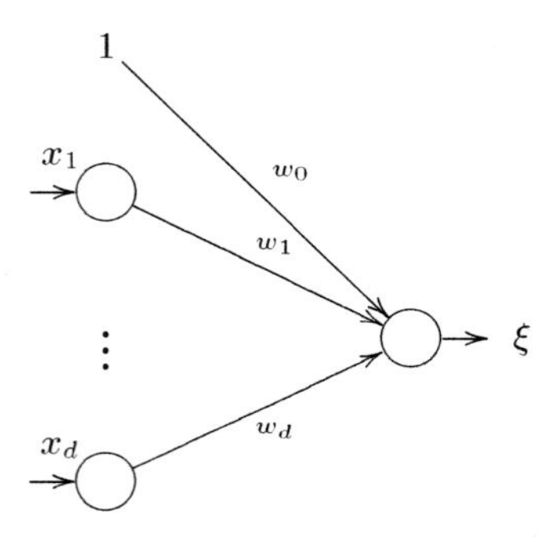

Fig. 3.1. A graphical representation of a McCulloch-Pitts neuron. A discontinuous step function $g(a)$ (Figure 3.2(a)) is applied to the weighted sum $a = w_0 + w_1 x_1 + \cdots + w_d x_d$ to produce the output ξ, where $-w_0$ is the *threshold.* (Reprinted with permission, Richard Dybowski and Vanya Gant, *Clinical Applications of Artificial Neural Networks*, 2001, Cambridge University Press.)

3.1.2 The Single-Layer Perceptron

In computing science, *pattern recognition* refers to the process where an algorithm or mathematical function f assigns (or *classifies*) a set of values $\mathbf{x}$ (a *feature vector*) to one of a finite number of classes κ. A classification can be represented by the expression

$$\widehat{\kappa} = f(\mathbf{x}),$$

where $\widehat{\kappa}$ is the class predicted by classifier f when it is presented with a set of values $\mathbf{x}$. Examples of pattern recognition include the diagnosis of diseases (where $\mathbf{x}$ is a set of symptoms and κ a possible disease), the recognition of characters written on a Personal Digital Assistant, and the assessment of the credit risk of customers.

One approach to pattern recognition is to build the classifier f manually; alternatively, one can devise a method by which f is somehow "learnt" from a set of past examples $(\mathbf{x}_1, \kappa_1), \ldots, (\mathbf{x}_n, \kappa_n)$, where κ_i is the class associated with $\mathbf{x}_i$.

In 1958, Rosenblatt [22] proposed that the McCulloch-Pitts neuron could be the basis of a pattern recognition system called a perceptron. A *(single-layer) perceptron* has the same structure as a McCulloch-Pitts neuron except that the discontinuous step function at the output node (Figure 3.2(a)) is replaced by a continuous sigmoidal logistic function (Figure 3.2(b)). Suppose that the classification made by a perceptron from an example $(\mathbf{x}_i, \kappa_i)$ is denoted by

$$\widehat{\kappa}_i = f(\mathbf{x}_i, \mathbf{w}),$$

where $\mathbf{w}$ is the set of weights in the perceptron. Here, the prediction made by the perceptron is $\widehat{\kappa}_i$, which, if correct, should equal κ_i. Rosenblatt's *perceptron learning rule* [23] was able to automatically adjust $\mathbf{w}$ iteratively based on a set of examples until the mismatches between the predictions $\widehat{\kappa}_i$ and the correct target values κ_i were minimized. This development by Rosenblatt was motivated by Hebb's hypothesis that learning is based on the reinforcement of active neuronal connections [10]; however, although the perceptron was able to learn from examples, it was limited in the type of classification problems to which it could be applied successfully.

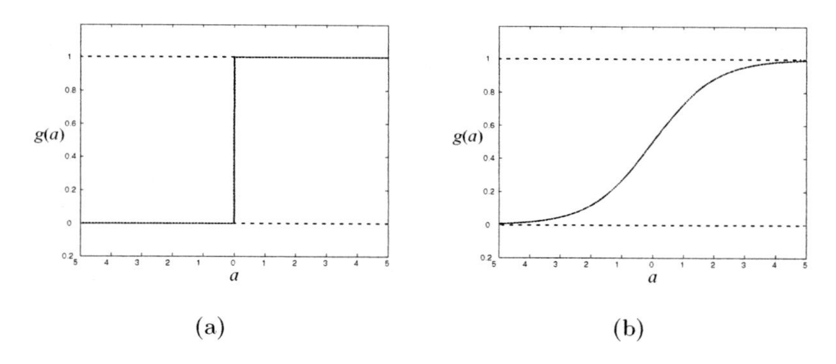

Fig. 3.2. Two activation functions: (a) a step function and (b) a logistic function.

A feature vector of values $\mathbf{x}$ consisting of d values can be represented as a point $\mathbf{x}$ in a d-dimensional space (*feature space*), and an example $(\mathbf{x}_i, \kappa_i)$ can be represented as the point $\mathbf{x}_i$ labelled with its associated class κ_i. Consequently, a set of examples $(\mathbf{x}_1, \kappa_1), \ldots, (\mathbf{x}_n, \kappa_n)$ can be depicted as a set of class-labelled points distributed in feature space.

A *decision boundary* partitions a feature space into a set of regions (*decision regions*), each region being associated with one of the classes of interest. If a new feature vector $\mathbf{x}^*$ happens to appear in the region associated with a particular class $\tilde{\kappa}$ then that vector is automatically assigned to $\tilde{\kappa}$.

The problem with the single-layer perceptron was that it could represent only planar decision boundaries (Figure 3.3(a)); however, for many real-world classification problems, such simple decision boundaries were inadequate. In many situations, a planar decision boundary would fail to segregate the points labelled with one class from the points associated with another class, possibly resulting in high rates of misclassification (Figure 3.3(b)).

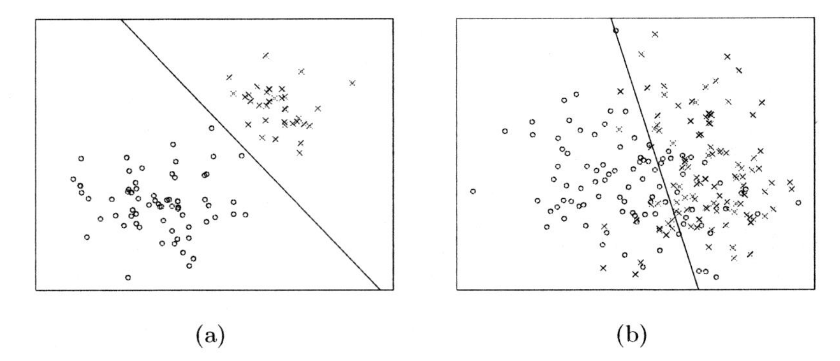

Fig. 3.3. Decision boundaries obtained from single-layer perceptrons. In (a), the samples from classes α_1 and α_2 (distinguished by symbols $\circ$ and $\times$) can be separated completely by a line; whereas in (b) they are not linearly separable. Each decision boundary corresponds to the contour line where posterior probability $p(\alpha_1|\mathbf{x})$ equals 0.5.

3.1.3 Enter the Multi-Layer Perceptron

Whereas a perceptron contains a single layer of weights, a *multi-layer perceptron* (MLP) has two or more layers of weights, each layer being separated by a layer of nodes called *hidden nodes.*

An MLP with two layers of weights is shown in Figure 3.4.[1] The first layer of nodes, which receives the inputs $x_1, \ldots, x_d$, is called the *input layer.* The layer of nodes producing the output values $\xi_1, \ldots, \xi_c$ is called the *output layer.* Layers of nodes between the input and output layers are referred to as *hidden layers.* The weighted sum a_j ($j = 1, \ldots, m$) at the jth hidden node h_j is given by $w_{(1 \to h_j)} + w_{(x_1 \to h_j)} x_1 + \cdots + w_{(x_d \to h_j)} x_d$, where $w_{(1 \to h_j)}$ is a *bias.* The value output by h_j is a function g_1 of a_j, and the output ξ_k ($k = 1, \ldots, c$) from the kth output node is a function g_2 of the weighted sum $w_{(1 \to \xi_k)} + w_{(h_1 \to \xi_k)} g_1(a_1) + \cdots + w_{(a_m \to \xi_k)} g_1(h_m)$, where $w_{(1 \to \xi_k)}$ is a bias. Activation function g_1 at the hidden nodes is typically sigmoidal; for example, it could be the hyperbolic tangent (tanh). Activation function g_2 at the output nodes can be either linear for regression or sigmoidal for classification. In the latter case, the logistic function is usually used (Figure 3.2 (b)).[2]

Although it was realized that the MLP architecture enabled the production of nonlinear decision boundaries, Minsky and Papert [17] pointed out in 1969 that the perceptron learning rule could not adjust the weights of an MLP. It was not until the

[1] To avoid ambiguity, the number of layers in a perceptron should refer to the layers of weights and not to the layers of nodes, as this avoids a single-layer perceptron also being referred to as a two-layer perceptron.

[2] An MLP can have more than one layer of hidden nodes, but one layer usually suffices for most tasks. In fact, an MLP with one hidden layer can approximate arbitrarily well any continuous function with inputs $x_1, \ldots, x_d$, provided that the number of hidden nodes is sufficiently large and that there are enough data to estimate the network weights [11]; however, for some tasks, the use of additional hidden weights can ease the representation of decision boundaries [7].

mid-1980s that the research community became aware of an algorithm for training MLPs: the *back-propagation algorithm* (Section 3.4).[3] The existence of the back-propagation algorithm meant that MLPs could be applied to real-world problems, which resulted in an explosion of interest in ANNs.

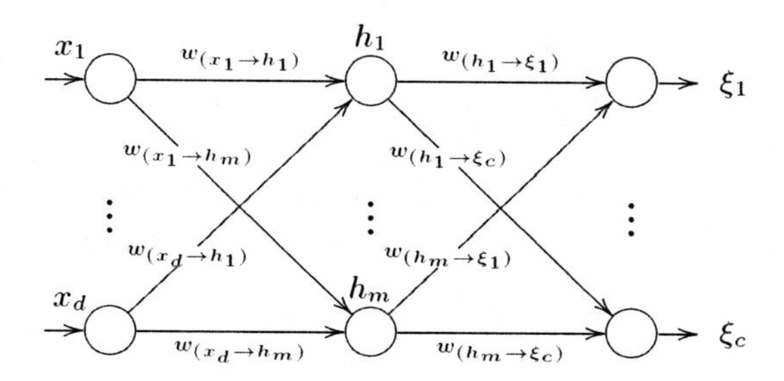

Fig. 3.4. A multi-layer perceptron with two layers of weights. In addition to the weights shown in the diagram, each hidden node and output node ◯ has an associated weight w called a *bias*: $1 \xrightarrow{w}$ ◯ . See text in Section 3.1.3 for details. (Reprinted with permission, Richard Dybowski and Vanya Gant, *Clinical Applications of Artificial Neural Networks*, 2001, Cambridge University Press.)

3.1.4 A Statistical Perspective

Initially, ANNs were regarded as constructs for computer scientists and cognitive scientists interested in Artificial Intelligence [e.g., 1, 3], but a statistical interpretation of ANNs emerged by the mid-1990s [e.g., 5, 21]. This statistical view of ANNs proved to be very powerful because it provided a sound theoretical framework for neural computation.

The 1990s saw an increasing interest in the application of Bayesian statistics to ANNs, initiated by the works of MacKay [14] and Neal [19], which brought the benefits of Bayesian reasoning to neural computation (Chaps. 10 and 12).

Today, ANNs are firmly regarded as statistical tools by both computer scientists and statisticians.

3.2 Regression

In order to understand how an ANN such as an MLP can act as a probability model, we need to be clear about the statistical concept called regression.

Suppose that we are given a sheet of graph paper upon which a set of points have been plotted. The points $(x_1, y_1), \ldots, (x_n, y_n)$ on the graph paper were obtained by

[3] It was later found that the first description of the back-propagation algorithm was contained in the 1974 doctorial dissertation by Werbos [26].

observing the values $y_1, \ldots, y_n$ for variable Y found to be associated with a set of values $x_1, \ldots, x_n$ for variable X. We are given a ruler and are asked to draw a straight line through the points. If the points lie exactly along a line, we could fit the straight line to the points accurately by eye. Even if the points were nearly in a line, fitting a straight line to the points by eye could be done reasonably satisfactorily. But, if the points were more scattered, fitting by eye would become too subjective and inaccurate; a better, objective method is required.

Starting with the set of values $x_1, \ldots, x_n$, we can imagine that the points $(x_1, y_1), \ldots, (x_n, y_n)$ came into existence by the following *generative* process. For each value x_i of X, there exists a conditional probability distribution $p(Y|x_i)$ with mean $\mathcal{E}[Y|x_i]$, and the value y_i was sampled randomly from this distribution.[4]

The mean $\mathcal{E}[Y|x]$ can be considered as a function of x, and the generative model can be applied to any structure of this function; for example, $\mathcal{E}[Y|x]$ could be related linearly to x (Figure 3.5(a)) or it could be a nonlinear polynomial of x (Figure 3.5(b)).

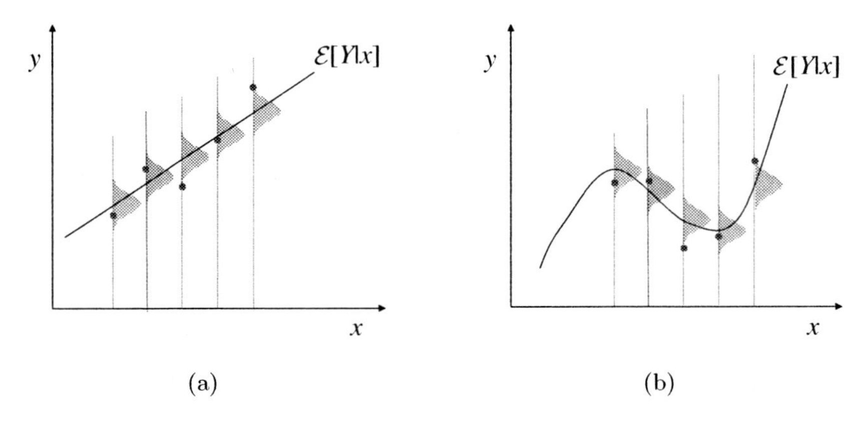

Fig. 3.5. Examples of (a) linear regression and (b) polynomial regression. Each point has been sampled from a Gaussian distribution (gray region) centered on a mean defined by $\mathcal{E}[Y|x]$.

The aim of *regression* is to estimate $\mathcal{E}[Y|x]$ from the set $\mathcal{D}$ of points $(x_1, y_1), \ldots, (x_n, y_n)$ in the context of the above generative model. This is done by assuming a general structure for a function f that relates $\mathcal{E}[Y|x]$ to x (the *regression function*). The function has a set of parameters $\boldsymbol{\theta}$ that modify the mapping of x to $\mathcal{E}[Y|x]$,

$$\mathcal{E}[Y|x] = f(x, \boldsymbol{\theta}), \tag{3.1}$$

and the parameters $\boldsymbol{\theta}$ are adjusted until the regression function "fits" to the data. For example, in the case of *linear regression*, $\mathcal{E}[Y|x]$ is assumed to be related linearly to x (Figure 3.5(a)):

$$\mathcal{E}[Y|x] = \beta_0 + \beta_1 x,$$

[4] The concept of a *conditional probability*, such as $p(Y|x_i)$, is explained in Chapter 1.

where the regression coefficients β_0 and β_1 are the parameters of the linear function.

3.2.1 Maximum Likelihood Estimation

The conventional approach to adjusting the parameters $\boldsymbol{\theta}$ of $f(x, \boldsymbol{\theta})$ with respect to data $\mathcal{D}$ is to use *maximum likelihood estimation*. This is based on the intuitive idea that the best estimate of $\boldsymbol{\theta}$ is that set of parameters $\hat{\boldsymbol{\theta}}$ for which the observed data have the highest probability of arising. This probability is given by the likelihood $p(\mathcal{D}|\boldsymbol{\theta})$; therefore, the aim is to find the set of parameters $\hat{\boldsymbol{\theta}}$ that maximize $p(\mathcal{D}|\boldsymbol{\theta})$:

$$\hat{\boldsymbol{\theta}} \equiv \arg\max_{\boldsymbol{\theta}} p(\mathcal{D}|\boldsymbol{\theta}).$$

This expression can be rewritten as

$$\hat{\boldsymbol{\theta}} = \arg\max_{\boldsymbol{\theta}} \prod_{i=1}^{n} p(y_i|x_i, \boldsymbol{\theta}).$$

if the points in $\mathcal{D}$ are sampled independently of each other.

If $\hat{\boldsymbol{\theta}}$ maximizes the likelihood $p(\mathcal{D}|\boldsymbol{\theta})$, it will also maximize the log-likelihood $\log p(\mathcal{D}|\boldsymbol{\theta})$. In other words,

$$\hat{\boldsymbol{\theta}} = \arg\max_{\boldsymbol{\theta}} \ \log \mathcal{L}(\boldsymbol{\theta}),$$

where

$$\begin{aligned} \log \mathcal{L}(\boldsymbol{\theta}) &\equiv \log p(\mathcal{D}|\boldsymbol{\theta}) \\ &= \sum_{i=1}^{n} \log p(y_i|x_i, \boldsymbol{\theta}) + const. \end{aligned} \tag{3.2}$$

3.3 From Regression to Probabilistic Classification

When Y is binary valued (i.e., equal only to 0 or 1),[5] the traditional choice for the regression function f in (3.1) is the sigmoidal *logistic regression* function

$$\mathcal{E}[Y|x] = \frac{1}{1 + \exp[-(\beta_0 + \beta_1 x)]}$$

(Figure 3.6(b)). Furthermore, because Y is binary valued, we have that[6]

[5] Because Y is binary-valued, $p(Y|x_i)$ is a binomial distribution, not a Gaussian distribution.

[6] By definition

$$\mathcal{E}[Y|x] \equiv \sum_{Y} Y p(Y|x)$$

when Y is discrete valued.

$$\mathcal{E}[Y|x] = \sum_{Y=0}^{1} Y p(Y|x)$$
$$= 0 \cdot p(Y=0|x) + 1 \cdot p(Y=1|x)$$
$$= p(Y=1|x);$$

thus, the logistic regression function acts as a *probability model* for $p(Y = 1|x, \boldsymbol{\theta})$:

$$p(Y = 1|x, \boldsymbol{\theta}) = \frac{1}{1 + \exp[-(\beta_0 + \beta_1 x)]}, \qquad (3.3)$$

where $\boldsymbol{\theta} = \{\beta_0, \beta_1\}$. For brevity, we will abbreviate $p(Y = \kappa|\mathbf{x}_i, \boldsymbol{\theta})$ to $\tilde{\pi}_{(\kappa),i}$, and sometimes to $\tilde{\pi}_i$ when $\kappa = 1$.

When Y is binary valued, we can write

$$p(y_i|x_i, \boldsymbol{\theta}) = \tilde{\pi}_i^{y_i}(1 - \tilde{\pi}_i)^{1-y_i};$$

therefore, from Equation (3.2), we have

$$\log \mathcal{L}(\boldsymbol{\theta}) = \sum_{i=1}^{n} \{y_i \log \tilde{\pi}_i + (1 - y_i)\log(1 - \tilde{\pi}_i)\} + const,$$

and the MLE $\hat{\boldsymbol{\theta}}$ corresponds to

$$\hat{\boldsymbol{\theta}} = \arg\max_{\boldsymbol{\theta}} \sum_{i=1}^{n} \{y_i \log \tilde{\pi}_i + (1 - y_i)\log(1 - \tilde{\pi}_i)\}.$$

From probability model (3.3), we can compute decision regions. If we ignore misclassification costs [e.g., 13],[7] a previously unclassified feature x^* is assigned to the most probable class; therefore, if x^* lies in the region R_1 of x values where $p(Y = 1|x, \hat{\boldsymbol{\theta}}) > 0.5$ we can assume that $Y = 1$ for x^*. Consequently, R_1 is the decision region for $Y = 1$. Similarly, the region R_0 of x values where $p(Y = 0|x, \hat{\boldsymbol{\theta}}) > 0.5$ is the decision region for $Y = 0$. The decision boundary between R_0 and R_1 is the region where $p(Y = 1|x, \hat{\boldsymbol{\theta}}) = 0.5$.

In sum, we assume that $Y = 1$ if x^* is in R_1 or $Y = 0$ if x^* is in R_0. This assignment is a type of *classification*; furthermore, because it is based on the conditional probability $p(Y = 1|x, \hat{\boldsymbol{\theta}})$, it is a *probabilistic classification*.

The above discussion pertained to a univariate logistic function, but an analogous discussion can be made for a multivariate logistic function, such as the bivariate function shown in Figure 3.7. In this case, decision region R_1 is the region of feature vectors $\mathbf{x}$ where $p(Y = 1|\mathbf{x}, \hat{\boldsymbol{\theta}}) > 0.5$, and the decision boundary is the region where $p(Y = 1|\mathbf{x}, \hat{\boldsymbol{\theta}}) = 0.5$.

[7] In addition to allowing for misclassification costs and regions of low classification confidence ("reject regions" or "doubt regions"), a classification system should also allow for the possibility that a future case may not belong to any of the predefined classes (an "outlier") [e.g., 21].

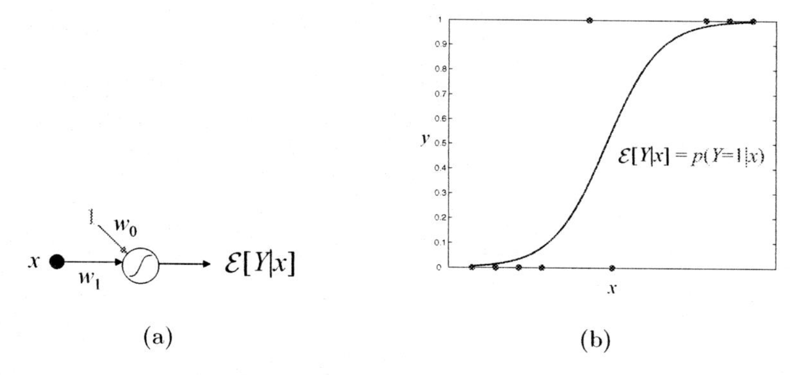

Fig. 3.6. (a) A graphical representation of a univariate logistic regression model with regression coefficients w_0 and w_1. (b) The output $\mathcal{E}[Y|x]$ of the model when fitted to nine binary-valued data points.

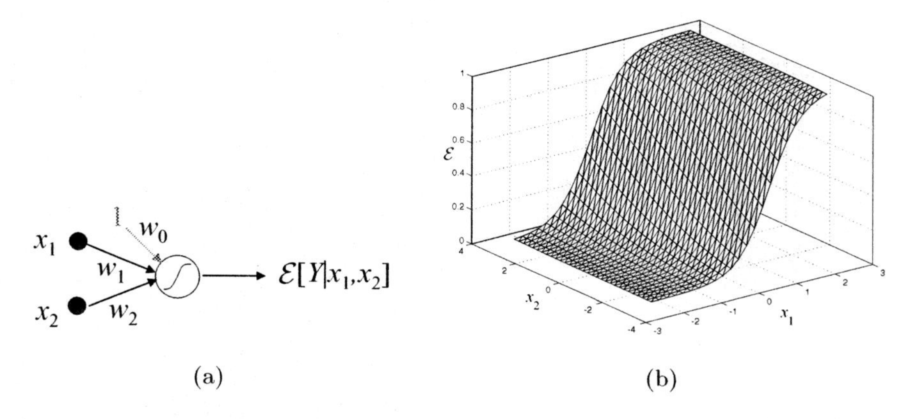

Fig. 3.7. (a) A graphical representation of a bivariate logistic regression model with regression coefficients w_0, w_1 and w_2. (b) Output from the model.

3.3.1 Multi-Layer Perceptrons

The type of decision boundary that can be achieved with the bivariate logistic probability model is limited (e.g., Figure 3.3(b)); however, consider the case where the outputs of two logistic functions are the inputs to a third logistic function (Figure 3.8(a)). From Figure 3.8(b), it can be seen that this arrangement, which is structurally equivalent to an MLP (Figure 3.4), enables a much more complex output to be achieved. This observation motivates the use of an MLP as a flexible regression model $f(\mathbf{x}, \hat{\mathbf{w}})$ and, thus, as a probability model capable of making complex decision boundaries (Figure 3.9):

$$p(Y = 1|\mathbf{x}, \hat{\mathbf{w}}) = \mathcal{E}[Y|\mathbf{x}] = f(\mathbf{x}, \hat{\mathbf{w}}).$$

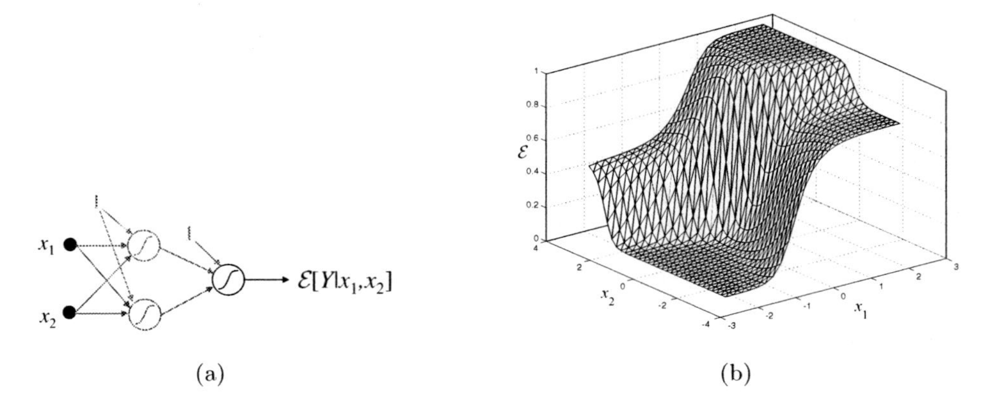

(a) (b)

Fig. 3.8. (a) A multi-layer perceptron represented as nested logistic functions. The outputs from the first two functions are the inputs to the third function. (b) Output from the multi-layer perceptron.

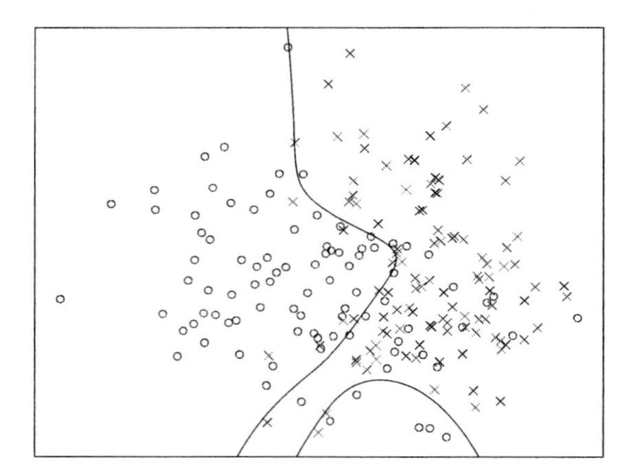

Fig. 3.9. The decision boundary obtained from an MLP. The data points are the same as those used in Figure 3.3(b). The MLP had six hidden nodes and was trained with the quasi-Newton optimization algorithm. Overfitting was penalized by weight decay with the weight-decay coefficient set at 0.2 (see Equation (3.11)).

The concept of maximum-likelihood estimation described earlier can also be used to determine weights $\mathbf{w}$ for an MLP. In other words, the weights are adjusted to a set of values $\hat{\mathbf{w}}$ that maximize the likelihood $p(\mathcal{D}|\mathbf{w})$,

$$\hat{\mathbf{w}} = \arg\max_{\mathbf{w}} p(\mathcal{D}|\mathbf{w}),$$

and thus the log-likelihood

$$\hat{\mathbf{w}} = \arg\max_{\mathbf{w}} \log p(\mathcal{D}|\mathbf{w}).$$

The standard practice within the neural-network community is to think in terms of minimizing error functions rather than maximizing log-likelihoods, where an *error function* $E(\mathbf{w})$ is defined as

$$E(\mathbf{w}) \equiv -\log p(\mathcal{D}|\mathbf{w}), \tag{3.4}$$

and maximization of a log-likelihood is equivalent to the minimization of the corresponding error function:

$$\hat{\mathbf{w}} = \arg\min_{\mathbf{w}} E(\mathbf{w}).$$

If the points in $\mathcal{D}$ are sampled independently, Equation (3.4) can be simplified to

$$E(\mathbf{w}) \equiv -\sum_{i=1}^{n} \log p(y_i|x_i, \mathbf{w}). \tag{3.5}$$

Furthermore, analogous to our treatment of the log-likelihood for logistic regression, we can replace (3.5) with

$$E(\mathbf{w}) = -\sum_{i=1}^{n} \{y_i \log \tilde{\pi}_i + (1 - y_i) \log(1 - \tilde{\pi}_i)\}, \tag{3.6}$$

which is the (two-class) *cross-entropy error function.*[8]

When there are only two classes of interest, there is no need to have an output node for $\tilde{\pi}_{(0)}$ in addition to a node for $\tilde{\pi}_{(1)}$ since $\tilde{\pi}_{(0)} = 1 - \tilde{\pi}_{(1)}$.

What if we have more than two classes, say, c classes? In this situation, we use a network with an output ξ_κ to represent $\tilde{\pi}_{(\kappa)}$ for each class κ. We also replace each target value y_i with a set of *binary dummy variables* $y_{(1),i}, \ldots, y_{(c),i}$, where $y_{(\kappa),i} = 1$ if $y_i = \kappa$ and 0 otherwise. This is called *1-in-c coding.* To ensure that $\sum_\kappa \tilde{\pi}_{(\kappa)} = 1$, the *softmax* activation function is used,

$$\tilde{\pi}_{(\kappa)} = \frac{\exp(a_\kappa)}{\sum_{\kappa'=1}^{c} \exp(a_{\kappa'})},$$

where a_k is the weighted sum to the κth output node, and the summation in the denominator is over all the output nodes. For the error function, (3.6) is replaced by its multi-class analogue:

$$E(\mathbf{w}) = -\sum_{i=1}^{n} \sum_{\kappa=1}^{C} y_{(\kappa),i} \log \tilde{\pi}_{(\kappa),i}.$$

3.4 Training a Multi-Layer Perceptron

Training an MLP with the exemplars present in a data set (*training set*) $\mathcal{D}$ means finding the set of weights $\hat{\mathbf{w}}$ that minimize the error $E(\mathbf{w})$.

---

[8] When Y is continuous-valued, the *sum-of-squares error function* is the standard choice:

$$E(\mathbf{w}) = \frac{1}{2} \sum_{i=1}^{n} \{f(\mathbf{x}_i, \mathbf{w}) - y_i\}^2.$$

If we were able to observe a plot of $E(\mathbf{w})$ over the set of all possible $\mathbf{w}$, we would see a landscape (the *error surface*) consisting typically of several maxima and minima (Figure 3.10). The problem is to locate a weight vector $\hat{\mathbf{w}}$ such that $E(\hat{\mathbf{w}})$ is a global minimum, but how do we search for this global minimum across the error surface? A simple approach is to use *gradient descent*. In gradient descent, we start with some initial (usually random) guess for the weight vector, $\mathbf{w}^{(0)}$. We then iteratively alter the weight vector such that, if the current weight vector is $\mathbf{w}^{(\tau)}$, we move a short distance $\triangle\mathbf{w}^{(\tau)}$ in the direction of the greatest rate of descent along the error surface (Figure 3.11). In vector notation, this is written as

$$\triangle\mathbf{w}^{(\tau)} = -\eta\nabla E(\mathbf{w})|_{\mathbf{w}^{(\tau)}}, \tag{3.7}$$

where η is a constant (the *learning rate*), and $\nabla E(\mathbf{w})|_{\mathbf{w}^{(\tau)}}$ is the gradient

$$(\partial E(\mathbf{w})/\partial w_1 \cdots \partial E(\mathbf{w})/\partial w_{|\mathbf{w}|})^{\mathsf{T}}$$

evaluated at $\mathbf{w}^{(\tau)}$. So, in order to implement (3.7), we have to calculate $\nabla E(\mathbf{w})|_{\mathbf{w}^{(\tau)}}$ from an MLP with weights $\mathbf{w}^{(\tau)}$. This can be achieved with the *error back-propagation algorithm*.

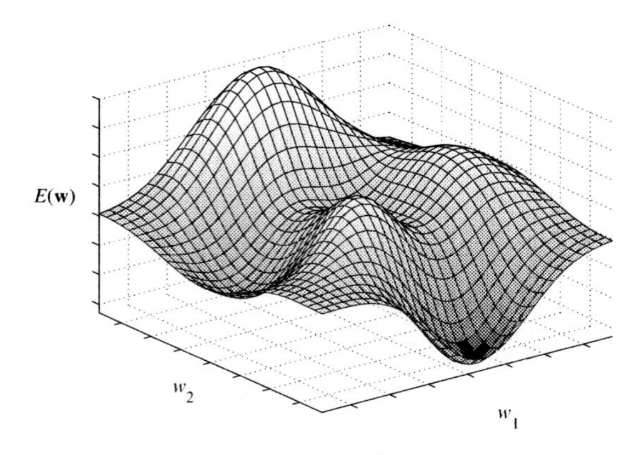

Fig. 3.10. Simulation of an error surface $E(\mathbf{w})$ with local maxima and minima. The error surface sits above weight space.

3.4.1 The Error Back-Propagation Algorithm

An error function $E(\mathbf{w})$ on a data set $\mathcal{D}$ can be written as the sum of errors on each pattern in $\mathcal{D}$:[9]

[9] For example, if $E(\mathbf{w})$ is the cross-entropy error function (3.6) then

$$E_i(\mathbf{w}) = -\{y_i \log \tilde{\pi}_i + (1 - y_i)\log(1 - \tilde{\pi}_i)\}.$$

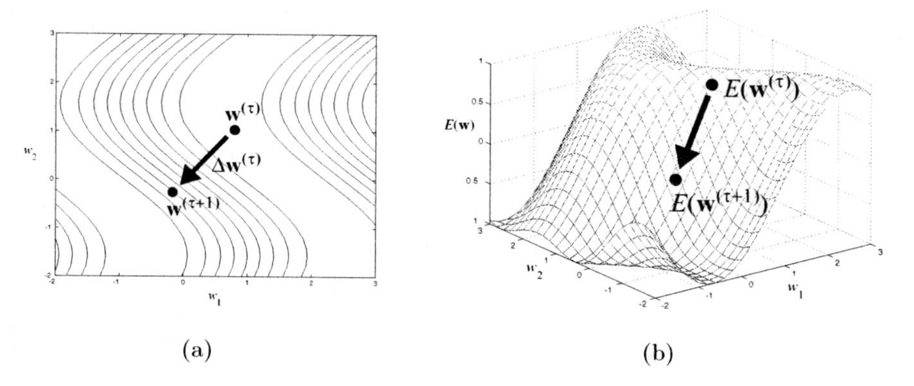

Fig. 3.11. (a) A step $\Delta\mathbf{w}^{(\tau)}$ in weight space from weight vector $\mathbf{w}^{(\tau)}$ to $\mathbf{w}^{(\tau+1)}$ during a search for the global minimum $E(\hat{\mathbf{w}})$. (b) The corresponding changes on the error function over weight space.

$$E(\mathbf{w}) = \sum_{i=1}^{n} E_i(\mathbf{w});$$

therefore, for each $\partial E(\mathbf{w})/\partial w$ in $\nabla E(\mathbf{w})$, we have

$$\frac{\partial E(\mathbf{w})}{\partial w} = \sum_{i=1}^{n} \frac{\partial E_i(\mathbf{w})}{\partial w}. \tag{3.8}$$

Each term within the sum in (3.8) can be determined as follows.

Suppose that we have the following three nodes within an MLP,

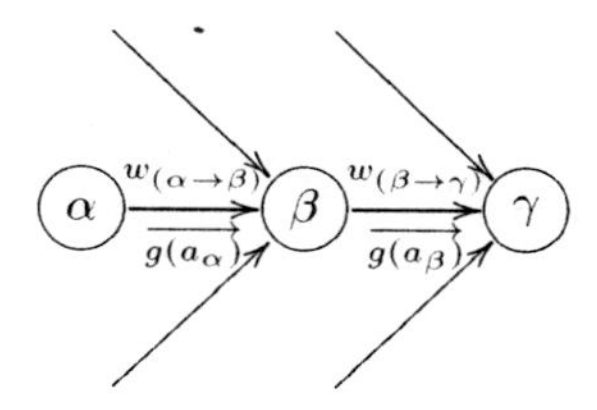

where $w_{(\alpha\to\beta)}$ is the weight on the link from node α to node β. For a given $\mathbf{x}$, node α receives the sum a_α and outputs the value $g(a_\alpha)$, where g is an activation function. Note that these three nodes can be *any* three successive nodes within an MLP containing *one or more* hidden layers. For example, if an MLP has only one hidden layer then node α is an input node, node β is a hidden node, and node γ is an output node. On the other hand, if an MLP has at least two hidden layers then α could be in input node and β and γ two successive hidden nodes; alternatively, α and β could be two successive hidden nodes and γ an output node.

For the element $\partial E_i(\mathbf{w})/\partial w_{(\alpha\to\beta)}$ in (3.8), the chain rule of partial derivatives gives the relationship

$$\frac{\partial E_i(\mathbf{w})}{\partial w_{(\alpha\to\beta)}} = g(a_\alpha)\frac{\partial E_i(\mathbf{w})}{\partial a_\beta}, \tag{3.9}$$

where $g(a_\alpha)$ is one of the values resulting from the *forward propagation* of values within the MLP from the input nodes to the output node(s); for example,

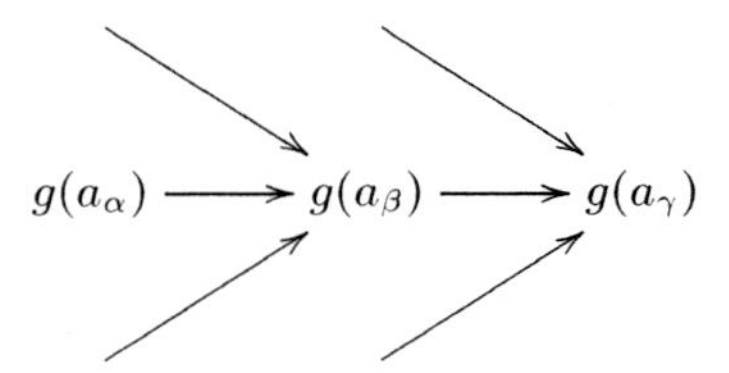

If node α is the input node that receives value x_i then $g(a_\alpha) = x_i$.

The *back-propagation formula* provides the relationship

$$\frac{\partial E_i(\mathbf{w})}{\partial a_\beta} = \frac{\mathrm{d}g(a_\beta)}{\mathrm{d}a_\beta}\sum_{\gamma'} w_{(\beta\to\gamma')}\frac{\partial E_i(\mathbf{w})}{\partial a_{\gamma'}},$$

where the sum is over all the nodes linked from node β, which includes γ. Note that this relationship enables $\partial E_i(\mathbf{w})/\partial a_\beta$, which is associated with node β, to be calculated from $\partial E_i(\mathbf{w})/\partial a_\gamma$, which is associated with a subsequent node γ; thus, the back-propagation formula allows the computational sequence

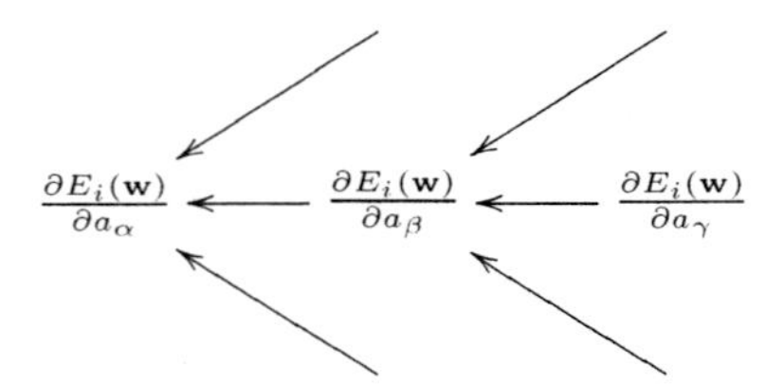

to take place, which starts at the output node(s) and finishes at the input nodes. This sequence is often referred to as a *backward propagation of errors*. If node γ is the output node that produces value ξ_κ then

$$\frac{\partial E_i(\mathbf{w})}{\partial a_\gamma} = \frac{\mathrm{d}g(a_\gamma)}{\mathrm{d}a_\gamma}\frac{\partial E_i(\mathbf{w})}{\partial \xi_\kappa}.$$

With forward propagation giving $g(a_\alpha)$, and backward propagation of errors producing $\partial E_i(\mathbf{w})/\partial a_\beta$, both factors on the right-hand side of (3.9) are available; consequently, $\partial E_i(\mathbf{w})/\partial w$ in (3.8) can be determined, and thus $\nabla E(\mathbf{w})$ for (3.7).

The computation of step $\Delta\mathbf{w}^{(\tau)}$ using (3.7) requires a single pass through the entire training set (an *epoch*). Because it involves the entire training set, it is called *batch learning*. An alternative is to perform a step as each pattern is encountered in the training set (*pattern-based learning*):

$$\Delta\mathbf{w}^{(\tau)} = -\eta\nabla E_i(\mathbf{w})|_{\mathbf{w}^{(\tau)}},$$

where

$$\nabla E_i(\mathbf{w}) = (\partial E_i(\mathbf{w})/\partial w_1 \cdots \partial E_i(\mathbf{w})/\partial w_{|\mathbf{w}|})^\mathsf{T}.$$

In pattern-based learning, the exemplars are used either sequentially or randomly. In practice, pattern-based learning is almost always used in preference to batch learning.

3.4.2 Alternative Training Strategies

The gradient descent rule (3.7) was one of the first training algorithms applied to ANNs. In fact, when applied to single-layer perceptrons, it is equivalent to the perceptron learning rule.

Unfortunately, the gradient descent algorithm is generally inefficient, resulting in very lengthy search times through weight space. Numerous attempts have been made to improve the basic gradient descent approach; for example, one approach is to add a *momentum* term to dampen unnecessary oscillations in the search trajectory within weight space,

$$\triangle \mathbf{w}^{(\tau)} = -\eta \nabla E(\mathbf{w})|_{\mathbf{w}^{(\tau)}} + \mu \triangle \mathbf{w}^{(\tau-1)}, \tag{3.10}$$

but the algorithm remains relatively inefficient, and arbitrary choices for parameters η and μ have to be made.

A number of algorithms that are substantially more efficient than gradient descent have been developed. These include the *conjugate-gradients* and *quasi-Newton* methods. It is beyond the scope of this chapter to go into details about these alternative search strategies (see Bishop [5]), but an empirical comparison of the gradient-descent and quasi-Newton methods is shown in Figure 3.12.

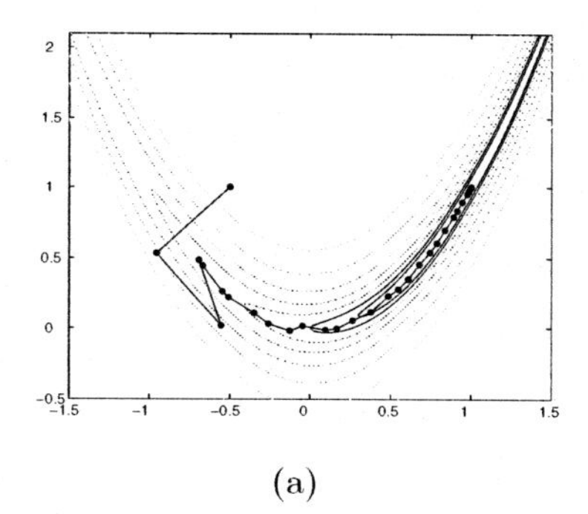

(a)

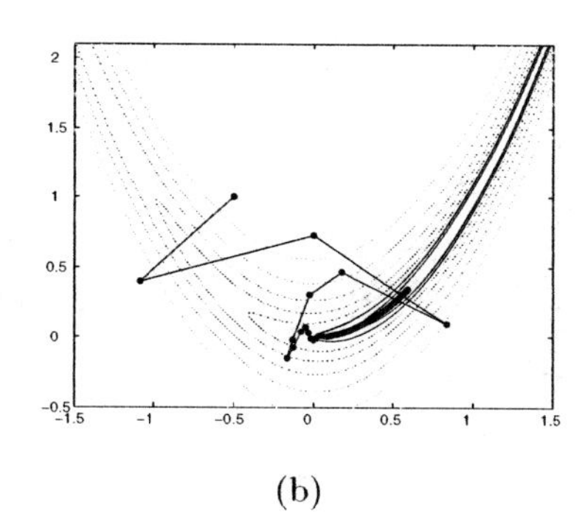

(b)

Fig. 3.12. Simulation of the trajectory of a weight vector $\mathbf{w}$ over an error surface $E(\mathbf{w})$. The search begins at (−0.5,1), and the minimum is at (1,1). Two types of optimization algorithms were used: (a) the quasi-Newton method; (b) the gradient-descent method with learning rate $\eta = 0.004$ and momentum $\mu = 0.5$ (Equation (3.10)). With the quasi-Newton method, the minimum was reached in 28 steps; whereas, with gradient descent, the minimum had not been reached by 100 steps. (Reprinted with permission, Ian T. Nabney, *NETLAB: Algorithms for Pattern Recognition*, 2002, Springer Verlag, London.)

3.5 Some Practical Considerations

We conclude with some important points concerning the use of MLPs, which include the potential of over-fitting, the problem of local minima, and the importance of data pre-processing. Software packages for neural computation are discussed in Section 16.4.

3.5.1 Over-Fitting

As stated earlier, the purpose of regression is to estimate the conditional expectation $\mathcal{E}[Y|\mathbf{x}]$ from a training set (*generalization*) rather than an exact representation of the data; however, because of the intrinsic flexibility of MLPs, the output from an MLP could fit the data too closely (referred to as *over-fitting*). Over-fitting (Figure 3.13(a)) will result in a high predictive performance with respect to the training set but a poor performance with respect to an independent *test set.*

If an MLP is too flexible then, for a given $\mathbf{x}_i$, $\tilde{\pi}_i$ could vary too much from one data set to the next (large *variance*). We can control the flexibility exhibited by an MLP but, if we curtail the flexibility too much, the MLP may have insufficient flexibility to model $\mathcal{E}[Y|\mathbf{x}]$ adequately from a data set (Figure 3.13(b)). In other words, $\tilde{\pi}_i$ will tend to be too far from $\mathcal{E}[Y|\mathbf{x}_i]$ (high *bias*).

The extremes of over-fitting (high variance but low bias) and insufficient flexibility (low variance but high bias) are detrimental to network performance. What we require is a compromise between the conflicting requirements of low bias and low variance: the *bias–variance trade-off.* Both bias and variance can be reduced by increasing the number of data points, but, in practice, the amount of data available is often limited.

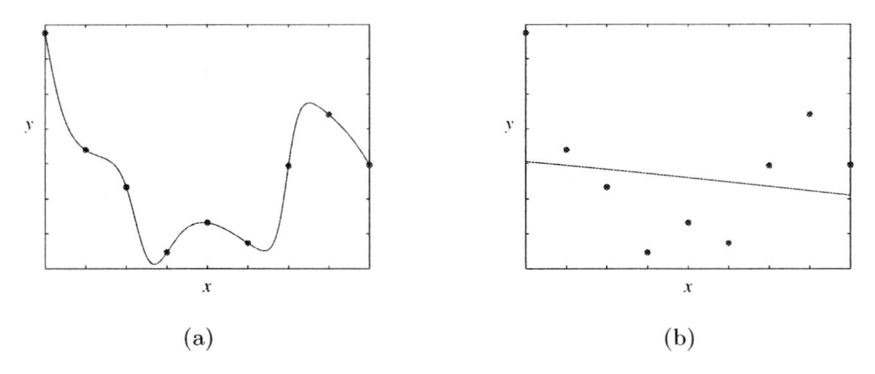

Fig. 3.13. An example of the effect of regularization on an MLP with a linear activation function at the output node. (a) The regularization coefficient ν of Equation (3.11) was set to zero, and the MLP over-fitted the data points. This MLP is expected to exhibit low bias but high variance. (b) The regularization coefficient was set to 2, and the MLP had insufficient flexibility to generalize from the same data points used in (a). This MLP is expected to exhibit low variance but high bias. (Reprinted with permission, Christopher Bishop, *Neural Networks for Pattern Recognition*, 1995, Clarendon Press, Oxford.)

The flexibility of an MLP can be controlled by a technique called *regularization* (Figure 3.13). In this approach, an error function $E(\mathbf{w})$ is augmented with a *regu-*

larization term, which penalizes against high flexibility. The most commonly-used regularization term is the *weight-decay term*:

$$E'(\mathbf{w}) = E(\mathbf{w}) + \frac{\nu}{2} \sum_{j=1}^{|\mathbf{w}|} w_j^2, \tag{3.11}$$

where ν is the *regularization coefficient*. The weight-decay term exploits the fact that large curvature (which can result in over-fitting) is associated with relatively large weights. The presence of such weights increases the weight-decay term and thus the penalized error function $E'(\mathbf{w})$. The optimal value for ν can be determined either by cross-validation or automatically through the *evidence framework* (see Section 10.7.2 and Chapter 12).

Another approach to controlling over-fitting is the procedure called *early stopping*. Suppose we plot $E(\mathbf{w})$ against the number of steps τ used to train an MLP. At first, $E(\mathbf{w})$ decreases as $\tilde{\pi}$ approaches $\mathcal{E}[Y|\mathbf{x}]$, but $E(\mathbf{w})$ continues to decrease whilst the MLP increasingly over-fits to the training set. If we now plot $E(\mathbf{w})$ against τ, but compute $E(\mathbf{w})$ on a data set that is independent of the training set (the *validation set*), we expect to see $E(\mathbf{w})$ first decrease as $\tilde{\pi}$ approaches $\mathcal{E}[Y|\mathbf{x}]$ but then increase as over-fitting takes place; therefore, we should stop the training of the MLP when the minimum of this second plot is reached (*early stopping*). However, a word of warning about early-stopping: Ripley [21] has observed cases when, after a minimum has been reached, the plot with respect to the validation set increased but then fell to a substantially lower minimum. This second minimum would be missed if early stopping had been implemented.

Model assessment

When assessing the efficacy of a trained MLP, the assessment should be done with respect to a data set that played no part whatsoever in the development of the model; therefore, this *test set* should be independent of both the training set and the validation set. Unfortunately, a number of authors have made the mistake of using the validation set as the test set, an error than can make an MLP appear to be more effective than it really is.[10]

When there is insufficient data for it to be permanently partitioned into a training set, a validation set, and a test set, ν-fold *cross-validation* can be used (Figure 3.14).

Hand [9] discusses in detail the various performance metrics that are available for the assessment of classifiers such as MLPs.

3.5.2 Local Minima

As stated in Section 3.4, the training of an MLP involves a search across an error surface that starts at some point $\mathbf{w}^{(0)}$ in weight space and hopefully finishes at the global minimum $E(\hat{\mathbf{w}})$. The trajectory of this search in weight space involves

[10] Amazingly, there have also been cases where the training set has been used as the test set.

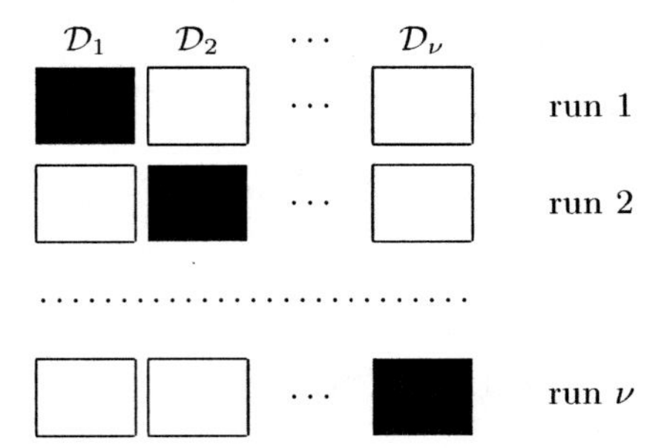

Fig. 3.14. Schematic illustration of ν-fold cross-validation. The entire data set $\mathcal{D}$ is randomly partitioned into ν subsets $\mathcal{D}_1, \mathcal{D}_2, \ldots, \mathcal{D}_\nu$. Each subset $\mathcal{D}_i (i = 1, \ldots, \nu)$ takes its turn to act as a temporary test set (black region) whilst the remaining $\nu - 1$ subsets (white regions) are first combined and then randomly partitioned into a training set and a validation set. The results from the ν test sets are averaged (Reprinted with permission, Christopher Bishop, *Neural Networks for Pattern Recognition*, 1995, Clarendon Press, Oxford.).

a succession of weight vectors $\mathbf{w}^{(0)}, \mathbf{w}^{(1)}, \ldots, \hat{\mathbf{w}}$, the direction taken from $\mathbf{w}^{(\tau)}$ to $\mathbf{w}^{(\tau+1)}$ being dictated by an optimization algorithm.

Optimization algorithms such as gradient descent always decrease the error function, so that $E(\mathbf{w}^{(\tau+1)}) < E(\mathbf{w}^{(\tau)})$, but this creates a potential problem. Error surfaces often consist of many minima, and the attempt by an algorithm to always decrease the error function at each step can result in a weight vector reaching a minimum that is not the global minimum (a *local minimum*). Furthermore, because the algorithm does not have a mechanism to increase the error function, the weight vector remains stuck at the local minimum. Consequently, the optimum weight vector $\hat{\mathbf{w}}$ is not reached (Figure 3.15).

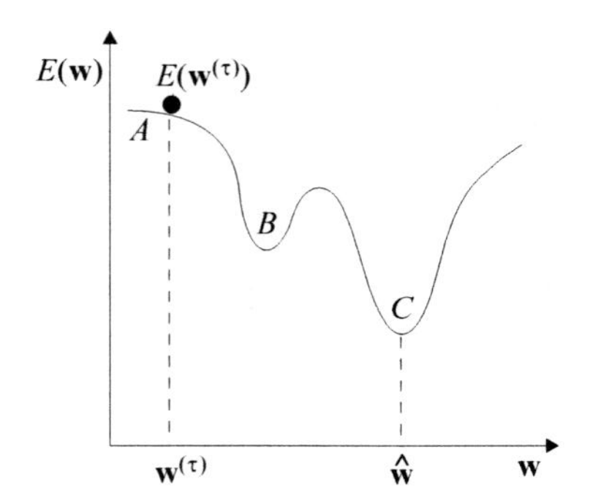

Fig. 3.15. A is the current location of $E(\mathbf{w})$ on an error surface during a search for the global minimum C. During the search, weight vector $\mathbf{w}$ arrives at a local minimum (B) from which it cannot escape.

We can increase our chance of locating $E(\hat{\mathbf{w}})$ by repeating our search from an entirely different starting point. Of course, the new search may also finish at a local minimum, but if we use many (at least ten) starting points, each chosen at random, our chance of finding the global maximum increases. This strategy is known as the *method of random restarts.*

Each random restart will result in an MLP. We could select the best-performing network from the resulting set of MLPs and discard the rest; alternatively, we could retain all the MLPs and average the outputs from each network. The set of MLPs used in the latter approach is called a *committee of networks*, and the theoretical justification for this approach is given in Section 10.7.3.

3.5.3 Number of Hidden Nodes

There is no theory that tells us what the optimal number of hidden nodes will be for a given classification or regression problem, although some rough guidelines have been proposed.[11] The optimal number can be determined empirically by successively increasing the number of hidden nodes in an MLP. The performance of each resulting MLP is assessed with respect to a validation set possibly via cross-validation. Tarassenko [24] gives an example of this approach.

3.5.4 Preprocessing Techniques

With most MLP-based applications, the feature vectors $\mathbf{x}$ used as input are derived from associated vectors of raw data. This conversion of a raw-data vector $\mathbf{v}$ to a feature vector $\mathbf{x}$ is referred to as *preprocessing*, and, in many cases, it is crucial to the success of a neural-computational task.

One reason for the importance of preprocessing is the so-called *curse of dimensionality* [e.g., 5]. An MLP with fewer inputs requires fewer weights, which are more likely to be properly constrained by a data set of limited size. A way of reducing the size of $\mathbf{v}$ is to select a subset of the original variables (*variable subset selection*). This can be achieved with a stepwise variable-selection procedure [12, 6].

Another approach to dimensionality reduction is to perform *principal component analysis (PCA)* on the raw data set $\{(\mathbf{v}_1, \kappa_1), \ldots, (\mathbf{v}_n, \kappa_n)\}$ [e.g., 13]. This technique linearly maps $\mathbf{v}$ to a lower-dimensional space. However, because principal components analysis ignores class labels, it may not provide any discrimination of the classes.

The use of background knowledge to derive features from $\mathbf{v}$ is another type of preprocessing. Tarassenko [24] gives a good example of this for the analysis of sleep electroencephalograms, which focused on the selection of known dominant frequencies.

Another important form of data preprocessing is the replacement of categorical variables with binary dummy variables (i.e., 1-of-d encoding). In addition, if the means and/or ranges of the continuous-valued input variables differ greatly, training can be facilitated by normalizing these values to have zero mean and unit variance.

[11] One guideline is to set the number of hidden nodes in a two-layer MLP equal to the geometric mean of the number d of input nodes and the number c of output nodes: $\sqrt{dc}$ [e.g., 15].

3.5.5 Training Sets

To ensure that each class is equally represented during the training of an MLP, a *balanced* data set should be used. If the number of exemplars from each class is not the same, and N_γ is the number of exemplars from the least represented class, Tarassenko [24] recommends randomly selecting enough exemplars from the other classes until a data set is produced with N_γ exemplars from each class.

If a balanced data set is produced by the above approach, $\tilde{\pi}$ must be adjusted to take account of the fact that the relative frequencies of the classes in the balanced training set differ from the true prior class probabilities. The adjusted value of $\tilde{\pi}_{(\kappa),i}$ is given by

$$\varpi_{(\kappa),i} = \frac{\tilde{\pi}_{(\kappa),i} p(\kappa)/\psi(\kappa)}{\sum_{\kappa'} \tilde{\pi}_{(\kappa'),i} p(\kappa')/\psi(\kappa')}, \tag{3.12}$$

where $p(\kappa)$ is the true prior probability of class κ, and $\psi(\kappa)$ is the relative frequency of class κ in the balanced data set. Tarassenko [24] points out that expression (3.12) should not be used if the differences between the true prior probabilities are very large; for example, $p(\kappa_1) = 0.001$ and $p(\kappa_2) = 0.999$. In such a situation, a *novelty detection* method should be used instead [4, 25].

How many exemplars should we have in a training set? If we wish to correctly classify $100(1-\epsilon)\%$ of all future feature vectors $\mathbf{x}$ (where $\epsilon < 1/8$), Baum and Haussler [2] recommend that at least $|\mathbf{w}|/\epsilon$ exemplars should be present in the training set, where $|\mathbf{w}|$ is the number of weights (including biases) in a two-layer, one-output-node MLP. For example, if we want to classify 90% of $\mathbf{x}$ correctly, we need about 10 times as many training exemplars as there are weights in the MLP.

3.6 Further Reading

A variety of books have been written on artificial neural networks. One of the more useful introductions is *Introduction to Neural Networks* by Gurney [8], which clearly describes the basic principles.

To many who use neural networks, the definitive work is *Neural Networks for Pattern Recognition* by Bishop [5]. This excellent text is one of the first to place neural nets in a statistical framework. We strongly recommend *NETLAB: Algorithms for Pattern Recognition* [18] as a source of algorithms (written in Matlab) to accompany Bishop's text.

A useful guide to the practicalities of neural-network development is Tarassenko's *A Guide to Neural Computing Applications* [24], which contains many helpful guidelines.

Acknowledgments

We would like to thank Ian Nabney and Peter Weller for their careful reading and constructive comments on an earlier draft of this chapter.

Figure 3.12 was inspired by Nabney [18], whereas Figures 3.13 and 3.14 were inspired by Bishop [5].

References

[1] I. Aleksander and H. Morton. *An Introduction to Neural Computing.* Chapman & Hall, London, 1990.

[2] E.B. Baum and D. Haussler. What size net gives valid generalization? *Neural Computation*, 1(1):151–215, 1989.

[3] R. Beale and T. Jackson. *Neural Computing: An Introduction.* IOP Publishing, Bristol, 1990.

[4] C.M. Bishop. Novelty detection and neural network validation. *IEE Proceedings: Vision, Image & Signal Processing*, 141:217–222, 1994.

[5] C.M. Bishop. *Neural Networks for Pattern Recognition.* Clarendon Press, Oxford, 1995.

[6] A. Blum and P. Langley. Selection of relevant features and examples in machine learning. *Artificial Intelligence*, 97(1-2):245–271, 1997.

[7] S.E. Fahlman and C. Lebiere. The cascade-correlation learning architecture. In D.S. Touretzky, editor, *Advances in Neural Information Processing Systems 2*, pages 524–532, Los Altos, CA, 1990. Morgan Kaufmann.

[8] K. Gurney. *An Introduction to Neural Networks.* UCL Press, London, 1997.

[9] D.J. Hand. *Construction and Assessment of Classification Rules.* John Wiley, Chichester, 1997.

[10] D. Hebb. *Organization of Behaviour.* Wiley, New York, 1949.

[11] K. Hornik. Approximation capabilities of multilayer feedforward networks. *Neural Networks*, 4(2):251–257, 1991.

[12] R. Kohavi and G. John. Wrappers for feature selection. *Artificial Intelligence*, 97(1-2):273–324, 1997.

[13] W.J. Krzanowski. *Principles of Multivariate Analysis.* Oxford University Press, Oxford, 1988.

[14] D.J.C. MacKay. A practical Bayesian framework for back-propagation networks. *Neural Computation*, 4(3):448–472, 1992.

[15] T. Masters. *Practical Neural Network Recipes in C++.* Academic Press, London, 1993.

[16] W. McCulloch and W. Pitts. A logical calculus of the ideas immanent in nervous activity. *Bulletin of Mathematical Biophysics*, 5:115–133, 1943.

[17] M.L. Minsky and S.A. Papert. *Perceptrons.* MIT Press, Cambridge, 1969.

[18] I.T. Nabney. *NETLAB: Algorithms for Pattern Recognition.* Springer, London, 2002.

[19] R.M. Neal. *Bayesian Learning for Neural Networks.* PhD thesis, University of Toronto, 1994.

[20] N. Rashevsky. Topology and life: In search of general mathematical principles in biology and sociology. *Bulletin of Mathematical Biophysics*, 16:317–348, 1954.

[21] B.D. Ripley. *Pattern Recognition and Neural Networks.* Cambridge University Press, Cambridge, 1996.

[22] F. Rosenblatt. The perceptron: A probabilistic model for information storage and organization in the brain. *Psychological Review*, 65:386–408, 1958.

[23] F. Rosenblatt. On the convergence of reinforcement procedures in simple perceptrons. Technical report VG-1196-G-4, Cornell Aeronautical Laboratory, Buffalo, NY, 1960.

[24] L. Tarassenko. *A Guide to Neural Computing Applications.* Arnold, London, 1998.

[25] L. Tarassenko, P. Hayton, N. Cerneaz, and M. Brady. Novelty detection for the identification of masses in mammograms. In *Proceedings of the 4th IEE International Conference on Artificial Neural Networks*, pages 442–447, Cambridge, 1995. Cambridge University Press.
[26] P.J. Werbos. *Beyond Regression: New Tools for Prediction and Analysis in the Behavioral Sciences.* PhD thesis, Harvard University, Cambridge, MA, 1974.

Part II

Bioinformatics

4

Introduction to Statistical Phylogenetics

Dirk Husmeier

Biomathematics and Statistics Scotland (BioSS)
JCMB, The King's Buildings, Edinburgh EH9 3JZ, UK
dirk@bioss.ac.uk

Summary. The objective of molecular phylogenetics is to reconstruct the evolutionary relationships among different species or strains from biological sequence alignments and present them in an appropriate, usually tree-structured, graph. Besides being of fundamental importance in itself – aiming to estimate, for instance, the ancestry of the human race or to infer the whole tree of life – phylogenetics has recently become of heightened interest in epidemiology, where it promises to provide increased insight into the emergence and evolution of infectious diseases, and in forensic science. Evolution is driven by stochastic forces that act on genomes, and phylogenetics essentially tries to discern significant similarities between diverged sequences amidst a chaos of random mutation and natural selection. Faced with noisy data resulting from intrinsically stochastic processes, the most powerful methods make use of probability theory. This chapter first discusses the shortcomings of the older non-probabilistic methods of clustering and parsimony and then describes the more recent probabilistic approach. Based on an explicit mathematical model of nucleotide substitution in terms of a homogeneous Markov chain, a phylogenetic tree can be interpreted as a Bayesian network. This interpretation allows the application of the inference methods introduced in Chapters 1 and 2. Two particular optimization algorithms that have been implemented in widely used software packages will be described. The chapter then discusses the question of statistical significance of the inference results, and it contrasts the two methods of significance estimation: the frequentist approach of bootstrapping versus the Bayesian method of Markov chain Monte Carlo.

Notation. The notation used in this chapter is described in the *Notation and Conventions* section of the Appendix. The symbol t is used with two different meanings: (1) physical time and (2) position in a DNA sequence alignment; see Table 4.1 on page 111. It becomes clear from the respective context which of the two interpretations applies. The notation does not distinguish between random variables and their values. It does, however, distinguish between observed and hidden nodes in a Bayesian network. The symbol y_i represents the random variable associated with an observed node i. On making an observation, y_i becomes a value. The symbol z_i represents the random variable associated with a hidden node i, that is, a node for which no data are available. For generic representation, x_i is used.

4.1 Motivation and Background on Phylogenetic Trees

In 1990 a young woman in Florida contracted AIDS without having previously been exposed to the established risks of HIV infection. Scientists at the Centers for Disease Control in Atlanta launched an extensive investigation to establish the cause of the infection. Eventually they uncovered that a dentist suffering from AIDS himself had infected several of his patients with HIV [26]. This finding was the result of applying two recent scientific methodologies: the experimental method of *DNA sequencing*, and the mathematical method of *phylogenetic analysis.*

The objective of phylogenetics is to reconstruct the evolutionary relationships among different species or strains (generic name *taxa*[1]) and to display them in a binary or bifurcating tree-structured graphical model called a *phylogenetic tree.* An example is given in Figure 4.1. The leaves of a phylogenetic tree represent contemporary species, like chicken, frog, mouse, etc. The inner or hidden nodes represent hypothetical ancestors, where a splitting of lineages occurs. These so-called speciation events lead to a diversification in the course of evolution, separating, for instance, warm-blooded from cold-blooded animals, birds from mammals, primates from rodents, and so on.

Figure 4.1 shows a so-called *rooted tree.* The node at the bottom of the tree represents the most recent common ancestor, from which ultimately all other nodes descended. The edges are directed, related to the direction of time: the closer a node is to the root of the tree, the older it is in time. Inferring this direction of evolutionary processes, however, is difficult and not amenable to the modelling and inference methods discussed in this introductory tutorial. Consequently, phylogenetic trees will be displayed as *unrooted trees*, shown in Figure 4.2. As opposed to a rooted tree, the edges in an unrooted tree are undirected, and no node is in the distinguished position of a root.[2]

A phylogenetic tree conveys two types of information. The *topology* defines the branching order of the tree and the way the contemporary species are distributed among the leaves. For example, from Figures 4.1 and 4.2 we learn that the mammals – human, chicken, mouse, and opossum – are grouped together and are separated from the group of animals that lay eggs – chicken and frog. Within the former group, opossum is grouped out because it is a

---

[1] In bacteria and viruses it is difficult to distinguish between *species* and *strains.* This chapter is rather sloppy in the use of these terms, and occasionally uses both terms synonymously.

[2] We can regain a rooted from an unrooted tree by including an *outgroup* in the analysis. An outgroup is a (set of) species that is known *a priori* to be less related to any of the other taxa used in the study, and the root will therefore be located on the branch between the other taxa and the outgroup. For example, in Figure 4.2, *frog* is the outgroup, because it is the only cold-blooded animal among a set of warm-blooded animals. By positioning the root on the branch leading to frog, we regain the rooted tree of Figure 4.1 (although the exact position of the root on this branch is not known).

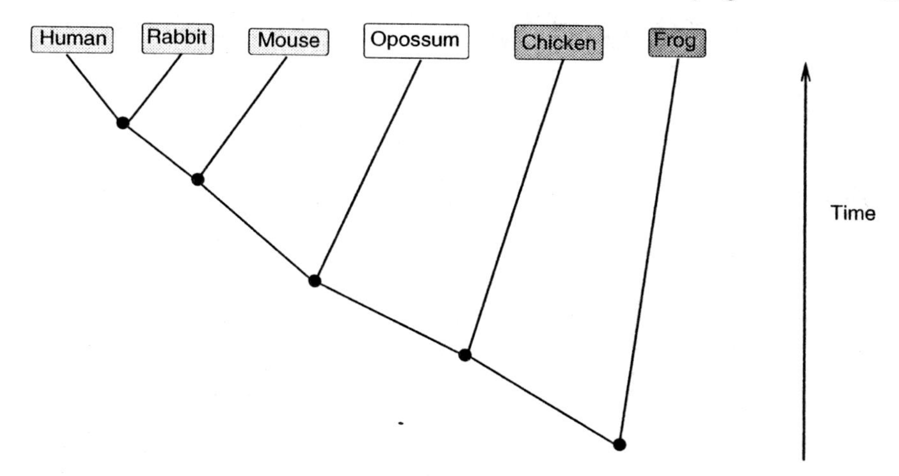

Fig. 4.1. Rooted phylogenetic tree. Leaf nodes represent extant or contemporary species. Hidden nodes represent hypothetical ancestors, where lineages bifurcate (so-called *speciation* events).

marsupial and therefore less closely related to the other "proper" mammals. Exchanging, for instance, the leaf positions of opossum and rabbit changes the branching order and thus leads to a different tree topology. For n species there are, in total, $(2n-3)!!$ different rooted, and $(2n-5)!!$ different unrooted tree topologies, where !! denotes double factorial: $(2n-5)!! = (2n-5)(2n-7)...1$. A proof is given in the appendix at the end of this chapter. In what follows, we will use the integer variable $S \in \{1, 2, \ldots, (2n-5)!!\}$ to label the different unrooted tree topologies.

The second type of information we obtain from a phylogenetic tree is given by the *branch lengths*, which represent *phylogenetic time*,[3] measured by the average amount of mutational change. For example, Figure 4.2 shows a comparatively long branch leading to the leaf with *frog*. This long branch indicates that a comparatively large number of mutations separates *frog* from the other animals, and that a large amount of phylogenetic time has passed since the lineage leading to *frog* separated from the remaining tree. This conjecture is reasonable because *frog* is the only cold-blooded animal, whereas all the other animals are warm-blooded. Note that the mutation rate is usually unknown, and we can therefore not infer *physical time* from the branch lengths. This distinction between *physical* time and *phylogenetic* time will be discussed in more detail in Section 4.4.2.

An unrooted tree for n species has $n-2$ inner nodes, and thus $m = n + (n-2) - 1 = 2n - 3$ branches. In what follows, individual branch lengths

[3] Throughout this chapter, *phylogenetic time* is (unconventionally) used with the meaning *evolutionary change*, which is given by the product of *physical time* and a *nucleotide substitution rate*. See Equation (4.21) for an exact definition.

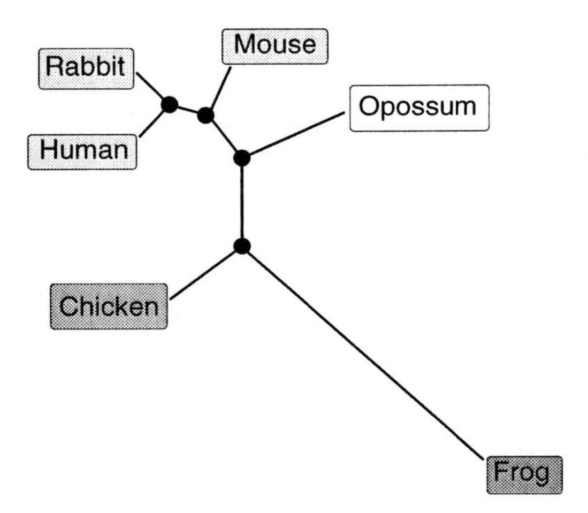

Fig. 4.2. Unrooted phylogenetic tree. Leaf nodes represent contemporary species, hidden nodes represent hypothetical ancestors. The tree conveys two types of information. The *topology* defines the branching order of the tree and the way the contemporary species are distributed among the leaves. The *branch lengths* represent phylogenetic time, measured by the average amount of mutational change.

will be denoted by w_i, and the total vector of branch lengths will be denoted by $\mathbf{w} = (w_1, \ldots, w_{2n-3})$.

Two further examples of phylogenetic trees are shown in Figures 4.3 and 4.4. Since the start of the AIDS epidemic in the early 1980s, there has been an increased interest in the emergence and evolution of infectious diseases. The reconstruction of the evolutionary relationships among extant strains of a virus or bacterium may help us to understand the origin and spread of an infection. Figure 4.3, for instance, shows a phylogenetic tree for various strains of HIV-1, HIV-2, and SIV. SIV, which stands for *simian immunodeficiency virus*, is an HIV-like virus that is commonly found in many African monkeys. While the HIV-1 strains are grouped together in a clade that is well separated from the rest of the tree, HIV-2 strains are closely related to SIV strains. This finding suggests that the virus may have crossed species boundaries, and that there may have been cross-infection between humans and monkeys. Figure 4.4 shows a phylogenetic tree that was reconstructed from the envelope gene of various HIV-1 strains during the Florida dentist investigation, mentioned at the beginning of this section. The tree reveals that several patients had been infected with strains that are closely related to those of the dentist. Also, both the strains of the dentist and those of his patients are grouped in a clade that is clearly separated from a set of independent control strains. This finding suggests that the patients had, in fact, been infected by their dentist [26].

The objective of the present chapter is to discuss methods for reconstructing phylogenetic trees. Since the driving forces of evolution are *mutations*, that is, errors in the *replication* of DNA, it seems reasonable to base our infer-

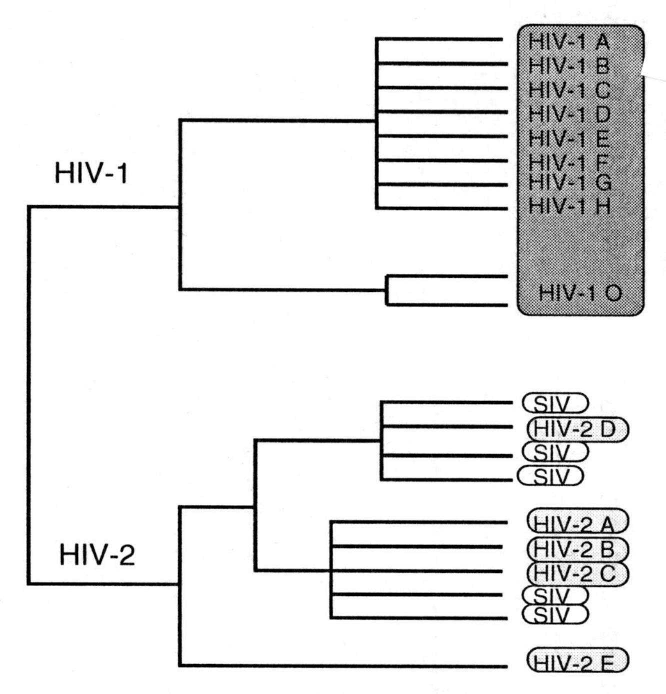

Fig. 4.3. Phylogenetic tree of HIV and SIV strains. HIV-1 strains are grouped together, whereas HIV-2 strains are closely related to SIV strains (HIV-like viruses found in many African monkeys), suggesting that there might have been cross-infection between humans and monkeys. Adapted in a slightly simplified form from [27], by permission of Blackwell Science.

ence on a comparison of DNA sequences[4] obtained from the different species or strains of interest. This approach has recently become viable by major breakthroughs in DNA sequencing techniques. In July 1995, the first complete genome of a free-living organism was published – the entire 1.8 million base pairs of the bacterium *Haemophilus influenzae* [13]. In June 2000, a working draft of the complete 3.3 billion base-pair DNA sequence of the entire human genome was pre-released. Since then, the amount of DNA sequence data in publicly accessible data bases has been growing exponentially.

DNA is composed of an alphabet of four *nucleotides*, which come in two families: the purines *adenine* (A) and *guanine* (G), and the pyrimidines *cytosine* (C) and *thymine* (T). DNA sequencing is the process of determining the

[4] Earlier approaches to phylogenetics were based on the analysis of non-molecular data, for instance, morphological characters. This chapter focuses on phylogenetic analysis based on molecular sequence data, mainly DNA sequences. The advantages of this more recent approach of *molecular phylogenetics* over classical *non-molecular phylogenetics* are discussed in [27].

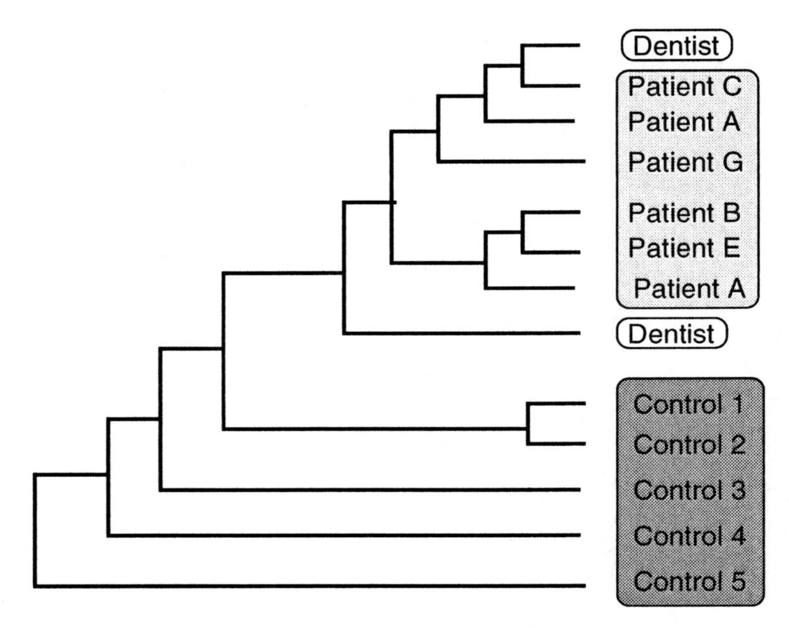

Fig. 4.4. The case of the Florida dentist. The figure shows a phylogenetic tree inferred from a sequence alignment of the envelope gene of various HIV-1 strains. The strains of several patients are closely related to those of the dentist and well separated from the strains of an independent control group. This finding suggests that the dentist had infected several of his patients with AIDS. Note that because HIV-1 is so variable, two different sequences are included for the dentist and for patient A. Adapted in a slightly simplified form from [27], by permission of Blackwell Science.

order of these nucleotides. After obtaining the DNA sequences of the taxa of interest, we need to compare *homologous* subsequences, that is, corresponding regions of the genome that code for the same protein. More precisely, we have to compare homologous nucleotides, that is, nucleotides which have been acquired directly from the common ancestor of the taxa of interest. The process of establishing which regions of a set of DNA sequences are homologous and should be compared is called *DNA sequence alignment*. Throughout this chapter we will assume that the sequence alignment is given. A brief introduction to the alignment problem was given in Section 2.3.4. For a more comprehensive review, see [4].

The top of Figure 4.5 shows a small section of the DNA sequence alignment obtained from the β-globin encoding genes in six species (four mammals, one bird, and one amphibian). Rows represent different species, columns represent different sites or positions in the DNA sequence. At the majority of sites, all nucleotides are identical, reflecting the fact that the sequences compared are homologous. At certain positions, however, differences occur, resulting from

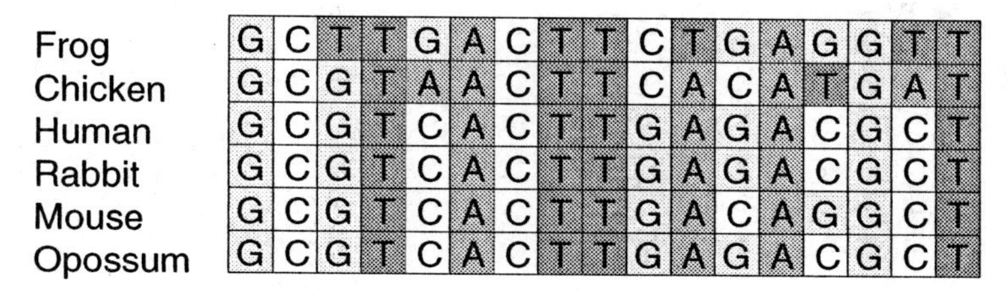

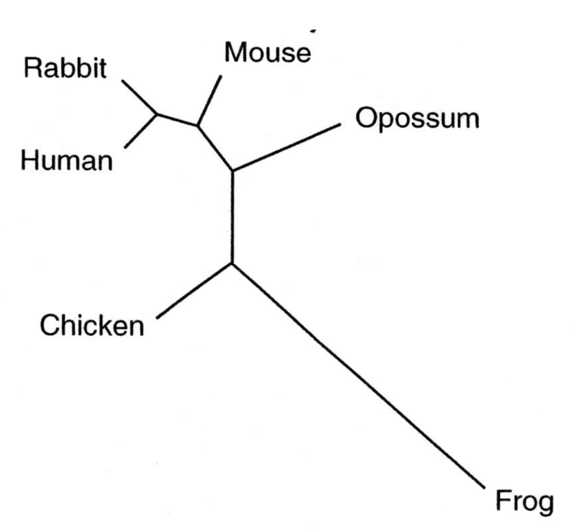

Fig. 4.5. Phylogenetic inference from DNA sequence alignments. The *top* figure shows a section of the DNA sequence alignment for the β-globin encoding gene in six species. The total alignment has a length of 444 nucleotides. The *bottom* figure shows a phylogenetic tree inferred from this alignment with DNAML, to be discussed in Section 4.4.5.

mutational changes during evolution. In the fifth column, for instance, human, rabbit, mouse, and opossum have a C, chicken has an A, and frog has a G. This reflects the fact that the first four species are mammals and therefore more closely related to each other than to the two remaining species. Obviously, however, nucleotide substitutions are not as deterministically related to the phylogenetic tree as in this example. Evolution is driven by stochastic forces that act on genomes, and our objective is to discern significant similarities between diverged sequences amidst a chaos of random mutation and natural selection. Faced with noisy data resulting from intrinsically stochastic processes, the most powerful methods make use of probability theory. This chapter will start with a brief summary of the older non-probabilistic methods – *genetic distance-based clustering*, discussed in Section 4.2, and *parsimony*, discussed in Section 4.3 – which will then be contrasted with the newer *probabilistic approach*, discussed in Section 4.4. Based on a mathematical model of nucleotide substitution in terms of a homogeneous Markov chain, a phylogenetic tree can be interpreted as a probabilistic generative model, which allows us to compute the likelihood of an observed DNA sequence alignment. The practical computation draws on well-established inference algorithms for Bayesian networks, discussed in Section 2.3.6. This result allows the application of standard inference procedures from statistics and machine learning, as reviewed in Chapter 1: maximum likelihood (Section 4.4.5), bootstrapping (Section 4.4.6), and Bayesian MCMC (Section 4.4.7).

4.2 Distance and Clustering Methods

4.2.1 Evolutionary Distances

Figure 4.6 shows the small section of an alignment of β-globin encoding DNA sequences from human, rabbit, and chicken. For the majority of sites the nucleotides of the different species are identical, which reflects the homology of the sequences. However, for a small proportion of sites, the nucleotides differ as a consequence of past mutations. For example, the nucleotide at the fourth site of the human sequence is an A, while the homologous sequence in rabbit has a G in this position. A comparison of the sequence pairs human versus chicken and rabbit versus chicken reveals three differences, respectively. A naive approach to phylogenetics is to count all the pairwise differences between the sequences, here shown in the table at the bottom left of Figure 4.6, and to derive a tree from them, as explained shortly and displayed in the bottom of Figure 4.6. Note that in this particular example, the tree we obtain in this way is intuitively plausible in that it groups human with rabbit, which is another mammal, rather than chicken, which is a bird.

A problem of this naive approach is that the pairwise difference between two taxa, that is, the observed number of sites in which two sequences differ, is not necessarily the same as the actual number of nucleotide substitutions that have occurred during evolution. Figure 4.7 gives an illustration. In the tree in the top left, the contemporary species have nucleotides A and G at a given site in the alignment, and the most recent common ancestor had an A at the corresponding position. This means that one nucleotide substitution event has occurred during evolution, along the right branch of the tree, and one nucleotide substitution is observed in the alignment of the extant sequences. Consequently, the estimated and actual numbers of nucleotide substitutions are the same, and the naive approach outlined above provides the right answer. However, in the tree in the middle of the top row of Figure 4.7, a separate nucleotide substitution event has occurred in each of the two branches, and the total number of nucleotide substitutions on the path connecting the two extant species is 2. The number of nucleotide substitutions observed from the DNA sequence alignment, on the other hand, is 1 and thus misses out one of the nucleotide substitution events. In fact, in all the other

Human ... T G T **A** T C G C T C ...
Rabbit ... T G T **G** T C G C T C ...

Human ... **T** G T **A** T C G **C** T C ...
Chicken ... **A** G T **C** T C G **T** T C ...

Rabbit ... **T** G T **G** T C G **C** T C ...
Chicken ... **A** G T **C** T C G **T** T C ...

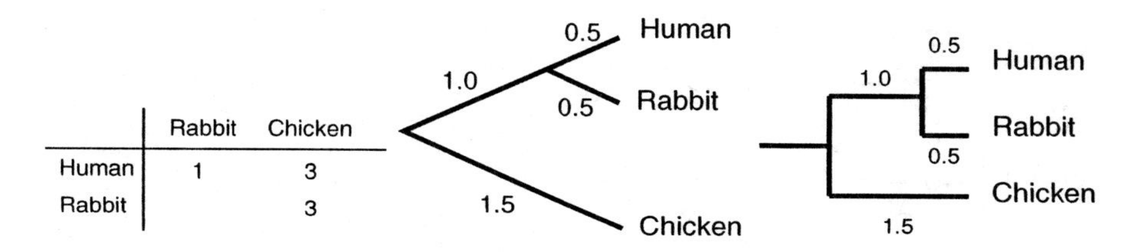

	Rabbit	Chicken
Human	1	3
Rabbit		3

Fig. 4.6. Genetic distances. The top figure shows a small section of an alignment of homologous β-globin encoding DNA sequences from human, rabbit, and chicken. Counting the number of nucleotide substitutions by which the sequences differ leads to the table in the bottom left, from which the phylogenetic trees in the bottom centre and right are obtained. The two trees are equivalent ways of displaying the same information. For the tree in the middle, information about pairwise genetic distances is contained in the branch lengths, indicated by the numbers on the branches. For the cladogram on the right, all the information is contained in the horizontal branch lengths, whereas the vertical branch lengths are arbitrary and do not convey any information. Note that the pairwise genetic distances, shown in the table on the left, are recovered by summing over the lengths of all the branches separating two sequences. Also, note that this example is given for illustration purposes only, and that real phylogenetic inference is based on much longer DNA sequences.

evolutionary scenarios depicted in Figure 4.7, we find that the observed number of nucleotide substitutions systematically underestimates the true number of nucleotide substitutions that have occurred during evolution. Consequently, the naive approach to measuring evolutionary distances by just counting the number of differences between two sequences is flawed and does not properly reflect the real amount of evolutionary change.

The failure of the naive approach to determining evolutionary distances can be understood from the following consideration. Assume that two lineages separated t time units ago, and that the nucleotide substitution rates for these lineages are constant during evolution. Then, the actual number of nucleotide substitutions along these lineages is proportional to time: the more time has passed, the more nucleotide substitution events will have occurred. In the limit of an infinite amount of time, $t \to \infty$, an infinite number of nucleotide substitutions will have occurred, which implies that the DNA sequences of

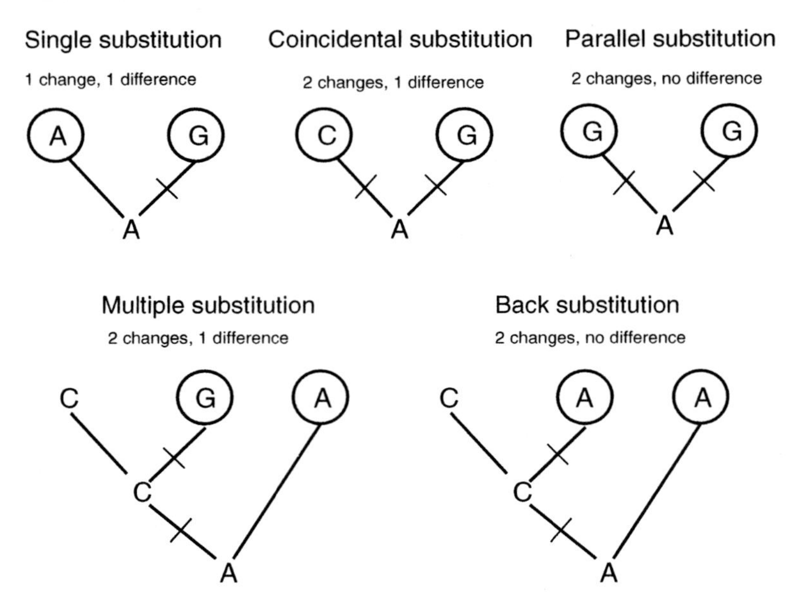

Fig. 4.7. Hidden and multiple nucleotide substitutions. The figure contains several phylogenetic trees, which display different nucleotide substitution scenarios. In each tree, the circles at the leaf level represent contemporary sequences from a DNA sequence alignment, for which a pairwise distance is to be computed. The letters inside these circles represent nucleotides at a given site in the alignment. Nodes further down in the tree hierarchy (that is, below the leaf nodes) represent (usually extinct) ancestors. The letters at these nodes show nucleotides at the corresponding site in the ancestral DNA sequence. For the tree in the top left, the observed number of nucleotide substitutions is identical to the actual number of substitutions that have occurred during evolution. However, in all the other cases, the actual number of nucleotide substitutions is larger than the observed number, hence a naive approach to computing pairwise evolutionary distances systematically underestimates their true values. Adapted from [27], by permission of Blackwell Science.

the corresponding extant species will be completely unrelated. However, since DNA is composed of a four-nucleotide alphabet, two unrelated sequences will still show, on average, an accidental nucleotide concurrence for 25% of the sites. This means that the naive distance measure shows a saturation effect and converges, for $t \to \infty$, towards a limit value of 75% difference, as opposed to the true evolutionary distance, which, for $t \to \infty$, diverges to infinity. Figure 4.8 illustrates this effect.

To correct for this effect, we need to apply a nonlinear transfer function that maps the interval $[0, 0.75]$ onto the positive real line, $[0, \infty)$. One such function is given by

$$d = -\frac{3}{4} \log(1 - \frac{4}{3} d_o) \tag{4.1}$$

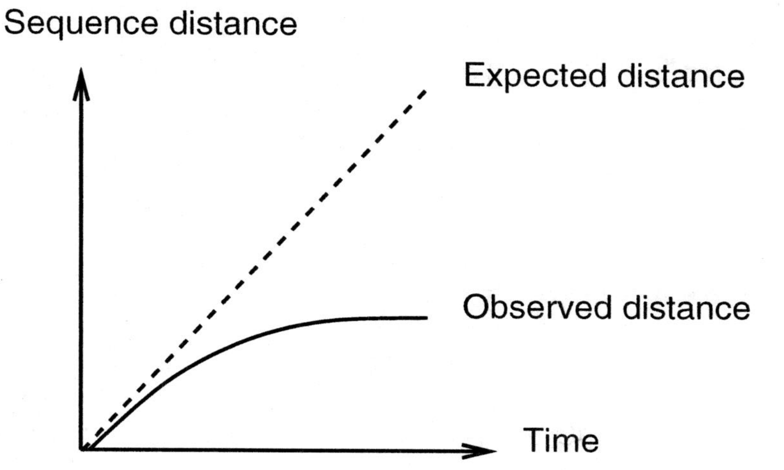

Fig. 4.8. Saturation of pairwise distance estimation. While the true evolutionary distance between two sequences is proportional to time, the average fraction of nucleotide differences observed in a DNA sequence alignment shows a saturation effect and converges towards a limit value of 0.75. Adapted from [27], by permission of Blackwell Science.

where d_o is the naive, observed evolutionary distance between two sequences, and d is the corrected distance. For small phylogenetic times, $t \to 0$, the fraction of observed differences is small, $d_o \to 0$, and a first-order Taylor series expansion of the log, $\log(1 - \frac{4}{3}d_o) = -\frac{4}{3}d_o$, shows that the observed and corrected pairwise distances are identical: $d = d_o$. However, for large times, $t \to \infty$, which implies $d_o \to \frac{3}{4}$, we have $d \to \infty$. Consequently, as opposed to the observed distances d_o, the corrected distances d of (4.1) avoid the saturation. Note that the choice of transfer function is not unique, and that there are several alternatives to equation (4.1). For more details, see, for instance, Section 8.6 in [4], and Section 5.2 in [27].

4.2.2 A Naive Clustering Algorithm: UPGMA

Given corrected pairwise distances, d_{ik}, we can think of applying a standard clustering algorithm. A simple approach is to use hierarchical average linkage clustering, which in the phylogenetics literature is usually referred to as *unweighted pair group method using arithmetic averages* (UPGMA). The name of the algorithm reflects the way the distance between two clusters is defined. If d_{ab} is the distance between two sequences a and b, then the distance d_{AB} between two clusters, that is, groups of sequences A and B, is defined as follows:

$$d_{AB} = \frac{1}{|A||B|} \sum_{a \in A} \sum_{b \in B} d_{ab} \tag{4.2}$$

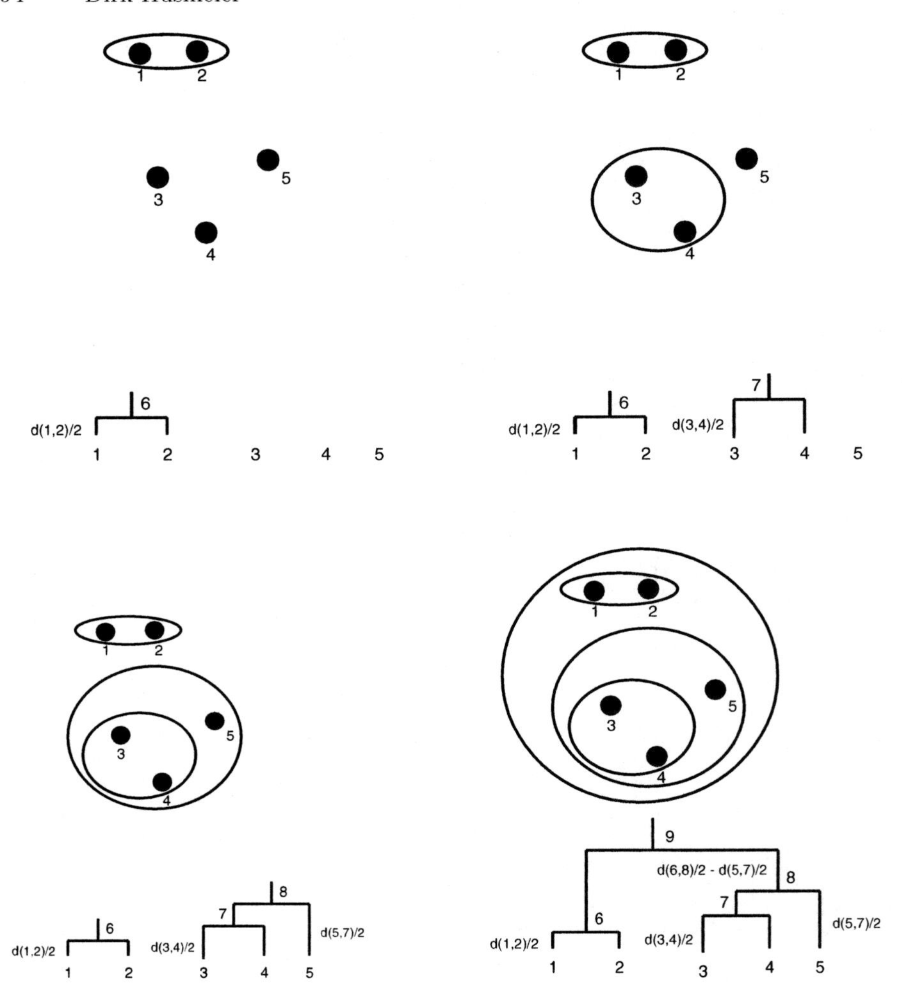

Fig. 4.9. Illustration of clustering with UPGMA. Sequences correspond to the black dots in the plane and form the leaves of the tree, placed at height zero. *Top left:* The sequences with the smallest distance d_{ij} are grouped together, and a new node representing this cluster is introduced at height $d_{ij}/2$. *Top right* and *bottom left*: The algorithm continues in this way, defining the distance between clusters by (4.2). *Bottom right:* The algorithm terminates when only one cluster, corresponding to the root of the tree, remains. Adapted from [4], by permission of Cambridge University Press.

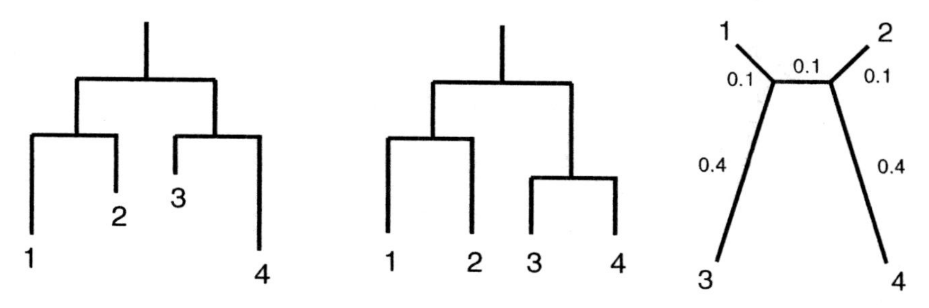

Fig. 4.10. Failure of UPGMA. The tree in the middle satisfies the molecular clock constraint: the distance between the root and a leaf node is the same for all lineages, which implies that DNA sequences evolve at a constant rate throughout the tree and that all lineages have experienced, on average, the same number of nucleotide substitutions. This constraint on the branch lengths usually does not hold, and a real tree tends to resemble more the example on the left. When the molecular clock constraint is violated, the naive UPGMA clustering algorithm may lead to systematically wrong results, as demonstrated on the right. The evolutionary distance between two taxa is obtained by summing the lengths of all the branches on the connecting path. Consequently, UPGMA will erroneously group taxa 1 and 2 together, since their distance is $0.1 + 0.1 + 0.1 = 0.3$, which is smaller than that of the true neighbouring pairs, taxa 1 and 3, and taxa 2 and 4, which both have an evolutionary distance of $0.1 + 0.4 = 0.5$. Adapted from [4], by permission of Cambridge University Press.

where $|A|$ and $|B|$ are the numbers of sequences in clusters A and B, respectively. Drawing on this definition, the clustering algorithm can be defined as follows (adapted from [4], Chapter7):

Initialization
- Assign each sequence i to its own cluster C_i. Define one leaf for each sequence, and place it at height zero.

Iteration
- Determine the two clusters C_i and C_j for which d_{ij} is minimal.
- Define a new cluster $C_k = C_i \cup C_j$.
- Add C_k to the current clusters and remove C_i and C_j.
- Define a new node k with daughter nodes i and j and place it at height $d_{ij}/2$.

Termination
- When only two clusters C_i, C_j remain, place the root at height $d_{ij}/2$.

Figure 4.9 illustrates this algorithm.

UPGMA is fast and easy to use. It has, however, serious drawbacks. Recall from Section 4.1 that it is difficult to infer the root position of a phylogenetic tree from a DNA sequence alignment. However, the tree we obtain with UPGMA, shown in Figure 4.9, does contain a well-defined root. This ability to root the tree is a consequence of imposing a constraint on the branch lengths:

as seen from Figure 4.9, the distances between the root and the leaf nodes are the same for all lineages. This so-called *molecular clock* constraint implies that DNA sequences evolve at a constant rate throughout the tree of life and that the average number of nucleotide substitutions is the same for all lineages. For many species, this assumption has been proved wrong (see, for instance, [27], Chapter 7, and [40]). Figure 4.10 shows that UPGMA may lead to systematically wrong results when the molecular clock constraint is violated. Consequently, it should not be used in phylogenetic analysis.

4.2.3 An Improved Clustering Algorithm: Neighbour Joining

Figure 4.10 shows that UPGMA may give wrong results when two neighbouring taxa have branches with very different lengths. To overcome this shortcoming, consider the following "distance-like" function introduced in [32] and [39]:

$$D_{ij} = d_{ij} - \bar{d}_i - \bar{d}_j; \qquad \bar{d}_i = \frac{1}{|L|-2} \sum_{l \in L} d_{il} \tag{4.3}$$

where the d_{ij} are the original[5] corrected pairwise distances, L is the set of leave nodes, and $|L|$ is the number of leaves in the tree. The idea is to subtract, from the original distances d_{ij}, the average distances to all other leaves. This correction compensates for long edges. Note, however, that D_{ij} may take negative values and is therefore not a distance measure. Applying (4.3) to the tree on the right of Figure 4.10, we obtain:

$$\begin{aligned}
\bar{d}_1 &= \frac{1}{2}(0.3 + 0.6 + 0.5) = 0.7 = \bar{d}_2 \\
\bar{d}_3 &= \frac{1}{2}(0.5 + 0.6 + 0.9) = 1.0 = \bar{d}_4 \\
D_{12} &= d_{12} - \bar{d}_1 - \bar{d}_2 = 0.3 - 0.7 - 0.7 = -1.1 \\
D_{13} &= d_{13} - \bar{d}_1 - \bar{d}_3 = 0.5 - 0.7 - 1.0 = -1.2 < D_{12}
\end{aligned}$$

On selecting the taxa pair (i, j) for which D_{ij} is minimal, we now obtain the true pairs $(1, 3)$ and $(2, 4)$ and avoid the false pair $(1, 2)$ that we would obtain with UPGMA. A general proof is given in [39]. To proceed, recall the standard axioms a set of numbers $\{d_{ij}\}$ has to satisfy in order to form a metric:

1) Non-negativity: $d_{ij} \geq 0$
2) Symmetry: $d_{ij} = d_{ji}$
3) Distinctness: $d_{ij} = 0$ if and only if $i = j$
4) Triangle inequality: $d_{ij} \leq d_{ik} + d_{kj}$

Obviously, a distance cannot be negative (axiom 1) and is independent of the direction in which it is measured (axiom 2). Moreover, the distance between

[5] "Original" means "not modified according to (4.3)." However, the raw distances from the sequence alignment have to be corrected according to (4.1).

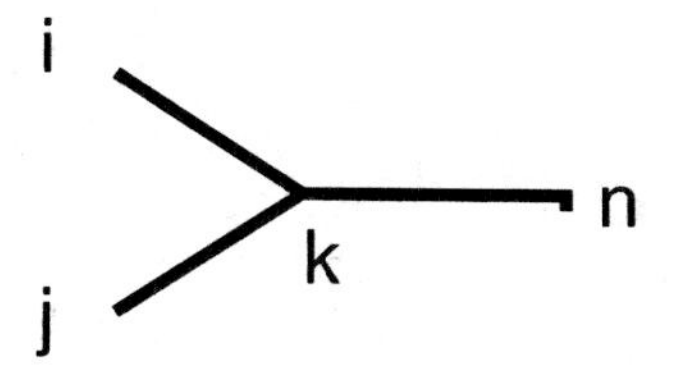

Fig. 4.11. Illustration of the additivity of a tree metric. Nodes i, j, and n are leaf nodes, while k is a hidden node. See text for details.

two points is zero if and only if these two points are the same (axiom 3). Axiom 4 states that the distance between two points cannot exceed the sum of the distances between each point and a third. This so-called triangle inequality is illustrated in Figure 4.11. The sum of the distances d_{ik} and d_{kj} is greater than the distance d_{ij}, which expresses the trivial fact that by travelling from i to j via k we make a detour and therefore have to cover a longer distance than when following the direct path "as the crow flies." However, for a tree, such a shortcut does not exist, and a path from i to j has to pass through k. Consequently, while being a metric is a *necessary* condition for being a valid measure of evolutionary change, it is not a *sufficient* condition, and we need a further axiom to define a tree. This so-called additivity constraint can be formulated in different equivalent ways (see, for instance, [27], Chapter 2). The simplest formulation is as follows [4]:

> A set of distances $\{d_{ij}\}$, $i, j \in L$, is said to be *additive* if there is a tree with a set of leaves L such that the distance d_{ij} between any pair of leaves $(i, j) \in L^2$ is the sum of the lengths of the edges on the path connecting them.

Applied to Figure 4.11 this additivity constraint implies that axiom 4 has to be replaced by a more stringent condition:

$$d_{ij} = d_{ik} + d_{kj} \tag{4.4}$$

For the edge configuration of Figure 4.11 we thus obtain:

$$\begin{aligned} d_{in} &= d_{ik} + d_{kn} \\ d_{jn} &= d_{jk} + d_{kn} \\ \Rightarrow\ 2d_{kn} &= d_{in} + d_{jn} - d_{ik} - d_{kj} \\ \Rightarrow\ d_{kn} &= \frac{1}{2}(d_{in} + d_{jn} - d_{ij}) \end{aligned} \tag{4.5}$$

Note that in the third line we have made use of the symmetry condition, axiom 2, and in the last line, we have applied (4.4). The upshot of this calculation is that we can compute the distance between the hidden node k and the leaf node n from the distances between the leaf nodes i, j, and n. This property can be exploited to obtain an improved clustering algorithm, which is called *neighbour joining* and was introduced in [32]. Start from a set L of leaf nodes, one for each sequence, and then iterate:

- Find the pair of nodes (i, j) that minimizes D_{ij}, defined by (4.3).
- Replace (i, j) by a new node k with new distances $d_{kn} = \frac{1}{2}(d_{in} + d_{jn} - d_{ij})$, for all remaining nodes n in L. Note that the expression for d_{kn} follows from (4.5).
- Remove the old leaves i and j from L, and add k as a new leaf to L.
- Add k to the tree, joining it to nodes i and j with edge lengths $d_{ik} = \frac{1}{2}(d_{ij} + \bar{d}_i - \bar{d}_j)$ and $d_{jk} = \frac{1}{2}(d_{ij} + \bar{d}_j - \bar{d}_i)$, respectively, where $\bar{d}_i$ and $\bar{d}_j$ are defined by (4.3).

The algorithm terminates when only two nodes i, k remain, which are connected by an edge of length d_{ik}. The expressions for the new distances d_{ik} and d_{jk} in the last step of the iteration are obtained as follows. From (4.5) we have (changing the indices $i \leftrightarrow n$ and using the symmetry of a metric):

$$d_{ik} = d_{ki} = \frac{1}{2}(d_{ni} + d_{ji} - d_{nj}) = \frac{1}{2}(d_{ij} + d_{in} - d_{jn}) \tag{4.6}$$

If the additivity constraint is satisfied, then (4.6) holds for all the remaining leaf nodes $n \in L \setminus \{i, j\}$, and we could compute d_{ik} from any n. To allow for violations of the additivity constraint, Studier and Keppler [39] proposed summing over all n. Dividing by $|L| - 2$ and applying definition (4.3) leads to the expression stated in the iteration. The derivation for d_{jk} is analogous.

It can be shown that if the distances $\{d_{ij}\}$, $i, j \in L$, satisfy the tree metric axioms, that is, the metric axioms *and* the additivity constraint, then the true tree will be correctly reconstructed with neighbour joining [32], [39]. However, real evolutionary distances usually do not exactly satisfy the additivity constraint, which compromises the reconstruction of the phylogenetic tree. Figure 4.12 shows a simple application of the neighbour joining algorithm, taken from [27]. The upper triangle of the table shows the pairwise distances between five hominoids. These distances were obtained from an alignment of mitochondrial DNA sequences, using a correction function similar to (4.1). Applying the neighbour joining algorithm to these pairwise distances, we obtain the phylogenetic tree shown in the bottom of Figure 4.12. The lower triangle of the table in Figure 4.12 shows the pairwise distances obtained from this tree. Note that these distances deviate to a certain extent from the observed distances. This deviation is a consequence of the fact that for evolutionary distances obtained from real DNA sequences, the tree metric axioms are not exactly satisfied, as mentioned above.

4.2.4 Shortcomings of Distance and Clustering Methods

Figure 4.13 illustrates the inherent shortcoming of distance methods: by mapping the high-dimensional space of sequences into the low-dimensional space

	Human	Chimp	Gorilla	Orang-utan	Gibbon
Human		0.0919	0.1083	0.1790	0.2057
Chimp	0.0919		0.1134	0.1940	0.2168
Gorilla	0.1068	0.1151		0.1882	0.2170
Orang-utan	0.1816	0.1898	0.1893		0.2172
Gibbon	0.2078	0.2160	0.2155	0.2172	

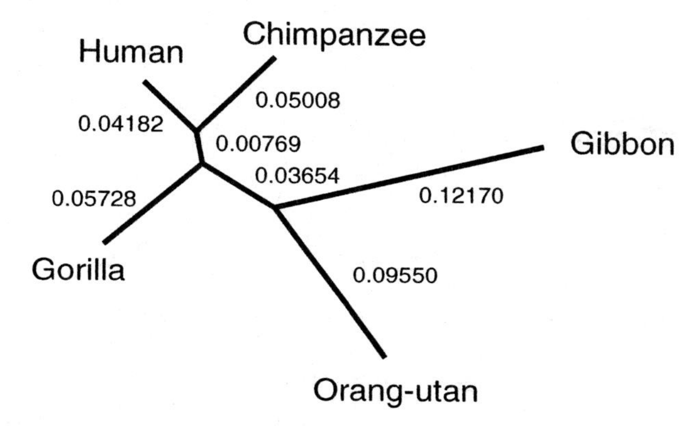

Fig. 4.12. Phylogenetic analysis with distance methods. The upper triangle of the table shows the pairwise evolutionary distances between five hominoids, obtained from an alignment of mitochondrial DNA sequences. Applying the neighbour joining algorithm to these distances gives the phylogenetic tree shown in the bottom. The pairwise distances obtained from this tree are shown in the lower triangle of the table. These estimated distances show some deviation from the distances obtained from the alignment, which reflects the fact that the true evolutionary distances do not satisfy the additivity constraint of a tree metric. Adapted from [27], by permission of Blackwell Science.

of pairwise distances, a considerable amount of information inevitably gets lost. Another way of describing this shortcoming is that once converted into pairwise distances, we can no longer reconstruct the original sequences. Now, as discussed above, pairwise distances need to satisfy the additivity constraint of a tree metric in order to define a tree. Sequences that satisfy this additivity constraint live in a low-dimensional submanifold in sequence space. Due to the intrinsic stochasticity of evolutionary processes, real DNA sequences are not confined to this submanifold, that is, the pairwise distances computed from the sequence alignment usually violate the additivity constraint. The consequence is that the tree distances, d_{ij}^{tree}, deviate systematically from the observed distances, d_{ij}, as shown in Figure 4.12, and the neighbour joining algorithm is no longer guaranteed to reconstruct the correct tree.

The attractive feature of clustering algorithms, like neighbour joining, is their low computational cost. This comes with the deluding feature of pseudo-

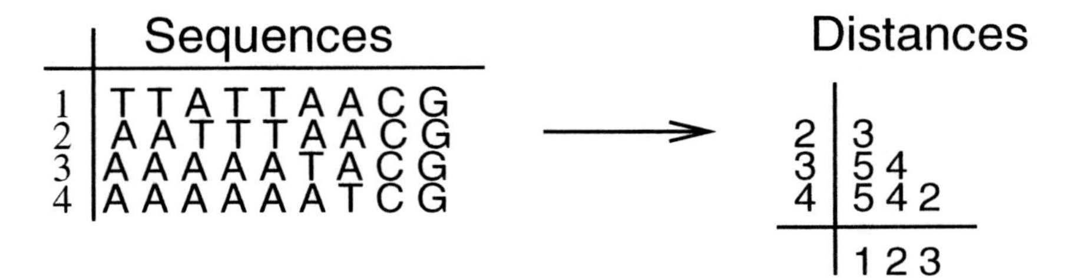

Fig. 4.13. Information loss of distance methods. By computing pairwise evolutionary distances from a DNA sequence alignment, the high-dimensional space of DNA sequences is mapped into the low-dimensional space of pairwise distances. This drastic reduction of dimension results in an inevitable loss of information.

determinism: the algorithm has no parameters to be tuned, it avoids the need to search through the space of all trees, and it is not troubled by the existence of local optima known from many iterative optimization methods. The price to pay for this computational convenience is the fact that neighbour joining does not optimize any objective function. Consequently, there is no guarantee that the algorithm finds the best tree, according to some optimality criterion. In a critical application, like the Florida court case described in Section 4.1, this shortcoming is obviously unacceptable. A better approach, therefore, is to search for the tree that optimizes some optimality criterion, as proposed by Fitch and Margoliash [12]. Such a procedure comes at higher computational costs, but with the power and speed of modern computers continuously increasing, this drawback becomes increasingly less important. Note, however, that any optimality function based on pairwise distances still suffers from the inherent information loss of the mapping from the sequence space into the space of pairwise distances, as discussed above and depicted in Figure 4.13. We will therefore, in the remainder of this chapter, look at methods that base the inference on the DNA sequences themselves.

4.3 Parsimony

4.3.1 Introduction

The basic idea behind *parsimony*, introduced in [11], is that the optimal phylogenetic tree is the one requiring the smallest number of nucleotide substitutions along its branches. Take, as an example, Figure 4.14, which shows an alignment of four DNA sequences and a hypothetical phylogenetic tree, in which strain 1 is grouped with strain 2, and strain 3 is grouped with strain 4. We pick a column of the alignment and distribute the nucleotides across the leaf nodes. Next, we try to reconstruct the evolutionary history by assigning nucleotides to the hidden nodes, which correspond to ancestral, unobserved sequences. For the first column of the alignment, strains 1 and 2 have an A,

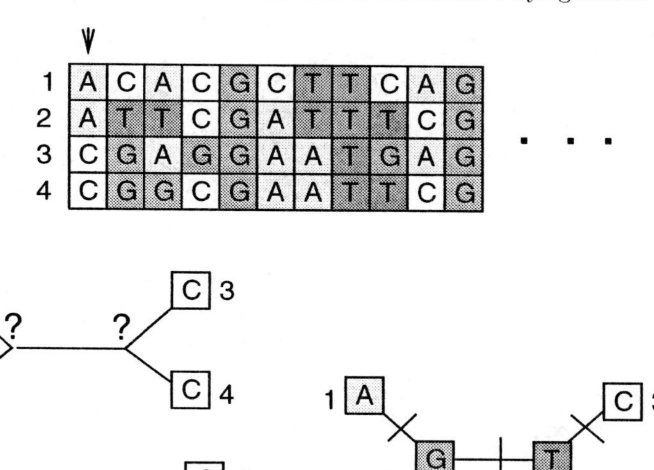

Fig. 4.14. Illustration of parsimony: single tree. For each column of nucleotides in the alignment, the evolutionary history is to be reconstructed by assigning nucleotides to the hidden nodes. An arbitrary assignment, shown on the right, can give up to five nucleotide substitutions needed for a reconstruction of evolution. A more skilful choice, shown at the bottom, reduces this number to a single substitution. Under the principle of parsimony this reconstruction is preferred over the less parsimonious reconstruction that requires five substitutions.

while strains 3 and 4 have a C. If we assign nucleotides to the hidden nodes arbitrarily, say a G to the first hidden node, and a T to the second, as shown on the right of Figure 4.14, we can get up to five nucleotide substitution events needed for a reconstruction of evolution. However, a more skilful choice, shown at the bottom of Figure 4.14, can reduce this number to a single nucleotide substitution. Under the principle of parsimony this reconstruction is preferred over the less parsimonious reconstruction that requires five substitutions.

Next, we have to compare different trees. With four taxa, we have three unrooted tree topologies: strain 1 can either be grouped with strain 2, with strain 3, or with strain 4. For a given column of nucleotides from the alignment, we repeat the previous process of assigning nucleotides to the hidden nodes in the most parsimonious way. This is repeated for each of the possible tree topologies in turn. We then count the number of nucleotide substitutions needed. An example is given in Figure 4.15 where, for the first column in the alignment, the tree that groups strains 1 and 2 against strains 3 and 4 requires the smallest number of substitutions and is therefore preferred by parsimony.

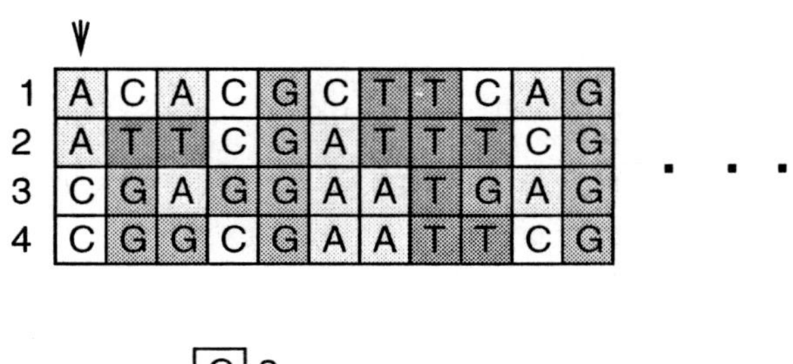

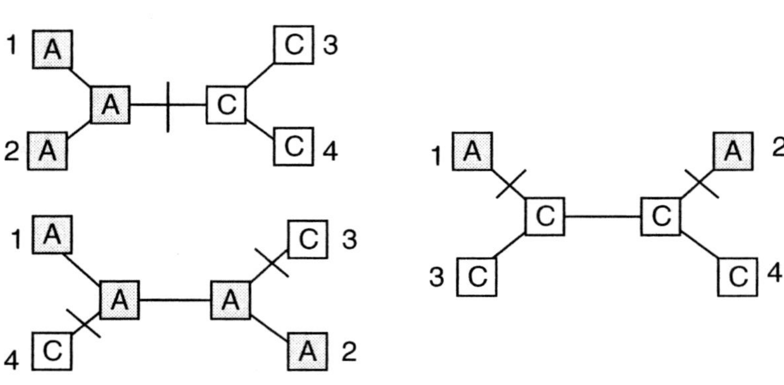

Fig. 4.15. Illustration of parsimony: tree selection. The figure shows the three unrooted tree topologies that can be obtained with four taxa (where the taxa are represented by numbers). For a given site in the DNA sequence alignment, and for each of the possible tree topologies in turn, nucleotides are assigned to the hidden nodes in the most parsimonious way; compare with Figure 4.14. The tree in the top left, which invokes only a single substitution, is preferred over the other, less parsimonious trees, which require at least two substitutions. The whole process is repeated for all sites in the alignment, and the total number of nucleotide substitutions is counted, for each tree in turn. Then, the tree that invokes the least total number of nucleotide substitutions is selected as the best candidate for the true evolutionary tree.

In fact, the whole process is repeated for all sites in the alignment. The total number of nucleotide substitutions is determined for each tree, and the tree that invokes the least total number of nucleotide substitutions is selected as the best candidate for the true evolutionary tree.

Parsimony is not limited in the number of taxa, and the restriction to four sequences in the previous example was chosen for illustration purposes only. Note, however, that the number of tree topologies grows super-exponentially with the number of taxa (see Table 4.2 on page 121), and that the optimization problem is NP–hard [36]. Consequently, iterative and approximate methods are needed for large sequence alignments of many taxa.

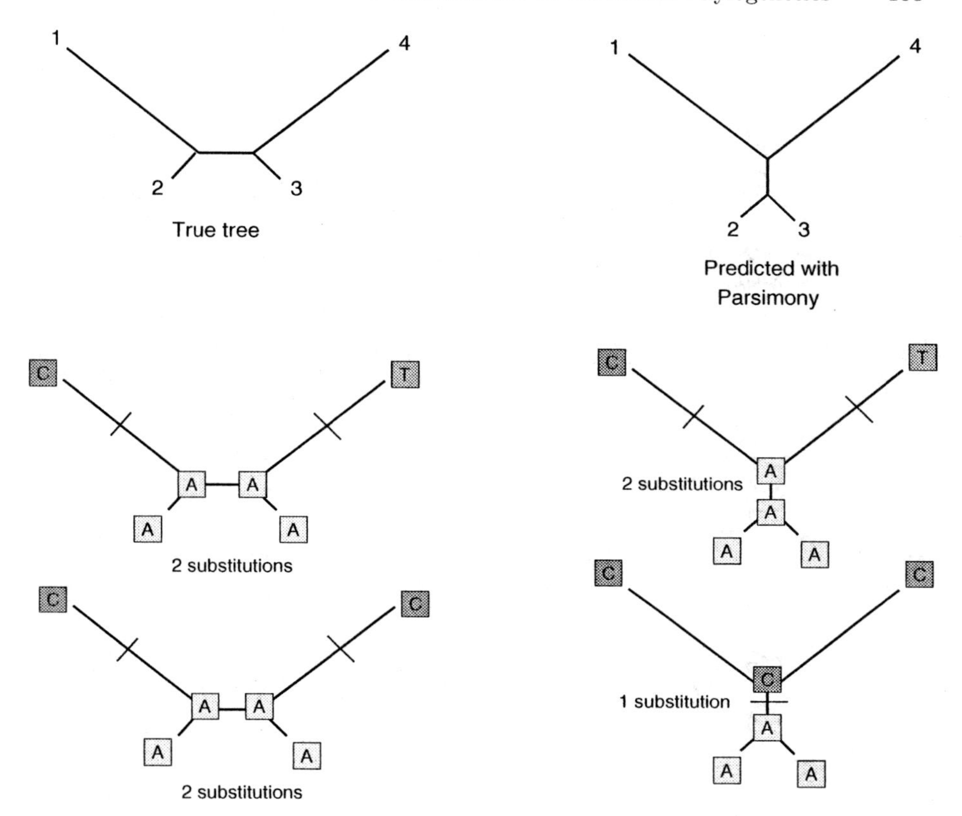

Fig. 4.16. Failure of parsimony. The plot in the *top left* shows the true tree, in which the branch lengths of related taxa differ significantly. When the ratio of the long and short branch lengths exceeds a certain threshold, parsimony systematically predicts the wrong tree, shown in the *top right*. For an explanation, consider the tree in the *middle left*, which shows two nucleotide substitutions, one on either long branch. When these nucleotide substitutions are different, both tree topologies give the same score of 2 substitutions. Such nucleotide configurations are uninformative in that they do not prefer one tree over the other. When the nucleotide substitutions are identical, which happens, on average, in 25% of the cases, the tree on the right has a parsimony score of 1. This score is lower than that of the true tree, which is 2. Hence, such so-called homoplasious substitutions support the wrong tree. When the ratio of the external branch lengths exceeds a critical threshold, these "bad" substitutions outweigh, on average, the "good" substitutions that support the true tree. Consequently, parsimony will obtain the wrong tree.

4.3.2 Objection to Parsimony

As opposed to the clustering methods discussed in the previous section, parsimony is an optimality method that minimizes a well-defined objective function: the total number of nucleotide substitutions along the tree branches. This approach shows a certain resemblance to minimum description length [31] in information theory and allows, unlike clustering methods, an evaluation of the quality of a reconstructed tree.

However, as opposed to the methods to be described in the next section, parsimony is not based on a probabilistic generative model. Proponents of parsimony used to consider this model-free inference an advantage [9], but it has now become clear that it is, in fact, the limiting case of a model-based approach – for the limit of a highly implausible evolutionary scenario. We will revisit this aspect later, in Section 4.4.4.

The fundamental objection to parsimony is that it is not *consistent*. *Consistency* is the desirable feature of a method to converge on the right answer given enough data. In certain evolutionary scenarios, however, parsimony gives the wrong tree even if we add more and more data [6], [8]. The classic scenario where this might happen has been termed *long branch attraction* and is illustrated in Figure 4.16.

4.4 Likelihood Methods

Likelihood methods are based on an explicit mathematical model of nucleotide substitution, which allows the formulation of the inference process in terms of a probabilistic generative model. This fact renders likelihood methods considerably more powerful than clustering and parsimony, discussed in Sections 4.2 and 4.3. As opposed to clustering, inference is based on an optimality function, which allows us to objectively compare different trees and to test hypotheses about evolutionary scenarios. Inference is based on the whole DNA sequence alignment, which avoids the information loss inherent in distance methods. By basing our inference on an explicit mathematical model of nucleotide substitution, the shortcomings of "model-free" inference are avoided. In particular, likelihood methods subsume parsimony as a limiting case for a rather unrealistic evolutionary scenario.

4.4.1 A Mathematical Model of Nucleotide Substitution

The driving forces for evolution are nucleotide substitutions, which can be modelled as transitions in a 4-element state space, shown in Figure 4.17. $P(y|x, w)$, where $x, y \in \{A, C, G, T\}$, denotes the probability of a transition from nucleotide x into nucleotide y, conditional on the elapsed phylogenetic time w. The latter is given by the product of an unknown mutation rate λ with physical time t: $w = \lambda t$. To rephrase this: $P(y|x, w)$ is the probability

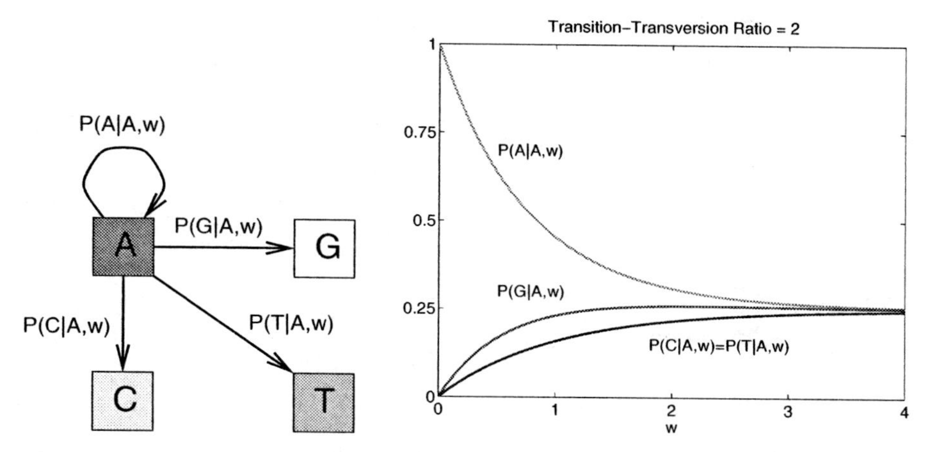

Fig. 4.17. Mathematical model of nucleotide substitution. *Left:* Nucleotide substitutions are modelled as transitions in a 4-element state space. The transition probabilities depend on the phylogenetic time $w = \lambda t$, where t is physical time, and λ is an unknown nucleotide substitution rate. *Right:* Dependence of the transition probabilities (vertical axis) on w (horizontal axis). The graphs were obtained from the Kimura model (4.16) with a transition–transversion ratio of 2.

that nucleotide y is found at a given site in the DNA sequence given that w phylogenetic time units before the same site was occupied by nucleotide x.

An intuitively plausible functional form for these probabilities is shown on the right of Figure 4.17. For $w = 0$, there is no time for nucleotide substitutions to occur. Consequently, $P(A|A, w = 0) = 1$, and $P(C|A, w = 0) = P(G|A, w = 0) = P(T|A, w = 0) = 0$. As w increases, nucleotide substitutions from A into the other states lead to an exponential decay of $P(A|A, w)$ and, concurrently, an increase of $P(C|A, w)$, $P(G|A, w)$, and $P(T|A, w)$. The rate of this decay or increase depends on the type of nucleotide substitution. Nucleotides are grouped into two families: purines (A and G), and pyrimidines (C and T). Nucleotide substitutions within a nucleotide class (purine $\rightarrow$ purine, pyrimidine $\rightarrow$ pyrimidine), so-called *transitions*,[6] are more likely than substitutions between nucleotide classes (purine $\leftrightarrow$ pyrimidine), so-called *transversions*. For $w \rightarrow \infty$, the system forgets its initial configuration as the result of the mixing caused by an increasing number of nucleotide substitutions (including backsubstitutions and multiple substitutions). Consequently,

[6] Unfortunately this terminology, which is used in molecular biology, leads to a certain ambiguity in the meaning of the word *transition*. When we talk about transitions between *states*, where the states are associated with nucleotides, as in Figure 4.17, a transition can be any nucleotide substitution event. When we talk about *transitions* as opposed to *transversions*, a transition refers to a certain type of nucleotide substitution.

$P(y|x,w) \rightarrow \Pi(y)$ for $w \rightarrow \infty$, where $x, y \in \{A, C, G, T\}$, and $\Pi(y)$ is the equilibrium distribution (here: $\Pi(y) = 1/4 \; \forall \; y$).

4.4.2 Details of the Mathematical Model of Nucleotide Substitution

This section provides the details of the mathematical model outlined in the preceding section and may be skipped at a first reading. Let $y_i(t) \in \{A, C, G, T\}$ denote the nucleotide at site i and time t, that is, the subscript refers to the position in the alignment, while the expression in brackets denotes physical or (later) phylogenetic time. (Note that this notation deviates from that of the other sections in this chapter; see Table 4.1.) The total length of the alignment is N, that is, $i \in \{1, \ldots, N\}$. The derivation of the aforementioned results is based on the theory of *homogeneous Markov chains* and the following assumptions:

1. The process is Markov:
   $P\Big(y_i(t + \Delta t)|y_i(t), y_i(t - \Delta t), \ldots\Big) = P\Big(y_i(t + \Delta t)|y_i(t)\Big)$
2. The Markov process is homogeneous in time:
   $P\Big(y_i(s + t)|y_i(s)\Big) = P\Big(y_i(t)|y_i(0)\Big)$
3. The Markov process is the same for all positions:
   $P\Big(y_i(t)|y_i(0)\Big) = P\Big(y_k(t)|y_k(0)\Big) \; \forall \; i, k \in \{1, \ldots, N\}$
4. Substitutions at different positions are independent of each other:
   $$P\Big(y_1(t), \ldots, y_N(t)|y_1(0), \ldots, y_N(0)\Big) = \prod_{i=1}^{N} P\Big(y_i(t)|y_i(0)\Big)$$

These assumptions imply that the probability of a nucleotide substitution does not depend on earlier substitutions (1), is site-independent (3), unaffected by substitutions at other sites (4), and does not change in the course of evolution (2). We will discuss later, in Sections 4.4.9–4.4.11, the implications of these approximations and how they can be relaxed. For now, note that as a consequence of approximations 1–4, the nucleotide substitution process at a given site is completely specified by the following 4-by-4 transition matrix:

$$\mathbf{P}(t) = \begin{pmatrix} P(y(t) = A|y(0) = A) & \ldots & P(y(t) = A|y(0) = T) \\ P(y(t) = G|y(0) = A) & \ldots & P(y(t) = G|y(0) = T) \\ P(y(t) = C|y(0) = A) & \ldots & P(y(t) = C|y(0) = T) \\ P(y(t) = T|y(0) = A) & \ldots & P(y(t) = T|y(0) = T) \end{pmatrix} \tag{4.7}$$

Because of the site independence, the site label has been dropped to simplify the notation. Equation (4.7) obviously implies that

$$\mathbf{P}(0) = \mathbf{I} \tag{4.8}$$

where $\mathbf{I}$ is the unit matrix. For an infinitesimally small time interval dt we make the ansatz

$$\mathbf{P}(dt) = \mathbf{P}(0) + \mathbf{R}dt \tag{4.9}$$

where $\mathbf{R}$ is a constant matrix, the so-called *rate matrix*. Now, a homogeneous Markov chain satisfies the Chapman–Kolmogorov equation:

$$\mathbf{P}(t_1 + t_2) = \mathbf{P}(t_1)\mathbf{P}(t_2) = \mathbf{P}(t_2)\mathbf{P}(t_1) \tag{4.10}$$

for arbitrary $t_1, t_2 \geq 0$; see, for instance, [19] or [28]. Setting $t_1 = t$ and $t_2 = dt$, we get:

$$\mathbf{P}(t + dt) = \mathbf{P}(dt)\mathbf{P}(t) \tag{4.11}$$

Inserting equations (4.8) and (4.9) into (4.11) gives

$$\mathbf{P}(t + dt) = (\mathbf{I} + \mathbf{R}dt)\mathbf{P}(t) \tag{4.12}$$

and, by a simple transformation,

$$\frac{d\mathbf{P}(t)}{dt} = \mathbf{R}\mathbf{P}(t) \tag{4.13}$$

Equation (4.13) describes a system of linear differential equations with initial condition (4.8). The solution is:

$$\mathbf{P}(t) = e^{\mathbf{R}t} \tag{4.14}$$

To ensure that $\mathbf{P}$(t) is a proper transition matrix, that is, has columns that sum to 1, the columns of the rate matrix $\mathbf{R}$ have to sum to 0. The proof follows from (4.9):

$$1 = \sum_i P_{ik}(dt) = 1 + dt \sum_i R_{ik} \iff \sum_i R_{ik} = 0 \tag{4.15}$$

A possible design for $\mathbf{R}$, the so-called Kimura model [21], is of the form

$$\mathbf{R} = \begin{pmatrix} -2\beta - \alpha & \beta & \alpha & \beta \\ \beta & -2\beta - \alpha & \beta & \alpha \\ \alpha & \beta & -2\beta - \alpha & \beta \\ \beta & \alpha & \beta & -2\beta - \alpha \end{pmatrix} \tag{4.16}$$

Here, the rows (from top to bottom) and columns (from left to right) correspond to the nucleotides A, C, G, T (in the indicated order). The positive parameters α and β denote the rates of transitions and transversions, respectively. An illustration is given in Figure 4.18. Inserting (4.16) into (4.14) leads to [21]:

$$\mathbf{P}(t) = e^{\mathbf{R}t} = \begin{pmatrix} \tilde{d}(t) & \tilde{f}(t) & \tilde{g}(t) & \tilde{f}(t) \\ \tilde{f}(t) & \tilde{d}(t) & \tilde{f}(t) & \tilde{g}(t) \\ \tilde{g}(t) & \tilde{f}(t) & \tilde{d}(t) & \tilde{f}(t) \\ \tilde{f}(t) & \tilde{g}(t) & \tilde{f}(t) & \tilde{d}(t) \end{pmatrix} \tag{4.17}$$

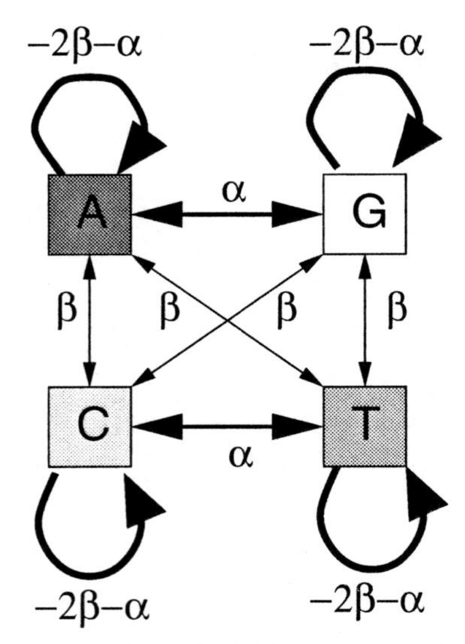

Fig. 4.18. Kimura model of nucleotide substitution. The figure presents a graphical display of the Kimura rate matrix (4.16). The positive parameter α denotes the transition rate, while the positive parameter β denotes the transversion rate. The thickness of a line is related to the size of the respective rate parameter, indicating that transitions are more likely than transversions: $\alpha > \beta$.

where

$$\tilde{f}(t) = \frac{1}{4}(1 - e^{-4\beta t}) \tag{4.18}$$

$$\tilde{g}(t) = \frac{1}{4}(1 + e^{-4\beta t} - 2e^{-2(\alpha+\beta)t}) \tag{4.19}$$

$$\tilde{d}(t) = 1 - 2\tilde{f}(t) - \tilde{g}(t) \tag{4.20}$$

Define

$$\tau = \frac{\alpha}{\beta}, \qquad \lambda = 4\beta, \qquad w = \lambda t \tag{4.21}$$

where w represents *phylogenetic time* – as opposed to *physical time* t – and τ is called the *transition–transversion ratio.* With these definitions, equations (4.18)–(4.20) simplify:

$$f(w) = \frac{1}{4}(1 - e^{-w}) \tag{4.22}$$

$$g(w) = \frac{1}{4}(1 + e^{-w} - 2e^{-\frac{\tau+1}{2}w}) \tag{4.23}$$

$$d(w) = 1 - 2f(w) - g(w) \tag{4.24}$$

Denote by $P(y|x, w)$ the probability that a given site in the DNA sequence is occupied by nucleotide y conditional on the fact that w phylogenetic time units before, this site was occupied by nucleotide x. We can then rewrite $\mathbf{P}$, the transition matrix of (4.7), as follows:

$$\mathbf{P}(w) = \begin{pmatrix} P(A|A,w) & P(A|C,w) & P(A|G,w) & P(A|T,w) \\ P(G|A,w) & P(G|C,w) & P(G|G,w) & P(G|T,w) \\ P(C|A,w) & P(C|C,w) & P(C|G,w) & P(C|T,w) \\ P(T|A,w) & P(T|C,w) & P(T|G,w) & P(T|T,w) \end{pmatrix}$$

$$= \begin{pmatrix} d(w) & f(w) & g(w) & f(w) \\ f(w) & d(w) & f(w) & g(w) \\ g(w) & f(w) & d(w) & f(w) \\ f(w) & g(w) & f(w) & d(w) \end{pmatrix} \quad (4.25)$$

where $d(w)$, $f(w)$, and $g(w)$ are given by (4.22)–(4.24). Setting $\tau = 2$ leads to the graphs shown in Figure 4.17. Note that all these graphs converge to the same value of 1/4. Hence in equilibrium, for $w \to \infty$, all nucleotides occur with equal probability $P(A) = P(C) = P(G) = P(T) = 1/4$. We can prove that this uniform distribution is an immediate consequence of the Kimura model (4.16). Define the column vector $\mathbf{u}$ to represent the time-dependent marginal distribution over the nucleotides,

$$\mathbf{u}(w) = \Big(P(y[w] = A), P(y[w] = C), P(y[w] = G), P(y[w] = T)\Big)^{\dagger} \quad (4.26)$$

which evolves in a homogeneous Markov chain determined by the transition matrix $\mathbf{P}$ of (4.25):

$$\mathbf{u}(w_0 + w) = \mathbf{P}(w)\mathbf{u}(w_0) \quad (4.27)$$

Now, an ergodic Markov chain is known to converge to its stationary distribution irrespective of its initial condition[7] (see, for instance, [19], Chapter 6):

$$\lim_{w \to \infty} \mathbf{u}(w) = \boldsymbol{\pi} \quad (4.28)$$

where the stationary distribution

$$\boldsymbol{\pi} = (\Pi_A, \Pi_C, \Pi_G, \Pi_T)^{\dagger} \quad (4.29)$$

is characterized by its invariance with respect to the Markov operator $\mathbf{P}$:

$$\mathbf{P}(w)\boldsymbol{\pi} = \boldsymbol{\pi} \quad (4.30)$$

Recall that $w = \lambda t$ represents phylogenetic time. Equation (4.30) holds true for all $t > 0$, which includes the limiting case $t \to 0$. Replacing w by dt in (4.30) and making use of (4.8) and (4.9) gives:

$$\mathbf{R}\boldsymbol{\pi} = 0 \quad (4.31)$$

[7] Compare with Section 2.2.2. The only difference is that the Markov process discussed in Section 2.2.2 was discrete in time, whereas the Markov chain we are dealing with in the present chapter is continuous in time.

For the Kimura model (4.16), the distribution $\boldsymbol{\pi}$ satisfying (4.31) can easily be shown to be the uniform distribution, $\boldsymbol{\pi} = (\frac{1}{4}, \frac{1}{4}, \frac{1}{4}, \frac{1}{4})^\dagger$, which completes the proof. To model a non-uniform stationary distribution over the nucleotides, the rate matrix of (4.16) has to be extended:

$$\mathbf{R} = \begin{pmatrix} . & \Pi_A\beta & \Pi_A\alpha & \Pi_A\beta \\ \Pi_C\beta & . & \Pi_C\beta & \Pi_C\alpha \\ \Pi_G\alpha & \Pi_G\beta & . & \Pi_G\beta \\ \Pi_T\beta & \Pi_T\alpha & \Pi_T\beta & . \end{pmatrix} \tag{4.32}$$

where the diagonal elements are given by the constraint that columns have to sum to zero. It can easily be shown that this rate matrix satisfies (4.31) for arbitrary distributions $\boldsymbol{\pi} = (\Pi_A, \Pi_C, \Pi_G, \Pi_T)^\dagger$. The rate matrix of (4.32) was proposed by Hasegawa, Kishino and Yano [20] and is called the HKY85 model of nucleotide substitution. Obviously, it subsumes the Kimura model (4.16) as a limiting case for $\Pi_A = \Pi_C = \Pi_G = \Pi_T = \frac{1}{4}$. A different parameterization was proposed by Felsenstein and Churchill [10]. More general models have been studied, as discussed in Section 6.3. Posada and Crandall [30] compared different rate matrices and applied statistical hypothesis tests to decide which model is most appropriate in a given evolutionary context. A similar comparison, following a Bayesian approach, was carried out by Suchard et al. [40]. Given a nucleotide substitution model, its parameters can be inferred from the sequence alignment by applying the methods to be discussed in the remainder of this chapter. However, to keep both the notation and the exposition of the methodology sufficiently simple, as appropriate for an introductory tutorial, this inference will not be covered in the present chapter. For the remainder of this chapter we will therefore assume that the rate matrix $\mathbf{R}$ and its parameters are fixed and known. This assumption will be relaxed later, in Chapters 5 and 6.

Note that by the *homogeneity* hypothesis, the rate matrix $\mathbf{R}$ is assumed to be constant over the whole phylogenetic tree. Consequently, DNA sequences converge towards the same equilibrium distribution $\boldsymbol{\pi}$ in all lineages, where $\boldsymbol{\pi}$ is given by (4.31). Furthermore, if the assumed distribution of nucleotides is equal to the equilibrium distribution $\boldsymbol{\pi}$ over the whole tree, the Markov model is called *stationary*. In what follows, we will assume that both the *homogeneity* and *stationarity* assumptions are satisfied. A relaxation of these restrictions will be discussed in Section 4.4.11.

Finally, note that Π_x, $x \in \{A, C, G, T\}$, constitutes both a parameter of the nucleotide substitution model, by (4.32), and a component of the stationary distribution over the nucleotides, by (4.29). In what follows, the notations Π_x and $\Pi(x)$ will be used synonymously, with the former alternative emphasizing more the parameter aspect, and, conversely, the latter alternative stressing more the distribution aspect.

Section 4.4.2	$x_i(t)$: Nucleotide at site i and time t.
Other sections	$x_i(t)$: Nucleotide associated with node i at site t.

Table 4.1. Conflicting notation. The table shows two different ways the symbols $x_i(t)$, $y_i(t)$, and $z_i(t)$ are used in this chapter.

4.4.3 Likelihood of a Phylogenetic Tree

A phylogenetic tree is a particular example of a Bayesian network, and we can therefore draw on the inference methods introduced in Chapters 1 and 2. In particular, we can expand the joint probability of the random variables associated with the tree nodes in terms of a product of transition probabilities (4.25) by applying the factorization rule (2.1). Denote by pa[i] the parent of node i, which is the node with an arrow feeding into node i. Note that for a tree there is only one such node, as opposed to the more general scenario discussed in Section 2.1. Let x_i denote the random variable or value[8] associated with node i, with $x_i \in \{A, C, G, T\}$; see Table 4.1. Then

$$P(x_1, \ldots, x_M) = \Pi(x_r) \prod_{i \in \mathcal{N}/\{r\}} P(x_i | x_{\mathrm{pa}[i]}, w_i) \tag{4.33}$$

by equation (2.1), where w_i is the length of the branch or edge feeding into node i, $\mathcal{N}$ is the set of all nodes, and r is the root node. Note that the marginal distribution over nucleotides at the root node has been set to the equilibrium distribution, $\Pi(x_r)$. This follows from the *stationarity* hypothesis, which assumes that the base composition in the ancestral sequence is equal to the equilibrium base composition and remains unchanged. Consider Figure 4.19, left. Observed nodes, drawn as filled circles and labelled by y_1, y_2, y_3, and y_4, represent contemporary species. Hidden nodes, drawn as empty circles and labelled by z_1 and z_2, represent hypothetical ancestors. We are interested in the joint probability $P(y_1, y_2, y_3, y_4, z_1, z_2 | \mathbf{w}, S)$, where $y_1, y_2, \ldots, z_2 \in \{A, C, G, T\}$ represent nucleotides at the nodes, $\mathbf{w}$ is the vector of all branch lengths, and S is a label defining the tree topology. To proceed, we first transform the undirected graph of Figure 4.19, left, into the directed graph of Figure 4.19, right, by setting, arbitrarily, the root of the tree to z_1. Then, application of (4.33) gives:

$$\begin{aligned} &P(y_1, y_2, y_3, y_4, z_1, z_2 | \mathbf{w}, S) = \\ &P(y_1|z_1, w_1) P(y_2|z_1, w_2) P(z_2|z_1, w_5) P(y_3|z_2, w_3) P(y_4|z_2, w_4) \Pi(z_1) \end{aligned} \tag{4.34}$$

The equilibrium distribution over the four nucleotides, $\Pi(z_1)$, $z_1 \in \{A, C, G, T\}$, is defined by (4.29) and (4.31) and is a parameter vector of the nucleotide substitution model, as discussed in Section 4.4.2. For the Kimura

[8] Recall that the notation does not distinguish between random variables and their values.

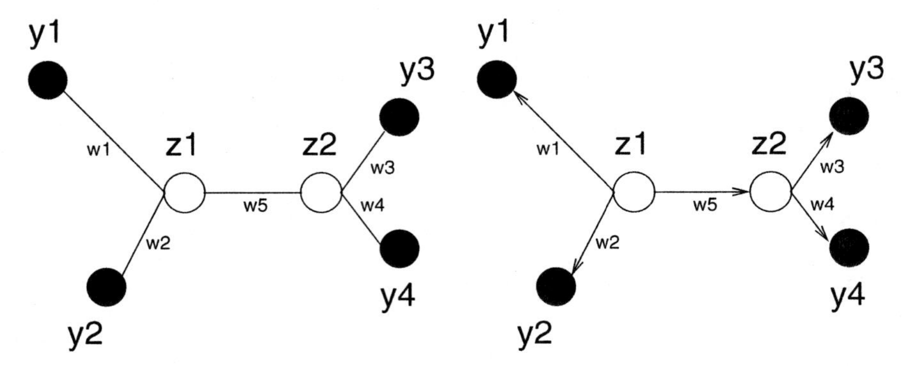

Fig. 4.19. Phylogenetic trees. Black nodes represent contemporary or extant species. White nodes represent hypothetical ancestors, where lineages bifurcate (speciation). *Left:* Undirected graph. *Right:* Directed graph. Node z_1 is the root of the tree, and arrows are directed.

model, for instance, we have $\Pi(A) = \Pi(C) = \Pi(G) = \Pi(T) = \frac{1}{4}$. The other factors represent transition probabilities, which are given by (4.25). Note that these transition probabilities depend on the branch lengths, w_i, which are defined in (4.21) and thus have an obvious and intuitively plausible interpretation: they represent phylogenetic time.

In transforming the undirected graph into a DAG,[9] we have arbitrarily rooted the tree. This is possible for a reversible nucleotide substitution model. Recall from Section 4.1 that we do not infer the direction of evolutionary change from a DNA sequence alignment. Mathematically this fact is expressed by the following *reversibility* condition:

$$P(y|x, w)\Pi(x) = P(x|y, w)\Pi(y) \tag{4.35}$$

where $x, y \in \{A, C, G, T\}$. Obviously, (4.35) is satisfied for the Kimura model, where $\Pi(x) = \Pi(y) = \frac{1}{4}$, and the symmetry of $\mathbf{R}$, expressed in (4.16), implies that $\mathbf{P}$ is also symmetric, by (4.14). For the HKY85 rate matrix, we see from (4.32) that

$$R_{yx}\Pi(x) = R_{xy}\Pi(y) \tag{4.36}$$

where R_{yx} is the element in the yth row and xth column[10] of the rate matrix $\mathbf{R}$. This identity implies that[11]

$$[R^n]_{yx}\Pi_x = [R^n]_{xy}\Pi_y \tag{4.37}$$

[9] DAG stands for *directed acyclic graph*; see Section 2.1.1.

[10] Recall that the rows and columns of the rate matrix $\mathbf{R}$ are associated with nucleotides, that is, the first row corresponds to A, the second to C, the third to G, and the fourth to T. The same applies to the columns. For example, for $x = A$ and $y = C$, R_{xy} represents the element in the first row and second column of $\mathbf{R}$.

[11] Recall that the notations Π_x and $\Pi(x)$ are used interchangeably.

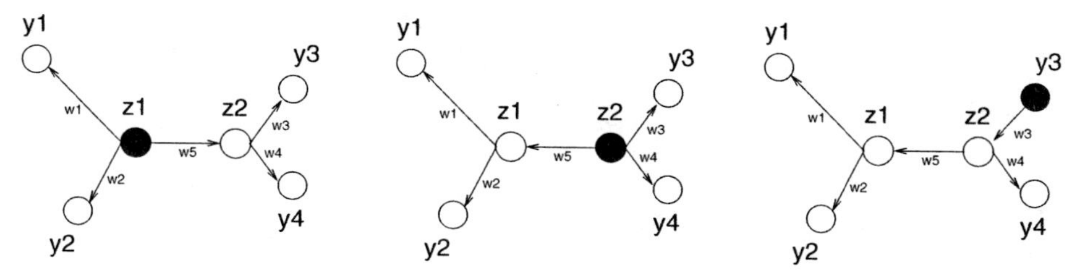

Fig. 4.20. Different root positions. The figure shows three directed graphs with different root positions (shown in black).

where $[R^n]_{yx}$ is the element in the yth row and xth column of matrix $\mathbf{R}^n$. The proof is given by induction. Assume that (4.36) and (4.37) for fixed n are true. Then

$$\begin{aligned}[R^{n+1}]_{yx}\Pi_x &= \sum_z R_{yz}[R^n]_{zx}\Pi_x = \sum_z R_{yz}[R^n]_{xz}\Pi_z \\ &= \sum_z [R^n]_{xz}R_{yz}\Pi_z = \sum_z [R^n]_{xz}R_{zy}\Pi_y = [R^{n+1}]_{xy}\Pi_y\end{aligned}$$

where the second equation follows from (4.37), and the fourth equation has applied (4.36). Consequently, starting from (4.36), (4.37) holds true for all n, and (4.35) is proved true by Taylor series expansion of (4.14). From (4.35), it can then be shown that the expansion of the joint probability $P(y_1, y_2, y_3, y_4, z_1, z_2|\mathbf{w}, S)$ is independent of the root position. Compare, for instance, the three directed graphs in Figure 4.20. We have already derived the expansion for the tree on the left; see (4.34). Applying the expansion rule (4.33) to the tree in the middle, we obtain:

$$\begin{aligned}&P(y_1, y_2, y_3, y_4, z_1, z_2|\mathbf{w}, S) = \\ &P(y_1|z_1, w_1)P(y_2|z_1, w_2)P(z_1|z_2, w_5)P(y_3|z_2, w_3)P(y_4|z_2, w_4)\Pi(z_2)\end{aligned} \quad (4.38)$$

Now, reversibility (4.35) implies that $P(z_1|z_2, w_5)\Pi(z_2) = P(z_2|z_1, w_5)\Pi(z_1)$, hence the expansions in (4.34) and (4.38) are equivalent. By the same token, expanding the joint probability $P(y_1, y_2, y_3, y_4, z_1, z_2|\mathbf{w}, S)$ according to the tree on the right of Figure 4.20 gives

$$\begin{aligned}&P(y_1, y_2, y_3, y_4, z_1, z_2|\mathbf{w}, S) = \\ &P(y_1|z_1, w_1)P(y_2|z_1, w_2)P(z_1|z_2, w_5)P(y_4|z_2, w_4)P(z_2|y_3, w_3)\Pi(y_3)\end{aligned} \quad (4.39)$$

By the reversibility condition (4.35), we have $P(z_2|y_3, w_3)\Pi(y_3) = P(y_3|z_2, w_3)\Pi(z_2)$. Consequently, the expansion in (4.39) is equivalent to (4.38), and hence to (4.34). In the terminology of Bayesian networks, discussed in Section 2.1, the three structures in Figure 4.20 are *equivalent*, that is, they represent the same joint probability distribution. In fact, we can even add a root node anywhere on the edge connecting two nodes and thereby transform

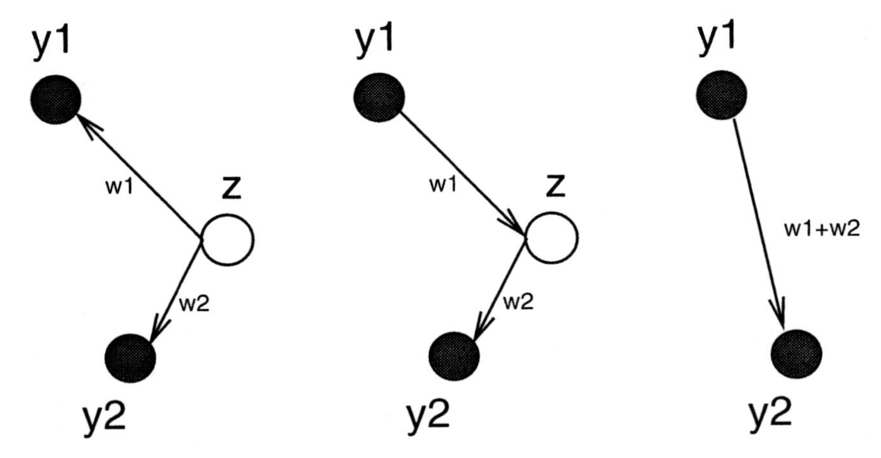

Fig. 4.21. Equivalent tree structures. Filled circles represent observed nodes. They correspond to extant species, for which DNA sequence data are available. The empty circle represents an ancestral species, for which we do not have any data. In the terminology of Bayesian networks, this node is hidden. The three Bayesian network structures shown in the figure are equivalent, as proved in the text. Note that the Bayesian network on the left is a rooted tree, with the ancestral node acting as a root.

an unrooted tree with $(n-1)$ nodes into a rooted tree with n nodes. This equivalence is illustrated in Figure 4.21. Recall that

$$\mathbf{P}(w_1 + w_2) = \mathbf{P}(w_1)\mathbf{P}(w_2) \tag{4.40}$$

by the Chapman–Kolmogorov equation (4.10). Rewriting this matrix equation in scalar form for the matrix *components* gives:

$$P(y|x, w_1 + w_2) = \sum_z P(y|z, w_2)P(z|x, w_1) \tag{4.41}$$

where $x, y, z \in \{A, C, G, T\}$. Now, the three Bayesian networks of Figure 4.21 lead to the following factorizations, by (4.33):

$$\text{Left}: \; P(y_1, y_2, z) = P(y_2|z, w_2)P(y_1|z, w_1)\Pi(z) \tag{4.42}$$

$$\text{Middle}: \; P(y_1, y_2, z) = P(y_2|z, w_2)P(z|y_1, w_1)\Pi(y_1) \tag{4.43}$$

$$\text{Right}: \; P(y_1, y_2) = P(y_2|y_1, w_1 + w_2)\Pi(y_1) \tag{4.44}$$

For the ancestral node, z, we do not have any DNA sequence data. Consequently, this node is hidden and has to be marginalized over:

$$\text{Left}: \; P(y_1, y_2) = \sum_z P(y_2|z, w_2)P(y_1|z, w_1)\Pi(z) \tag{4.45}$$

$$\text{Middle}: \; P(y_1, y_2) = \sum_z P(y_2|z, w_2)P(z|y_1, w_1)\Pi(y_1) \tag{4.46}$$

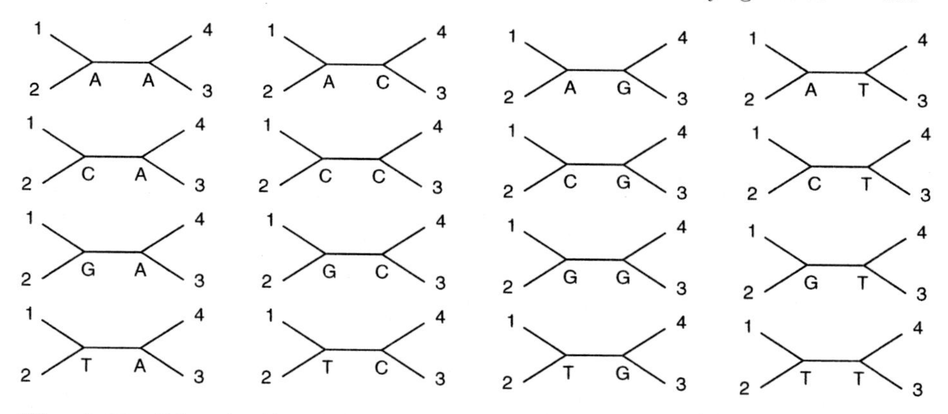

Fig. 4.22. Marginalization over hidden nodes. Leaf nodes represent extant taxa, which are observed, that is, for which DNA sequence data are available. Inner nodes represent hypothetical ancestors, which are *hidden*, that is, for which no observations exist. To obtain the probability of an observation, that is, the probability of observing a given column of nucleotides at a given position in the DNA sequence alignment, we have to sum over all possible configurations of hidden nodes. Reprinted from [27], by permission of Blackwell Science.

By the reversibility condition (4.35), the expressions on the right of (4.45) and (4.46) are equal. By the Chapman–Kolmogorov equation (4.41), the expressions on the right of (4.44) and (4.46) are also equal. Consequently, all three expressions are equal, and the three structures of Figure 4.21 are equivalent. This equivalence proves the conjecture true that we may transform an unrooted tree into a rooted tree by adding an extra root node anywhere on any arbitrary edge connecting two nodes. A more rigorous proof [7] generalizes this to any phylogenetic tree: if the transition matrix is reversible, trees that only differ with respect to the position of the root and the directions of the edges are equivalent. Consequently, we can choose the position of the root arbitrarily.

The factorization (4.34) allows us to compute the probability of a complete configuration of nucleotides. However, while we obtain the nucleotides of the extant species, y_i, from the DNA sequence alignment, the nucleotides at the inner nodes, z_i, are never observed. This requires us to marginalize over them, as illustrated in Figure 4.22:

$$P(\mathbf{y}|\mathbf{w}, S) = P(y_1, y_2, y_3, y_4|\mathbf{w}, S) = \sum_{z_1} \sum_{z_2} P(y_1, y_2, y_3, y_4, z_1, z_2|\mathbf{w}, S) \tag{4.47}$$

This marginalization seems to be hampered by excessive computational complexity. An unrooted tree with n leaves contains $n-2$ hidden nodes, and each hidden node can be in four different states, corresponding to the nucleotides A, C, G, T. Consequently, it seems that, for an alignment of n sequences, we have to sum over $4^{(n-2)}$ terms, which is obviously computationally intractable

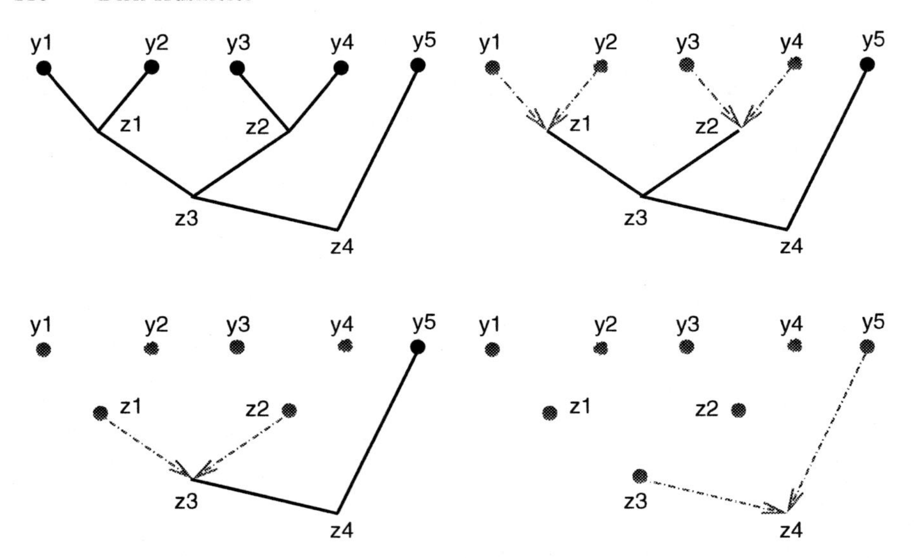

Fig. 4.23. Illustration of the peeling algorithm. The various peeling steps correspond to the rearrangement of the sums in (4.49) so as to obtain the following iterative steps. Top right: computing the evidence for z_1 and z_2, (4.50) and (4.51). Bottom left: computing the evidence for z_3, (4.52). Bottom right: computing the evidence for z_4, (4.53). In general, this procedure reduces the computational complexity of the marginalization from 4^H terms down to at most $4^3H + 4$ terms, where H is the number of hidden nodes.

for large alignments. Fortunately, we can exploit the sparseness of the connectivity of the tree-structured Bayesian network to reduce the computational complexity from exponential to polynomial time. The underlying idea is similar to the dynamic programming procedure known from hidden Markov models, discussed in Section 2.3.4, and applies Pearl's *message passing algorithm* [29], which in the context of phylogenetics is referred to as the *peeling algorithm* [7]. An illustration is given in Figure 4.23, which shows a rooted tree with 5 leaves and 4 hidden nodes. By the factorization rule (4.33) we can expand the joint probability as follows:

$$
\begin{aligned}
&P(y_1, y_2, y_3, y_4, y_5, z_1, z_2, z_3, z_4) = \qquad (4.48)\\
&\quad P(y_1|z_1)P(y_2|z_1)P(z_1|z_3)P(y_3|z_2)P(y_4|z_2)P(z_2|z_3)P(z_3|z_4)P(y_5|z_4)\Pi(z_4)
\end{aligned}
$$

where the dependence on the branch lengths has been dropped to simplify the notation. When marginalizing over the hidden nodes, the sums can be rearranged:

$$\sum_{z_1}\sum_{z_2}\sum_{z_3}\sum_{z_4} P(y_1, y_2, y_3, y_4, y_5, z_1, z_2, z_3, z_4) =$$
$$\sum_{z_4} \Pi(z_4)P(y_5|z_4)\sum_{z_3} P(z_3|z_4)\sum_{z_1} P(y_1|z_1)P(y_2|z_1)P(z_1|z_3)$$
$$\sum_{z_2} P(y_3|z_2)P(y_4|z_2)P(z_2|z_3) \quad (4.49)$$

This rearrangement can be rewritten in the following recursive manner:

$$e(z_1) = P(y_1|z_1)P(y_2|z_1) \quad (4.50)$$
$$e(z_2) = P(y_3|z_2)P(y_4|z_2) \quad (4.51)$$
$$e(z_3) = \sum_{z_1}\sum_{z_2} e(z_1)e(z_2)P(z_1|z_3)P(z_2|z_3) \quad (4.52)$$
$$e(z_4) = \sum_{z_3} e(z_3)P(z_3|z_4)P(y_5|z_4) \quad (4.53)$$
$$P(\mathbf{y}) = \sum_{z_4} e(z_4)\Pi(z_4) \quad (4.54)$$

where $\mathbf{y} = (y_1, y_2, \ldots, y_5)^\dagger$. In (4.50) and (4.51), we compute the "evidence" for nodes z_1 and z_2, respectively, which corresponds to the first peeling step in the top right of Figure 4.23. Since both z_1 and z_2 can take on four values, $z_1, z_2 \in \{A, C, G, T\}$, we have to compute 2×4 terms. Next, in (4.52), we compute the evidence for node z_3, which corresponds to the bottom left of Figure 4.23. For a fixed value of z_3, this computation requires a summation over $4^2 = 16$ terms, which has to be repeated for each possible value of $z_3 \in \{A, C, G, T\}$. Hence overall, we have to compute $4^3 = 64$ terms. We continue with the evidence for node z_4, (4.53) and Figure 4.23, bottom right, which invokes 4 further sums over 4 terms each. Finally, in (4.54), we finish off by summing over all four possible terms of $e(z_4)$, $z_4 \in \{A, C, G, T\}$. In total, this computation involves a summation over 4 terms from (4.50), 4 terms from (4.51), 64 terms from (4.52), 16 terms from (4.53), and 4 terms from (4.54), that is $4 + 4 + 64 + 16 + 4 = 92$ terms altogether, which is considerably cheaper than the brute force summation over $4^4 = 256$ terms. To generalize this procedure to arbitrary trees, introduce a hidden random variable $z_l \in \{A, C, G, T\}$ associated with leaf node l and define its evidence as

$$e(z_l) = \delta_{z_l, y_l} = \begin{bmatrix} 1 \text{ if } z_l = y_l \\ 0 \text{ if } z_l \neq y_l \end{bmatrix} \quad (4.55)$$

where $y_l \in \{A, C, G, T\}$ is the nucleotide observed for leaf node l at the corresponding position in the DNA sequence alignment. In generalization of (4.50)–(4.53), the evidence for any hidden node i with associated random variable $z_i \in \{A, C, G, T\}$ is

$$e(z_i) = \sum_{z_{c1}}\sum_{z_{c2}} e(z_{c1})e(z_{c2})P(z_{c1}|z_i)P(z_{c2}|z_i) \quad (4.56)$$

where $c1$ and $c2$ are the two children of node i, and their associated random variables are $z_{c1}, z_{c2} \in \{A, C, G, T\}$. Finally, in generalization of (4.54), we have

$$P(\mathbf{y}) = \sum_{z_r} e(z_r)\Pi(z_r) \tag{4.57}$$

where r is the root node with associated random variable $z_r \in \{A, C, G, T\}$. Equation (4.56) shows that for each hidden node, we have to compute 4 sums over at most 4^2 terms each, which is followed by another sum over 4 terms in (4.57). The peeling algorithm thus reduces the computational complexity from a summation over 4^H terms by the brute-force method to at most $4^3 H + 4$ terms, where $H = n - 1$ is the number of hidden nodes in the corresponding rooted tree, and n is the number of leaf nodes. Consequently, the computational complexity is reduced from an exponential to a linear dependence on H. For further details, see [7] and [29].

The upshot of this procedure is that we can compute, for the tth column $\mathbf{y}_t$ in the sequence alignment (meaning a vector with the nucleotides in the tth column), the probability $P(\mathbf{y}_t|\mathbf{w}, S)$. Note that this probability depends on the tree topology, S, and the vector of branch lengths, $\mathbf{w}$, as illustrated in Figure 4.24. The respective computation can be repeated for every site, $1 \leq t \leq N$. Under the assumption that mutations at different sites t are independent of each other – see page 106 – the likelihood $P(\mathcal{D}|\mathbf{w}, S)$ of the whole DNA sequence alignment $\mathcal{D} = \{\mathbf{y}_1, \dots, \mathbf{y}_N\}$ factorizes:

$$P(\mathcal{D}|\mathbf{w}, S) = \prod_{t=1}^{N} P(\mathbf{y}_t|\mathbf{w}, S) \tag{4.58}$$

Equation (4.58) gives us an objective score or optimality function that opens the way to standard statistical inference and hypothesis tests. In what follows, we will apply the two alternative statistical inference methods outlined in Chapter 1: (1) the frequentist approach of maximum likelihood (Section 4.4.5) and bootstrapping (Section 4.4.6), and (2) the Bayesian approach (Section 4.4.7). First, however, let us make a brief comparison with the parsimony method of Section 4.3.

4.4.4 A Comparison with Parsimony

Maximum parsimony, summarized in Section 4.3, aims to minimize the total number of nucleotide substitutions, which is equivalent to minimizing the cost function

$$C = \sum_{t=1}^{N} \sum_{i \in \mathcal{N}/\{r\}} \delta\Big(x_i(t), x_{\mathrm{pa}[i]}(t)\Big) \tag{4.59}$$

where N is the length of the alignment, $\mathcal{N}$ is the set of all nodes in the tree, including both extant species and their extinct ancestors, r is the root

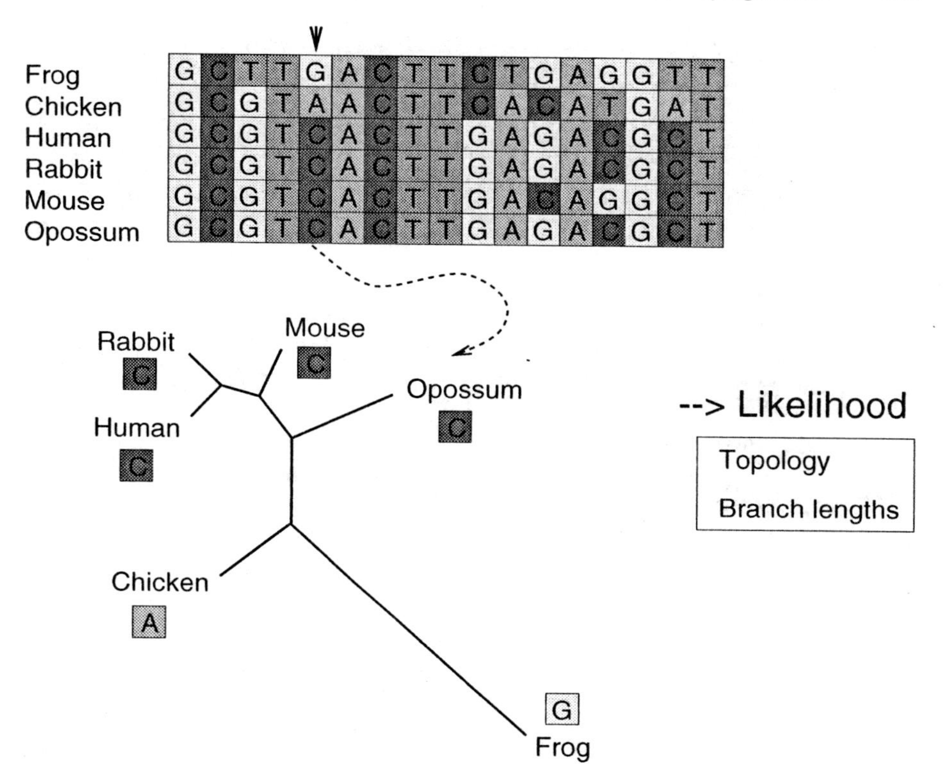

Fig. 4.24. Probabilistic approach to phylogenetics. For a given column $\mathbf{y}_t$ in the DNA sequence alignment, a probability $P(\mathbf{y}_t|\mathbf{w}, S)$ can be computed, which depends on the tree topology, S, and the vector of branch lengths, $\mathbf{w}$. This can be done for every site, $1 \leq t \leq N$, which allows the computation of the likelihood $P(\mathcal{D}|\mathbf{w}, S)$ of the whole DNA sequence alignment $\mathcal{D} = \{\mathbf{y}_1, \ldots, \mathbf{y}_N\}$.

node, $x_i(t) \in \{A, C, G, T\}$ represents the nucleotide at node i in position t of the alignment (see Table 4.1 on page 111), $\text{pa}[i]$ is the parent of node i, and δ denotes the Kronecker delta, which is 1 if the two arguments are identical, and 0 if they are different. Consider a hypothetical alignment of both the extant species, $\mathcal{D}$, and their ancestors, $\mathcal{H}$. From (4.33), and under the assumption of independent nucleotide substitution (see page 106), we have

$$\log P(\mathcal{D}, \mathcal{H}) = \sum_{t=1}^{N} \sum_{i \in \mathcal{N}/\{r\}} \log P\Big(x_i(t)|x_{\text{pa}[i]}(t)\Big) + \sum_{t=1}^{N} \log \Pi\Big(x_r(t)\Big) \quad (4.60)$$

A maximization of the log likelihood (4.60) with respect to the tree topology is equivalent to a minimization of the parsimony cost function (4.59) if we define

$$P\Big(x_i(t)|x_{\text{pa}[i]}(t)\Big) = a\delta\Big(x_i(t), x_{\text{pa}[i]}(t)\Big) + b\Big[1 - \delta\Big(x_i(t), x_{\text{pa}[i]}(t)\Big)\Big] \quad (4.61)$$

where a and b are two constants chosen such that $P(\mathcal{D}, \mathcal{H})$ is a proper probability ([1], Chapter 10). Equations (4.59)–(4.61) imply that parsimony can be viewed as a special case of the likelihood method, where two approximations have been made. First, a proper maximum likelihood approach, to be discussed in the next section, is based on the likelihood $P(\mathcal{D}) = \sum_{\mathcal{H}} P(\mathcal{D}, \mathcal{H})$, which implies a marginalization over the hidden variables $\mathcal{H}$, as demonstrated in the previous section. Parsimony replaces this marginalization, $\sum_{\mathcal{H}} P(\mathcal{D}, \mathcal{H})$, by an optimization, $\max_{\mathcal{H}} P(\mathcal{D}, \mathcal{H})$. This replacement is a fast, but suboptimal approximation to the true likelihood. Second, as opposed to the nucleotide substitution probabilities discussed in Section 4.4.1 and derived in Section 4.4.2, the nucleotide substitution probabilities of equation (4.61) do not depend on the branch lengths w_i, that is, they are independent of phylogenetic time. This assumption is obviously implausible, and it explains the failure of parsimony in certain evolutionary scenarios, as discussed in Section 4.3.2. Note that weighted parsimony [33], which replaces the Kronecker delta in (4.59) by some more general nucleotide-dependent, but still branch length-independent function, does not overcome these shortcomings.

4.4.5 Maximum Likelihood

Given a DNA sequence alignment $\mathcal{D}$, we want to optimize the tree topology S and the branch lengths $\mathbf{w}$ in a maximum likelihood sense:[12]

$$(\hat{S}, \hat{\mathbf{w}}) = \text{argmax}_{S,\mathbf{w}} \{P(\mathcal{D}|\mathbf{w}, S)\} \tag{4.62}$$

More accurately, we should also state the dependence of the likelihood on the nucleotide substitution model and its parameters, which also need to be estimated from the data. For the Kimura model (4.16) we have one parameter: the transition–transversion ratio τ. The more general HKY85 model (4.32) has three further parameters: the equilibrium probabilities for the nucleotides, $\Pi_A, \Pi_C, \Pi_G, \Pi_T$ (due to the constraint $\Pi_A + \Pi_C + \Pi_G + \Pi_T = 1$, there are three rather than four free parameters). More complex nucleotide substitution models are reviewed in [30]. In order to keep the amount of detail in this introductory tutorial limited, we will assume that the nucleotide substitution parameters are given and fixed, and they will not be made explicit in the notation. The optimization procedure for the branch lengths, outlined below, can readily be extended to include the nucleotide substitution parameters.

A practical difficulty of maximum likelihood applied to phylogenetics is that (4.62) has no analytic solution, and the numerical optimization problem is NP–hard. For a given tree topology S, we can (locally) optimize the branch lengths $\mathbf{w}$ in an iterative, greedy way by following some *gradient ascent* scheme, $\mathbf{w} \rightarrow \mathbf{w} + \triangle\mathbf{w}$ with

[12] Recall from Section 1.2 that the maximum likelihood estimator satisfies several optimality criteria.

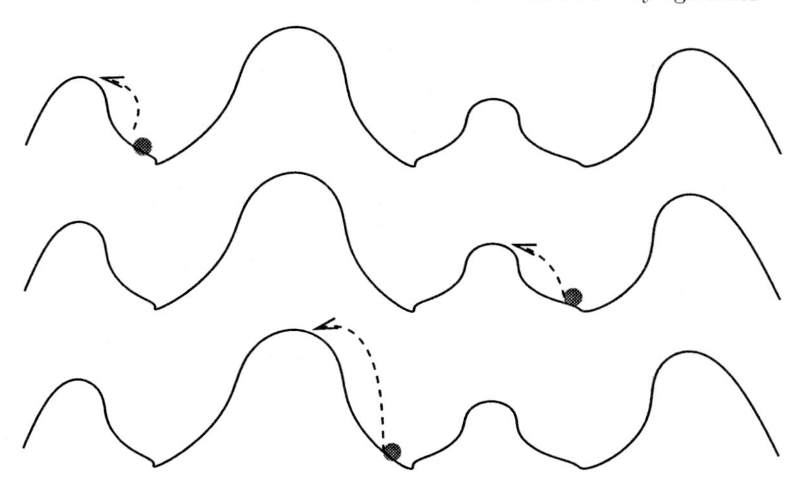

Fig. 4.25. Illustration of greedy, iterative optimization. The graphs represent the likelihood over the space of tree topologies and branch lengths. *Top:* For a given tree topology, the branch lengths are optimized by some gradient ascent scheme (4.63), as illustrated by the dashed arrows. *Middle and bottom:* This optimization has to be repeated for different tree topologies. Note that the true log likelihood surface defined by (4.58) is spanned over the high-dimensional space of all tree topologies and associated vectors of branch lengths, and that the one-dimensional analogy shown in this figure is merely given as an illustration.

n	4	6	10	20
M	3	105	2×10^6	2×10^{20}

Table 4.2. Number of different unrooted tree topologies, M, as a function of the number of taxa, n. The general relation is $M = (2n-5)!!$, that is, M increases super-exponentially with n. A proof is given in the appendix to this chapter.

$$\triangle \mathbf{w} \; = \; \mathbf{A}\nabla_{\mathbf{w}} \log P(\mathcal{D}|\mathbf{w}, S) \tag{4.63}$$

for some positive definite matrix $\mathbf{A}$. This optimization of the branch lengths has to be repeated for every possible tree topology S, as illustrated in Figure 4.25. For n taxa there are $(2n-5)!!$ different (unrooted) tree topologies, as shown in the appendix to this chapter. The number of different tree topologies increases thus super-exponentially with the number of taxa, as demonstrated in Table 4.2. Consequently, an exhaustive search is impossible for all but very small sequence numbers n, and heuristic search procedures have to be adopted. Two such procedures that have been implemented in widely applied software packages will be described next.

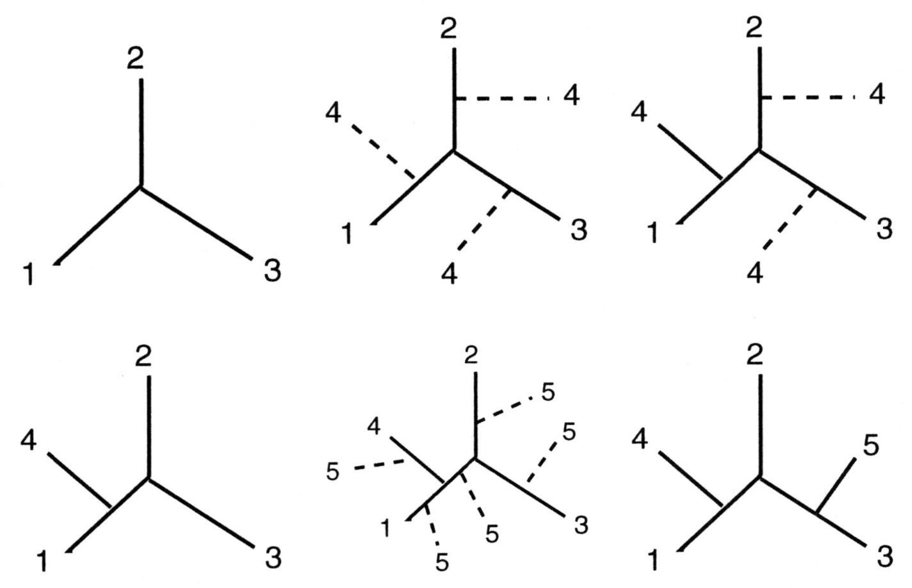

Fig. 4.26. Iterative insertion of new branches in DNAML. Starting from an unrooted tree of three species (*top left*), a new branch, corresponding to the fourth sequence in the alignment, is inserted at every possible position (*top centre*), and the tree with the highest likelihood is kept (*top right*). Taking this tree as the new starting position (*bottom left*), a new branch, corresponding to the fifth sequence in the alignment, is inserted at every possible position (*bottom centre*), and the tree with the highest likelihood is selected. This procedure is continued for all sequences in the alignment. Note that whenever a branch has been inserted or repositioned, the branch lengths are optimized with an iterative, gradient ascent procedure (4.63).

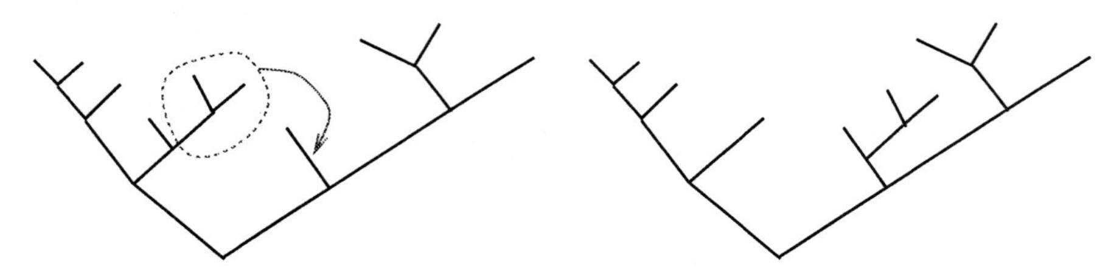

Fig. 4.27. Tree manipulation by branch regrafting in DNAML. If the likelihood after branch regrafting increases, the new tree is accepted; otherwise, it is rejected. Note that whenever a branch has been repositioned, the branch lengths have to be reoptimized with an iterative, gradient ascent procedure (4.63).

DNAML

The idea of DNAML, proposed in [7] and [10], and implemented in Felsenstein's software package PHYLIP [5], is to incrementally build a tree from a DNA sequence alignment. The algorithm starts with the first three sequences

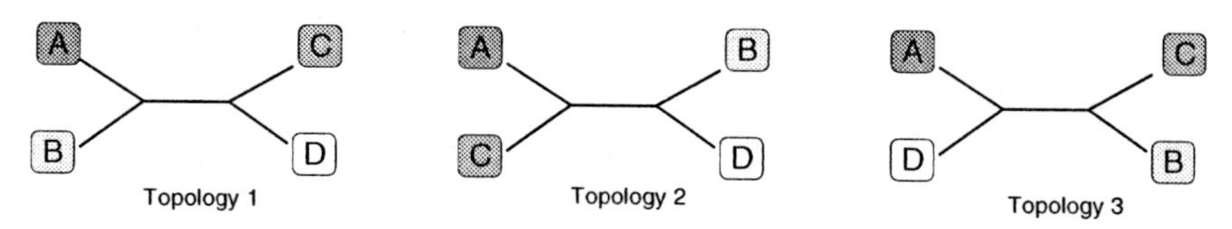

Fig. 4.28. Unrooted tree topologies for an alignment of four sequences, A, B, C, and D. The figure shows the three possible topologies. Note that the letters refer to taxa, not nucleotides.

in the alignment, for which there is only one unrooted tree topology. It then adds each new branch, corresponding to the next sequence in the alignment, at the location where it maximizes the likelihood of the current tree. This process is illustrated in Figure 4.26. Note that an unrooted tree with n leaves contains $(2n-3)$ edges. Consequently, the total number of tree topologies visited in this way is $\sum_{i=3}^{n-1}(2i-3) = (n-3)(n-1)$, which is considerably smaller than the total number of tree topologies, $(2n-5)!!$. The hope is that this restricted search space contains the true phylogenetic tree, or at least a very similar one, with a high probability. However, the result of the heuristic procedure described depends on the rather arbitrary sequence order, and this dependence usually makes the search method described above too restrictive. It is therefore advisable to repeat the whole process for different sequence orders and then to select the tree with the highest likelihood. Also, the neighbourhood of the final tree should be searched for a tree with a higher likelihood score, as illustrated in Figure 4.27: the tree is manipulated by selecting and regrafting a branch or a subtree at random, and the new tree is accepted if the likelihood increases. Such tree manipulations are repeated a few times. Note that whenever the tree topology has been changed by inserting or repositioning a branch, all branch lengths $\mathbf{w}$ have to be reoptimized with the iterative, gradient ascent procedure of equation (4.63). This optimization is computationally expensive, which has called for a faster, alternative search procedure.

Quartet puzzling

For a DNA sequence alignment of four sequences, say A, B, C, and D, there are three distinct unrooted tree topologies: sequence A can either be grouped with sequence B, ((A,B),(C,D)), or with sequence C, ((A,C),(B,D)), or with sequence D, ((A,D),(B,C)). The possible tree topologies are shown in Figure 4.28. The idea of *quartet puzzling*, proposed by Strimmer and von Haeseler [38], is to reconstruct all possible $\binom{n}{4}$ quartet trees with maximum likelihood (where n is the number of sequences) and then, in a subsequent puzzling step, to combine these quartet trees to an overall tree. This puzzling step is based on incrementally augmenting the penalty scores for the tree branches and is illustrated in Figure 4.29. A more recent version of quartet puzzling, which replaces the binary penalty scores by likelihood-dependent scores, is described

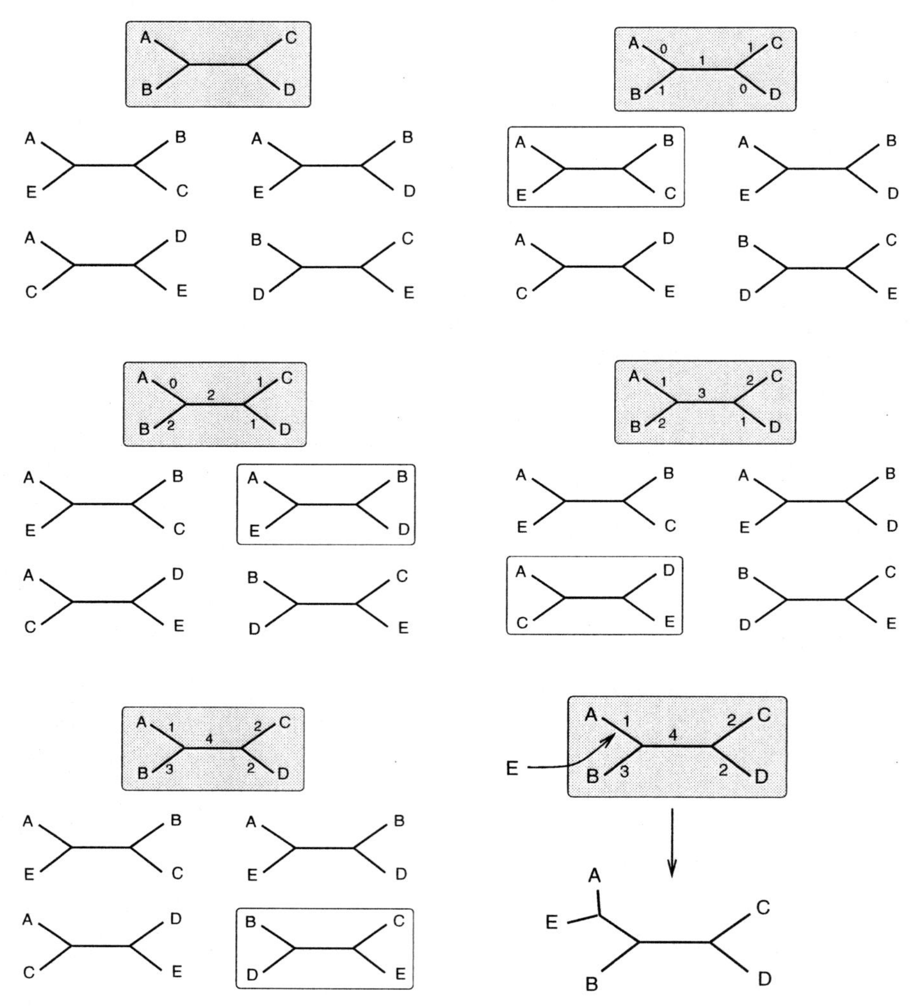

Fig. 4.29. **Quartet puzzling**, illustrated for a hypothetical alignment of five sequences A, B, C, D, and E. For each of the five possible quartets, the maximum likelihood tree is determined (*top left*). Starting from the tree obtained for the first four sequences A, B, C, and D (shaded), the other four trees are "puzzled in" as follows. *Top right:* The topology ((A,E),(B,C)) suggests that E should not be positioned on the path from B to C, so the penalty scores of the edges on this path, initialized to 0, are augmented by 1. *Middle left:* The topology ((A,E),(B,D)) suggests that E should not be positioned on the path from B to D, so the penalty scores of the edges on this path are augmented by 1. This procedure is continued. *Middle right:* The topology ((A,C),(D,E)) augments the penalty scores of the edges on the path from A to C. *Bottom left:* The topology ((B,D),(C,E)) augments the penalty scores of the edges on the path from B to D. *Bottom right:* The edge corresponding to sequence E is inserted at the branch with the minimal penalty score. A more recent version of this algorithm [37] replaces the binary penalty scores by likelihood-dependent scores.

in [37]. As for DNAML, the outcome of the algorithm may depend on the order of sequences in the alignment, and the tree puzzling procedure should therefore be repeated for different, reshuffled, sequence orders.

Following the initial branch length optimization in $3\binom{n}{4} < 3n^4$ quartet trees, by application of (4.63), the puzzling steps do not require any further branch length optimization. This renders quartet puzzling a much faster algorithm than DNAML, where each tree manipulation requires a separate optimization of $\mathbf{w}$.

Strimmer et al. [38], [37] compared the accuracy of quartet puzzling with DNAML and neighbour joining (described in Section 4.2.3). The results are shown in Figure 4.30. DNAML tends to give better results than quartet puzzling at the expense of increased computational costs. However, quartet puzzling achieves a consistent improvement on neighbour joining, which suggests that despite the required heuristic approximations, likelihood methods systematically outperform the distance-based clustering approaches of Section 4.2. For a software implementation of quartet puzzling, see [34].

The structural EM algorithm

Friedman et al. [14] applied the structural EM algorithm, which was briefly described in Section 2.3.6, to the maximum likelihood optimization problem. Assume we want to apply a local tree manipulation operation to the tree of Figure 4.23 by exchanging the two upper branches that lead to the extant species y_1 and y_3. If the hidden nodes z_1, z_2, z_3 and z_4 were observed, we would only need to compute the conditional probabilities $P(y_1|z_2)$ and $P(y_3|z_1)$. By computing these probabilities for all sequence positions and replacing

$$P(y_1|z_1) \to P(y_3|z_1), \qquad P(y_3|z_2) \to P(y_1|z_2) \tag{4.64}$$

in (4.48), we could easily compute the likelihood of the new tree. The upshot is that for complete observation, a local tree manipulation only requires us to re-compute the conditional probabilities of those nodes that are immediately affected by this local operation. Consequently, the computational costs are comparatively low. However, for incomplete observation, where we do not observe any sequence data for the ancestral species corresponding to the hidden nodes z_i, the marginalization (4.49) causes global dependencies between all the terms in the expansion (4.48). These dependencies destroy the modularity of (4.48). The upshot is that for incomplete observation, even a *local* tree manipulation requires us to re-compute the likelihood with a *global* computation that involves all the conditional probabilities $p(y_i|z_k)$ and $p(z_i|z_k)$ – irrespective of whether or not these conditional probabilities correspond to branches that have been affected by the local tree manipulation. Obviously, this requirement increases the computational costs substantially.

In a nutshell, the idea of the structural EM algorithm is as follows (see Section 2.3.3 for a revision of the standard EM algorithm). In the E-step,

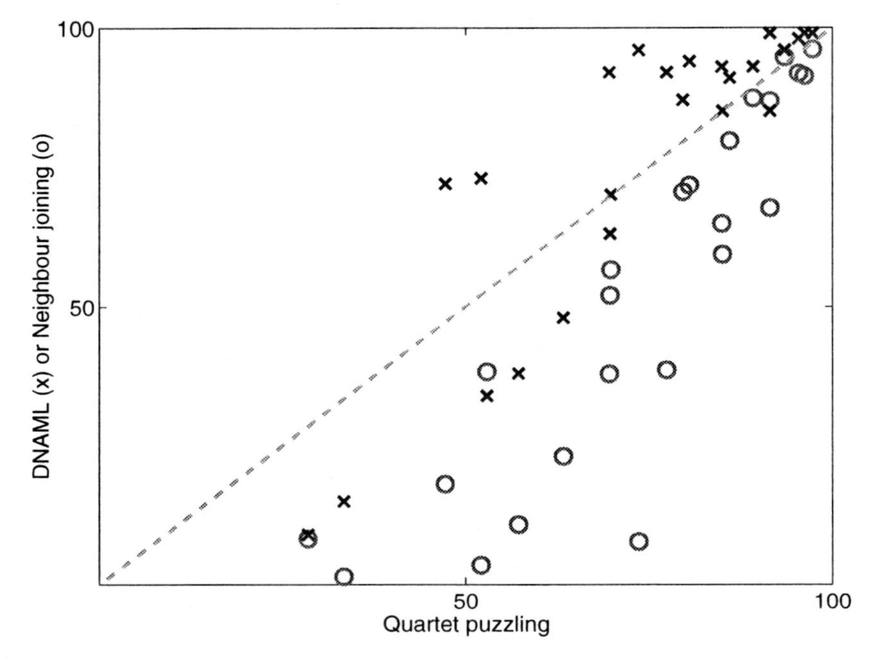

Fig. 4.30. Comparison between quartet puzzling, DNAML, and neighbour joining. The figure visualizes the results of a simulation study reported in [38] and [37]. The authors generated synthetic 8-taxa DNA sequence alignments of different length (500 and 1000 nucleotides) and from different phylogenetic trees (with and without molecular clock constraint, and with different branch lengths). Three phylogenetic inference methods were compared: DNAML, quartet puzzling, and neighbour joining. For each of these algorithms, the inference accuracy, that is, the percentage recovery of the true phylogenetic tree topology, was determined from repeated simulations. The figure plots the accuracy scores obtained with DNAML (crosses) and neighbour joining (circles) against those obtained with quartet puzzling (using the version described in [37]). The dashed, diagonal line indicates equal performance, entries above this line indicate a performance better than obtained with quartet puzzling, for entries below this line the respective method is outperformed by quartet puzzling. The figure suggests that while quartet puzzling tends, in general, to be outperformed by DNAML, it performs consistently better than neighbour joining.

impute the hidden variables with their expectation values. In the M-step, search for a tree with a higher score, where the score is given by the complete likelihood (4.60) with the hidden variables replaced by their imputed values.[13]

[13] More accurately, the score is given by (2.48), that is, the expectation value of the complete log likelihood with respect to the distribution of the hidden nodes. This distribution of the hidden nodes is computed in the E-step. The imputation step is, in general, an approximation, where the expectation value of a nonlinear

This search exploits the modular structure of the complete likelihood and is therefore considerably faster than a search that requires a re-computation of the true (or "incomplete") likelihood, as in DNAML. Like the standard EM algorithm, this procedure has to be iterated. However, if the computational costs of the E-step can be kept sufficiently low, the increased speed of the M-step may lead to a reduction of the computational costs of the overall tree optimization. For further details, see [14].

The structural EM-algorithm [14] has not been widely applied in phylogenetics. This is partly due to the lack of a user-friendly software implementation,[14] and partly due to the absence of a convincing benchmark study comparing its performance with that of DNAML and quartet puzzling. This tutorial will therefore not provide a more detailed introduction to this subject.

4.4.6 Bootstrapping

Recall from the discussion of the *frequentist approach* to statistical learning in Section 1.2 that a parameter and/or model estimation with maximum likelihood has to be substantiated with a separate hypothesis test. The objective of this hypothesis test is to ensure that the structures we have learned from the data reflect true features of the evolutionary speciation process rather than chance fluctuations inherent in the intrinsically stochastic events of mutation and selection. In an ideal scenario, depicted in Figure 1.3, we would be able to repeatedly generate new data from the same data-generating process, and then to estimate the intrinsic uncertainty of our inference procedure by repeating the estimation process on each of the replicated data sets. Obviously, this approach is not applicable because we cannot set the clock back by 4.5 billion years to restart the process of evolution. We therefore resort to bootstrapping as a computational approximation, discussed in Section 1.2, where we mimic the intrinsic stochasticity of the data-generating processes – in our case the processes of mutation and selection – by drawing new data with replacement from the true data, as illustrated in Figure 1.5. If we accept the fourth approximation on page 106, namely that nucleotide substitutions at different sites of the alignment are independent of each other, we can generate bootstrap replicas by repeatedly drawing new columns with replacement from the original alignment such that each replicated alignment has the same length as the original one. In Section 4.4.9, we will discuss how the assumption of independent nucleotide substitutions can be relaxed, and the required modifications have to be reflected in the bootstrap replication. For instance,

---

function is replaced by the function of the expectation value. As opposed to the standard EM-algorithm, described in Section 2.3.3, the M-step of the *structural EM algorithm* is with respect to structures (topologies) rather than parameters (branch lengths).

[14] It is indicative of contemporary computational molecular biology that the degree of popularity of an algorithm seems to depend critically on the user–friendliness of the software package in which it is implemented.

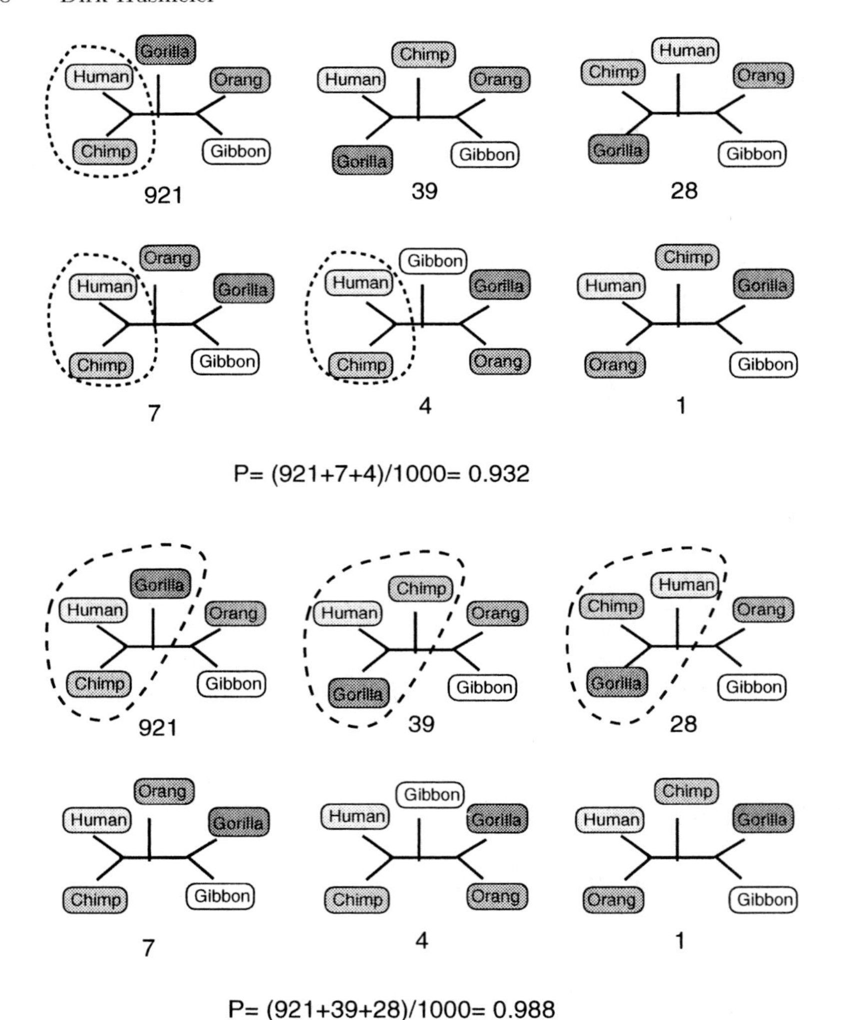

Fig. 4.31. Bootstrapping phylogenetic trees. The figure shows the tree topologies obtained from 1000 bootstrap replicas of a mitochondrial DNA sequence alignment of five hominoids and demonstrates how to compute the bootstrap support values for clade formations.

if we use a codon position specific approach, where we use different nucleotide substitution parameters for the three codon positions, the label that indicates the codon position of a nucleotide needs to be conserved in each bootstrap replica.

Given a set of bootstrap replicated DNA sequence alignments, the tree estimation procedure is repeated on each of these bootstrap replicas in the same way as it was performed on the true sequence alignment. This repeated

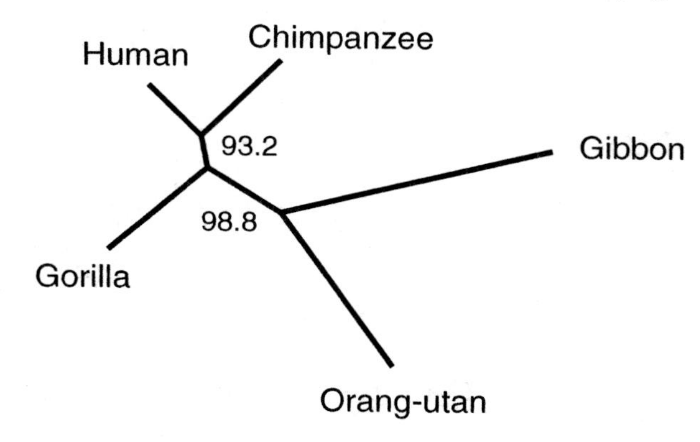

Clade	Probability
(Human Chimp)	0.932
(Human Chimp Gorilla)	0.988

Fig. 4.32. Bootstrap support values for clade formations in a phylogenetic tree of five hominoids, obtained from 1000 bootstrap replicas, as illustrated in Figure 4.31.

estimation results in a collection of bootstrap trees, from which we can estimate the confidence we have in the clades, that is, subtrees. An illustration is given in Figures 4.31 and 4.32. The tree itself can be chosen to be the tree obtained with maximum likelihood from the original sequence alignment. A more sophisticated approach is the consensus tree method, described in Section 6.4.

An inherent shortcoming of bootstrapping is its inability to detect model misspecifications. Take, for instance, the UPGMA clustering method, described in Section 4.2.2, and recall from Figure 4.10 that UPGMA always leads to a tree that satisfies the molecular clock constraint. Applying UPGMA to bootstrap replicas of the original alignment will result in an ensemble of trees that all satisfy the molecular clock constraint. Consequently, the validity of this constraint will be backed by a bootstrap support value of 100%. Also, recall from Figure 4.10 that UPGMA may lead to systematically wrong clade formations. This flawed inference is an intrinsic weakness of UPGMA, and it will therefore show up in most of the bootstrap replicas. Consequently, a wrong clade formation, like the one described in the caption of Figure 4.10, will obtain a large bootstrap support value, and the bootstrap procedure will substantiate the prediction from an inherently flawed inference method.

A practical difficulty of bootstrapping is its large computational cost. Recall, from the discussion of the preceding section, that a maximum likelihood estimation of a phylogenetic tree is an NP–hard optimization problem, which, in general, requires us to adopt an expensive iterative search procedure on the high-dimensional, multimodal likelihood surface. This search has to be repeated for each bootstrap replica. For five sequences, as in the example of Figures 4.31 and 4.32, this approach is feasible. However, when increasing the number of sequences in the alignment, bootstrapping soon becomes computationally intractable. Several heuristic simplifications have been proposed in the literature. They will not be reported here, because they are either not particularly powerful [22], [35], or not supported by a mathematical theory [38]. Instead, we will turn to a principled alternative to the frequentist approach, which is mathematically sound and computationally much more economical than bootstrapping.

4.4.7 Bayesian Inference

Recall, from the discussion in Section 1.3, that *Bayesian inference* is entirely based on the observed data $\mathcal{D}$, which in our case is the given DNA sequence alignment. Also, recall that the entities of interest, the tree topology S and the branch lengths $\mathbf{w}$, are treated as random variables. An illustration of the Bayesian paradigm is given in Figure 1.7. The inference procedure is similar to that of Sections 2.2.1 and 2.2.2. Given a DNA sequence alignment, we first want to find the posterior distribution of tree topologies S and, from this distribution, the topology $\hat{S}$ that is most supported by the data:

$$\hat{S} = \text{argmax}_S \Big\{ P(S|\mathcal{D}) \Big\} \tag{4.65}$$

Then, given the topology $\hat{S}$ and the data, we want to find the posterior probability of the branch lengths $\mathbf{w}$, and the best branch lengths:

$$\hat{\mathbf{w}} = \text{argmax}_{\mathbf{w}} \Big\{ P(\mathbf{w}|\hat{S}, \mathcal{D}) \Big\} \tag{4.66}$$

From the distribution $P(\mathbf{w}|S, \mathcal{D})$ we can estimate the credible intervals[15] for the branch lengths, and from $P(S|\mathcal{D})$ we can compute the set of posterior probabilities of the clade formations, which is the Bayesian equivalent to the bootstrap support values discussed in the previous section.

Unfortunately, the implementation of this approach is not as straightforward as it might seem. Recall from Table 4.2 on page 121 that the number of tree topologies increases super-exponentially with the number of sequences in the alignment. Consequently, the naive approach – computing $P(S|\mathcal{D})$ for every possible tree topology S – is computationally intractable for all but very small numbers of taxa. We therefore have to resort to *Markov chain Monte Carlo* (MCMC), introduced in Section 2.2.2, and illustrated in Figure 4.33, so

[15] A *credible interval* is the Bayesian equivalent to a *confidence interval* in classical statistics.

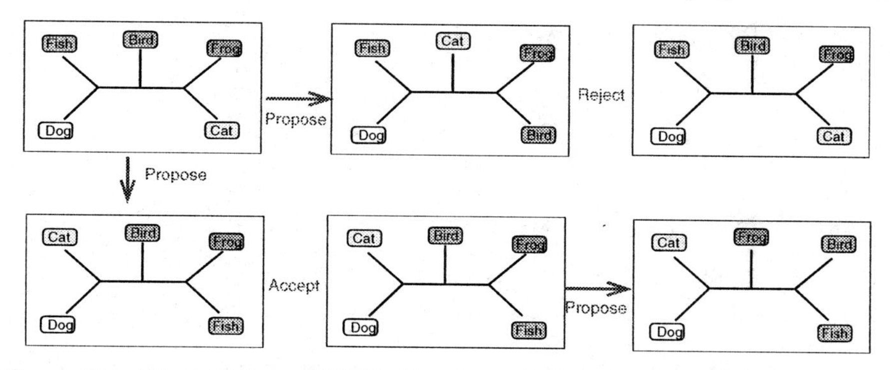

Fig. 4.33. Illustration of MCMC in phylogenetic analysis. Given a phylogenetic tree, a new tree is sampled from a proposal distribution. This new tree, which is usually similar to the previous one, is then accepted with an acceptance probability given by (4.71).

as to obtain a representative sample of topologies S from $P(S|\mathcal{D})$. However, as opposed to the inference problem of Sections 2.2.1 and 2.2.2, the integral over the parameters $\mathbf{w}$:

$$P(\mathcal{D}|S) = \int P(\mathcal{D}, \mathbf{w}|S)d\mathbf{w} \tag{4.67}$$

is analytically intractable, which implies that we can *not* get a closed form solution for $P(S|\mathcal{D}) \propto P(\mathcal{D}|S)P(S)$. Consequently, we have to sample both the topologies S and the branch lengths $\mathbf{w}$ from the joint posterior probability $P(S, \mathbf{w}|\mathcal{D})$, and then obtain $P(S|\mathcal{D})$ by marginalization:

$$P(S|\mathcal{D}) = \int P(S, \mathbf{w}|\mathcal{D})d\mathbf{w} \tag{4.68}$$

Now, from the MCMC simulation we obtain a sample of topologies and parameter vectors, $\{S_i, \mathbf{w}_i\}_{i=1}^M$, which give us the following empirical distribution:

$$P(S, \mathbf{w}|\mathcal{D}) \approx \frac{1}{M}\sum_{i=1}^{M} \delta_{S,S_i}\delta(\mathbf{w} - \mathbf{w}_i) \tag{4.69}$$

where δ_{S,S_i} denotes the Kronecker delta symbol, which is one if $S = S_i$, and zero otherwise, and $\delta(\mathbf{w} - \mathbf{w}_i)$ is the delta function,[16] which is normalized: $\int \delta(\mathbf{w} - \mathbf{w}_i)d\mathbf{w} = 1$. Inserting (4.69) into (4.68) thus gives:

$$P(S|\mathcal{D}) = \frac{1}{M}\sum_{i=1}^{M} \delta_{S,S_i} = \frac{M_S}{M} \tag{4.70}$$

[16] Recall that $\delta(0) = \infty$, $\delta(x) = 0$ if $x \neq 0$, and $\int_{-\infty}^{\infty} \delta(x)dx = 1$.

where M_S denotes the number of trees in the MCMC sample that have topology S.

Note that the dimension of the vector of branch lengths $\mathbf{w}$ does not change when changing the tree topology.[17] This invariance results from the fact that the number of species remains unchanged, hence we do not need to consider the dimension-changing reversible jumps of [18]. Consequently, we can apply the standard Metropolis–Hastings algorithm, described in Section 2.2.2. Given a tree with topology S and branch lengths $\mathbf{w}$, we sample a new tree with topology S' and branch lengths $\mathbf{w}'$ from the proposal distribution $Q(S', \mathbf{w}'|S, \mathbf{w})$, to be discussed shortly, and accept this new tree with the following acceptance probability, in generalization of (2.33):

$$A(S', \mathbf{w}'|S, \mathbf{w}) = \min\left\{\frac{P(S', \mathbf{w}'|\mathcal{D})}{P(S, \mathbf{w}|\mathcal{D})}\frac{Q(S, \mathbf{w}|S', \mathbf{w}')}{Q(S', \mathbf{w}'|S, \mathbf{w})}, 1\right\}$$
$$= \min\left\{\frac{P(\mathcal{D}|S', \mathbf{w}')}{P(\mathcal{D}|S, \mathbf{w})}\frac{P(S', \mathbf{w}')}{P(S, \mathbf{w})}\frac{Q(S, \mathbf{w}|S', \mathbf{w}')}{Q(S', \mathbf{w}'|S, \mathbf{w})}, 1\right\} \quad (4.71)$$

Here, $P(\mathcal{D}|S, \mathbf{w})$ is the likelihood of a tree with topology S and branch lengths $\mathbf{w}$, obtained from (4.58), and $P(S, \mathbf{w})$ denotes the prior probability on tree topologies and branch lengths. In the absence of true prior knowledge about the nature of evolutionary processes, we just choose the uniform distribution,[18] as in [23].

The Bayesian approach to phylogenetics, outlined above, was proposed and tested in [23], [24], and [46]. The practical problem of implementation is to design proposal probabilities Q of the moves in tree space efficiently so as to ensure effective mixing and fast convergence of the Markov chain; compare with the discussion in Section 2.2.2, especially Figure 2.14. Also, one has to make sure that the Hastings ratios, $\frac{Q(S', \mathbf{w}'|S, \mathbf{w})}{Q(S, \mathbf{w}|S', \mathbf{w}')}$, are computed properly. Take, for instance, one of the moves proposed in [23], which is illustrated in Figure 4.34 and which can be described algorithmically as follows:

1. Select a backbone consisting of three consecutive branches at random. Denote the length of this backbone, given by the sum of these three branch lengths, by m.
2. Select a random variable U from a uniform distribution over the unit interval $[0, 1]$, and multiply the lengths of the three selected branches by $\exp[\lambda(U - 0.5)]$. Here, $\lambda > 0$ is a tuning parameter, corresponding to the

[17] It would have been more accurate to make the association of the branch lengths $\mathbf{w}$ with the tree topology S explicit in the notation and to write $\mathbf{w}_S$ rather than $\mathbf{w}$. The stated invariance can then be written as follows: $\dim[\mathbf{w}_S] = \dim[\mathbf{w}_{S'}]$, for different tree topologies S, S'. However, for the sake of reduced opacity of the notation, the subscript S is suppressed in this chapter.

[18] In order to have a proper prior, the branch lengths have to be restricted to a finite interval, that is, the prior is uniform over some (large) interval, and zero otherwise; compare with Section 5.10.3.

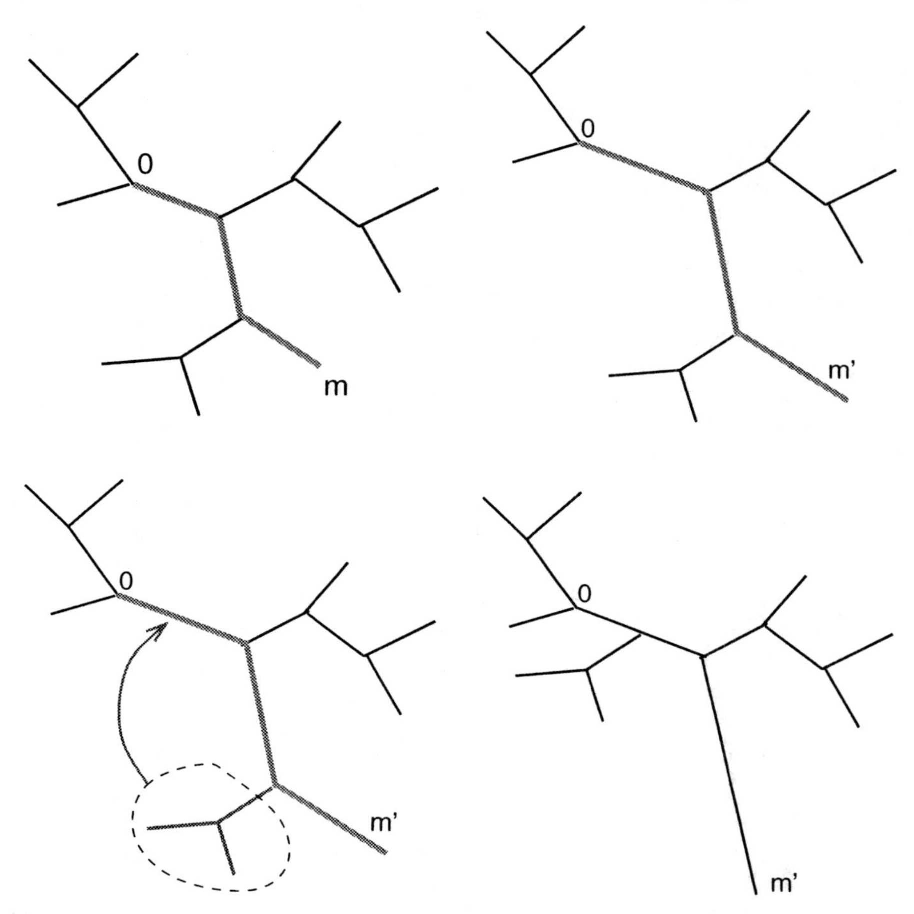

Fig. 4.34. MCMC moves in tree space. The figure illustrates a possible move in tree space, proposed in [23]. First, a backbone connecting four nodes is selected (*top left*) and extended or shrunk randomly (*top right*). Second, one of the two centre branches is randomly selected (*bottom left*) and then repositioned randomly on the backbone (*bottom right*). The first step changes the branch lengths $\mathbf{w}$. The second step may or may not change the tree topology S; in the present example, it does change the topology. Adapted from [23], by permission of Oxford University Press.

step size λ in the example of Figure 2.14. The length of the new backbone is given by $m' = m \exp[\lambda(U - 0.5)]$.

3. Select one of the two centre branches at random, with probability 1/2.
4. Regraft the selected branch on the backbone, choosing its new position uniformly from the interval $[0, m']$, where 0 corresponds to the left end of the backbone, and m' to the right end.

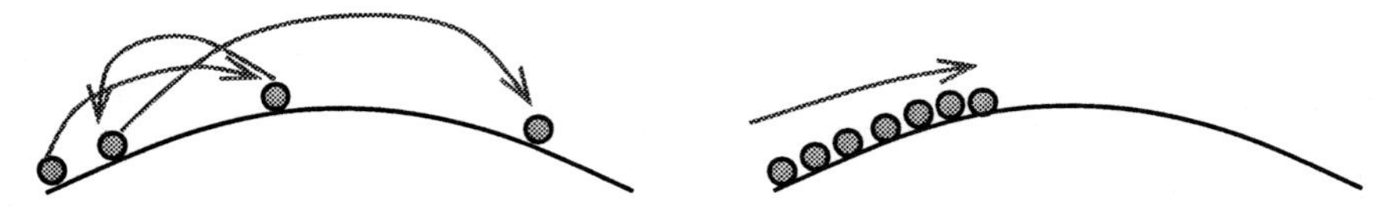

Fig. 4.35. A comparison between Bayesian MCMC and bootstrapping. The objective of both Bayesian MCMC and bootstrapping is to explore the uncertainty of inference, which is related to the curvature of the log likelihood surface. This figure gives an illustration for a simple one-dimensional case. The Bayesian MCMC approach, shown on the left, explores the log likelihood (or, in the case of a non-uniform prior, the log posterior) surface with a Markov chain. New configurations are first generated from a proposal distribution, and then accepted with a certain acceptance probability. Each accepted configuration is stored, and it contributes to the information about the curvature of the log likelihood surface. The frequentist approach, shown on the right, aims to find the maximum of the log likelihood surface. This maximum is a point estimate devoid of any information on uncertainty; consequently, this optimization is repeated several times for different bootstrap replicas. Information about estimation uncertainty is contained in the spread of the bootstrap maxima, that is, in the average deviation of the peak in response to resampling the data. Each optimization, however, is time-consuming, and all the information gathered along the trajectory leading to the peak of the log likelihood surface is eventually discarded. This waste of information renders bootstrapping much more computationally expensive than the Bayesian approach, where all the information along the MCMC trajectory is kept.

The second step changes the branch lengths $\mathbf{w}$. The fourth step may or may not change the tree topology S, depending on the new position to which the selected centre branch is moved. To compute the Hastings ratio, think of the selected backbone as a continuous line of length m, so the positions of the two centre branches can be defined by random variables $x \in [0, m]$ and $y \in [0, m]$. Let y be the position of the centre branch that gets regrafted. Since the new position is chosen from the uniform distribution, the probability of the forward move is $Q(y') = \frac{1}{m'}$, where m' is the new length of the backbone, resulting from step 2 of the move. The probability of the backward move is $Q(y) = \frac{1}{m}$. The probability to find the other branch at its given position before the move is $Q(x)$. The relative position of this branch does not change, but the extension or shrinkage of the backbone, $[0, m] \to [0, m']$, implies a coordinate transformation, $x \to x' = \frac{m'}{m}x$, with a concomitant probability transformation, $Q(x') = Q(x)\frac{dx}{dx'} = Q(x)\frac{m}{m'}$. The proposal probabilities of backbone selection in step 1, selection of U in step 2, and centre branch selection in step 3 are symmetric and thus cancel out. Consequently, the Hastings ratio, that is, the ratio of the probabilities of the forward and backward moves, is given by $\frac{Q(S',\mathbf{w}'|S,\mathbf{w})}{Q(S,\mathbf{w}|S',\mathbf{w}')} = \frac{Q(y')Q(x')}{Q(y)Q(x)} = \left(\frac{m}{m'}\right)^2$.

The outcome of a Bayesian MCMC simulation is similar to maximum likelihood with bootstrapping. The clade support scores are computed from the MCMC trajectory in the same way as they are computed from a collection of bootstrap replicas; see Figure 4.31 for a demonstration of this computation, and Figure 4.32 for a representation of the resulting tree. Again, a consensus tree can be obtained from the clade support scores, as described in Section 6.4. The clade support scores are now to be interpreted as Bayesian posterior probabilities, which in practice may differ little from the bootstrap support values of the previous section; see, however, the discussion at the end of Section 6.5. The main advantage of Bayesian MCMC over bootstrapping is the considerable reduction in the computational costs. Larget and Simon [23] applied the Bayesian MCMC scheme outlined above to a DNA sequence alignment of 14 whales and 17 artiodactyles (sheep, goat, deer etc.). The computation took about 7 hours (on a 300-MHz Pentium II PC), whereas the equivalent application of maximum likelihood and bootstrapping would have taken about 175 days. An explanation for this reduction in the computational cost is given in Figure 4.35.

In the previous exposition we have assumed, for the sake of notational and conceptual simplicity, that the parameters of the nucleotide substitution model are known and fixed. In practical applications they should be included in the inference procedure. This extension of the MCMC scheme is straightforward; see Chapters 5 and 6, and references therein. Note, however, that a change between different nucleotide substitution models, for instance, between the Kimura model (4.16) and the HKY85 model (4.32), incurs a change of the dimension of the parameter space. This change of dimension calls for the application of the reversible jump procedure of Section 2.3.7. A detailed discussion is beyond the scope of this introductory tutorial, and the interested reader is referred to [40].

4.4.8 Gaps

Given a sequence alignment, we have to decide how to deal with gaps. A straightforward approach is to treat gaps as missing values, in the same way as the intrinsically hidden ancestral nodes (see Figure 4.22), and marginalize over them. Consequently, we have to replace the evidence for an *observed* leaf node, (4.55), by the following modified evidence for an *unobserved* leaf node:

$$e(z_l) \;=\; \Pi(z_l) \tag{4.72}$$

where l is a leaf node with associated random variable $z_l \in \{A, C, G, T\}$, and $\Pi(z_l)$ is the equilibrium distribution over nucleotides, given by (4.29)–(4.31); note that this choice of $\Pi(z_l)$ follows from the stationarity hypothesis. This method is not entirely satisfactory because it does not capture evolutionary information that is potentially contained in the gaps. More recent approaches, like [25], extend the nucleotide substitution model, described in Section 4.4.2, by explicitly including gaps. Again, this active area of current research is beyond the scope of the present chapter.

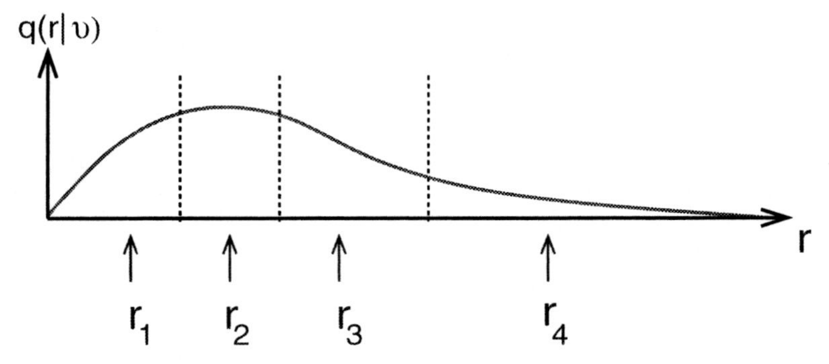

Fig. 4.36. Discrete gamma distribution, introduced by Yang [45] to model rate heterogeneity. The interval $[0, \infty)$ is subdivided into K (here: $K = 4$) intervals such that each interval contains an equal area of the gamma distribution.

4.4.9 Rate Heterogeneity

A critical weakness of the mathematical nucleotide substitution model assumed so far is the third assumption on page 106, according to which the Markov process is position independent. This assumption is strongly violated in real DNA. First, DNA sequences contain *coding* and *non-coding* regions. Nucleotide substitutions in the coding regions may lead to a changed amino acid sequence, which may result in a disfunctional protein. Consequently, nucleotide substitutions in the coding region may lead to organisms that are not viable. This effectively reduces the nucleotide substitution rate: sequences encoding disfunctional proteins are essentially discarded as organisms containing these sequences do not contribute to the next generation. How much the substitution rate is effectively reduced depends on the protein structure. Mutations in loop regions are less likely to be fatal than mutations in helical or functional regions, and the effective substitution rate varies accordingly. For non-coding regions, which are not translated into proteins, nucleotide substitutions are mostly unaffected by any selection pressure, unless the region is involved in controlling gene expression. In this case mutations are often lethal and the nucleotide substitution rate in the respective part of the sequence is considerably reduced. Second, amino acids are encoded by triplets of nucleotides. Mutations in the third codon position are usually less critical than those in the first or second codon position in that the mutated triplet either encodes the same amino acid – as a consequence of the redundancy of the genetic code – or an amino acid with similar physiochemical properties.

To model the second cause of rate variation, we can use three different nucleotide substitution rates, one for each codon position. To allow for rate heterogeneity at the first level, we introduce a site-dependent variable r_t with which the nucleotide substitution rates are multiplied. As seen from (4.21),[19] r_t effectively rescales the branch lengths at site t, and we can therefore replace (4.58) by

$$P(\mathcal{D}|\mathbf{w}, \mathcal{R}, S) = \prod_{t=1}^{N} P(\mathbf{y}_t|r_t\mathbf{w}, S) \tag{4.73}$$

Since the site-dependent rate variations are unknown, $\mathcal{R} = \{r_t\}$ is a set of hidden variables that need to be integrated out:

$$P(\mathcal{D}|\mathbf{w}, S) = \int_0^\infty \cdots \int_0^\infty \prod_{t=1}^{N} P(\mathbf{y}_t|r_t\mathbf{w}, S) P(r_1, \ldots, r_N) dr_1 \ldots dr_N \tag{4.74}$$

where $P(r_1, \ldots, r_N)$ is the joint prior distribution over the scaling variables. To reduce (4.74) to a form that is analytically tractable, Yang [44] replaced the joint distribution $P(r_1, \ldots, r_N)$ by the product of its marginals

$$P(r_1, \ldots, r_N) = \prod_{t=1}^{N} q(r_t|\upsilon) \tag{4.75}$$

where $q(r_t|\upsilon)$ is a distribution that depends on the hyperparameter(s) υ. Inserting (4.75) into (4.74) gives the simplified expression

$$P(\mathcal{D}|\mathbf{w}, \upsilon, S) = \prod_{t=1}^{N} \int_0^\infty P(\mathbf{y}_t|r_t\mathbf{w}, S) q(r_t|\upsilon) dr_t \tag{4.76}$$

If we adopt the maximum likelihood approach of Section 4.4.5, we now have to maximize, for a fixed tree topology S, the likelihood with respect to both $\mathbf{w}$ and υ. When following the Bayesian approach of Section 4.4.7, we have to sample both $\mathbf{w}$ and υ from the respective posterior distributions. Yang [44] chose $q(r_t|\upsilon)$ to be a gamma distribution with mean 1 and variance $\frac{1}{\upsilon}$, which renders the integral in (4.76) analytically tractable. However, the cost for the computation of the likelihood grows exponentially with the number of sequences, and the approach thus becomes inviable for large alignments. Yang [45] therefore approximated the integral by a discrete sum as follows. The interval $[0, \infty)$ is subdivided into K intervals such that each interval contains an equal area of the gamma distribution $q(r_t|\upsilon)$. Define r_k^υ to be the (υ-dependent) mean of the gamma distribution in the kth interval, as illustrated in Figure 4.36. Then

$$P(\mathcal{D}|\mathbf{w}, \upsilon, S) = \frac{1}{K} \prod_{t=1}^{N} \sum_{k=1}^{K} P(\mathbf{y}_t|r_k^\upsilon\mathbf{w}, S) \tag{4.77}$$

[19] Note that the symbol t in (4.21) has a different meaning and represents physical time rather than sites in a DNA sequence alignment; see Table 4.1 on page 111.

is a good approximation to (4.76) for values of K as small as 3 or 4. Note that this approximation only requires K times as much computation as is required for the non-varying site model.

A shortcoming of Yang's approach is the assumption of independently and identically distributed rate parameters r_t, as expressed in (4.75). This assumption is obviously flawed: when a site t lies in a coding region, for example, then the adjacent sites $t-1$ and $t+1$ will, most likely, lie in the same coding region, and the rate parameters r_{t-1}, r_t, and r_{t+1} will therefore not be independent. To introduce spatial correlations at the lowest possible order, Felsenstein and Churchill [10] chose discrete rates r_t, as for Yang's discrete gamma distribution [45], but they replaced (4.75) by

$$P(r_1, \ldots, r_N) = q(r_1) \prod_{t=2}^{N} q(r_t | r_{t-1}, \upsilon) \tag{4.78}$$

This approach is effectively a hidden Markov model (HMM), introduced in Section 2.3.4, where the rates r_t correspond to hidden states, and the transition probabilities are given by $q(r_t|r_{t-1}, \upsilon)$. We will discuss similar combinations of HMMs with phylogenetic trees in Section 5.10.

4.4.10 Protein and RNA Sequences

So far we have entirely focused on DNA sequences. In principle the methods described in the present chapter can equally be applied to protein sequences. The difference is that the four-letter alphabet of nucleotides has to be expanded into an alphabet of twenty amino acids. For the distance and parsimony methods, described in Sections 4.2 and 4.3, this makes little difference in terms of computational costs. However, for the probabilistic approach of Section 4.4, the computational costs increase dramatically as a consequence of the required marginalization, described in Section 4.4.3 and illustrated in Figure 4.22, which now has to cover 20 rather than 4 possible values at every hidden node. Moreover, the number of parameters of a reasonable amino acid substitution matrix is considerably higher than for the nucleotide substitution matrices of equations (4.16) and (4.32), rendering parameter inference a much more formidable problem. The interested reader is referred to [42].

RNA sequences are similar to DNA sequences in that they also use a four-letter alphabet, with the letter T for *thymine* replaced by U for *uracil.* However, RNA sequences show characteristic single-strand secondary structure formations that are conserved by base-pairing interactions. The substitution of a base involved in such an interaction is usually compensated for by a corresponding change at the interacting site. This process of *compensatory substitution* or *covariation* maintains structural stability and biological function. Since interacting base pairs may involve sites that are remote in the sequence, the fourth assumption on page 106 is violated, and the standard approach outlined in this chapter will lead to suboptimal results. An improved

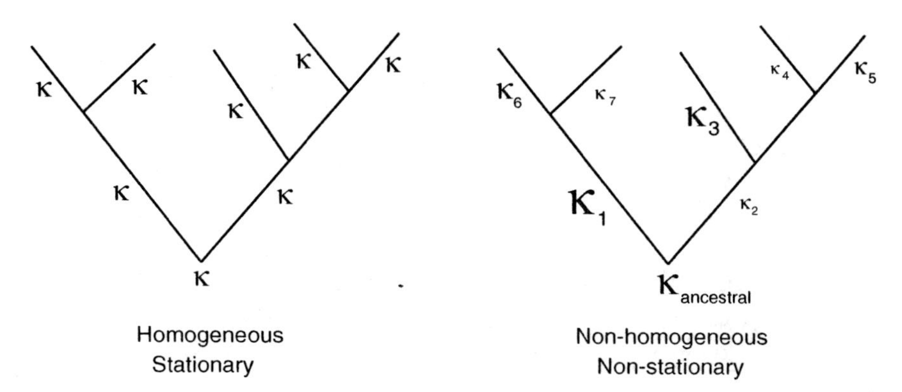

Fig. 4.37. Non-homogeneous, non-stationary nucleotide substitution model. *Left:* The homogeneity and stationarity assumptions imply that the equilibrium G+C content κ is the same for all lineages and equal to the ancestral G+C content. *Right:* In the non-homogeneous, non-stationary nucleotide substitution model of Galtier and Gouy [16], the equilibrium G+C-content κ may vary among lineages, and it may deviate from the ancestral G+C content.

approach, which relaxes the assumption of independent nucleotide substitutions and therefore becomes applicable to RNA sequences, will be discussed in Chapter 6.

4.4.11 A Non-homogeneous and Non-stationary Markov Model of Nucleotide Substitution

The Markov model of nucleotide substitution, discussed in Section 4.4.2, has been assumed to be *homogeneous*; see page 106. This assumption implies that in any lineage, DNA sequences converge towards a common equilibrium base composition, $\boldsymbol{\pi}$, given by (4.29)–(4.31). Furthermore, it has been assumed that the actual base composition is equal to the equilibrium base composition $\boldsymbol{\pi}$ over the whole tree. We have made use of this *stationarity* hypothesis in the computation of the likelihood, by assuming that the base composition in the ancestral sequence – $\Pi(x_r)$ in (4.33) – is equal to the equilibrium base composition $(\Pi_A, \Pi_C, \Pi_G, \Pi_T)$ in the assumed rate matrix (4.32).

If the homogeneity and stationarity assumptions were true, equal nucleotide frequencies would be expected in extant sequences. However, many sequence alignments were found to deviate from this principle, and it seems that compositional changes are a major feature of genome evolution [15]. Galtier and Gouy showed that a violation of the homogeneity and stationarity assumptions may lead to biased results in phylogenetic analysis in that sequences with similar base composition tend to be grouped together irrespective of their actual phylogenetic relationships [15].

An approach that relaxes the homogeneity and stationarity assumptions was proposed by Galtier and Gouy [16]. The focus of their model is variation in the G+C content in time and between lineages. When the dinucleotide GC occurs in a genome, cytosine (C) is typically chemically modified by methylation with the consequence that it mutates, with a high probability, into a T. For certain biological reasons the methylation process is occasionally suppressed, which leads to an increased concentration of GC dinucleotides, and in fact to more C and G nucleotides in general ([4], Chapt. 3). Clary and Wolstenholme [2] found that the G+C content at the third-codon position varies across genomes, and that it is, for instance, significantly suppressed in mitochondrial DNA of *Drosophila*. The ribosomal G+C content has been found to be highly correlated with physiological traits in bacteria, which provides important clues about the origin of life on Earth, as discussed shortly.

Tamura [41] proposed a nucleotide substitution model that allows for transition–transversion and G+C-content biases. Effectively, the Tamura rate matrix is equal to the HKY85 rate matrix (4.32), with the constraints $\Pi_A = \Pi_T$ and $\Pi_C = \Pi_G$. The Tamura model can therefore be thought of as a 2-parameter model, whose parameters are the transition–transversion ratio τ, and the equilibrium G+C content κ. Based on this approach, Galtier and Guoy [16] proposed a Markovian nucleotide substitution model where κ is allowed to vary from branch to branch, and the ancestral G+C content is a separate parameter of the nucleotide substitution model; see Figure 4.37 for an illustration. This modification has two implications. First, the base composition in a given lineage is, in general, different from the equilibrium base composition, hence the model is no longer *stationary*. Second, the rate matrix varies among lineages (because κ varies among lineages), hence the model is no longer *homogeneous*. This non-homogeneity implies that the application of the Chapman–Kolmogorov equation (4.10) in (4.40) is no longer valid. Consequently, (4.40) does not hold true, the three structures in Figure 4.21 are no longer equivalent, and the symmetry between different rooted trees, discussed in Section 4.4.3, is broken. The location of the root in its branch has therefore to be specified as a separate parameter of the model, and an optimization algorithm, as discussed in Section 4.4.5, will recover a *rooted* rather than an *unrooted* tree.

Besides overcoming the bias in phylogenetic analysis incurred as a consequence of compositional G+C changes, the method of Galtier and Gouy [16] has led to new insight into the origin of life on Earth.

According to an earlier tree of life reconstructed from ribosomal RNA (rRNA) sequence alignments by Carl Woese [43], hyperthermophiles – bacteria that thrive in high temperatures – are found near or at the root of the tree. This finding has led to the widely accepted hypothesis that life originated in a hot environment, like in submarine volcanic vents, where the seawater can reach temperatures well above the normal boiling point [3].

Galtier et al. [17] applied their non-homogeneous, non-stationary Markov model of nucleotide substitution to an alignment of rRNA sequences from different species distributed throughout the universal tree of life. A maximum-likelihood estimation, as described in Section 4.4.5, gave an ancestral G+C content of about 55%, with the upper limit of a 95% confidence interval obtained with bootstrapping hardly exceeding the 60% mark. However, hyperthermophiles are characterized by a significantly higher G+C content of about 65%. The reason is that in prokaryotic rRNA, G-C pairs are more stable than A-U pairs at high temperatures because of an additional hydrogen bond (see Chapter 6). Consequently, the nucleotide makeup of rRNA in the earliest ancestral organisms is incompatible with life at high temperatures, in contrast with standard conjectures about the origin of life on Earth.

4.5 Summary

This chapter has provided a brief introduction to statistical phylogenetics, with a focus on the mathematical methodology. We have compared two older non-probabilistic approaches – clustering and parsimony – with the more recent probabilistic approach.

Besides incurring an inevitable loss of information by mapping the sequence alignment down to pairwise distances, *clustering* (Section 4.2) is an algorithmic approach that does not aim to optimize an objective function. Consequently, clustering is not guaranteed to find the best or even a good tree according to a pre-specified evaluation criterion, and a discrimination between competing phylogenetic hypotheses is impossible.

Parsimony (Section 4.3) is based on an objective function and thereby overcomes the principal objection to clustering. An optimization algorithm searches for the best tree with the lowest parsimony cost, and different trees can be evaluated on the basis of this cost function. However, parsimony is a “model-free” approach in that its cost function is not derived from any explicit mathematical model. In principle, this lack of an explicit model renders the assessment of the merits and shortcomings of an inference method difficult. Moreover, the *model-free* approach of parsimony can, in fact, be interpreted within the *model-based* likelihood framework, where it turns out to be a special case obtained for an over-simplified and implausible nucleotide substitution model (Section 4.4.4). The fact that parsimony is implicitly based on such a flawed model explains its inherent shortcoming of inconsistency (Section 4.3.2), whereby in certain evolutionary scenarios the wrong tree is inferred irrespective of the length of the sequence alignment.

Likelihood methods (Section 4.4) are based on an objective function derived from an explicit probabilistic model of nucleotide substitution. This model-based approach overcomes the shortcomings of the non-probabilistic methods described above, and it is only due to the increased computational cost of likelihood methods that the application of non-probabilistic methods to *large* sequence alignments may still be justified. Obviously, any mathematical model is an abstraction and simplification of reality. The fundamental advantage of model-based over model-free inference is the fact that we are aware of these limitations, as discussed at the beginning of Section 4.4.2, and we can therefore systematically work on improved, more general models that gradually overcome known shortcomings – see Sections 4.4.9–4.4.11. Also, besides inferring a phylogenetic tree from a sequence alignment, the use of an explicit mathematical model of nucleotide substitution allows us to gain deeper insight into the nature of evolution itself – and to test, for instance, hypotheses about the origin of life on Earth (Section 4.4.11).

Appendix

For n species there are, in total, $(2n-3)!!$ different rooted, and $(2n-5)!!$ different unrooted tree topologies. We can prove this proposition by induction. For $n=3$ taxa we have 1 unrooted and 3 different rooted tree topologies. Since $3!!=3$ and $1!!=1$, the proposition holds true for $n=3$. Next, we have to show that the truth of the proposition for n taxa implies that it also holds true for $n+1$ taxa. A rooted tree with n leaves has $n-1$ hidden nodes, that is, $2n-1$ nodes altogether, which implies that there are $2n-2$ edges. For an unrooted tree, the number of inner nodes is reduced by 1, which also reduces the number of edges by 1; so we have $2n-3$ edges. We assume that the statement holds true for n taxa, so we have $(2n-5)!!$ different unrooted tree topologies. We now add a further sequence to the alignment. The branch leading to the new species can be added to any of the $2n-3$ existing branches, giving us $(2n-3)(2n-5)!!=(2n-3)!!=(2[n+1]-5)!!$ new tree topologies. Consequently, the proposition holds true for $n+1$ taxa, which completes the proof for the unrooted tree topologies. To obtain a rooted tree from an unrooted tree, note that the root can be added to any of its $2n-3$ edges. Consequently, we can get $2n-3$ different rooted tree topologies from a given unrooted tree topology. Given that the number of unrooted tree topologies for n taxa is $(2n-5)!!$, as has just been proved, the number of different rooted tree topologies is $(2n-3)(2n-5)!!=(2n-3)!!$. This completes the proof.

Acknowledgments

I would like to thank Isabelle Grimmenstein, Anja von Heydebreck, Jochen Maydt, Magnus Rattray, and Vivek Gowri-Shankar for critical feedback on a first draft of this chapter. Also, I am indebted to Frank Wright for several stimulating discussions on phylogenetics in the last few years, which have substantially shaped my view and understanding of this subject. Last but not least, I am grateful to Philip Smith for his help with proofreading.

References

[1] P. Baldi and P. Brunak. *Bioinformatics – The Machine Learning Approach.* MIT Press, Cambridge, MA, 1998.

[2] D. O. Clary and D. R. Wolstenholme. The mitochondrial DNA molecule of *drosophila yakuba*: nucleotide sequence, gene organization and genetic code. *Journal of Molecular Evolution*, 22:252–271, 1985.

[3] P. Davies. *The Fifth Miracle: The Search for the Origin of Life*. Penguin Books, Middlesex, England, 1999.

[4] R. Durbin, S. R. Eddy, A. Krogh, and G. Mitchison. *Biological sequence analysis. Probabilistic models of proteins and nucleic acids*. Cambridge University Press, Cambridge, UK, 1998.

[5] J. Felsenstein. Phylip. Free package of programs for inferring phylogenies, available from http://evolution.genetics.washington.edu/phylip.html.

[6] J. Felsenstein. Cases in which parsimony or compatibility methods will be positively misleading. *Systematic Zoology*, 27:401–440, 1978.

[7] J. Felsenstein. Evolution trees from DNA sequences: A maximum likelihood approach. *Journal of Molecular Evolution*, 17:368–376, 1981.

[8] J. Felsenstein. Phylogenies from molecular sequences: Inference and reliability. *Annual Review of Genetics*, 22:521–565, 1988.

[9] J. Felsenstein. The troubled growth of statistical phylogenetics. *Systems Biology*, 50(4):465–467, 2001.

[10] J. Felsenstein and G. A. Churchill. A hidden Markov model approach to variation among sites in rate of evolution. *Molecular Biology and Evolution*, 13(1):93–104, 1996.

[11] W. M. Fitch. Towards defining the course of evolution: Minimum change for a specific tree topology. *Systematic Zoology*, 20:406–416, 1971.

[12] W. M. Fitch and E. Margoliash. Construction of phylogenetic trees. *Science*, 155:279–284, 1987.

[13] R. Fleischmann, M. Adams, O. White, R. Clayton, E. Kirkness, A. Kerlavage, C. Bult, J. Tomb, B. Dougherty, J. Merrick, K. McKenny, G. Sutton, W. Fitzhugh, C. Fields, J. Gocayne, J. Cott, R. Shirley, L. Liu, A. Glodek, J. Kelley, J. Weidman, C. Phillips, T. Spriggs, E. Hedblom, M. Cotton, T. Utterback, M. Hanna, D. Guyen, D. Saudek, R. Brandon, L. Fine, J. Fritchmann, N. Geoghagen, C. Gnehm, L. McDonald, K. Small, C. Fraser, H. Smith, and J. Venter. Whole-genome random sequencing and assembly of *Haemophilus influenzae*. *Science*, 269:496–512, 1995.

[14] N. Friedman, M. Ninio, I. Pe'er, and T. Pupko. A structural EM algorithm for phylogentic inference. *Journal of Computational Biology*, 9:331–353, 2002.

[15] N. Galtier and M. Gouy. Eubacterial phylogeny: a new multiple-tree analysis method applied to 15 sequence data sets questions the monophyly of gram-positive bacteria. *Research in Microbiology*, 145:531–541, 1994.

[16] N. Galtier and M. Gouy. Inferring patterns and process: Maximum-likelihood implementation of a nonhomogeneous model of DNA sequence evolution for phylogenetic analysis. *Molecular Biology and Evolution*, 15(7):871–879, 1998.

[17] N. Galtier, N. J. Tourasse, and M. Gouy. A nonhyperthermophilic common ancestor to extant life forms. *Science*, 283:220–221, 1999.

[18] P. Green. Reversible jump Markov chain Monte Carlo computation and Bayesian model determination. *Biometrika*, 82:711–732, 1995.

[19] G. R. Grimmett and D. R. Stirzaker. *Probability and random processes.* Oxford University Press, New York, 3rd edition, 1985.

[20] M. Hasegawa, H. Kishino, and T. Yano. Dating the human-ape splitting by a molecular clock of mitochondrial DNA. *Journal of Molecular Evolution*, 22:160–174, 1985.

[21] M. Kimura. A simple method for estimating evolutionary rates of base substitutions through comparative studies of nucleotide sequences. *Journal of Molecular Evolution*, 16:111–120, 1980.

[22] H. Kishino and M. Hasegawa. Evaluation of the maximum likelihood estimate of the evolutionary tree topology from DNA sequence data, and the branching order in hominoidea. *Journal of Molecular Evolution*, 29:170–179, 1989.

[23] B. Larget and D. L. Simon. Markov chain Monte Carlo algorithms for the Bayesian analysis of phylogenetic trees. *Molecular Biology and Evolution*, 16(6):750–759, 1999.

[24] B. Mau, M. A. Newton, and B. Larget. Bayesian phylogenetic inference via Markov chain Monte Carlo methods. *Biometrics*, 55:1–12, 1999.

[25] G. McGuire, C. D. Denham, and D. J. Balding. Models of sequence evolution for DNA sequences containing gaps. *Molecular Biology and Evolution*, 18(4):481–490, 2001.

[26] C. Ou, C. Ciesielski, G. Myers, C. Bandea, C. Luo, B. Korber, J. Mullins, G. Schochetman, R. Berkelman, A. Economou, J. Witte, I. Furman, G. Satten, K. MacInnes, J. Curran, and H. Jaffe. Molecular epidemiology of HIV transmission in a dental practice. *Science*, 256:1165–1171, 1992.

[27] R. D. M. Page and E. C. Holmes. *Molecular Evolution – A Phylogenetic Approach.* Blackwell Science, Cambridge, UK, 1998.

[28] A. Papoulis. *Probability, Random Variables, and Stochastic Processes.* McGraw-Hill, Singapore, 3rd edition, 1991.

[29] J. Pearl. *Probabilistic Reasoning in Intelligent Systems: Networks of Plausible Inference.* Morgan Kaufmann, San Francisco, CA, 1988.

[30] D. Posada and K. A. Crandall. Selecting the best-fit model of nucleotide substitution. *Systematical Biology*, 50(4):580–601, 2001.

[31] J. J. Rissanen. Modeling by shortest data description. *Automatica*, 14:465–471, 1978.

[32] N. Saitou and M. Nei. The neighbor-joining method: a new method for reconstructing phylogenetic trees. *Molecular Biology and Evolution*, 4:406–425, 1987.

[33] D. Sankoff and R. J. Cedergren. Simultaneous comparison of three or more sequences related by a tree. In D. Sankoff and J. B. Kruskal, editors,

Time Warps, String Edits, and Macromolecules: the Theory and Practice of Sequence Comparison, pages 253–264. Addison-Wesley, 1983.
[34] H. A. Schmidt, K. Strimmer, M. Vingron, and A. von Haeseler. TREE-PUZZLE: maximum likelihood phylogenetic analysis using quartets and parallel computing. *Bioinformatics*, 18(3):502–504, 2002.
[35] H. Shimodaira and M. Hasegawa. Multiple comparisons of log-likelihoods with applications to phylogenetic inference. *Molecular Biology and Evolution*, 16(8):1114–1116, 1999.
[36] M. A. Steel. The complexity of reconstructing trees from qualitative characters and subtrees. *Journal of Classification*, 9:91–116, 1992.
[37] K. Strimmer, N. Goldman, and A. von Haeseler. Bayesian probabilities and quartet puzzling. *Molecular Biology and Evolution*, 14:210–211, 1997.
[38] K. Strimmer and A. von Haeseler. Quartet puzzling: A quartet maximum likelihood method for reconstructing tree topologies. *Molecular Biology and Evolution*, 13:964–969, 1996.
[39] J. A. Studier and K. J. Keppler. A note on the neighbor-joining algorithm of Saitou and Nei. *Molecular Biology and Evolution*, 5:729–731, 1988.
[40] M. A. Suchard, R. E. Weiss, and J. S. Sinsheimer. Bayesian selection of continuous-time Markov chain evolutionary models. *Molecular Biology and Evolution*, 18(6):1001–1013, 2001.
[41] K. Tamura. Estimation of the number of nucleotide substitutions when there are strong transition-transversion and G+C-content biases. *Molecular Biology and Evolution*, 9(4):678–687, 1992.
[42] S. Whelan and N. Goldman. A general empirical model of protein evolution derived from multiple families using a maximum-likelihood approach. *Molecular Biology and Evolution*, 15(5):691–699, 2001.
[43] C. R. Woese. Bacterial evolution. *Microbiology Review*, 51:221–271, 1987.
[44] Z. Yang. Maximum likelihood estimation of phylogeny from DNA sequences when substitution rates differ over sites. *Molecular Biology and Evolution*, 10:1396–1401, 1993.
[45] Z. Yang. Maximum likelihood phylogenetic estimation from DNA sequences with variable rates over sites: approximate methods. *Journal of Molecular Evolution*, 39:306–314, 1994.
[46] Z. Yang and B. Rannala. Bayesian phylogenetic inference using DNA sequences: a Markov chain Monte Carlo method. *Molecular Biology and Evolution*, 14:717–724, 1997.

5

Detecting Recombination in DNA Sequence Alignments

Dirk Husmeier[1] and Frank Wright[2]

[1] Biomathematics & Statistics Scotland (BioSS)
JCMB, The King's Buildings, Edinburgh EH9 3JZ, UK
dirk@bioss.ac.uk

[2] Biomathematics & Statistics Scotland (BioSS)
BioSS Office at the Scottish Crop Research Institute, Dundee DD2 5DA, UK
frank@bioss.ac.uk

Summary. The underlying assumption of the phylogenetic inference methods discussed in the previous chapter is that we have one set of hierarchical relationships among the taxa. While this approach is reasonable when applied to most DNA sequence alignments, it can be violated in certain bacteria and viruses due to sporadic recombination, which is a process whereby different strains exchange or transfer DNA subsequences. The present chapter discusses the implications of recombination for phylogenetic inference and describes various methods for detecting and identifying recombinant regions in sequence alignments.

5.1 Introduction

The recent advent of multiple-resistant pathogens has led to an increased interest in interspecific recombination as an important, and previously underestimated, source of genetic diversification in bacteria and viruses. The discovery of a surprisingly high frequency of mosaic RNA sequences in HIV-1 suggests that a substantial proportion of AIDS patients have been coinfected with HIV-1 strains belonging to different subtypes, and that recombination between these genomes can occur *in vivo* to generate new biologically active viruses [24]. A phylogenetic analysis of the bacterial genera *Neisseria* and *Streptococcus* has revealed that the introduction of blocks of DNA from penicillin-resistant non-pathogenic strains into sensitive pathogenic strains has led to new strains that are both pathogenic *and* resistant [17]. Thus interspecific recombination, illustrated in Figure 5.1, raises the possibility that bacteria and viruses can acquire biologically important traits through the exchange and transfer of genetic material.

In the last few years, several methods for detecting interspecific recombination have been developed – following up on the seminal paper by Maynard

Smith [17] – and it is beyond the scope of this chapter to provide a comprehensive overview. Instead, the focus will be on a few typical and representative methods so as to illustrate the underlying principles and to highlight the merits and shortcomings of each approach. For a broader overview of existing methods, see [22].

5.2 Recombination in Bacteria and Viruses

The underlying assumption of most phylogenetic tree reconstruction methods is that there is one set of hierarchical relationships among the taxa. While this is a reasonable approach when applied to most DNA sequence alignments, it can be violated in certain bacteria and viruses due to interspecific *recombination*. Recombination is a genetic process that results in the exchange or transfer of DNA/RNA subsequences and constitutes an important source of genetic diversification in certain bacteria and viruses. The resulting mixing of genetic material can lead to a change of the branching order (topology) of the phylogenetic tree in the affected region, which results in conflicting phylogenetic information from different regions of the alignment. Figure 5.1 demonstrates for a simple hypothetical scenario involving four strains how the transfer or exchange of genetic material between different strains may lead to a change of the phylogenetic tree topology in the region affected by recombination, which results in conflicting phylogenetic information stemming from different regions of the alignment. Figure 5.2 illustrates the effects of recombination on the analysis of phylogenetic relationships among different HIV-1 strains. Both figures demonstrate that the presence of mosaic sequences resulting from recombination can lead to systematic errors in phylogenetic tree estimation. Their detection, therefore, is a crucial prerequisite for consistently inferring the evolutionary history of a set of DNA/RNA sequences.

5.3 Phylogenetic Networks

An obvious approach to allow for recombination is to relax the constraint that the process of evolution has to be represented by a bifurcating tree, as assumed throughout Chapter 4. Figure 5.3 shows how the conflicting phylogenetic trees resulting from the recombination scenario of Figure 5.1 can be reconciled with a phylogenetic network. Figure 5.5, left, illustrates that recombination may lead to a network-like structure. A non-probabilistic approach to inferring phylogenetic networks from sequence alignments was introduced by Bandelt and Dress [1]: the method of *split decomposition*. Strimmer et al. [26], [27] put this method into a proper probabilistic framework. Their approach is based on the same nucleotide substitution model as described in Sections 4.4.1 and 4.4.2. The authors then show how to compute the likelihood of a general directed acyclic probabilistic network. In fact, this approach applies the method

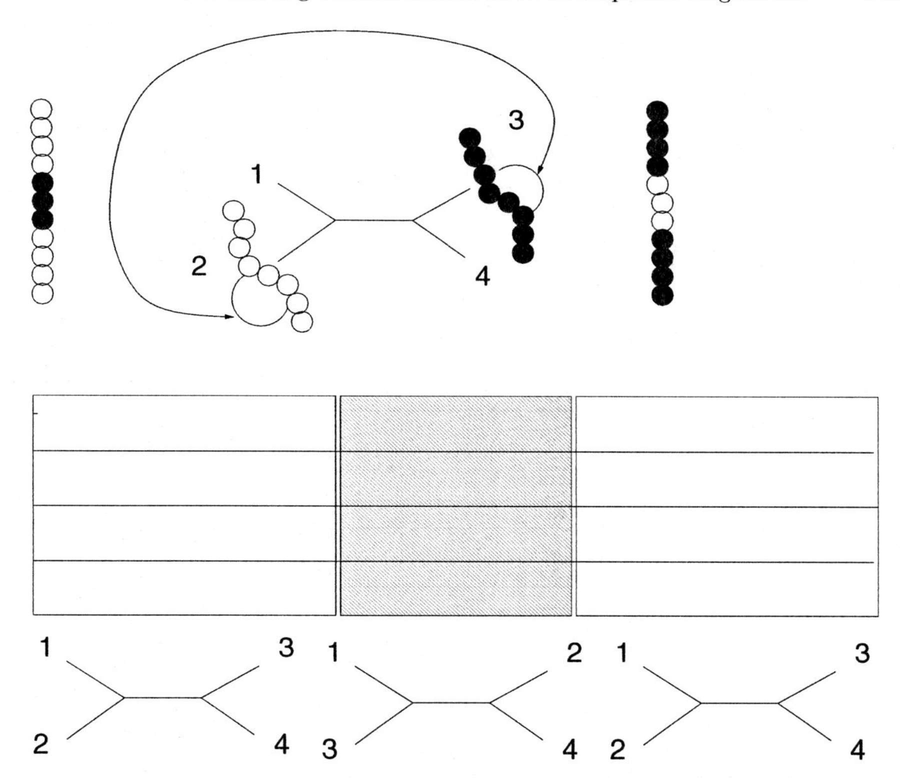

Fig. 5.1. Influence of recombination on phylogenetic inference. The figure shows a hypothetical phylogenetic tree of four strains. Recombination is the transfer or exchange of DNA subsequences between different strains (top diagram, middle), which results in two so-called mosaic sequences (top diagram, margins). The affected region in the multiple DNA sequence alignment, shown by the shaded area in the middle diagram, seems to originate from a different tree topology, in which two branches of the phylogenetic tree have been swapped (bottom diagram, where the numbers at the leaves represent the four strains). A phylogenetic inference algorithm that does not identify this region is likely to give suboptimal results, since the estimation of the branch lengths of the predominant tree will be adversely affected by the conflicting signal coming from the recombinant region. Reprinted from [12], by permission of Mary Ann Liebert.

of Bayesian networks, described in Chapter 2, to phylogenetic analysis, which subsumes the inference of tree-like structures as a limiting case. The structure of a phylogenetic network is a directed acyclic graph (DAG), whose conditional probabilities, parameterized by the edge lengths, are derived by modelling the nucleotide substitution process along an edge by a homogeneous Markov process, as discussed in Sections 4.4.1 and 4.4.2. The main difference is that in a network, as opposed to a tree, a node can have several parents, which calls

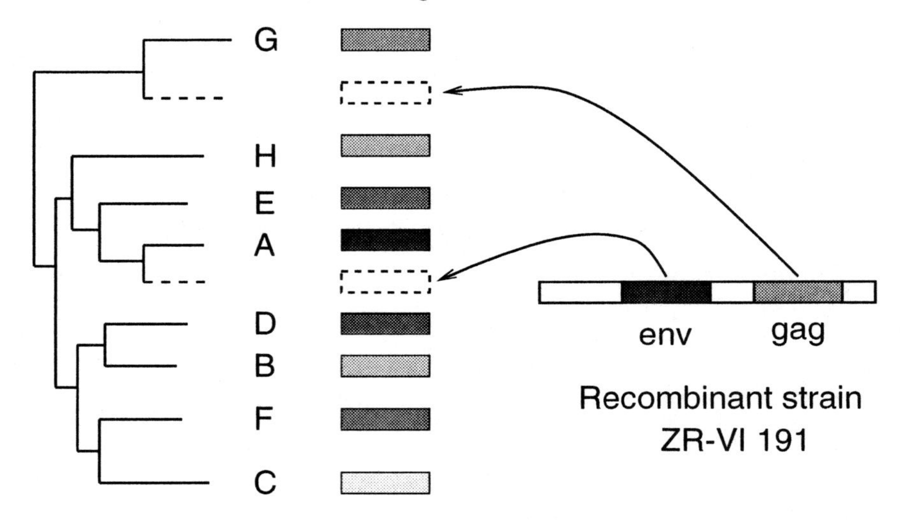

Fig. 5.2. Recombination in HIV-1. The left diagram shows a phylogenetic tree of eight established subtypes of HIV-1. The right diagram represents the sequence of a recombinant strain (RS). When the phylogenetic analysis is based on the *env* gene, the RS strain is found to be most closely related to the A subtype. When the phylogenetic analysis is repeated for the *gag* gene, the RS strain seems to be most closely related to the G subtype. A conventional phylogenetic analysis treats the RS sequence as a monolithic entity. This fails to resolve the conflicting phylogenetic signals stemming from different regions of the alignment, and leads to a distorted "average" tree that is in a "limbo" state between the two true trees mentioned above. It is therefore vital to identify the mosaic structure of the RS strain, and to infer different phylogenetic trees for the different regions. Adapted from [24], by permission of Macmillan Magazines Limited.

for a generalization of the assignment of local node probabilities, given by (4.25) for a tree, to the multi-parent case. Consider a node X with two parents, Y_1 and Y_2, on two branches, 1 and 2, that have edge lengths w_1 and w_2, respectively. An illustration is given in Figure 5.4. Strimmer et al. [26] define the probability $P(X|Y_1, Y_2)$ of observing state $X \in \{A, C, G, T\}$ given states $Y_1, Y_2 \in \{A, C, G, T\}$ to be

$$P(X|Y_1, Y_2; w_1, w_2, Q_1, Q_2) = Q_1 P(X|Y_1; w_1) + Q_2 P(X|Y_2; w_2) \qquad (5.1)$$

where $P(X|Y_1; w_1)$ and $P(X|Y_2; w_2)$ are given by (4.25), as for a tree, and Q_i, $i \in \{1, 2\}$, denotes the prior probability that the child node X is influenced by the parent in branch i, Y_i. Obviously, these prior probabilities are easily interpreted as recombination parameters: for a sequence of a given length, they denote the proportion of sites stemming from the respective parent. For a derivation of the complete likelihood of a phylogenetic network, see [26]. Note that when the likelihood is known, the inference and model selection algorithms of Chapters 1 and 2 can be applied. This especially implies the

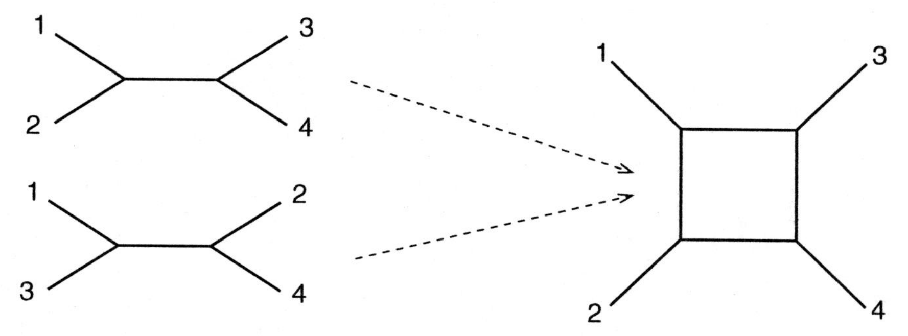

Fig. 5.3. Phylogenetic network. The left part of the figure shows the two phylogenetic trees of Figure 5.1. The right diagram shows a phylogenetic network that resolves the conflicting tree topologies. Strain 1, for instance, is grouped with both strain 2, as in the top tree on the left, and with strain 3, as in the bottom tree on the left.

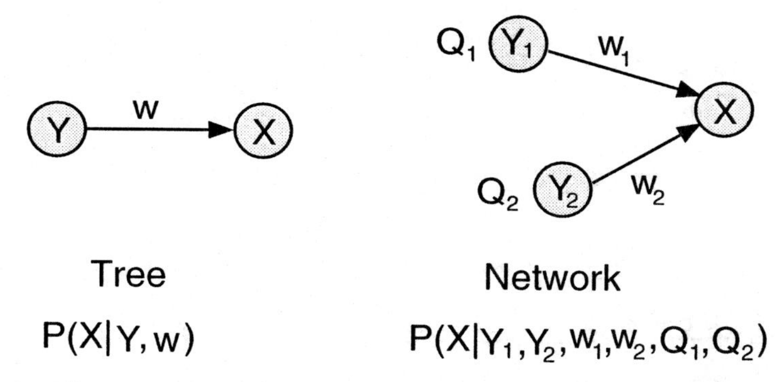

Fig. 5.4. Elementary components of a phylogenetic network. In a phylogenetic tree, each node has at most one parent, while in a phylogenetic network, a node can have more than one parent. The figure is an illustration for equation (5.1). See text for details.

test of the hypothesis that a phylogenetic network offers a significantly better description of the data than a bifurcating tree.

Shortcomings of phylogenetic networks

While a reticulated structure that strongly deviates from a tree indicates the presence of recombination, it does not easily allow the location of the recombinant regions in the sequence alignment. The methods described in the remainder of this chapter address this shortcoming and aim to detect the mosaic structure of a sequence alignment, that is, to locate the breakpoints and determine the nature of the sequence blocks that result from recombination.

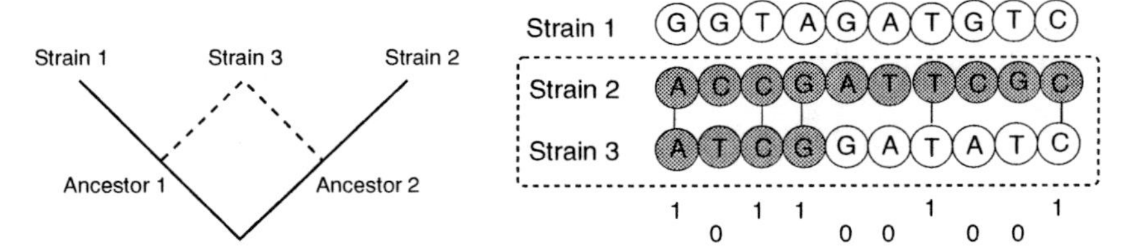

Fig. 5.5. Illustration of the maximum chi-squared method. The tree on the *left* depicts a hypothetical recombination scenario. Two contemporary taxa, strains 1 and 2, are derived from their respective ancestors without recombination. A third sequence, strain 3, results from a recombination event in which subsequences are transferred or exchanged between ancestors 1 and 2. The figure on the *right* shows the resulting sequence alignment, where the different shades pertain to the different lineages of the tree on the left. Strain 3 is a mosaic sequence, whose right subsequence is derived from ancestor 1, and whose left subsequence is derived from ancestor 2. When strains 2 and 3 are compared, the distribution of varying sites, symbolized by zeros, is inhomogeneous, with a higher concentration of zeros in the right than in the left block.

5.4 Maximum Chi-squared

One of the first methods to both detect the presence of recombination and find the location of the recombinant regions was proposed by John Maynard Smith [17]. His approach, the maximum chi-squared test, is illustrated in Figure 5.5. The tree on the *left* depicts a hypothetical recombination scenario. Two contemporary taxa, strains 1 and 2, are derived from their respective ancestors without recombination, that is, the difference between the ancestral and contemporary sequences is solely due to nucleotide substitutions. A third sequence, strain 3, results from a recombination event in which subsequences are transferred or exchanged between ancestors 1 and 2. The figure on the *right* shows a possible sequence alignment. Strain 3 is a mosaic. Its right subsequence is derived from ancestor 1; hence it is more similar to sequence 1. Its left subsequence is derived from ancestor 2; hence it is more similar to sequence 2. Suppose we compare sequences 2 and 3. We will find identical sites, represented by 1's in Figure 5.5, and varying or *polymorphic* sites, represented by 0's. Assume, for the moment, that nucleotide substitution rates do not vary. In the absence of recombination, we would expect the 0's and 1's to be homogeneously distributed across the alignment. However, when a recombination event has occurred, we expect to find different blocks with different distributions. For example, in Figure 5.5, we expect the average number of 0's to be smaller in the left block than in the right. To formalize this notion, suppose that on comparing two sequences of length N we find D polymorphic sites. We introduce an arbitrary breakpoint at position t, which leaves a block of t sites on the left, of which $x_1(t)$ are found to be polymorphic, and a block of $N-t$ sites on the right, of which $x_2(t)$ are polymorphic. Obviously, $x_1(t)+x_2(t)=D$. Define $e_1(t)$ and $e_2(t)$ to be the expectation values of $x_1(t)$

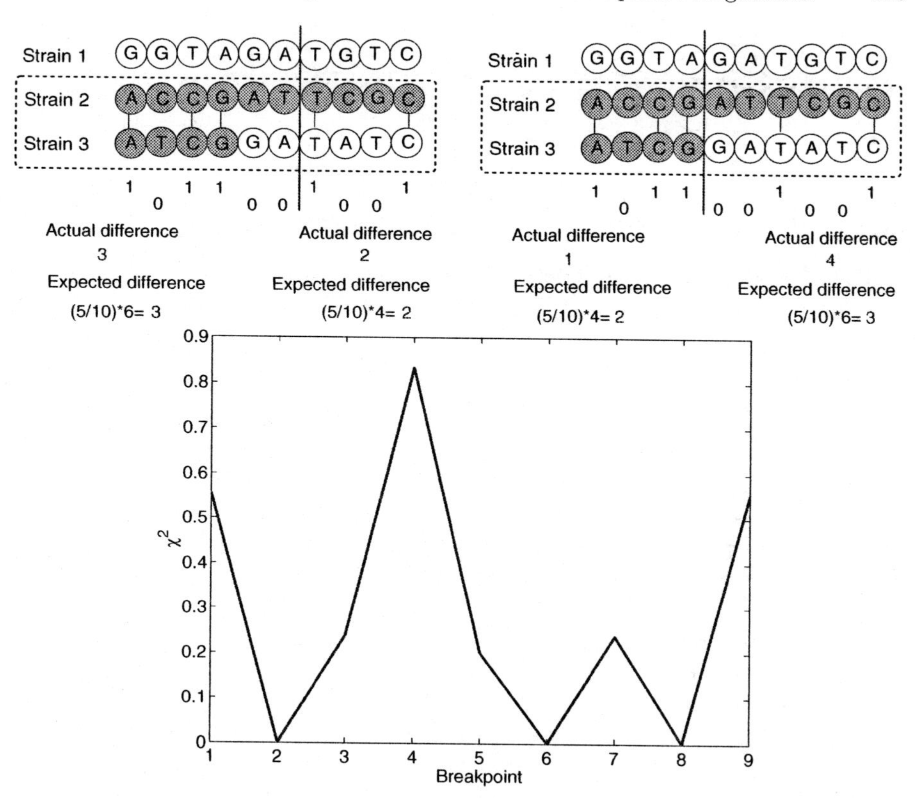

Fig. 5.6. Illustration of the maximum chi-squared method. The two subfigures in the top show a sequence alignment of three taxa, of which two are selected for comparison. The different shades of the circles represent different lineages; compare with Figure 5.5, left. The *top left* subfigure shows a breakpoint for which the chi-squared statistic is $\chi^2(t) = 0$. The *top right* subfigure shows the location of the true breakpoint. The value of the chi-squared statistic is $\chi^2(t) = 5/6$. The subfigure in the bottom shows a plot of $\chi^2(t)$ against all possible breakpoint positions t. Note that this statistic has its maximum at the true breakpoint: $t^* = 4$.

and $x_2(t)$ under the null hypothesis of no recombination, that is, $e_1(t) = \frac{D}{N}t$ and $e_2(t) = \frac{D}{N}(N - t)$. To measure the deviation of the observed from the expected number of polymorphic sites, we compute the chi-squared statistic:

$$\chi^2(t) = \frac{\left[x_1(t) - e_1(t)\right]^2}{e_1(t)} + \frac{\left[x_2(t) - e_2(t)\right]^2}{e_2(t)} \tag{5.2}$$

We then find the breakpoint t^* for which the value of $\chi^2(t)$ is maximal:

$$t^* = \operatorname{argmax}\left\{\chi^2(t)\right\}, \qquad \chi^2 = \max\left\{\chi^2(t)\right\} = \chi^2(t^*) \tag{5.3}$$

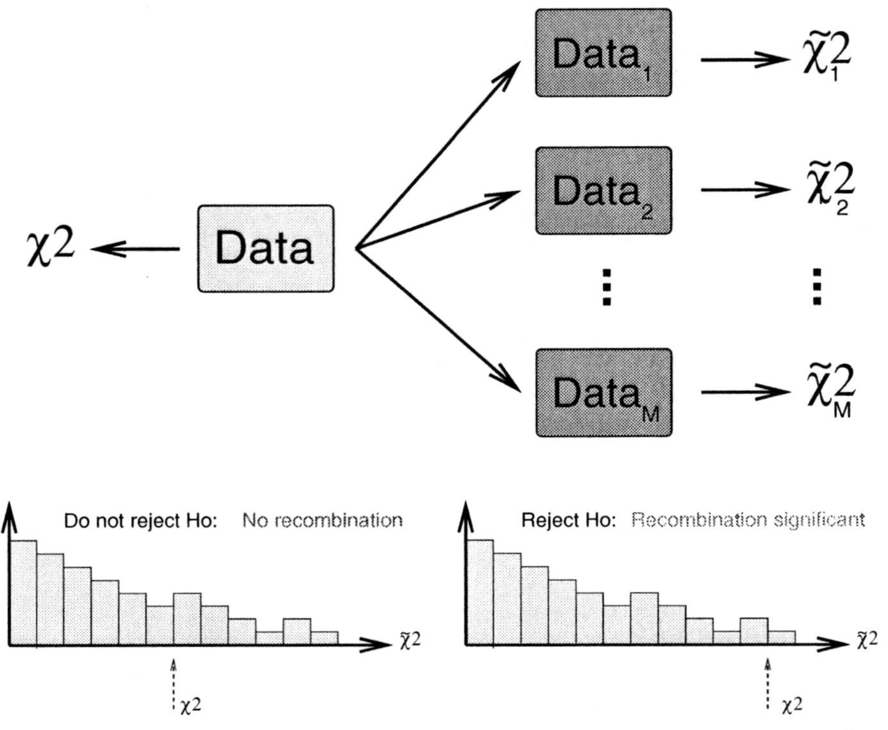

Fig. 5.7. Randomization test. *Top:* The maximum chi-squared statistic, χ^2, is computed from the original data, and for M exemplars of randomized data. This application to the randomized data leads to the sample $\{\tilde{\chi}_1^2, \ldots, \tilde{\chi}_M^2\}$. *Bottom:* The distribution of $\tilde{\chi}^2$ obtained from the randomized data is the empirical distribution of χ^2 under the null hypothesis H_0 that no recombination has occurred. The subfigure in the *bottom left* shows a scenario where the probability of the event $\tilde{\chi}^2 > \chi^2$ is rather large, suggesting that the observed value χ^2 could have occurred by chance and that the detected recombination event is not significant. Conversely, for the subfigure in the *bottom right*, the probability of the event $\tilde{\chi}^2 > \chi^2$ is small, which suggests that a maximum chi-squared value as large as χ^2 is unlikely to have occurred by chance. Consequently, the null hypothesis H_0 is rejected, and the recombination event is found to be significant.

This location is the best candidate for a recombinant breakpoint. An illustration is given in Figure 5.6. The top left subfigure shows an arbitrary breakpoint, $t = 6$, for which we get: $x_1(t) = 3$, $x_2(t) = 2$, $e_1(t) = 3$, $e_2(t) = 2$, and $\chi^2(t) = \frac{(3-3)^2}{3} + \frac{(2-2)^2}{2} = 0$. The top right subfigure shows the correct breakpoint, $t = 4$, which gives: $x_1(t) = 1$, $x_2(t) = 4$, $e_1(t) = 2$, $e_2(t) = 3$, and $\chi^2(t) = \frac{(1-2)^2}{2} + \frac{(4-3)^2}{3} = \frac{5}{6}$. The bottom figure shows a plot of $\chi^2(t)$ for all possible breakpoints t. Note that this statistic has its maximum at the true breakpoint: $t^* = 4$.

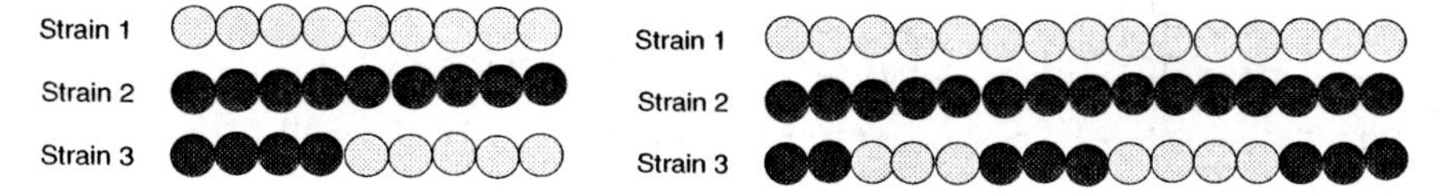

Fig. 5.8. Shortcoming of the chi-squared method. The figure shows two sequence alignments, where the colours of the circles pertain to different lineages of the tree in Figure 5.5. *Left:* Alignment in the two-block structure, where the application of the chi-squared method is straightforward. *Right:* A recombinant block in the middle of the alignment requires the data to be split into smaller subsets and each region to be analyzed separately.

Next, we have to test whether the deviation from the homogeneous distribution is significant, that is, whether the maximum value of $\chi^2(t)$ is greater than what one would expect to obtain by chance. Under the null hypothesis that no recombination event has occurred, χ^2 is asymptotically chi-squared distributed [9]. Unfortunately, however, most alignments are not sufficiently long for this asymptotic result to hold, and a test based on the chi-squared statistic would therefore be unreliable. To overcome the restrictions of asymptotic methods, a randomization test can be used, as illustrated in Figure 5.7. The objective is to simulate the distribution of χ^2 under the null hypothesis that no recombination event has occurred. To this end, the columns in the original sequence alignment, $\mathcal{D}$, are permuted randomly so as to destroy any order. For each of these randomized data sets, $\tilde{\mathcal{D}}_1, \dots, \tilde{\mathcal{D}}_M$, the maximum chi-squared value $\tilde{\chi}_i^2$, $i \in \{1, \dots, M\}$, is found. Define $m = \left|\{i|\tilde{\chi}_i^2 > \chi^2\}\right|$ to be the number of times we observe that $\tilde{\chi}_i^2 > \chi^2$. The empirical probability of this event, that is, the empirical *p-value*, is given by $p = \frac{m}{M}$. When this *p-value* is small, say less than 0.05 or 0.01, a chi-squared value as large as the observed one, χ^2, is unlikely to have occurred by chance. We would therefore reject the null hypothesis and accept the detected recombination as *significant*. Otherwise, there is not enough evidence in the data to reject the null hypothesis, and we would decide that the detected recombination event is *not significant*.

Shortcomings of the maximum chi-squared method

The maximum chi-squared method has several limitations. First, the alignment must be in the two-block form of Figure 5.8, left. When a recombination event occurs in the middle of a sequence alignment, as in Figure 5.8, right, then the maximum chi-squared method may fail to find the recombination event. It is possible to split the data up into smaller subsets, but this is tedious and requires some prior knowledge about the locations of putative recombinant regions.

The second limitation concerns rate heterogeneity, as discussed in Section 4.4.9. Suppose we have a sequence alignment of two sequences, where the nucleotide substitution rate in the left region is considerably higher than in the right region. Consequently, the distribution of polymorphic sites will not be homogeneous across the alignment, but we will rather get two different distributions: a low concentration of polymorphic sites on the right of the breakpoint, and a high concentration in the region to the left of the breakpoint. The chi-squared method, as described above, will only look for a breakpoint that separates two significantly different distributions, and it can therefore *not* distinguish between recombination and rate heterogeneity.

To remedy this shortcoming, Maynard Smith [17] suggested the following procedure. First, select an alignment of three sequences such that it contains the putative mosaic strain and both parental sequences. Here, parental sequences denote sequences in the lineage of the strains that were involved in the recombination event. An illustration is given in Figure 5.5. Next, keep only the *polymorphic sites*, where a polymorphic site in this context is defined as a site that varies within this set of three strains. Finally, select the putative mosaic sequence and one of the two parental sequences, and apply the chi-squared method as described above. This procedure ensures that the proportion of polymorphic sites no longer varies. Consequently, blocks and breakpoints that are caused by rate heterogeneity rather than recombination will effectively be suppressed. This remedy, however, suffers from two new problems. First, we need to know and have at our disposal both parental sequences of a given putative mosaic strain. Second, by discarding all but the polymorphic sites, we do not make the most efficient use of the information contained in the sequences. As a consequence, a recombinant breakpoint can only be located within the set of nucleotides lying between two polymorphic sites. At the heart of these problems is the fact that the maximum chi-squared method does not make use of explicit phylogenetic information, that is, it does not invoke a phylogenetic tree inferred from (subregions of) the sequence alignment. We will therefore look, in the forthcoming sections, at methods that do take this information into account.

5.5 PLATO

PLATO, an acronym for *Partial Likelihoods Assessed Through Optimization*, was introduced by Grassly and Holmes [6] and is illustrated in Figure 5.9. Suppose we know the predominant phylogenetic tree, that is, the tree that we would obtain if no recombination event had occurred. Also, recall from Section 4.4.3 and Figure 4.24 that we can compute, for a given tree, the probability for each column in the alignment. We can therefore systematically look for subsets with a low likelihood under the given tree model by computing the statistic

$$Q = \frac{\frac{1}{W+1}\sum_{t=b-W/2}^{b+W/2} L_t}{\frac{1}{N-W-1}\left(\sum_{t=1}^{b-W/2-1} L_t + \sum_{t=b+W/2+1}^{N} L_t\right)} \tag{5.4}$$

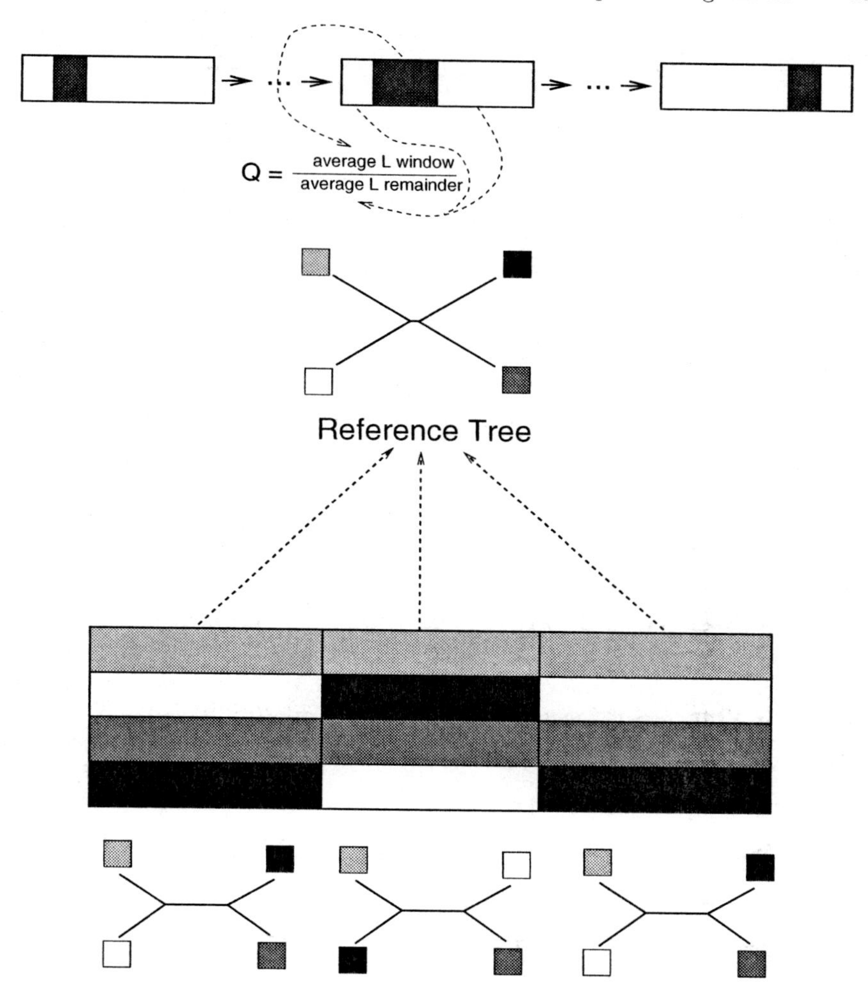

Fig. 5.9. Illustration of PLATO. A window of varying size is moved along the DNA sequence alignment. The average log likelihood is computed for both the window and the remainder of the sequence, and the Q-statistic is defined as the ratio of these values (top). If the reference model, from which the log likelihood scores are computed, were the predominant tree (meaning the tree one would obtain if no recombination event had occurred), large Q values would be a reliable indication for recombinant regions. However, the predominant tree is not known, and is approximated by a tree estimated from the whole sequence alignment. This includes the recombinant regions, which perturb the parameter estimation for the reference tree (bottom) and thus cause the test to lose power. Reprinted from [11], by permission of Oxford University Press.

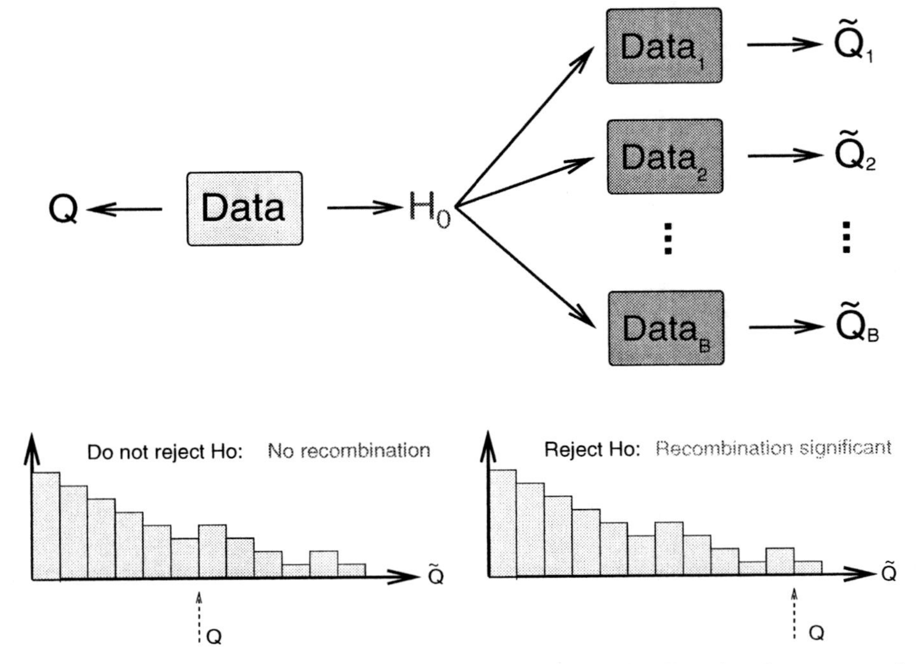

Fig. 5.10. Parametric bootstrapping and PLATO. *Top:* A reference tree is estimated from the original sequence alignment, Data. From this reference tree, the maximum Q-statistic is obtained. Then, an ensemble of new alignments is generated from the reference tree, that is, under the null hypothesis H_0 that no recombination has occurred. For each of these bootstrap replicas, $\{\mathsf{Data}_1, \ldots, \mathsf{Data}_B\}$, the process of finding the maximum Q-statistic is repeated. This gives an empirical distribution of the maximum Q-statistic under the null hypothesis of no recombination, $\{\tilde{Q}_1, \ldots, \tilde{Q}_B\}$. Based on a comparison of Q with this null distribution, the hypothesis of recombination is either rejected or accepted. Compare with Figure 5.7.

where L_t denotes the log likelihood of the tth column vector in the alignment, W is the size of the subset, and N is the length of the alignment (see Figure 5.9, top). This measure is calculated for all possible positions b along the sequence alignment and for varying subset sizes, typically $5 \leq W < N/2$. If the sequence alignment is homogeneous, the numerator and denominator in (5.4) can be expected to be similar in size, and Q tends to be close to 1. However, when a recombination event has occurred, as illustrated in the bottom of Figure 5.9, the average log likelihood for the recombinant region can be expected to be considerably smaller than for the non-recombinant regions. Since log likelihood scores are negative values, the respective value for the Q statistic will therefore be large. Consequently, we can identify putative recombinant regions by looking for regions with significantly increased Q values. To allow for rate heterogeneity, the likelihood scores are computed under a rate variation model, as described in Section 4.4.9. Parametric bootstrapping, illustrated in Figure 5.10, is applied to generate the null distribution of the maximized Q value under the null hypothesis of no recombination and thereby to decide whether the maximum Q value obtained from the original alignment is significantly larger than what could be obtained by chance.

Shortcomings of PLATO

If the reference model, from which the log likelihood scores are computed, were the predominant tree (meaning the tree one would obtain if no recombination event had happened), significantly large Q values would be a reliable indication for recombinant regions. However, the predominant tree is not known and is approximated by a tree estimated from the whole sequence alignment. This includes the recombinant regions, which perturb the parameter estimation for the reference tree (see Figure 5.9, bottom). Consequently, the method becomes increasingly unreliable as the recombinant regions grow in length.

5.6 TOPAL

TOPAL [19], [18], illustrated in Figure 5.11, replaces the global by a local reference tree. A window of typically 200–500 bases is slid along the DNA sequence alignment. The reference tree is estimated from the left half of the window and used to compute a goodness-of-fit score for both parts of the window. The difference between these goodness-of-fit scores, the so-called DSS statistic, is likely to be small within a homogeneous part of the alignment, but large as the window is moved into a recombinant region. Parametric bootstrapping, illustrated in Figure 5.10, is applied to compute a distribution of DSS peaks under the null hypothesis of no recombination, and significantly large DSS peaks are indicators of putative recombinant breakpoints.

The DSS statistic

Ideally, the reference tree would be obtained with maximum likelihood, as discussed in Section 4.4. In order to reduce the computational costs, TOPAL uses a distance method. From each of the two sub-alignments selected by the two halves of the window, a distance matrix is calculated, as described in Section 4.2. Denote by $\{d_i\}$ the set of pairwise distances obtained from the left half of the window, and by $\{\tilde{d}_i\}$ the set of pairwise distances obtained from the right half. From the first set of pairwise distances, $\{d_i\}$, a phylogenetic reference tree is obtained, either with the neighbour joining algorithm, described in Section 4.2, or with the Fitch–Margoliash optimization algorithm [4]. Denote by $\{e_i\}$ the set of pairwise distances obtained from this reference tree. The goodness of fit scores for the two window halves, SS_l and SS_r, are given by

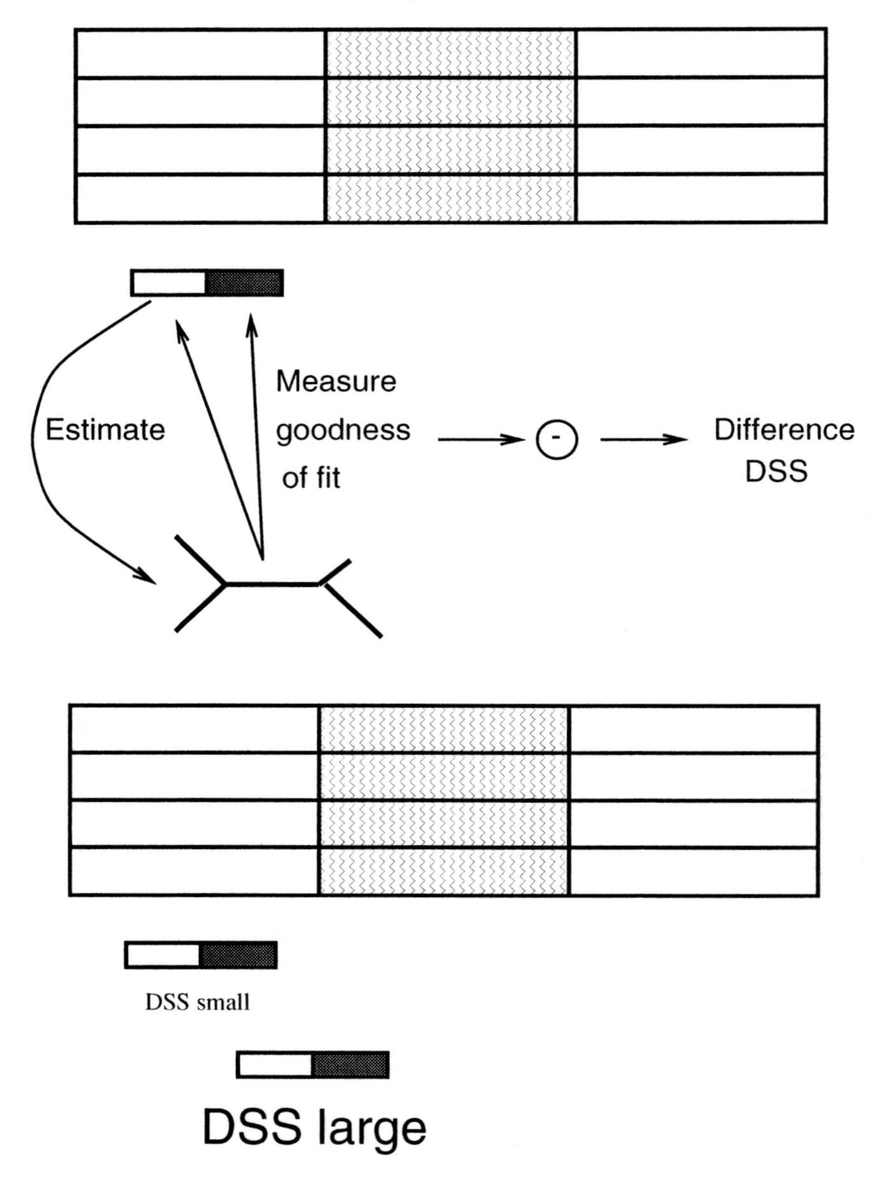

Fig. 5.11. Illustration of TOPAL. A window is moved along the DNA sequence alignment. A tree is estimated from the left part of the window, and a goodness-of-fit score is computed for both parts of the window. The DSS statistic is defined as the difference between these scores. When the window is centred on or near the breakpoint of a recombinant region, the tree estimated from the left subwindow is not an adequate description for the data on the right, which leads to a large DSS value. Reprinted from [11], by permission of Oxford University Press.

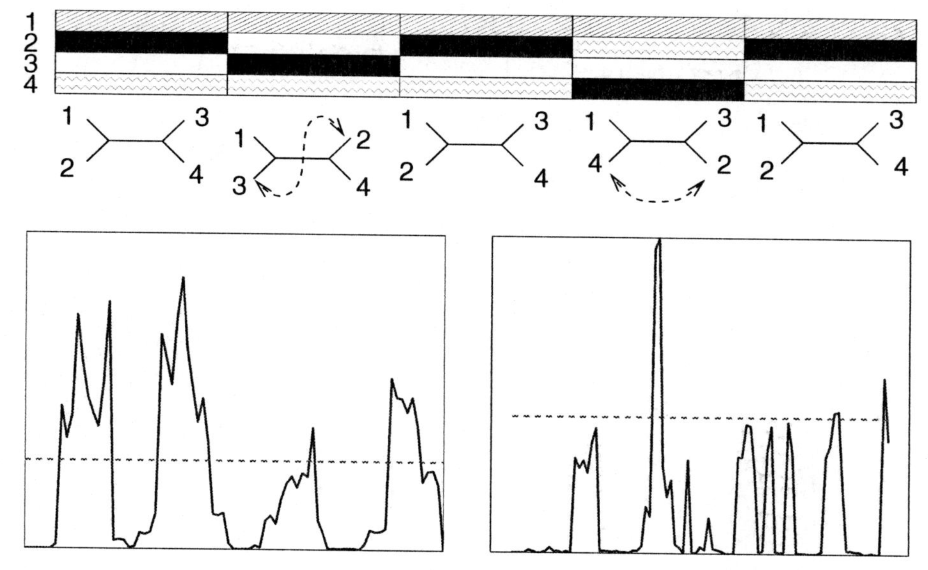

Fig. 5.12. Dependence of TOPAL on the window size. *Top:* Synthetic DNA sequences are obtained by simulating their evolution down a known phylogenetic tree, using the Kimura model of nucleotide substitution (4.16), as described in Section 4.4. Two recombination events are simulated by exchanging the indicated lineages. *Bottom left:* Application of TOPAL with a window size of 200 nucleotides. The solid line shows the DSS statistic (5.6) plotted against the sites in the DNA sequence alignment. The dashed line indicates the 95-percentile under the null hypothesis of no recombination, obtained with parametric bootstrapping. All four breakpoints of the recombinant regions are detected. The spatial resolution is of the order of the window size. *Bottom right:* Application of TOPAL with a window size of 100 nucleotides. The power of the detection method has significantly deteriorated, and only one of the four breakpoints is properly detected. Reprinted from [10], by permission of Oxford University Press.

$$SS_l = \sum_i (d_i - e_i)^2, \qquad SS_r = \sum_i (\tilde{d}_i - e_i)^2 \tag{5.5}$$

and the DSS statistic is given by the difference of these scores:

$$DSS = |SS_r - SS_l| \tag{5.6}$$

For a homogeneous sequence alignment, $SS_r \approx SS_l$, and DSS will be small. When the tree topology in the right part of the window has changed as a consequence of recombination, the tree estimated from the left subwindow is not an adequate model for the data on the right. Consequently, $SS_r \gg SS_l$, and DSS will be large. This is illustrated in Figure 5.11. However, when the effective branch lengths vary as a consequence of rate variation – discussed in Section 4.4.9 – the ensuing mismatch of the trees will also cause $SS_r \gg SS_l$, and thus DSS to become large. The method described above, therefore, cannot distinguish between recombination and rate variation. To redeem this shortcoming, a revised version of TOPAL [18] normalizes the pairwise distances prior to computing the DSS statistic. Denote by $\overline{D}$ the average pairwise distance obtained from the whole sequence alignment, and by $\overline{d}$ the average pairwise distance obtained from a given window. Then, all pairwise distances obtained from this window are rescaled:

$$d_i \rightarrow \frac{\overline{D}}{\overline{d}} d_i \tag{5.7}$$

This rescaling corrects for the effects of rate variation, and large DSS values can therefore be assumed to be indicative of real recombination events.

Shortcomings of TOPAL

By using a local rather than a global reference tree, TOPAL overcomes the inherent shortcoming of PLATO. However, the spatial resolution for the identification of the breakpoints is typically of the order of the window size and, consequently, rather poor. Figure 5.12 demonstrates that the spatial resolution cannot be improved by just selecting a smaller window: this renders the reference tree unreliable, and the detection method thus loses power and becomes unreliable. The problems associated with estimating a reference tree from a small subset of the sequence alignment is aggravated by the fact that TOPAL uses a distance-based rather than a likelihood-based estimation approach. As discussed in Section 4.2 and illustrated in Figure 4.13, this leads to an inevitable loss of information. Also, when estimating a reference tree from a short sequence alignment, this estimation is subject to intrinsic uncertainty, which is not captured by TOPAL.

5.7 Probabilistic Divergence Method (PDM)

Husmeier and Wright [13] introduced a method that is akin to TOPAL, but addresses some of its shortcomings. First, by using a likelihood score, the intrinsic information loss associated with a score based on pairwise distances is prevented. Second, a single optimized reference tree is replaced by a distribution over trees, which captures the intrinsic uncertainty of tree estimation from short sequence alignments. Third, the method focuses on topology changes, thereby overcoming possible difficulties with the distance rescaling scheme described above. An illustration of the concepts is given in Figures 5.13–5.15. For a formal introduction, consider a given alignment of DNA sequences, $\mathcal{D}$, from which we select a consecutive subset $\mathcal{D}_t$ of predefined width W, centred on the tth site of the alignment. Let S be an integer label for tree topologies, and define

$$P_S(t) := P(S|\mathcal{D}_t) = \int\int P(S, \mathbf{w}, \boldsymbol{\theta}|\mathcal{D}_t) d\mathbf{w} d\boldsymbol{\theta} \tag{5.8}$$

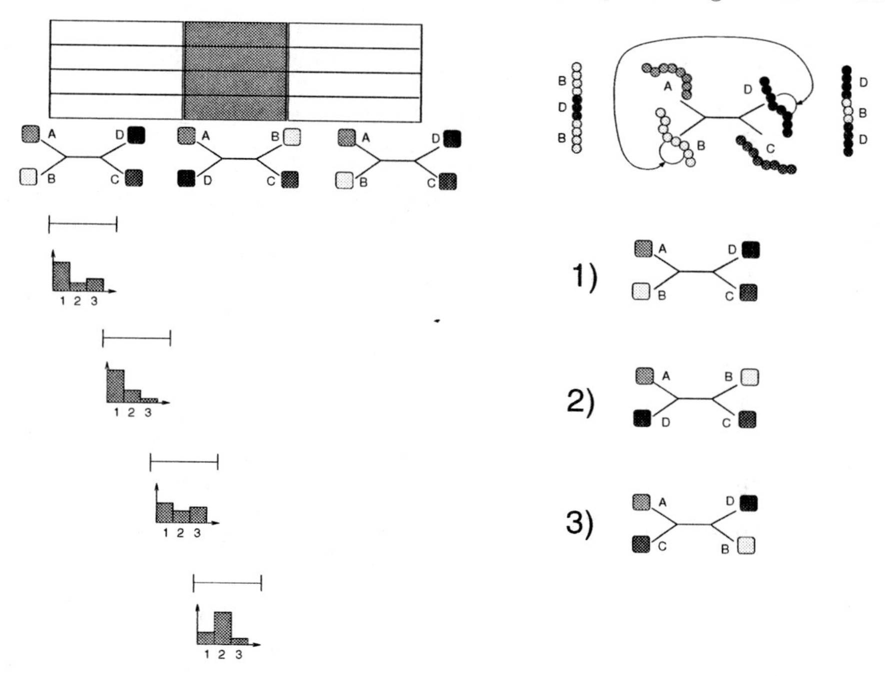

Fig. 5.13. Illustration of the probabilistic divergence method (PDM). The *top right* subfigure shows a recombination scenario in a four-species tree similar to Figure 5.1. The *top left* subfigure shows the resulting sequence alignment, where the tree topology in the centre block is different from the topology in the flanking regions as a consequence of recombination. The subfigure in the *bottom right* shows the three possible tree topologies. The *bottom left* subfigure shows the posterior distribution over tree topologies conditional on different subregions of the alignment, selected by a moving window. Obviously, when moving the window into a region that corresponds to a different tree topology, the posterior distribution usually changes markedly.

This is the marginal posterior probability of tree topologies S, conditional on the "window" $\mathcal{D}_t$, which includes a marginalization over the branch lengths $\mathbf{w}$ and the parameters of the nucleotide substitution model, $\boldsymbol{\theta}$ – see Section 4.4 for a revision of these concepts. In practice the integral in (5.8) is solved numerically by means of a Markov chain Monte Carlo (MCMC) simulation, as discussed in Section 4.4.7 and illustrated in Figures 4.33 and 4.34. This MCMC simulation yields a sample of triples $\{S_{ti}, \mathbf{w}_{ti}, \boldsymbol{\theta}_{ti}\}_{i=1}^{M}$ simulated from the joint posterior distribution $P(S, \mathbf{w}, \boldsymbol{\theta}|\mathcal{D}_t)$. We then replace the true posterior distribution by the empirical distribution

$$P(S, \mathbf{w}, \boldsymbol{\theta}|\mathcal{D}_t) \approx \frac{1}{M}\sum_{i=1}^{M} \delta_{S,S_{ti}}\delta(\mathbf{w}-\mathbf{w}_{ti})\delta(\boldsymbol{\theta}-\boldsymbol{\theta}_{ti}) \qquad (5.9)$$

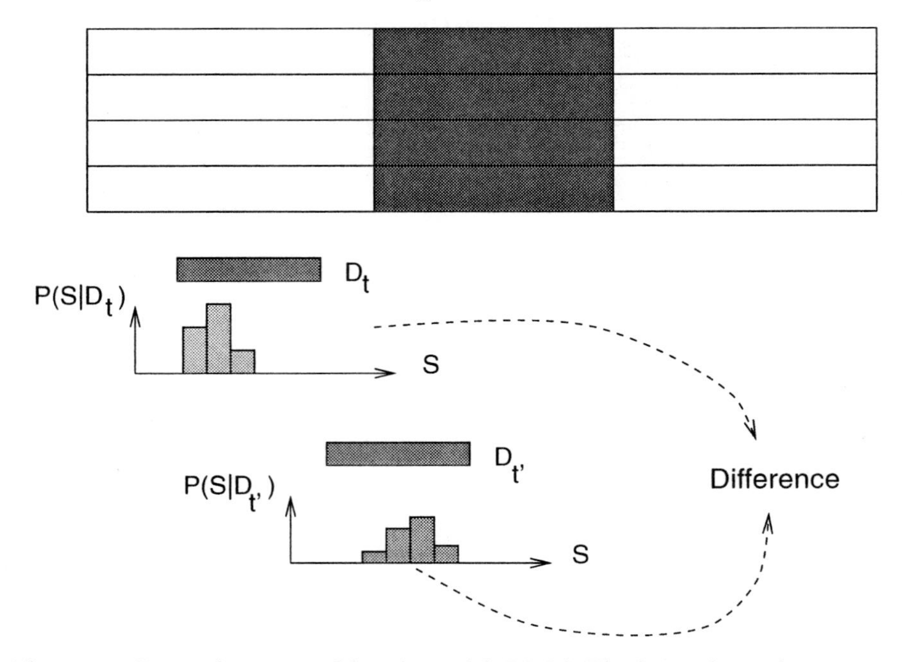

Fig. 5.14. Detecting recombination with PDM. The figure shows the posterior probability $P(S|D_t)$ of tree topologies S conditional on two subsets D_t and $D_{t'}$ selected by a moving window. When the window is moved into a recombinant region, the posterior distribution $P(S|D_t)$ can be expected to change significantly, and therefore to lead to a high PDM score.

where $\delta_{S,S_{ti}}$ denotes the Kronecker delta symbol, and $\delta(.)$ is the delta function.[3] Inserting (5.9) into (5.8) gives:

$$P_S(t) = \frac{1}{M}\sum_{i=1}^{M} \delta_{S,S_{ti}} = \frac{M_S(t)}{M} \tag{5.10}$$

where $M_S(t)$ denotes the number of times a tree has been found to have topology S.

The basic idea of the probabilistic divergence method (PDM) for detecting recombinant regions is to move the window $\mathcal{D}_t$ along the alignment and to monitor the distribution $P_S(t)$. We would then, obviously, expect a substantial change in the shape of this distribution as we move the window into a recombinant region, as illustrated in Figures 5.13 and 5.14. The question, then, is how to easily monitor such a change and how to estimate its significance. To this end we consider the Kullback-Leibler divergence (2.49) as the natural distance measure in probability space:

[3] Recall that $\delta(0) = \infty$, $\delta(x) = 0$ if $x \neq 0$, and $\int_{-\infty}^{\infty} \delta(x)dx = 1$.

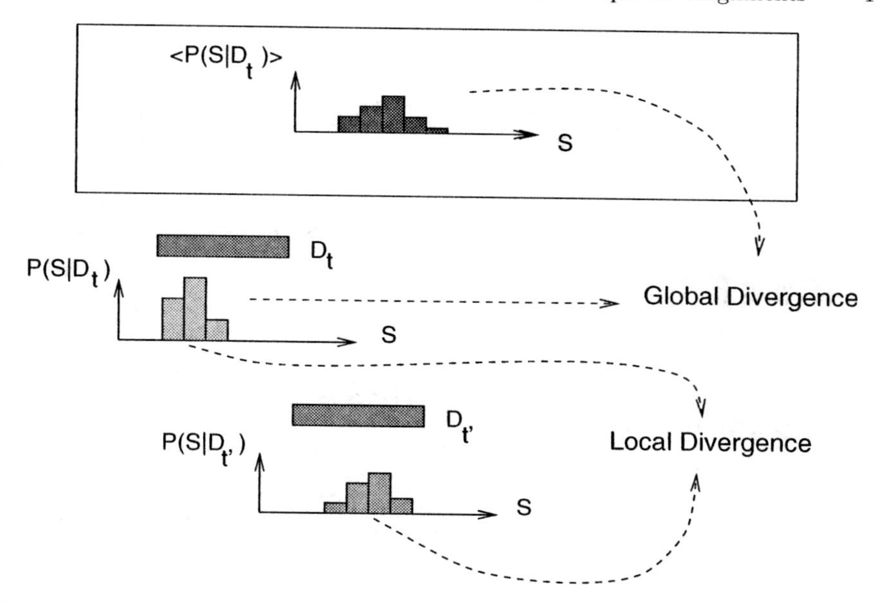

Fig. 5.15. Global and local PDM. The figure shows the posterior probability $P(S|D_t)$ of tree topologies S conditional on two subsets D_t and $D_{t'}$ selected by a moving window. The *local PDM* compares two distributions conditional on adjacent windows. This measure is a local divergence score. Alternatively, one can first obtain a reference distribution $\langle P(S|D_t) \rangle$ by averaging $P(S|D_t)$ over all window positions, and then compute a *global PDM* between $\langle P(S|D_t) \rangle$ and each local distribution $P(S|D_t)$.

$$K(P,Q) = \sum_S P_S \log \left(\frac{P_S}{Q_S} \right) \tag{5.11}$$

in which P and Q denote probability distributions. Recall from the discussion after (2.49) that $K(P,Q)$ is always non-negative, and zero if and only if $P = Q$. To estimate the divergence between the local and the global distribution, define P as in (5.10) and Q as the average distribution:

$$d[P(t), \overline{P}] = K[P(t), \overline{P}]; \qquad \overline{P}_S = \frac{1}{M_w} \sum_{t=1}^{M_w} P_S(t) \tag{5.12}$$

where M_w is the number of different window positions. This divergence score is the *global PDM*. Since Support$(P) \subseteq$ Support$(\overline{P})$, where Support(P) is the set of all topologies S for which $P_S \neq 0$, the non-singularity of the expression on the left-hand side of (5.12) is guaranteed. To determine the divergence between two local distributions $P(t)$ and $P(t + \Delta t)$ – conditional on two adjacent windows with centre positions t and $t + \Delta t$ – a slightly modified divergence measure[4] is used:

$$d[P(t), P(t+\Delta t)] = \qquad (5.13)$$
$$\frac{1}{2}\left[K\left(P(t), \frac{P(t)+P(t+\Delta t)}{2}\right) + K\left(P(t+\Delta t), \frac{P(t)+P(t+\Delta t)}{2}\right)\right]$$

Note again that $\text{Support}[P(t)], \text{Support}[P(t+\Delta t)] \subseteq \text{Support}\left[\frac{P(t)+P(t+\Delta t)}{2}\right]$ guarantees the non-singularity of $d[P(t), P(t+\Delta t)]$. To estimate whether the observed divergence measures are significantly different from zero, note that under the null hypothesis of no recombination, $P = Q$, the Kullback-Leibler divergence is asymptotically chi-squared distributed [9]. Denote by $\tilde{M}$ the number of independent samples from which P and Q are determined, and by $\nu = |\text{Support(P)}|$ the cardinality of the support of P. Then, for $P = Q$ and $\tilde{M} \gg \nu$, we have:

$$2\tilde{M}\,K(P,Q) \;\sim\; P\chi^2(\nu - 1) \qquad (5.14)$$

where $P\chi^2(\nu-1)$ denotes the chi-squared distribution with $\nu - 1$ degrees of freedom [9]. Note that consecutive samples of an MCMC simulation are usually not independent, so the observed sample size M has to be replaced by the effective *independent* sample size $\tilde{M}$. For example, if the autocorrelation function is exponential with an autocorrelation time $\tau \gg 1$, then $\tilde{M} = \frac{M}{2\tau}$, as shown in the appendix of [14].

The local PDM (5.13) depends on the distance between two windows, Δt. It seems natural to choose two consecutive windows, as in TOPAL. However, by allowing a certain overlap between the windows the spatial resolution of the detection method can be improved. Husmeier and Wright [13] found that the best results can be obtained by averaging over different degrees of window overlap:

$$\overline{d} \;=\; \frac{1}{A}\sum_{a=1}^{A} d[P(t), P(t+a\Delta t)] \qquad (5.15)$$

where $d(.)$ is defined in (5.13), and the average is over all window overlaps between 50% and 90%.

In summary, the method described above gives us two recombination detection scores: *PDM-global* (5.12) as a global measure akin to PLATO, and *PDM-local* (5.13), (5.15) as a local measure in the vein of TOPAL. An illustration is given in Figure 5.15.

Shortcomings of PDM

Like TOPAL, PDM is a window method. While TOPAL needs a sufficiently large subset to reliably estimate the reference tree, PDM needs a sufficiently

[4] The divergence measure of (5.13) was introduced by Sibson; see, for instance, [15], Chapter 14.

large window to obtain a sufficiently informative posterior distribution over tree topologies. For a small subset $\mathcal{D}_t$, the posterior distribution $P(S|\mathcal{D}_t)$ will be diffuse so that moving the window into a recombinant region, as illustrated in Figure 5.15, will only give a small divergence score, whose deviation from zero may not be significant. In [13], a window of 500 nucleotides was used, and the method was tested on alignments of eight sequences. For larger alignments, a larger window may have to be used, which will obviously compromise the spatial resolution. The simulation study described in the next section demonstrates that PDM clearly outperforms PLATO, and that it achieves a slightly better detection accuracy than TOPAL. This improvement, however, comes at a considerable increase in the computational costs because the fast optimization routines of TOPAL and PLATO have to be replaced by computationally expensive MCMC simulations.

5.8 Empirical Comparison I

Husmeier and Wright [13] carried out a simulation study to evaluate the detection accuracy of PLATO, TOPAL, and PDM. Synthetic DNA sequences were obtained by simulating their evolution down known phylogenetic trees, shown in Figure 5.16, using the Kimura model of nucleotide substitution (4.16), described in Section 4.4. The transition-transversion ratio was set to $\tau = 2$; compare with (4.21). A variety of different recombination scenarios was simulated. In experiment series 1, partial sequences were evolved down different topologies, as indicated in the left of Figure 5.16, and then spliced together. This process reflects the swapping of branches, that is, the *exchange* of DNA subsequences. In experiment series 2, the sequences were simulated along the branches of the phylogenetic tree as far as a particular depth, half the length of the indicated branch. At this point, a region from a sequence replaced the corresponding region in another sequence, as indicated in the right of Figure 5.16. The sequences were then evolved along the remaining part of the phylogeny. This process simulates the *transfer* of genetic material between different strains. In both experiment series, two recombination events of different detection difficulty were simulated, and the process was repeated for different branch lengths. In experiment series 2, a differently diverged region was included, where the branch lengths had effectively been increased by a factor of 3. This inclusion of a differently diverged region tests whether the detection methods can distinguish between rate variation and recombination. Details of the branch lengths and the location of the recombinant regions can be found in the caption of Figure 5.16.

For both TOPAL and PDM, a window of 500 nucleotides was moved along the alignment with a fixed step size of $\Delta t = 10$ nucleotides. For PLATO, the Q-statistic (5.4) was computed for all windows with a length between five nucleotides and half the sequence length. Further details of the application of

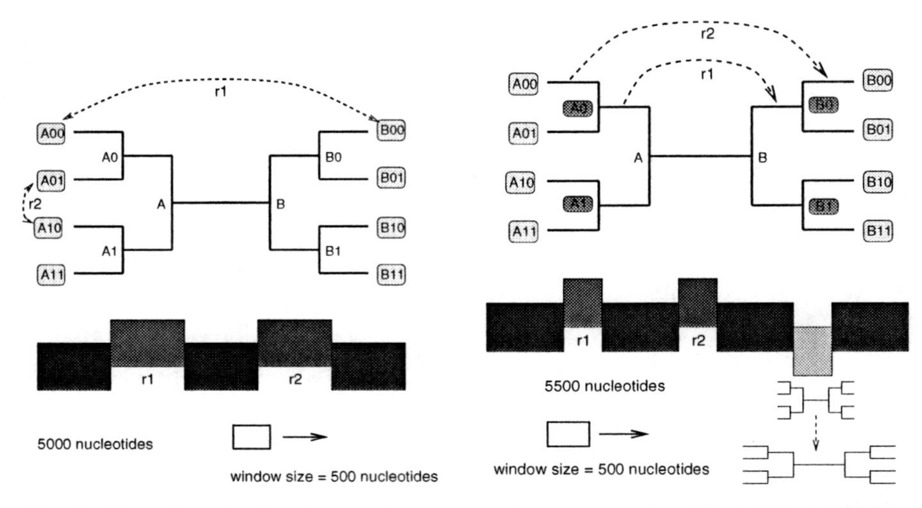

Fig. 5.16. Synthetic simulation study for comparing PLATO, TOPAL, and PDM. The phylogenetic tree on the left (simulation 1) shows two recent recombination events, between closely related taxa ($A01 \leftrightarrow A10$) and between distantly related taxa ($A00 \leftrightarrow B00$), where the indicated lineages are swapped. The phylogenetic tree on the right (simulation 2) shows a recent ($A00 \leftrightarrow B00$) and an ancient ($A0 \leftrightarrow B0$) recombination event between distantly related taxa, where DNA subsequences are transferred at a single point in time, half-way along the branches. The subfigures in the bottom indicate the locations of the recombinant regions in the sequence alignment. In simulation study 1, the total alignment is 5000 nucleotides long, and each recombinant region has a length of 1000 nucleotides. In simulation study 2, the total alignment is 5500 nucleotides long, and each recombinant region has a length of 500 nucleotides. The alignment also contains a differently diverged region of 500 nucleotides, where the effective branch lengths of the tree are increased by a factor of 3. The simulation was carried out for two different settings of branch lengths. *Long branch lengths:* The branch between ancestors A and B has the length $w = 0.2$, and all other branches have the length $w = 0.1$. *Short branch lengths:* The branch between ancestors A and B has the length $w = 0.02$, and all other branches have the length $w = 0.01$.

the methods, including the parameter settings and the software used, can be found in [13].

Figure 5.17 shows the results obtained with the various methods on the first benchmark problem. PLATO detects the first recombinant region, but fails to detect the second. TOPAL detects both recombinant regions when the branch lengths of the phylogenetic tree are large ($w = 0.1$), but fails to detect the second region when the branch lengths are small ($w = 0.01$). PDM detects both recombinant regions for all branch lengths, although the accuracy degrades as the branch lengths decrease. Note that the spatial resolution of the detection with PDM is similar to that with TOPAL, and typically of the

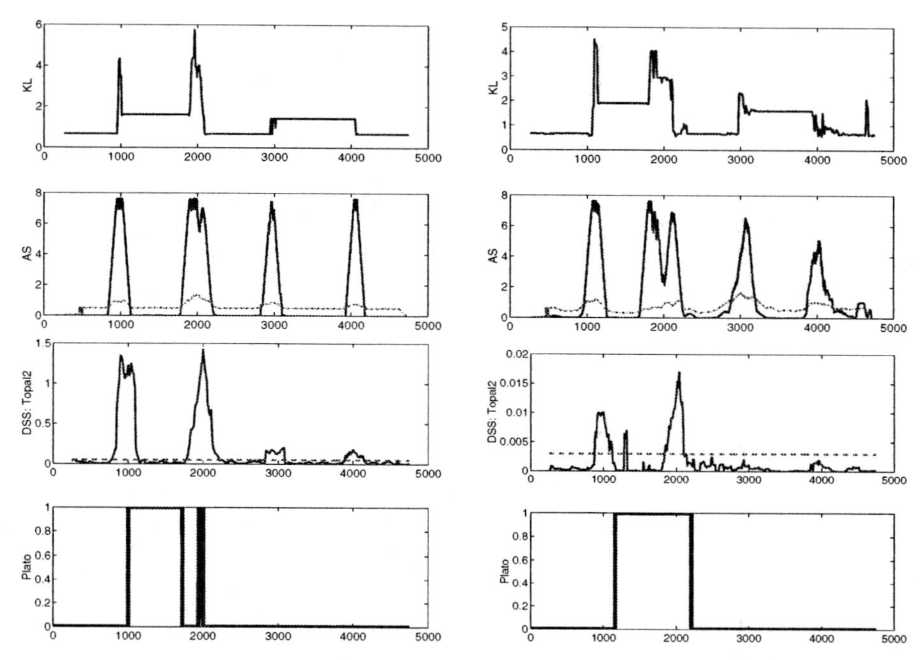

Fig. 5.17. Detection of recombination for the first synthetic problem, experiment series 1, as illustrated on the left of Figure 5.16. *Left column:* Long branch lengths. *Right column:* Small branch lengths. *Top row:* PDM-global (5.12). *2nd row:* PDM-local. The solid line shows the local PDM score (5.15), the dashed line indicates the asymptotic 95-percentile under the null hypothesis of no recombination. *3rd row:* TOPAL. The solid line shows the DSS statistic (5.6), the dashed line indicates the 95-percentile under the null hypothesis of no recombination. *Bottom row:* PLATO. The graph indicates critical regions in the alignment, for which the Q-statistic (5.4) is significantly larger than expected under the null hypothesis of no recombination. 1: critical region. 0: uncritical region. The true recombinant regions are situated between sites 1000 and 2000 (involving distantly related strains) and between sites 3000 and 4000 (involving closely related strains); compare with Figure 5.16, left. In all figures, the horizontal axis represents sites in the DNA sequence alignment. Reprinted from [13], by permission of Oxford University Press.

same size as the discrepancy between the prediction with PLATO and the true location of the recombinant regions.

Figure 5.18 demonstrates the performance of the various methods on the second synthetic problem. The level of difficulty is increased by a shortening of the recombinant blocks and the existence of a confounding region, which has evolved at a higher rate ("mutation hotzone") *without* being subject to recombination. PLATO, in fact, fails to detect the recombinant blocks and gets confounded by this differently diverged region. TOPAL and PDM suc-

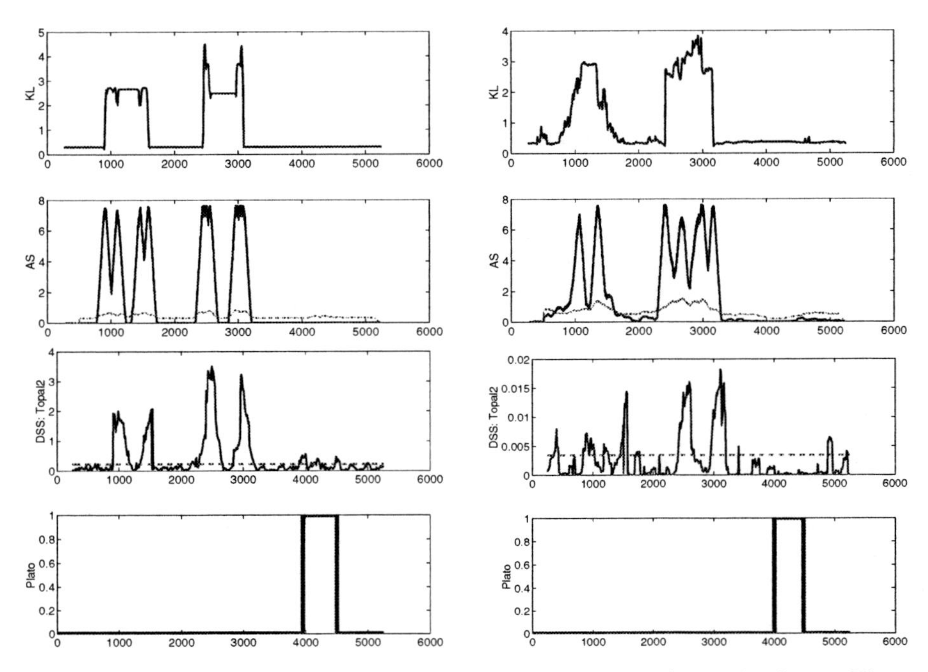

Fig. 5.18. Detection of recombination for the second synthetic problem, experiment series 2, as illustrated on the right of Figure 5.16. The recombinant regions are located between sites 1000 and 1500 (ancient recombination event) and between sites 2500 and 3000 (recent recombination event). The region between sites 4000 and 4500 has diverged at an increased evolution rate (factor 3) without being subject to recombination. Compare with Figure 5.16, right. The graphs are explained in the caption of Figure 5.17. Reprinted from [13], by permission of Oxford University Press.

ceed in distinguishing between recombination and rate variation.[5] However, TOPAL does not properly detect the first (ancient, and therefore more hidden) recombination event when the branch lengths of the phylogenetic tree are small. PDM, on the contrary, detects both recombination events irrespective of the branch lengths. The spatial resolution, however, deteriorates as the branch lengths decrease.

5.9 RECPARS

As discussed in the previous sections, window methods are inherently limited in the spatial resolution with which the breakpoints of recombinant regions

[5] In [13], one exception is reported, where TOPAL mistakes a differently diverged region for a recombinant region.

can be detected. A different approach, which does not resort to the use of a window, was proposed by Hein [8]. The idea is to introduce a hidden state S_t that represents the tree topology at a given site t in the DNA sequence alignment. A state transition from one topology into another corresponds to a recombination event. To model correlations between adjacent sites, a site graph is introduced, representing which nucleotides interact in determining the tree topology. Thus, the standard phylogenetic model of a tree, discussed in Chapter 4, is generalized by the combination of two graphical models: (1) a taxon graph (phylogenetic tree) representing the relationships between the taxa, and (2) a site graph representing interactions between the site-dependent hidden states. To keep the mathematical model tractable and the computational costs limited, the latter are reduced to nearest-neighbour interactions; compare with the discussion in Section 2.3.4. Breakpoints of mosaic segments correspond to state transitions in the optimal hidden state sequence. Hein [8] defined optimality in a parsimony sense. His algorithm, RECPARS, searches for the most parsimonious state sequence[6] $\mathcal{S} = (S_1, \ldots, S_N)$, that is, the one that minimizes a given parsimony cost function $E(\mathcal{S})$. Since the dependence structure between sites is restricted to nearest-neighbour interactions, as discussed above, the search can be carried out in polynomial time with dynamic programming, which is akin to the Viterbi algorithm described in Section 2.3.4.

Shortcomings of RECPARS

While RECPARS is faster than the HMM method described in the next section, it suffers from the shortcomings inherent to parsimony, discussed in Section 4.3. Moreover, $E(\mathcal{S})$ depends only on the topology-defining sites; thus the algorithm discards a substantial amount of information in the alignment. The most serious disadvantage is that the cost function $E(\mathcal{S})$ depends on certain parameters - the mutation cost C_{mut}, and the recombination cost C_{rec} - which can *not* be optimized within the framework of this method. Consequently, these parameters have to be chosen by the user in advance, and the predictions depend on this rather arbitrary prior selection.

5.10 Combining Phylogenetic Trees with HMMs

5.10.1 Introduction

To overcome the shortcomings of RECPARS, discussed in the previous section, McGuire et al. [20] translated the concept of RECPARS into a probabilistic framework. First, the parsimony approach to phylogenetics, discussed in Section 4.3, is replaced by the likelihood method, described in Section 4.4 and

[6] Note the difference in the notation: $\mathcal{S}$ denotes a state sequence, while S or S_t denotes an individual state (associated with site t).

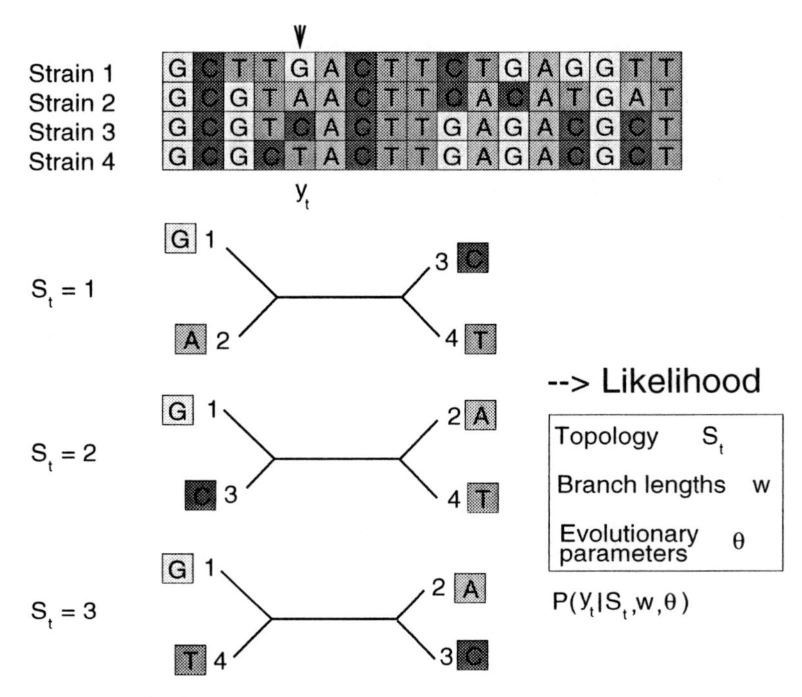

Fig. 5.19. Probabilistic approach to phylogenetics and modelling recombination. For a given column $\mathbf{y}_t$ in the sequence alignment, a probability $P(\mathbf{y}_t|S_t, \mathbf{w}, \boldsymbol{\theta})$ can be computed, which depends on the tree topology S_t, the vector of branch lengths $\mathbf{w}$, and the parameters of the nucleotide substitution model $\boldsymbol{\theta}$. In the presence of recombination, the tree topology can change and thus becomes a random variable that depends on the site label t. For four taxa, there are three different tree topologies. The vectors $\mathbf{w}$ and $\boldsymbol{\theta}$ are accumulated vectors, as defined in the paragraph above equation (5.17). Reprinted from [11], by permission of Oxford University Press.

illustrated in Figure 5.19. Second, the recombination cost in RECPARS is replaced by a recombination probability, illustrated in Figure 5.20, which turns the hidden state graph of RECPARS into a hidden Markov model; see Section 2.3.4. Figure 5.21, left, shows the corresponding Bayesian network. White nodes represent hidden states, S_t, which have direct interactions only with the states at adjacent sites, S_{t-1} and S_{t+1}. Black nodes represent columns in the DNA sequence alignment, $\mathbf{y}_t$. The squares represent the model parameters, which are the branch lengths of the phylogenetic trees, $\mathbf{w}$, the parameters of the nucleotide substitution model, $\boldsymbol{\theta}$, and the recombination parameter, ν; see Figures 5.19 and 5.20. The joint probability of the DNA sequence alignment, $\mathcal{D} = (\mathbf{y}_1, \ldots, \mathbf{y}_N)$, and the sequence of hidden states,[7] $\mathcal{S} = (S_1, \ldots, S_N)$,

[7] Note the difference between $\mathcal{S}$ (a state sequence) and S or S_t (an individual hidden state), as explained in the previous footnote.

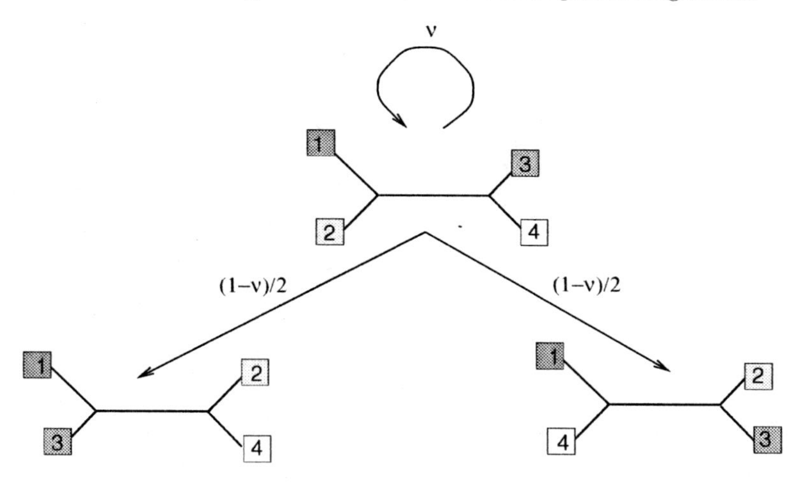

Fig. 5.20. Transition probabilities. The hidden states of the HMM represent different tree topologies, and state transitions correspond to recombination events. The transition probability ν is the probability that on moving from a site in the DNA sequence alignment to an adjacent site, no topology change occurs. If a topology change occurs, we assume that, *a priori*, all transitions are equally likely. Reprinted from [11], by permission of Oxford University Press.

factorizes, by the expansion rule for Bayesian networks (2.1):

$$P(\mathcal{D}, \mathcal{S}|\mathbf{w}, \boldsymbol{\theta}, \nu) = P(\mathbf{y}_1, \ldots, \mathbf{y}_N, S_1, \ldots, S_N|\mathbf{w}, \boldsymbol{\theta}, \nu)$$
$$= \prod_{t=1}^{N} P(\mathbf{y}_t|S_t, \mathbf{w}, \boldsymbol{\theta}) \prod_{t=2}^{N} P(S_t|S_{t-1}, \nu) P(S_1) \qquad (5.16)$$

Compare this equation with (2.51). $P(S_1)$ is the marginal distribution over the hidden states, that is, the K possible tree topologies. The $P(S_t|S_{t-1}, \nu)$ are the transition probabilities, which depend on the recombination parameter $\nu \in [0, 1]$, as illustrated in Figure 5.20. The functional form chosen in [10, 11] is given by (2.63), discussed in Section 2.3.5. The parameter ν defines the probability that on moving from a site in the DNA sequence alignment to an adjacent site, no topology change occurs. If a topology change occurs – corresponding to a recombination event – all transitions into other topologies are assumed to be equally likely. The $P(\mathbf{y}_t|S_t, \mathbf{w}, \boldsymbol{\theta})$ are the emission probabilities, which depend on the vector of branch lengths, $\mathbf{w}$, and the parameters of the nucleotide substitution model, $\boldsymbol{\theta}$. For example, for the Kimura model (4.16), $\boldsymbol{\theta}$ is given by the transition-transversion rate τ, defined in (4.21). For the HKY85 model, $\boldsymbol{\theta} = (\tau, \boldsymbol{\pi})$, where $\boldsymbol{\pi}$ was defined in (4.29). In fact, both $\mathbf{w}$ and $\boldsymbol{\theta}$ are dependent on the hidden state, so more precisely, the emission probabilities should be written as $P(\mathbf{y}_t|S_t, \mathbf{w}_{S_t}, \boldsymbol{\theta}_{S_t})$. To simplify the notation, this chapter uses the accumulated vectors $\mathbf{w} = (\mathbf{w}_1, \ldots, \mathbf{w}_K)$ and $\boldsymbol{\theta} = (\boldsymbol{\theta}_1, \ldots, \boldsymbol{\theta}_K)$ and defines: $P(\mathbf{y}_t|S_t, \mathbf{w}_{S_t}, \boldsymbol{\theta}_{S_t}) = P(\mathbf{y}_t|S_t, \mathbf{w}, \boldsymbol{\theta})$. This means that S_t indicates

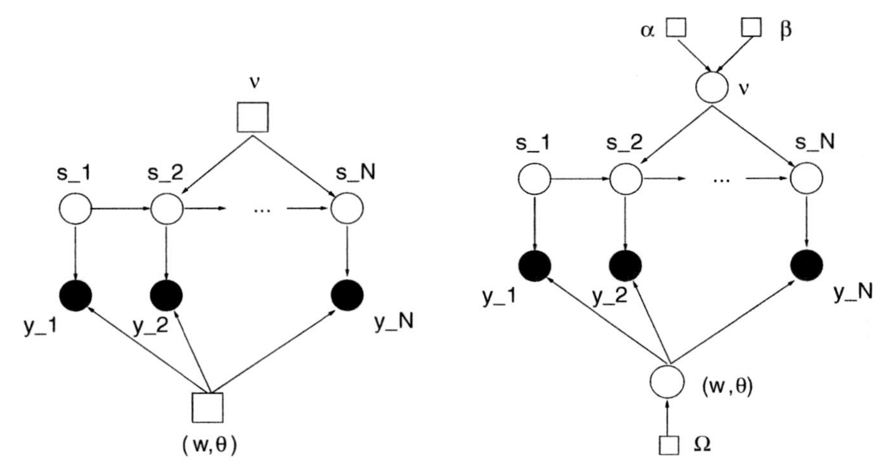

Fig. 5.21. Modelling recombination with hidden Markov models. Positions in the model, labelled by the subscript t, correspond to sites in the DNA sequence alignment. Black nodes represent observed random variables; these are the columns in the DNA sequence alignment. White nodes represent hidden states; these are the different tree topologies, shown (for four sequences) in Figure 5.19. Arrows represent conditional dependencies. Squares represent parameters of the model. The probability of observing a column vector $\mathbf{y}_t$ at position t in the DNA sequence alignment depends on the tree topology S_t, the vector of branch lengths $\mathbf{w}$, and the parameters of the nucleotide substitution model $\boldsymbol{\theta}$. The tree topology at position t depends on the topologies at the adjacent sites, S_{t-1} and S_{t+1}, and the recombination parameter ν. *Left:* In the maximum likelihood approach, ν, $\mathbf{w}$, and $\boldsymbol{\theta}$ are parameters that have to be estimated. *Right:* In the Bayesian approach, ν, $\mathbf{w}$, and $\boldsymbol{\theta}$ are random variables. The prior distribution for ν is a beta distribution with hyperparameters α and β. The prior distributions for the remaining parameters depend on some hyperparameters Ω, as discussed in the text. The parameters ν, $\mathbf{w}$, and $\boldsymbol{\theta}$ are sampled from the posterior distribution with Markov chain Monte Carlo. Reprinted from [11], by permission of Oxford University Press.

which subvectors of $\mathbf{w}$ and $\boldsymbol{\theta}$ apply. The computation of $P(\mathbf{y}_t|S_t, \mathbf{w}, \boldsymbol{\theta})$ makes use of the peeling algorithm, discussed in Section 4.4.3, and illustrated in Figure 4.23. Note that while the standard likelihood approach to phylogenetics, expressed in (4.58), assumes that one tree topology S applies to the whole sequence alignment, (5.16) allows for topology changes, corresponding to recombination events. The best prediction of the recombinant regions and their breakpoints is given by

$$\begin{aligned}\hat{\mathcal{S}} &= \text{argmax}_{\mathcal{S}} P(\mathcal{S}|\mathcal{D}, \mathbf{w}, \boldsymbol{\theta}, \nu) \\ &= \text{argmax}_{S_1,\ldots,S_N} P(S_1, \ldots, S_N|\mathbf{y}_1, \ldots, \mathbf{y}_N, \mathbf{w}, \boldsymbol{\theta}, \nu) \qquad (5.17)\end{aligned}$$

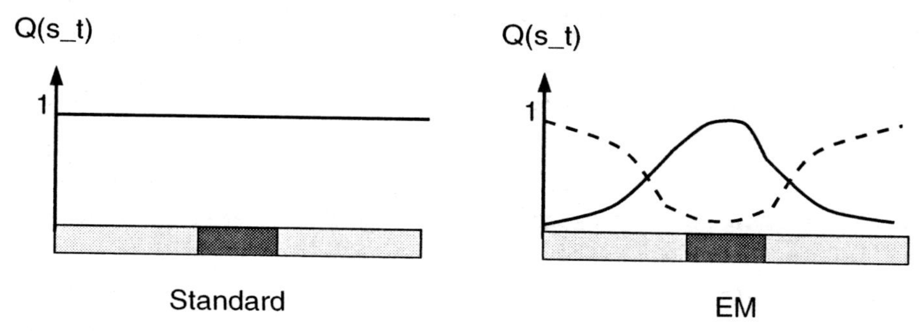

Fig. 5.22. Nucleotide weighting schemes. The bottom of each figure represents a multiple DNA sequence alignment with a recombinant zone in the middle. *Left:* The standard approach. The tree parameters are estimated from the whole sequence alignment, which corresponds to a uniform weight of 1 for all sites. *Right:* The EM algorithm. The solid line shows the site-dependent weights $Q(S_t = T_R)$ for the recombinant topology T_R, the dashed line represents the weights for the non-recombinant topology $T_0 : Q(S_t = T_0)$. Note that the weights $Q(S_t)$ are updated automatically in every iteration of the optimization procedure (in the E-step).

which is computed with the Viterbi algorithm, described in Section 2.3.4, especially equations (2.52) and (2.54). The marginal probability $P(S_1)$ and the parameters $\mathbf{w}$, $\boldsymbol{\theta}$, and ν need to be estimated.

5.10.2 Maximum Likelihood

Husmeier and Wright [12] optimized the parameters in a maximum likelihood sense with the EM algorithm (see Section 2.3.3.) This approach follows the procedure discussed in Section 2.3.5. The M-step for the marginal probabilities $P(S_t)$ is described in the paragraphs above and below (2.63) on page 51. The M-step for ν is given by (2.68). The M-step for $\mathbf{w}$ and $\boldsymbol{\theta}$ requires us to maximize the expression in (2.58):

$$A(\mathbf{w}, \boldsymbol{\theta}) = \sum_{t=1}^{N} \sum_{S_t} Q(S_t) \log P(\mathbf{y}_t | S_t, \mathbf{w}, \boldsymbol{\theta}) \tag{5.18}$$

where the distribution $Q(S_t)$ is obtained in the E-step, as described in the section after equation (2.62). Note that (5.18) does not have a closed form solution. Consequently, the parameters have to be optimized in an iterative procedure, as described in Section 4.4.5. Effectively, one can apply the optimization routines discussed in Section 4.4.5. The only modification required is a state-dependent weighting of the sites in the sequence alignment, as illustrated in Figure 5.22. These weights come out of the E-step of the EM algorithm, using the forward–backward algorithm, as described in the paragraph following (2.62). The cycles of E and M steps have to be iterated; see

Section 2.3.3. Note that as opposed to Section 4.4.3, the dependence of the emission probabilities on $\boldsymbol{\theta}$ has been made explicit in the notation, and in general these parameters should be optimized together with the branch lengths $\mathbf{w}$. However, in [12], where the Kimura model (4.16) of nucleotide substitution was employed, the single parameter[8] $\boldsymbol{\theta} = \tau$ (4.21) was estimated from the whole sequence alignment in advance, and only the branch lengths $\mathbf{w}$ were optimized with a gradient ascent scheme applied to (5.18).

The maximum likelihood approach has the disadvantage that the optimal sequence of hidden states, $\hat{\mathcal{S}}$, given by (5.17), depends on the parameters $\mathbf{w}$, $\boldsymbol{\theta}$. These parameters were estimated from the sequence alignment, which renders the approach susceptible to over-fitting. Within the frequentist paradigm of inference, discussed in Section 1.2, we have to test the null hypothesis of no recombination against the alternative hypothesis that a recombination event has occurred. For the practical implementation, we can use *nonparametric bootstrapping*, described in Sections 1.2 and 4.4.6, and illustrated in Figure 1.5, or *parametric bootstrapping*, illustrated in Figure 5.10. These approaches are computationally expensive because they require us to repeat the iterative optimization procedure of the EM algorithm on many (typically at least a hundred) bootstrap replicas of the sequence alignment; see Figure 4.35. An alternative would be to resort to asymptotic model selection scores, like the likelihood ratio test [9], or the BIC score, discussed in Section 2.3.2. However, for complex models and comparatively small data sets, these scores cannot be assumed to be reliable, and their use is therefore not recommended. Motivated by Figure 4.35, we will therefore look at a Bayesian approach, which is based on the principle described in Section 2.3.7, and was proposed by Husmeier and McGuire [10, 11].

5.10.3 Bayesian Approach

Within the Bayesian framework, summarized in Section 1.3, the prediction of the optimal state sequence $\mathcal{S}$ should be based on the posterior probability $P(\mathcal{S}|\mathcal{D})$, which requires the remaining parameters to be integrated out:

$$P(\mathcal{S}|\mathcal{D}) = \int P(\mathcal{S}, \mathbf{w}, \boldsymbol{\theta}, \nu|\mathcal{D}) d\mathbf{w} d\boldsymbol{\theta} d\nu \tag{5.19}$$

In principle this avoids the over-fitting scenario mentioned above and removes the need for a separate hypothesis test. The difficulty, however, is that the integral in (5.19) is analytically intractable. This intractability calls for a numerical approximation with Markov chain Monte Carlo (MCMC), as introduced in Section 2.2.2, and extended in Section 2.3.7. The subsections below will discuss (1) the choice of prior probabilities, (2) the implementation of the MCMC method, (3) convergence issues, and (4) the prediction resulting from this scheme. A test of the practical viability and a comparison with the other approaches introduced in this chapter is the subject of Section 5.11.

[8] The parameter τ was chosen to be the same for all states S_t.

Prior probabilities

Inherent in the Bayesian framework is the choice of prior probabilities for all model parameters, as illustrated in Figure 5.21, right. The approach in [10, 11] makes the common assumption of parameter independence (e.g., [7]), $P(\nu, \mathbf{w}, \boldsymbol{\theta}) = P(\nu)P(\mathbf{w})P(\boldsymbol{\theta})$. Thus, with (5.16), we obtain for the joint distribution:

$$P(\mathcal{D}, \mathcal{S}, \mathbf{w}, \boldsymbol{\theta}, \nu) = \prod_{t=1}^{N} P(\mathbf{y}_t|S_t, \mathbf{w}, \boldsymbol{\theta}) \prod_{t=2}^{N} P(S_t|S_{t-1}, \nu)P(S_1)P(\mathbf{w})P(\boldsymbol{\theta})P(\nu) \quad (5.20)$$

Due to the absence of specific biological knowledge about the nature of recombination processes, the prior distributions are chosen rather vague. Also, prior probabilities are chosen either conjugate, where possible, or uniform, but proper (that is, restricted to a finite interval). The conjugate prior for the recombination parameter ν is a beta distribution (1.12), whose shape is determined by two hyperparameters α and β; see Figure 1.8. In [10, 11], these hyperparameters were chosen such that the resulting prior is sufficiently vague, while incorporating the prior knowledge that recombination events are fairly rare. *A priori*, the branch lengths $\mathbf{w}$ are assumed to be uniformly distributed in the interval $[0, 1]$. Fixing an upper bound on the branch lengths is necessary to avoid the use of an improper prior, for which the MCMC scheme might not converge. Since for real DNA sequence alignments branch lengths are unlikely to approach values as large as 1, this restriction should not cause any difficulties. The prior on S_1 was chosen uniform in [10, 11].[9] Finally, the prior on $\boldsymbol{\theta}$ depends on the nucleotide substitution model and is discussed in [10, 11].

The MCMC scheme

Ultimately, we are interested in the marginal posterior probability of the state sequences, $P(\mathcal{S}|\mathcal{D})$, which requires a marginalization over the model parameters according to (5.19). The numerical approximation is to sample from the joint posterior distribution

$$P(\mathcal{S}, \mathbf{w}, \boldsymbol{\theta}, \nu|\mathcal{D}) \quad (5.21)$$

and then to discard the model parameters. Sampling from the joint posterior probability follows the Gibbs sampling scheme [2], which is illustrated in Figure 5.23. Applied to (5.21), this method samples each parameter group separately conditional on the others. So if the superscript (i) denotes the ith sample of the Markov chain, we obtain the $(i+1)$th sample as follows:

[9] One can also treat $P(S_1)$ itself as a parameter vector – see the text around (2.63) on page 51. The conjugate prior for these parameters is a Dirichlet distribution.

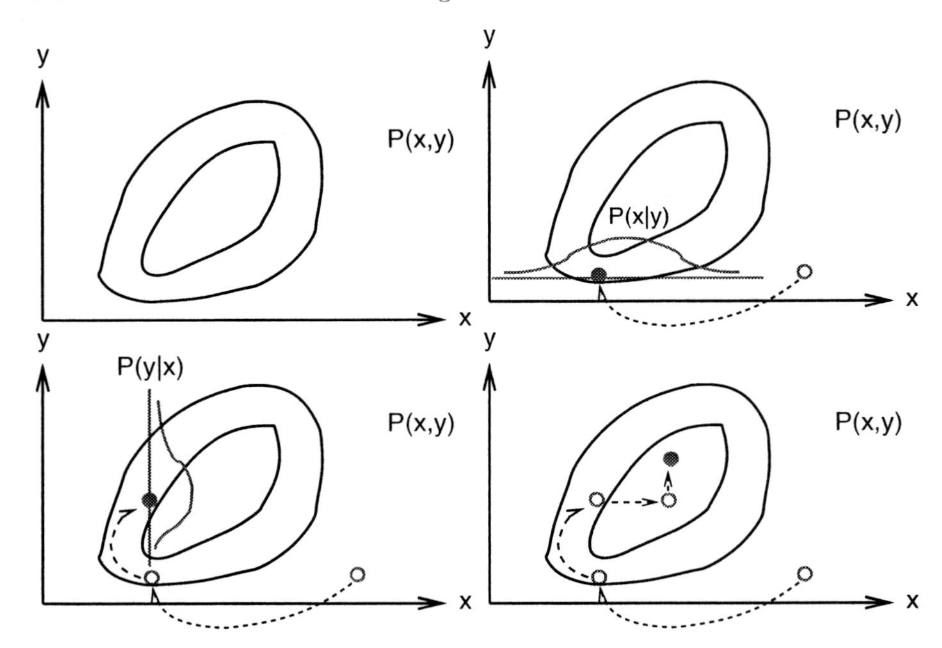

Fig. 5.23. Gibbs sampling. The subfigure in the *top left* shows a bivariate joint distribution $P(x, y)$. It is assumed that it is impossible to sample from $P(x, y)$ directly, but that we can draw samples from its univariate marginal distributions. Gibbs sampling then proceeds by iterating the following two steps: (1) *Top right:* Sample x from the conditional probability $P(x|y)$ for fixed y. (2) *Bottom left:* Sample y from the conditional probability $P(y|x)$ for fixed x. (3) *Bottom right:* Iterating these steps produces a Markov chain, which under fairly general conditions converges in distribution to the desired bivariate distribution $P(x, y)$. Adapted from [16], by permission of Kluwer Academic Publisher.

$$
\begin{aligned}
\mathcal{S}^{(i+1)} &\sim P(\cdot|\mathbf{w}^{(i)}, \boldsymbol{\theta}^{(i)}, \nu^{(i)}, \mathcal{D}) \\
\mathbf{w}^{(i+1)} &\sim P(\cdot|\mathcal{S}^{(i+1)}, \boldsymbol{\theta}^{(i)}, \nu^{(i)}, \mathcal{D}) \\
\boldsymbol{\theta}^{(i+1)} &\sim P(\cdot|\mathcal{S}^{(i+1)}, \mathbf{w}^{(i+1)}, \nu^{(i)}, \mathcal{D}) \\
\nu^{(i+1)} &\sim P(\cdot|\mathcal{S}^{(i+1)}, \mathbf{w}^{(i+1)}, \boldsymbol{\theta}^{(i+1)}, \mathcal{D})
\end{aligned}
\tag{5.22}
$$

The order of these sampling steps, which will be discussed in the remainder of this subsection, is arbitrary.

Define $\Psi = \sum_{t=1}^{N-1} \delta_{S_t, S_{t+1}}$. From (2.63) and the functional form of the prior on ν, (1.12), it is seen that writing the joint probability (5.20) as a function of ν gives:

$$
P(\mathcal{D}, \mathcal{S}, \mathbf{w}, \boldsymbol{\theta}, \nu) \;\propto\; \nu^{\Psi+\alpha-1}(1-\nu)^{N-\Psi+\beta-2} \tag{5.23}
$$

On normalization this gives

$$
P(\nu|\mathcal{D}, \mathcal{S}, \mathbf{w}, \boldsymbol{\theta}) \;=\; \mathcal{B}(\nu|\Psi+\alpha, N-\Psi+\beta-1) \tag{5.24}
$$

where $\mathcal{B}$ is the beta distribution (1.12), from which sampling is straightforward [25].

The sampling of the state sequences $\mathcal{S}$ can follow the approach suggested in [23], where each state S_t is sampled separately conditional on the others, that is, with a Gibbs-within-Gibbs scheme:

$$\begin{aligned}
S_1^{(i+1)} &\sim P(\cdot|S_2^{(i)}, S_3^{(i)}, \ldots, S_N^{(i)}, \mathcal{D}, \mathbf{w}^{(i)}, \boldsymbol{\theta}^{(i)}, \nu^{(i)}) \\
S_2^{(i+1)} &\sim P(\cdot|S_1^{(i+1)}, S_3^{(i)}, \ldots, S_N^{(i)}, \mathcal{D}, \mathbf{w}^{(i)}, \boldsymbol{\theta}^{(i)}, \nu^{(i)}) \\
&\vdots \\
S_N^{(i+1)} &\sim P(\cdot|S_1^{(i+1)}, S_2^{(i+1)}, \ldots, S_{N-1}^{(i+1)}, \mathcal{D}, \mathbf{w}^{(i)}, \boldsymbol{\theta}^{(i)}, \nu^{(i)})
\end{aligned} \tag{5.25}$$

The computational complexity of this approach is reduced considerably by the sparseness of the connectivity in the HMM. Recall from Section 2.1.1 that a node in a Bayesian network is only dependent on its Markov blanket, that is, the set of parents, children, and coparents. This fundamental feature of Bayesian networks implies that

$$\begin{aligned}
&P(S_t|S_1, \ldots, S_{t-1}, S_{t+1}, \ldots, S_N, \mathcal{D}, \mathbf{w}, \boldsymbol{\theta}, \nu) \\
&= P(S_t|S_{t-1}, S_{t+1}, \mathbf{y}_t, \mathbf{w}, \boldsymbol{\theta}, \nu) \\
&\propto P(S_{t+1}|S_t, \nu)P(S_t|S_{t-1}, \nu)P(\mathbf{y}_t|S_t, \mathbf{w}, \boldsymbol{\theta})
\end{aligned} \tag{5.26}$$

where $P(S_t|S_{t-1}, \nu)$ and $P(S_{t+1}|S_t, \nu)$ are given by (2.63). Note that the last expression in (5.26) is easily normalized to give a proper probability, from which sampling is straightforward (since $S_t \in \{1, \ldots, K\}$ is discrete).

Finally, the remaining parameters, $\mathbf{w}$ and $\boldsymbol{\theta}$, are sampled with the Metropolis–Hastings algorithm, described in Sections 2.2.2 and 4.4.7, especially equation (4.71). The overall algorithm is thus of the form of a Metropolis–Hastings and Gibbs-within-Gibbs scheme.

Improving the convergence of the Markov chain

In theory, the MCMC algorithm converges to the posterior distribution (5.21) irrespective of the choice of the proposal distribution (assuming ergodicity). In practice, a "good" choice of the proposal probabilities is crucial to achieve a convergence of the Markov chain within a reasonable amount of time. The dependence of the convergence and mixing properties on the proposal probabilities was demonstrated in Section 2.2.2, especially Figure 2.14. Tuning the proposal probabilities for the present MCMC study follows the same principles, albeit at a higher level of complexity. The details are beyond the scope of this chapter, and can be found in [11].

Prediction

Recall that the proposed Bayesian method samples topology sequences from the joint posterior distribution $P(\mathcal{S}|\mathcal{D}) = P(S_1, \ldots, S_N|\mathcal{D})$, where S_t represents the topology at site t. To display the results graphically, we can marginalize, for each site in turn, over all the remaining sites so as to return the marginal posterior probabilities $P(S_t|\mathcal{D})$. These probabilities can then be plotted, for each topology S_t, along the sequence alignment. For instance, if we have an alignment of four sequences, for which there are three different (unrooted) tree topologies, we get three different plots: $P(S_t = 1|\mathcal{D})$, $P(S_t = 2|\mathcal{D})$, and $P(S_t = 3|\mathcal{D})$. Examples will be shown in the next section, in Figures 5.27–5.29. Assigning each site t to the mode of the posterior distribution $P(S_t|\mathcal{D})$ gives a list of putative recombinant regions, identical to the output of RECPARS. Note, however, that the posterior probabilities $P(S_t|\mathcal{D})$ contain further, additional information, as they also indicate the uncertainty in the prediction.

5.10.4 Shortcomings of the HMM Approach

The method of combining a phylogenetic tree with an HMM – henceforth referred to as the *HMM method* – is restricted to DNA sequence alignments with small numbers of taxa. This is because each possible tree topology constitutes a separate state of the HMM, and the number of tree topologies increases super-exponentially with the number of sequences, as shown in Table 4.2 on page 121. In fact, in [10, 11], the HMM method was only applied to sequence alignments of four taxa. In practical applications, the HMM method has therefore to be combined with a low-resolution preprocessing method, using, for instance, RECPARS, Section 5.9, or the window methods, Sections 5.6 and 5.7. In a first, preliminary analysis, apply the preprocessing method to identify putative recombinant sequences and their approximate mosaic structures. In a second, subsequent step, apply the HMM approach to the tentative sets of four sequences that result from the preprocessing step. This will allow a more accurate analysis of the mosaic structure than can be obtained from the window methods with their inherently low resolution, and it will resolve contradictions that are likely to arise from different (arbitrary) settings of the parsimony cost parameters of RECPARS. In general, after identifying a small set of putative recombinant sequences with any fast low-resolution method, the exact nature of the recombination processes and the location of the breakpoints can be further investigated with the high-resolution HMM method.

A second limitation is the fact that the states of the HMM represent only different tree topologies, but do not allow for different rates of nucleotide substitution. A way to redeem this deficiency is to employ a factorial hidden Markov model (FHMM), as discussed in [5], and to introduce two different types of hidden states: one representing different topologies, the other representing different nucleotide substitution rates. This approach effectively combines the method in [10, 11], described in the present section, with the approach in [3], where the different states of the HMM correspond to different rates of nucleotide substitution. Implementing this FHMM approach is a project for future research.

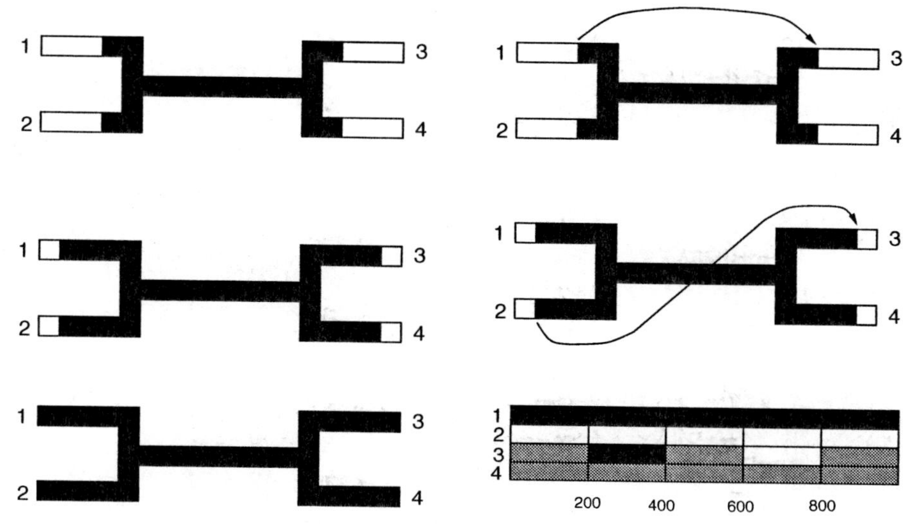

Fig. 5.24. Simulation of recombination. Four sequences are evolved along the interior branch and the first quarter of the exterior branches of a phylogenetic tree (top left). At this point, the subsequence between sites 201 and 400 in strain 3 is replaced by the corresponding subsequence in strain 1 (top right). The sequences then continue to evolve along the exterior branches until the branch length is 0.75 times the final exterior branch length (middle, left). This process is followed by a second recombination event, where the subsequence between sites 601 and 800 in strain 2 replaces the corresponding subsequence in strain 3 (middle right). The sequences then continue to evolve along the exterior branches for the remaining length (bottom left). Note that this model simulates a realistic scenario where an ancestor of strain 3 incorporates genetic material from ancestors of other extant strains, and the transfer of DNA subsequences is followed by subsequent evolution. The resulting mosaic structure is shown in the bottom right. Reprinted from [11], by permission of Oxford University Press.

5.11 Empirical Comparison II

Husmeier and McGuire [11] compared the performance of the Bayesian HMM method of Section 5.10.3 with PLATO, introduced in Section 5.5, TOPAL, discussed in Section 5.6, and RECPARS, described in Section 5.9. The present section gives a brief summary of their findings. For further details, see [11].

5.11.1 Simulated Recombination

DNA sequences, 1000 nucleotides long, were evolved along a 4-species tree, using the Kimura model of nucleotide substitution ($\tau = 2$), discussed in Section 4.4.2, and illustrated in Figure 4.18. Two recombination events were simulated, as shown in Figure 5.24. In the main part of the alignment, strain 3

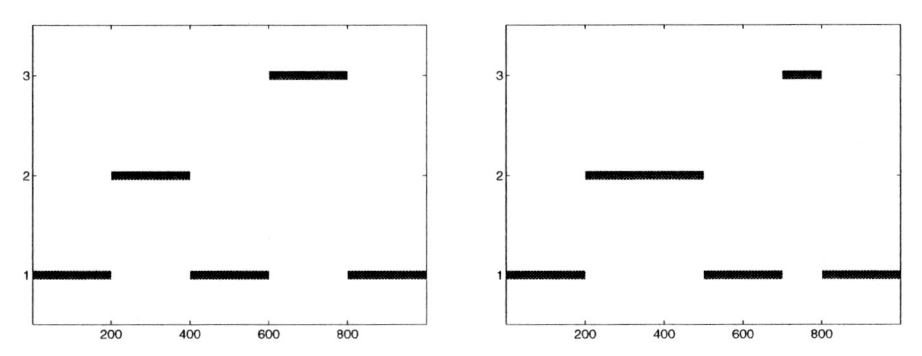

Fig. 5.25. True mosaic structures for the synthetic data. The recombination process was simulated according to Figure 5.24. The vertical axis represents the three different tree topologies. The horizontal axis shows sites in the DNA sequence alignment. Reprinted from [11], by permission of Oxford University Press.

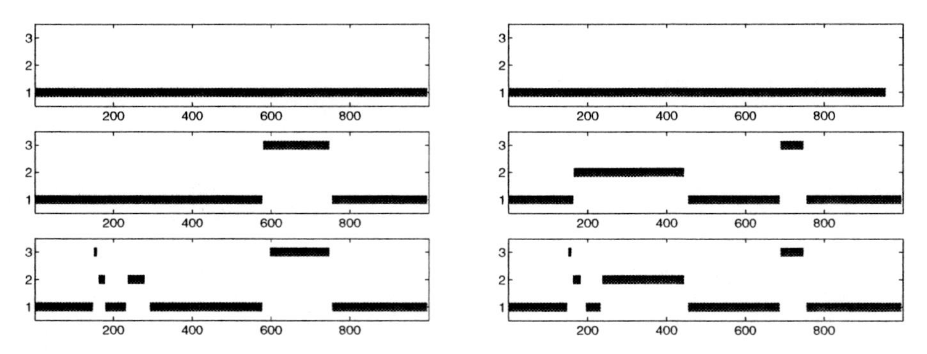

Fig. 5.26. Prediction with RECPARS on the synthetic sequence alignment, for which the true mosaic structures are shown in Figure 5.25. The left figure corresponds to the left figure in Figure 5.25, and the right figure corresponds to the right figure in Figure 5.25. Each figure contains three subfigures, which show the results for different recombination–mutation cost ratios, C_{recomb}/C_{mut}. *Top subfigure:* $C_{recomb}/C_{mut} = 10.0$; *middle subfigure:* $C_{recomb}/C_{mut} = 3.0$; *bottom subfigure:* $C_{recomb}/C_{mut} = 1.5$. The horizontal axis in each subfigure represents sites in the sequence alignment, while the vertical axis represents the three possible tree topologies. Reprinted from [11], by permission of Oxford University Press.

is most closely related to strain 4. However, in the first recombinant region, it is most closely related to strain 1, and in the second recombinant region, it is most closely related to strain 2. Thus, the first recombination event corresponds to a transition from topology 1 into topology 2. The second recombination event corresponds to a transition from topology 1 into topology 3. The simulation was repeated for different lengths of the recombinant regions. The true mosaic structure of the alignment is shown in Figure 5.25. For further details, see [11].

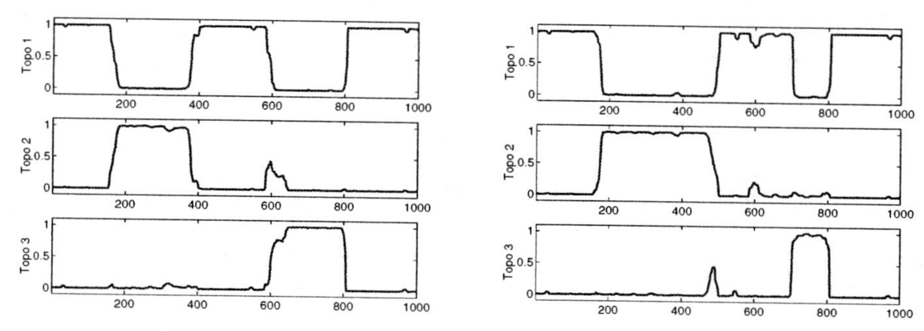

Fig. 5.27. Prediction with the HMM method on the synthetic sequence alignment, for which the true mosaic structures are shown in Figure 5.25. The left figure corresponds to the left figure in Figure 5.25, and the right figure corresponds to the right figure in Figure 5.25. Each figure contains three subfigures, which show the posterior probabilities of the three topologies, $P(S_t = 1|\mathcal{D})$ (top), $P(S_t = 2|\mathcal{D})$ (middle), $P(S_t = 3|\mathcal{D})$ (bottom), plotted against the site t in the DNA sequence alignment. Reprinted from [11], by permission of Oxford University Press.

The predictions with RECPARS are shown in Figure 5.26. The results depend critically on the recombination–mutation cost ratio, C_{recomb}/C_{mut}, which can *not* be optimized within the framework of this method, as discussed in Section 5.9, but rather has to be chosen arbitrarily in advance. With a value of $C_{recomb}/C_{mut} = 10.0$, no recombinant regions are found. As C_{recomb}/C_{mut} is decreased, an increasing number of recombinant regions are detected. The best results in the right subfigure of Figure 5.26 show a qualitative agreement with the true locations, but note that selecting C_{recomb}/C_{mut} in this way is not possible in real applications where the nature of the recombination processes is not known beforehand.

The prediction with the Bayesian HMM method is shown in Figure 5.27. The figure contains two subfigures, which correspond to the respective true mosaic structures depicted in Figure 5.25. Each subfigure contains three graphs, which show the posterior probabilities $P(S_t|\mathcal{D})$ for the three possible tree topologies, $S_t \in \{1, 2, 3\}$. These graphs show clear and pronounced transitions between the states, with a correct prediction of the topology change, and an accurate location of the breakpoints. Note that as opposed to RECPARS, this prediction does not depend on any arbitrary parameters that would have to be set in advance.[10]

The predictions with TOPAL were similar to Figure 5.12. With a short window of only 100 nucleotides, TOPAL only detected two of the four breakpoints. For a sufficiently large window size of 200 nucleotides, TOPAL detected all four breakpoints. However, the spatial resolution was similar to

[10] Recall from (5.19) that within the Bayesian paradigm, the parameters have effectively been integrated out.

that of Figure 5.12, that is, of the order of the window size and, consequently, rather poor.

PLATO failed to detect any recombinant region. This failure corroborates the discussion at the end of Section 5.5, which suggested that PLATO becomes unreliable when the recombinant regions are fairly long.

The next two subsections will describe two real-world applications. In both cases, the performance of PLATO was poor, and the predictions with RECPARS were found to depend critically on the arbitrary setting of the recombination–mutation cost ratio, C_{recomb}/C_{mut}. Therefore, only the predictions with TOPAL and the HMM method will be presented here. For the full results, see [11].

5.11.2 Gene Conversion in Maize

Gene conversion is a process equivalent to recombination, which occurs in multigene families, where a DNA subsequence of one gene can be replaced by the DNA subsequence from another. Indication of gene conversion between a pair of maize actin genes has been reported in [21] for the alignment of the sequences Maz56 (GenBank/EMBL accession number U60514), Maz63 (U60513), Maz89 (U60508), and Maz95 (U60507). An illustration is given in Figure 5.28, where the topologies are defined as follows. Topology 1: (Maz56,Maz63),(Maz89,Maz95); topology 2: (Maz56,Maz89),(Maz63,Maz95); topology 3: (Maz56,Maz95),(Maz63,Maz89). The total length of the alignment is 1008 nucleotides.

The predictions with TOPAL (for a window size of 200 nucleotides) and the HMM method are shown in the bottom of Figure 5.28. TOPAL gives a qualitatively correct prediction of the mosaic structure, detecting one significant breakpoint at about the correct position. However, an exact location of this breakpoint is impossible due to the rather large intrinsic uncertainty in the prediction. The HMM method achieves a considerable improvement on TOPAL by predicting the location of the breakpoint much more accurately – in agreement with the earlier findings reported in [21] – and by also giving a correct prediction of the nature of the recombination event, that is, the ensuing topology change of the phylogenetic tree. Recall, however, that as opposed to TOPAL, the HMM method is restricted to alignments of small numbers of sequences.

5.11.3 Recombination in *Neisseria*

One of the first indications for interspecific recombination was found in the bacterial genus *Neisseria* [17]. Zhou and Spratt [28] investigated the 787-nucleotide *argF* gene sequence alignment of the strains (1) *N.gonorrhoeae* (X64860), (2) *N.meningitidis* (X64866), (3) *N.cinerea* (X64869), and (4) *N.mucosa* (X64873); GenBank/EMBL accession numbers are given in brackets. There are three different tree topologies:

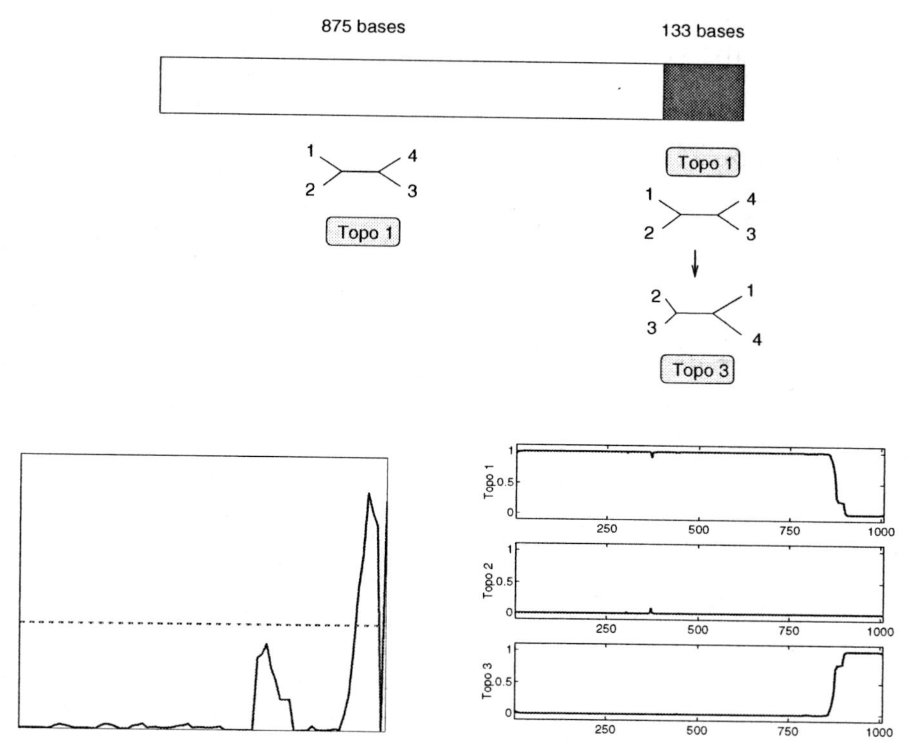

Fig. 5.28. Gene conversion between two maize actin genes. *Top:* Indication of gene conversion between a pair of maize actin genes, corresponding to a transition from topology 1 into topology 3 after the first 875 nucleotides of their coding regions, has been reported in [21]. *Bottom left:* Prediction with TOPAL. The DSS statistic (5.6), represented by the vertical axis, is plotted against the site t in the sequence alignment. The dashed horizontal line indicates the 95-percentile under the null-hypothesis of no recombination. Peaks over this line indicate significant breakpoints. *Bottom right:* Prediction with the Bayesian HMM method. The graphs are explained in the caption of Figure 5.27. Reprinted from [11], by permission of Oxford University Press.

Topology 1: (*N.meningitidis,N.gonorrhoeae*),(*N.cinerea,N.mucosa*); topology 2: (*N.meningitidis,N.mucosa*),(*N.gonorrhoeae,N.cinerea*); and topology 3: (*N.meningitidis,N.cinerea*),(*N.gonorrhoeae,N.mucosa*). In the main part of the alignment, *N.meningitidis* is grouped with *N.gonorrhoeae*, corresponding to topology $S_t = 1$. However, Zhou and Spratt [28] found two anomalous regions in the DNA alignment, which occur at positions $t = 1 - 202$ and $t = 507 - 538$. Between $t = 1$ and 202, *N.meningitidis* is grouped with *N.cinerea*, which corresponds to topology 3, that is, to a transition from state $S_t = 3$ into $S_t = 1$ at position $t = 202$. Zhou and Spratt [28] suggested that the region $t = 507 - 538$

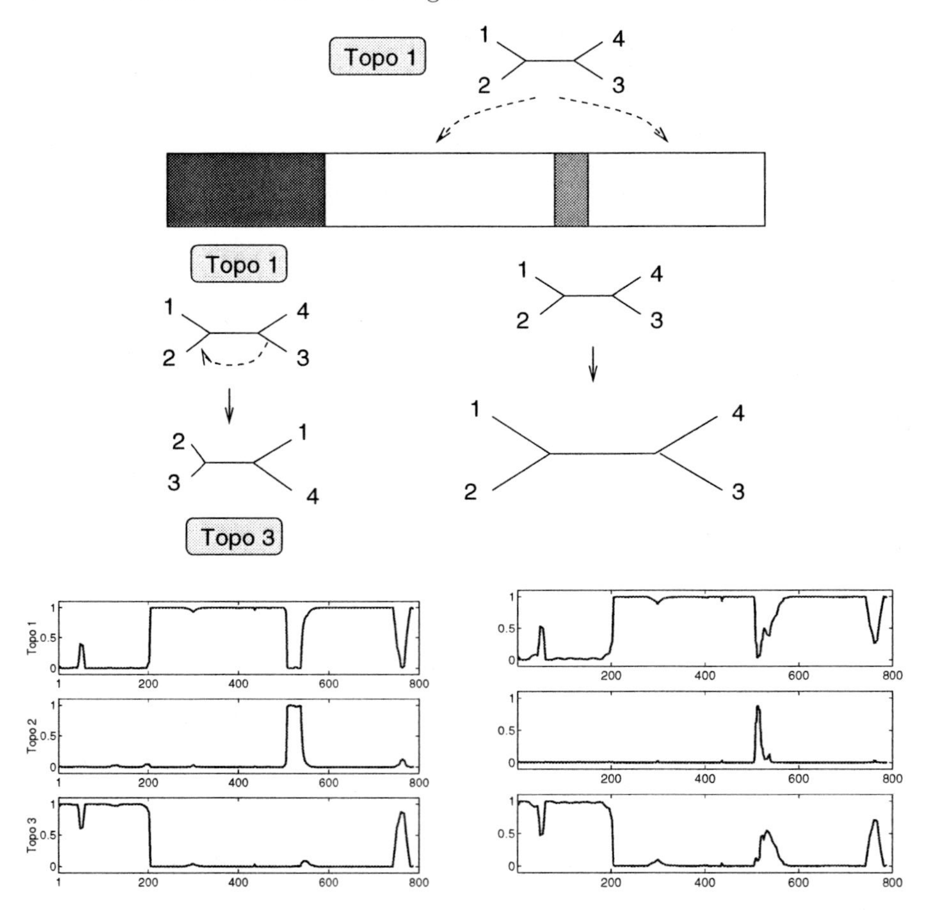

Fig. 5.29. Recombination in Neisseria. *Top:* According to Zhou and Spratt [28], a recombination event corresponding to a transition from topology 1 into topology 3 has affected the first 202 nucleotides of the DNA sequence alignment of four strains of *Neisseria*. A second more diverged region seems to be the result of rate variation. *Bottom:* Prediction with the HMM method. The figure contains two subfigures, where each subfigure is composed of three graphs, which are explained in the caption of Figure 5.27. *Left:* Prediction with the maximum likelihood method of Section 5.10.2. *Right:* Prediction with the Bayesian MCMC scheme of Section 5.10.3. Reprinted from [11], by permission of Oxford University Press.

seems to be the result of rate variation. The situation is illustrated in Figure 5.29.

Figure 5.29, bottom, shows the prediction of $P(S_t|\mathcal{D})$, where the subfigure in the bottom left was obtained with the maximum likelihood HMM method of Section 5.10.2, henceforth called HMM-ML, and the subfigure in the bottom right with the Bayesian HMM method of Section 5.10.3, henceforth referred to as HMM-Bayes. Both methods agree in predicting a sharp transition from topology $S_t = 3$ to $S_t = 1$ at breakpoint $t = 202$, which is in agreement with the findings in [28]. Both methods also agree in predicting a short recombinant region of the same topology change at the end of the alignment. This region was not reported in [28]. Since it is very short – only about 20 nucleotides long – it may not be detectable by other, less accurate methods.

Differences between the predictions of HMM-ML and HMM-Bayes are found in the middle of the alignment, where two further breakpoints occur at sites $t = 506$ and $t = 537$. This is in agreement with [28]. However, while [28] suggested that the region between $t = 506$ and $t = 537$ seems to be the result of rate heterogeneity, HMM-ML predicts a recombination event with a clear transition from topology $S_t = 1$ into $S_t = 2$. This seems to be the result of over-fitting: since the distribution of the nucleotide column vectors $\mathbf{y}_t$ in the indicated region is significantly different from the rest of the alignment, modelling this region with a different hidden state can increase the likelihood although the hidden state itself (topology $S_t = 2$) might be ill-matched to the data. This deficiency is redeemed with HMM-Bayes, whose prediction is shown in Figure 5.29, bottom right. The critical region between sites $t = 506$ and $t = 537$ is again identified, indicated by a strong drop in the posterior probability for the predominant topology, $P(S_t = 1|\mathcal{D})$. However, the uncertainty in the nature of this region is indicated by a distributed representation, where both alternative hidden states, $S_t = 2$ and $S_t = 3$, are assigned a significant probability mass. With the prediction of this uncertainty, HMM-Bayes also indicates a certain model misspecification inherent to the current scheme – the absence of hidden states for representing different evolutionary rates – and thus avoids the over-fitting incurred when applying HMM-ML.

5.12 Conclusion

The present chapter has reviewed various methods for detecting recombination in DNA sequence alignments. The focus has been on methods that identify the mosaic structure and the breakpoints of an alignment – different from Section 5.3 – and that make use of phylogenetic information – as opposed to Section 5.4. Note that each section in this chapter has a "shortcomings" subsection. This is indicative of the current state of the art, where a universally applicable and reliable off-the-shelf detection method does not yet exist. For practical applications it is therefore important to understand the strengths and weaknesses of the various approaches, and to possibly combine them in a way determined by the nature of the particular problem under investigation.

Finally, note that most of the methods discussed in this chapter focus on topology changes rather than recombination in general. If a recombination event only changes the branch lengths of a tree without affecting its topology, it will not be detected. However, the main motivation for the detection methods discussed in the present chapter is a pre-screening of an alignment for topology changes as a crucial prerequisite for a consistent phylogenetic analysis. Most standard phylogenetic methods, as discussed in Chapter 4, are based on the implicit assumption that the given alignment results from a single phylogenetic tree. In the presence of recombination they would therefore infer some "average" tree. If a recombination event leads to different trees with the same topology but different branch lengths, the wrong assumption of having only one tree is not too dramatic: the topology will still be correct (as it has not been changed by the recombination event), and the branch lengths will show some average value. This is still reasonable, since branch lengths are continuous numbers, and the mean of continuous numbers is well defined. If a recombination event, however, leads to a change of the topology, inferring an average tree is no longer reasonable: tree topologies are cardinal entities, for which an average value is *not* defined. In fact, it is well-known that in this case the resulting "average" tree will be in a distorted "limbo" state between the dominant and recombinant trees, which renders the whole inference scheme unreliable. Thus, by focusing on recombination-induced topology changes we focus on those events that cause the main problems with standard phylogenetic analysis methods.

5.13 Software

A free software package (TOPALi) that implements several of the methods discussed in this chapter can be obtained from `http://www.bioss.sari.ac.uk/~dirk/My_software.html`.

Acknowledgments

The work on this chapter was supported by the Scottish Executive Environmental and Rural Affairs Department (SEERAD). We would like to thank Isabelle Grimmenstein and Jochen Maydt for critical feedback on a draft version of this chapter, as well as Philip Smith for proofreading it.

References

[1] H. Bandelt and A. W. M. Dress. Split decomposition: a new and useful approach to phylogenetic analysis of distance data. *Molecular Phylogenetics and Evolution*, 1:242–252, 1992.

[2] G. Casella and E. I. George. Explaining the Gibbs sampler. *The American Statistician*, 46(3):167–174, 1992.

[3] J. Felsenstein and G. A. Churchill. A hidden Markov model approach to variation among sites in rate of evolution. *Molecular Biology and Evolution*, 13(1):93–104, 1996.

[4] W. M. Fitch and E. Margoliash. Construction of phylogenetic trees. *Science*, 155:279–284, 1987.

[5] Z. Ghahramani and M. I. Jordan. Factorial hidden Markov models. *Machine Learning*, 29:245–273, 1997.

[6] N. C. Grassly and E. C. Holmes. A likelihood method for the detection of selection and recombination using nucleotide sequences. *Molecular Biology and Evolution*, 14(3):239–247, 1997.

[7] D. Heckerman. A tutorial on learning with Bayesian networks. In M. I. Jordan, editor, *Learning in Graphical Models*, pages 301–354. Kluwer Academic Publishers, Dordrecht, The Netherlands, 1998. Reprinted by MIT Press in 1999.

[8] J. Hein. A heuristic method to reconstruct the history of sequences subject to recombination. *Journal of Molecular Evolution*, 36:396–405, 1993.

[9] P. G. Hoel. *Introduction to Mathematical Statistics*. John Wiley and Sons, Singapore, 1984.

[10] D. Husmeier and G. McGuire. Detecting recombination with MCMC. *Bioinformatics*, 18(Suppl.1):S345–S353, 2002.

[11] D. Husmeier and G. McGuire. Detecting recombination in 4-taxa DNA sequence alignments with Bayesian hidden Markov models and Markov chain Monte Carlo. *Molecular Biology and Evolution*, 20(3):315–337, 2003.

[12] D. Husmeier and F. Wright. Detection of recombination in DNA multiple alignments with hidden Markov models. *Journal of Computational Biology*, 8(4):401–427, 2001.

[13] D. Husmeier and F. Wright. Probabilistic divergence measures for detecting interspecies recombination. *Bioinformatics*, 17(Suppl.1):S123–S131, 2001.

[14] D. Husmeier and F. Wright. A Bayesian approach to discriminate between alternative DNA sequence segmentations. *Bioinformatics*, 18(2):226–234, 2002.

[15] W. J. Krzanowski and F. H. C. Marriott. *Multivariate Analysis*, volume 2. Arnold, 1995. ISBN 0-340-59325-3.

[16] D. J. C. MacKay. Introduction to Monte Carlo methods. In M. I. Jordan, editor, *Learning in Graphical Models*, pages 301–354. Kluwer Academic Publishers, Dordrecht, The Netherlands, 1998. Reprinted by MIT Press in 1999.

[17] J. Maynard Smith. Analyzing the mosaic structure of genes. *Journal of Molecular Evolution*, 34:126–129, 1992.

[18] G. McGuire and F. Wright. TOPAL 2.0: improved detection of mosaic sequences within multiple alignments. *Bioinformatics*, 16(2):130–134, 2000.

[19] G. McGuire, F. Wright, and M. Prentice. A graphical method for detecting recombination in phylogenetic data sets. *Molecular Biology and Evolution*, 14(11):1125–1131, 1997.

[20] G. McGuire, F. Wright, and M. Prentice. A Bayesian method for detecting recombination in DNA multiple alignments. *Journal of Computational Biology*, 7(1/2):159–170, 2000.

[21] M. Moniz de Sa and G. Drouin. Phylogeny and substitution rates of angiosperm actin genes. *Molecular Biology and Evolution*, 13:1198–1212, 1996.

[22] D. Posada, K. A. Crandall, and E. C. Holmes. Recombination in evolutionary genomics. *Annual Review of Genetics*, 36:75–97, 2002.

[23] C. P. Robert, G. Celeux, and J. Diebolt. Bayesian estimation of hidden Markov chains: A stochastic implementation. *Statistics & Probability Letters*, 16:77–83, 1993.

[24] D. L. Robertson, P. M. Sharp, F. E. McCutchan, and B. H. Hahn. Recombination in HIV-1. *Nature*, 374:124–126, 1995.

[25] R. Y. Rubinstein. *Simulation and the Monte Carlo Method.* John Wiley & Sons, New York, 1981.

[26] K. Strimmer and V. Moulton. Likelihood analysis of phylogenetic networks using directed graphical models. *Molecular Biology and Evolution*, 17(6):875–881, 2000.

[27] K. Strimmer, C. Wiuf, and V. Moulton. Recombination analysis using directed graphical models. *Molecular Biology and Evolution*, 18(1):97–99, 2001.

[28] J. Zhou and B. G. Spratt. Sequence diversity within the *argF*, *fbp* and *recA* genes of natural isolates of *Neisseria meningitidis*: interspecies recombination within the *argF* gene. *Molecular Microbiology*, 6:2135–2146, 1992.

6

RNA-Based Phylogenetic Methods

Magnus Rattray[1] and Paul G. Higgs[2]

[1] Department of Computer Science, University of Manchester, UK
magnus@cs.man.ac.uk

[2] Department of Physics and Astronomy, McMaster University, Canada
higgsp@mcmaster.ca

Summary. RNA molecules are used extensively in phylogenetic studies. Their strongly conserved secondary structure can be used to improve the alignment of highly diverged sequences, and this in turn can improve phylogenetic accuracy. The conservation of secondary structure in RNA molecules is a consequence of compensatory substitutions or covariation: when a base changes on one side of a helix this will usually be compensated for by a similar change on the opposite side, in order to maintain structural stability and biological function. The standard nucleotide substitution models for DNA, introduced in Chapter 4, ignore this covariation of base-paired sites, which leads to biased inference results and unreliable posterior probabilities of subtrees (clades). In the present chapter we discuss how these shortcomings can be overcome with a generalised substitution model that treats base-paired sites in the RNA helices, rather than single nucleotides, as a unit of evolution. We will present results from a study of mammalian evolution using Bayesian inference methods and explain why it is particularly important to include structure information when estimating Bayesian posterior probabilities.

6.1 Introduction

Ribonucleic Acid (RNA) is an important bio-molecule with a diverse set of functional roles. RNA consists of a linear polymer with a backbone of ribose sugar rings linked by phosphate groups. Each sugar has one of four bases, Adenine, Cytosine, Guanine and Uracil (A,C,G and U), and the sequence of bases determines the structure and function of the molecule. In this chapter we will mainly be concerned with transfer RNA and ribosomal RNA molecules. Transfer RNA (tRNA) is a relatively small RNA molecule that is involved in protein synthesis. There are many different tRNA molecules each of which corresponds to a specific amino acid in the protein being synthesised. Ribosomal RNA (rRNA) molecules exist in the ribosome which is a small intracellular particle that exists in multiple copies per cell. Each ribosome contains three RNA molecules which are called the small sub-unit rRNA (SSU or 16S rRNA), large sub-unit rRNA (LSU or 23S rRNA) and the smaller 5S rRNA.

The S numbers refer to the sedimentation coefficients of these molecules in Bacteria. The corresponding molecules are larger in eukaryotes and smaller in mitochondria, so that the same molecules can have different S numbers. We therefore prefer to use the less ambiguous SSU/LSU nomenclature.

RNA molecules are used extensively in phylogenetic analysis. Of particular importance is the SSU rRNA, which was used to establish the modern view of the early history of cellular life. Until the early 1970s it was thought that cellular organisms could be divided into two main categories: *eukaryotes*, which possess a cell nucleus and *prokaryotes*, which do not. Molecular phylogenies constructed using the SSU rRNA showed that the prokaryotes should actually be divided into two very different groups now referred to as Bacteria and Archea [1]. Bacterial phylogeny is still controversial because different genes can give rise to different trees. This could be due to errors in the methods or because there has been horizontal transfer of genes between organisms [2], as discussed in Chapter 5.

Nevertheless, the rRNA tree is still a standard to which most other phylogenetic hypotheses are compared [3]. The SSU rRNA is useful for obtaining resolution over long evolutionary times because it is a sufficiently long molecule to contain significant amounts of evolutionary information and because it evolves at a relatively slow rate, so that it still contains useful information about early evolutionary events. The SSU rRNA is also ubiquitous and occurs in all forms of cellular life as well as in the mitochondria and chloroplasts. RNA molecules have been used in a broad range of other important phylogenetic studies and provide resolution not only over very long evolutionary times, but also down to the evolutionary time-scales which are relevant for establishing intra-ordinal or intra-species relationships.

Although RNA molecules are used extensively in phylogenetic inference, the phylogenetic inference programs used in these studies typically ignore important features of the molecular evolution which are related to the molecular structure. The structure of RNA molecules is often highly conserved over long evolutionary times and this is advantageous as it allows highly accurate alignment of the sequences. Using RNA structure to improve alignments has been shown to significantly improve the accuracy of phylogenetic methods [4]. However, the conserved structure strongly influences evolution at the sequence level and this should be taken into account when developing phylogenetic methods.

In this chapter we will briefly introduce RNA secondary structure and structure prediction methods. We will explain how the evolution process in populations is affected by the conserved helical structures in RNA molecules and we will describe a class of evolutionary models that are specifically designed to model evolution in RNA helices. Finally, we will present results from a study of mammalian evolution using Bayesian inference methods and explain why it is particularly important to include structure information when estimating Bayesian posterior probabilities.

6.2 RNA Structure

Like proteins, RNA molecules form complex three-dimensional (tertiary) structures. The only way to obtain an accurate tertiary structure is through experimental methods such as X-ray crystallography. The secondary structure is a useful two-dimensional representation of certain key structural features. RNA molecules form helices when two parts of the same sequence are complementary, and the secondary structure shows which parts of the sequence form the helical regions of the molecule. Computational methods exist that provide an accurate secondary structure from sequence information, without resorting to time-consuming and expensive experimental methods. The secondary structure is therefore a very useful abstraction and provides us with an accurate representation of the structural features most relevant for improving phylogenetic methods. A discussion of the relationship between secondary and tertiary structures is given in [5].

The secondary structure

RNA molecules can form helical structures when two parts of the sequence are complementary. Hydrogen bonds can occur between G-C (3 bonds), A-U (2 bonds) and G-U (1 bond) base-pairs. The first two are know as *Watson–Crick base-pairs* since they are analogous to the pairings in DNA (with Thymine having been replaced by Uracil). The G-U base-pair is less stable and although it occurs at an appreciable frequency in the helices, it is less common than the Watson–Crick pairs. The three common types of base-pair are often referred to as canonical base-pairs. Some non-canonical or *mismatch (MM) base-pairs* do appear within helices, but these occur relatively rarely, typically at about 3–4% of sites in the helices.

In Figure 6.1 we show an example of a secondary structure diagram showing a small part of the SSU rRNA from *E. coli*. Examples of complete SSU and LSU rRNA secondary structures can be found on the Comparative RNA Website [6] (http://www.rna.icmb.utexas.edu). The secondary structure shows all of the base-paired helical regions in the molecule. As well as base-paired helical regions, there are also single stranded regions known as loops and bulges.

Secondary structure prediction

There has been a great deal of work on computational approaches to RNA structure prediction. As with protein structure prediction the only way to obtain a completely accurate tertiary structure is by experimental methods such as X-ray crystallography. However, unlike protein structure prediction we can make quite accurate secondary structure predictions using computational methods. The main approaches are the *minimum free energy methods* and *comparative methods*, which we will describe below. More detailed recent reviews of secondary structure prediction methods are provided in [5, 7].

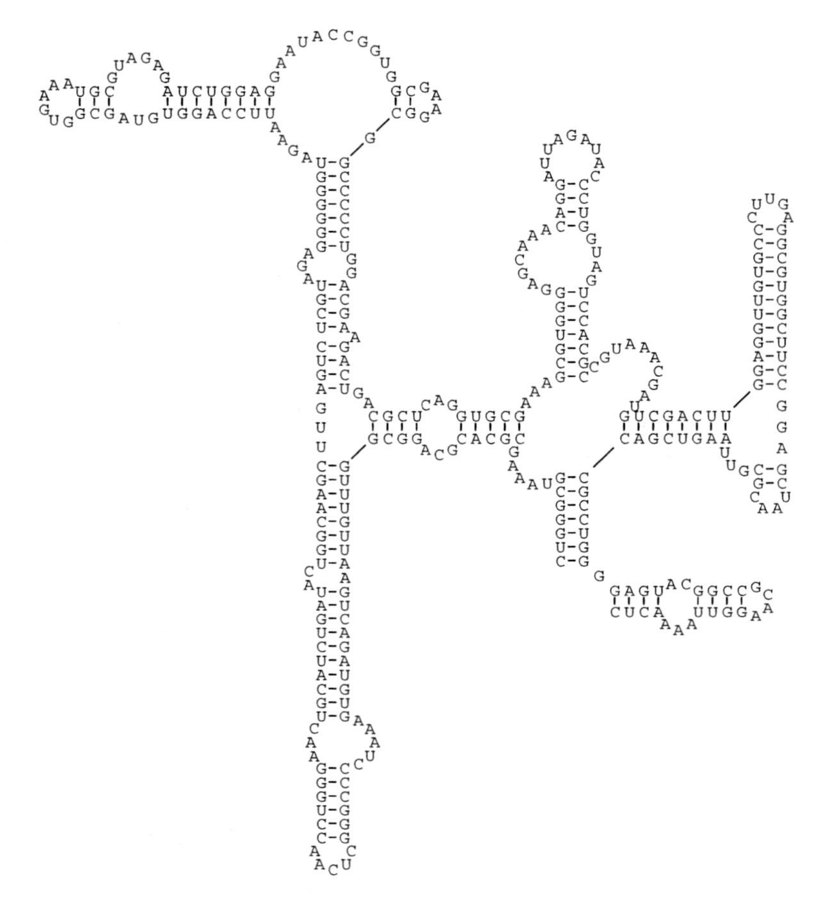

Fig. 6.1. Part of the secondary structure of the SSU rRNA from *E. coli*.

If a molecule exists in thermal equilibrium then it will spend most of its time in the minimum free energy (MFE) configuration. MFE methods use a simplified model of the free energy which can be determined from the secondary structure. Energy and entropy changes due to helix formation can be measured from experiments with short RNA sequences [8]. Much of the stability of a helix comes from the stacking interactions between successive base-pairs and the free energy is usually assumed to obey a nearest neighbour model, i.e. there is a free energy contribution from each two successive base-pairs. There are also free energy penalties associated with the loops due to the loss of entropy when the loop ends are constrained. It is usually assumed that the loop free energies depend only on the length of the loop and not on details of the sequence, although there are some specific exceptions to this rule.

In principle we could compute the free energy of every possible secondary structure in order to determine the MFE structure. However, the number of possible secondary structures grows exponentially with the sequence length and therefore this approach is not computationally feasible. Luckily there exist polynomial time dynamic programming algorithms to obtain the MFE structure [9, 10, 11]. These algorithms have $O(N^3)$ time complexity where N is the sequence length. Freely available software implementing the algorithms is available (e.g. mfold, available from http://www.ibc.wustl.edu/~zuker/rna). Remarkably, it is also possible to compute the entire partition function for these free energy models using a dynamic programming algorithm [12] and this allows the calculation of the probability of particular base-pairs occurring in the complete equilibrium ensemble of structures.

MFE methods work quite well for small molecules such as tRNAs where about 85% of paired sites are correctly predicted [13]. For large RNAs the performance can be quite variable, e.g. 10% to 81% accuracy in correctly predicted paired sites with an average of 46% for SSU rRNAs [14] and similar results for LSU rRNAs [15]. It is unclear exactly what the source of this inaccuracy is. It could be that the free energy models used are inaccurate but it has also been argued that molecules are not folding into the most thermodynamically stable state. In this case the folding kinetics should be considered. One hypothesis is that RNA folding happens in a hierarchical manner, with smaller structural domains forming first, followed by larger scale structures forming over progressively longer time-scales [16]. These folding pathways may not end up at the MFE structure, because there may be large energetic barriers which disallow large-scale rearrangement of the structure. Computational methods for modelling the folding kinetics are reviewed in [5].

When sequences are available for the same molecule from many different species then comparative methods are by far the most accurate [17]. This is typically the case for the RNA molecules used in phylogenetic studies and the structure predictions used in our analysis are therefore determined by the comparative method. The key observation used in the comparative method is that the RNA structure evolves much more slowly than the sequence. Therefore, when a base changes on one side of a helix this will usually be compensated for by a similar change on the opposite side, in order to maintain structural stability and therefore biological function. This process is known as *compensatory substitution* or *covariation*. The comparative method of structure prediction uses the covariation of base-paired sites in a set of sequences in order to infer the secondary structure.

The comparative method requires that sequences are sufficiently closely related that they can be reliably aligned, but that there is sufficient divergence for many sequence substitutions to have occurred in the helices [18]. This is not a fully automated method but rather there are a number of stages and the method requires a certain degree of hand-crafting to particular cases. The first step is to align the sequences using standard multiple alignment algorithms, usually refined by hand. Then one searches for sites which covary in such a way that the base-pairing is conserved. In order to match covarying sites it may then be necessary to modify the alignment iteratively. Structures derived by the comparative method have been found to predict base-pairs with close to 100% accuracy in comparison with high-resolution crystal structures [17] and are currently much more accurate than methods based on thermodynamics or kinetics [15].

Full probabilistic models of homologous RNA molecules have also been developed [19] which are analogous to profile hidden Markov models developed for modelling protein families. These models can represent the conserved sequence motifs which exist in related molecules and include an explicit model of the RNA secondary structure which allows them to take account of the covariation process. This provides a principled probabilistic framework for carrying out a comparative analysis. In practice these models are currently not practical for large-scale structure prediction and have mainly been applied to the detection of small RNA genes in genomic DNA.

6.3 Substitution Processes in RNA Helices

Sequence evolution and compensatory mutations

In phylogenetics we are usually interested in the properties of evolving populations of species, or of the genes carried by those species. The models used for phylogenetic inference therefore describe evolution in terms of substitutions at the population level, where substitutions are defined to be mutations that have become common (or *fixed*[3]) within the population. The idea is that the population is summarised by a consensus sequence that contains the most common version of each gene's DNA sequence (or of the sites within that gene's DNA). In practice we may only use the sequence of a single individual within the population, but this is a reasonable approximation to the consensus as long as the intra-species variation is much lower than the inter-species variation.

Mutations occur at the level of individuals within a population. It is therefore important to appreciate how these mutations become fixed or lost in populations and this is the subject of population genetics theory. Of particular interest to us is the process of *compensatory mutations* whereby a mutation on one side of an RNA helix is compensated by a mutation on the opposite side, thereby maintaining the molecule's stability [21, 22, 23]. Mutations are intrinsically stochastic in nature and we can model the process of fixation or loss as a diffusion process [24].

The specific case of compensatory mutations in the RNA helices was studied in [23]. A single base-pair in an RNA helix was considered in isolation, so that the state-space was 16-dimensional with each variable representing a different ordered pair of bases. Simplifying approximations were used to reduce

[3] A discussion of *fixation* in population genetics can be found in [20], Section 4.2.

this to a three-dimensional diffusion equation which was amenable to analysis. The model includes a parameter s determining the strength of selection against a non–Watson–Crick base-pair and a parameter u determining the mutation rate. In order to simplify the analysis the marginally stable GU/UG pairs were considered unstable, so that pairs were either stable Watson–Crick pairs or unstable mismatch pairs.

Of particular interest is the shape of the stationary distribution of base-pair frequencies, since this determines how the consensus sequence of the population will look. The behaviour of this distribution was found to be mainly determined by a quantity $\xi \propto Nu^2/s$ where N is the population size. When ξ is large (weak selection) the probability of unstable pairs can be significant, so that there is some probability of observing an unstable pair in the consensus sequence corresponding to a helix. However, when ξ is low (strong selection) then the stationary frequency distribution is peaked around the stable base pairs and it is very unlikely that we will observe an unstable pair in the consensus sequence. Also of interest is the dynamics of the stationary process as this determines how the consensus sequence changes over time. For large ξ the change from one Watson–Crick pair to another is most likely to occur via an unstable intermediate pair in the consensus sequence (e.g. AU$\rightarrow$ AG$\rightarrow$ CG) which we will call a *two-step process*. However, if ξ is small then the consensus sequence is more likely to change directly from one Watson–Crick pair to another directly (e.g. AU$\rightarrow$ CG) and we will call this a *one-step process*. In this latter case the unstable intermediate (AG) never obtains a high frequency within the population and is never represented in the consensus sequence. This can happen because the mutation (AG$\rightarrow$ CG) can occur to one of the rare AG mutants within the population. Being stable and selectively neutral, the resulting CG mutant may then become fixed in the population by chance.

Models of the substitution process

Models of the substitution process used in molecular phylogenetics are at the level of populations rather than individuals. However, results from the population genetics theory described above are important because they suggest certain features which we would expect to observe in the base-pair substitution process. The small ξ regime is probably of greatest relevance in practice, since unstable base-pairs occur with relatively low (3–4%) frequency in the helices of most RNA molecules. This means that the one-step process described above should be included in population level models of the substitution process. A number of existing models of the substitution process do not allow for substitutions requiring simultaneous changes on both sides of the helix [25, 26, 27]. Such a restriction is reasonable at the level of individuals, where two simultaneous compensatory mutations are vanishingly unlikely to occur. However, the population genetics theory demonstrates that such changes are quite likely in the consensus sequence of the population. Savill et al. [28] compared a large number of substitution models which either allowed or disallowed the one-step

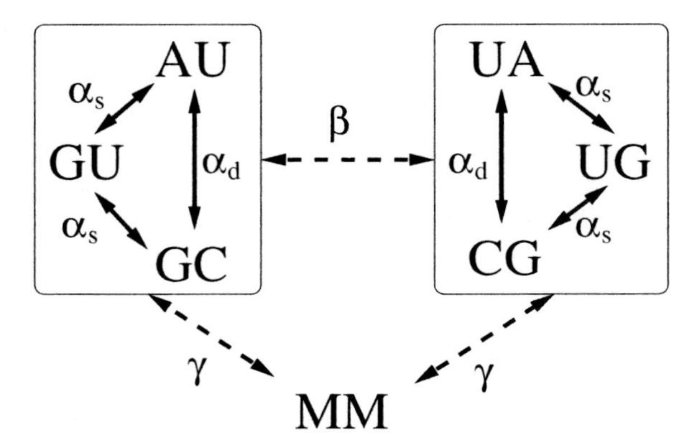

Fig. 6.2. We show the different types of substitution that can occur at paired sites of the RNA helix. The MM (mismatch) state corresponds to the ten unstable pairings that occur with low probability. Substitutions shown as solid lines occur more frequently than the other substitutions since they do not require pairs to enter an unstable configuration. Greek symbols denote different types of substitution: α_s for single transitions, α_d for double transitions, β for double transversions and γ for substitutions to and from mismatch states. These are the rate parameters in the Tillier and Collins substitution model [29] (see (6.4) in the main text). Adapted from [29], with permission.

process in RNA helices. Models which do allow the one-step process (e.g. [29]) appear to fit the data much better than those which do not.

As well as considering the one-step and two-step substitution processes described above, we must also consider the role of the GU/UG stable intermediate base-pairs which were not modelled in the population genetics theory. These pairs exist with appreciable probability within the population and are less selected against than the unstable non-canonical base-pairs. It is therefore much more likely to observe changes between Watson–Crick pairs that can occur via a stable intermediate (e.g. AU$\rightarrow$ GC via GU) than changes which cannot (e.g. AU $\rightarrow$ UA). The former substitutions are *double transitions* while the latter are *double transversions*[4]. Our results in Section 6.4 demonstrate that single or double transitions are indeed much faster than double transversions for the data set considered there. Figure 6.2 shows the different substitutions, with frequent substitutions shown as solid arrows and infrequent substitutions shown as dashed arrows. We emphasise again that substitutions that allow both sites to change simultaneously are quite common within a population and should be allowed in the particular substitution model used.

[4] Recall from Section 4.4.1 that DNA or RNA bases can be classified as purines (A,G) or pyrimidines (C,U/T). Transitions are substitutions within these groups (e.g. A$\rightarrow$G) and transversions are substitutions between them (e.g. A$\rightarrow$U).

Standard models of DNA substitution, discussed in Chapter 4, especially Section 4.4.2, assume a time-homogeneous and stationary Markov process. We denote the probability of a substitution[5] from base i to base j in time t as $P_{ij}(t)$. The matrix of probabilities $\mathbf{P}$ can be obtained from the rate matrix $\mathbf{R}$ according to (4.14):

$$\mathbf{P}(t) = \mathrm{e}^{\mathbf{R}t} \; . \tag{6.1}$$

Some examples of particular rate matrices are introduced in Section 4.4.2. We denote the frequency of each base as Π_i and there is clearly a constraint that these sum to one. Time-homogeneous, stationary Markov models satisfy the time-reversibility condition (4.36),

$$\Pi_i R_{ij} = \Pi_j R_{ji} \; , \tag{6.2}$$

where R_{ij} are elements of the rate matrix $\mathbf{R}$. We choose to define parameters α_{ij} such that $R_{ij} = \alpha_{ij}\Pi_j$ for a symmetric choice of α_{ij}. There is typically an additional constraint that the average rate of substitutions is one per unit time and this determines the unit of time measurement,

$$\sum_i \sum_{j \neq i} \Pi_i R_{ij} = 1 \; . \tag{6.3}$$

The most general time-reversible DNA substitution process (GTR4) has four frequency parameters Π_i and six rate parameters α_{ij}. With the constraint that frequencies sum to one and an additional constraint on the number of substitutions per unit time, the GTR4 model has eight free parameters. Simpler models have been developed which constrain certain parameters to be the same by appealing to symmetries (e.g. the Kimura and HKY85 models defined in Section 4.4.2). These models are useful because they allow a closed form solution of the rate equation (6.1). However, in practice these symmetries often do not hold and the data sets we consider are usually sufficiently large to provide support for the more general models. In this case the eigenvalues and eigenvectors of $\mathbf{R}$ must be obtained in order to solve (6.1). This only has to be done once for each particular choice of parameter values and is therefore a minor computational cost to pay in our applications.

Models of base-pair substitution are similar to standard DNA substitution models except that the states are now pairs of bases, rather than individual bases. In principle, there are 16 possible ordered pairs that can be formed from four bases and we would require a 16×16 substitution rate matrix to describe the evolutionary process. In practice there are only six frequently occurring pairs. Some models use only a 6×6 rate matrix and ignore mismatches completely, whereas other models group all the mismatches into a single MM state

[5] In Chapter 4, the probability of a substitution from base i to base j in time t is defined as $P_{ji}(t)$ rather than $P_{ij}(t)$, hence the matrices $\mathbf{P}$ and $\mathbf{R}$ in Chapter 4 are the transpositions of those used in this chapter.

and hence use a 7×7 substitution matrix. A number of 6, 7 and 16 state substitution models were compared using likelihood ratio tests and other model selection methods in [28]. It was confirmed there that models which included the one-step substitution process were significantly better than those which did not.

The most general time-reversible 7-state model (GTR7) has 7 frequency parameters and 21 rate parameters. With the same constraints described above for GTR4 the model has 26 free parameters. As with DNA substitution models, one can appeal to symmetries in the substitution process in order to reduce the number of free parameters and allow a closed form solution to (6.1). One example of this is the 7-state model due to Tillier and Collins [29]. They include all state frequencies but restrict the rates according to certain symmetries. They have four rate parameters: α_s for single transitions, α_d for double transitions, β for double transversions and γ for substitutions to and from mismatch states (see Figure 6.2). The rate matrix corresponding to this model is then

$$\mathbf{R} = \begin{array}{c} \\ AU \\ GU \\ GC \\ UA \\ UG \\ CG \\ MM \end{array} \begin{array}{c} \begin{array}{ccccccc} AU & GU & GC & UA & UG & CG & MM \end{array} \\ \begin{pmatrix} * & \Pi_2\alpha_s & \Pi_3\alpha_d & \Pi_4\beta & \Pi_5\beta & \Pi_6\beta & \Pi_7\gamma \\ \Pi_1\alpha_s & * & \Pi_3\alpha_s & \Pi_4\beta & \Pi_5\beta & \Pi_6\beta & \Pi_7\gamma \\ \Pi_1\alpha_d & \Pi_2\alpha_s & * & \Pi_4\beta & \Pi_5\beta & \Pi_6\beta & \Pi_7\gamma \\ \Pi_1\beta & \Pi_2\beta & \Pi_3\beta & * & \Pi_5\alpha_s & \Pi_6\alpha_d & \Pi_7\gamma \\ \Pi_1\beta & \Pi_2\beta & \Pi_3\beta & \Pi_4\alpha_s & * & \Pi_6\alpha_s & \Pi_7\gamma \\ \Pi_1\beta & \Pi_2\beta & \Pi_3\beta & \Pi_4\alpha_d & \Pi_5\alpha_s & * & \Pi_7\gamma \\ \Pi_1\gamma & \Pi_2\gamma & \Pi_3\gamma & \Pi_4\gamma & \Pi_5\gamma & \Pi_6\gamma & * \end{pmatrix} \end{array} \tag{6.4}$$

where the diagonals can be determined by the convention that the rows sum to zero. For this simplified rate matrix it is possible to solve the eigensystem explicitly. However, it was found in [28] that relaxing the symmetries provides a significant improvement in the likelihood and therefore GTR7 is usually preferred in practice.

The PHASE package

The most useful 6, 7 and 16-state base-pair substitution models have been implemented in the PHASE phylogenetic inference software (PHylogeny And Sequence Evolution, available from www.bioinf.man.ac.uk/resources/). The package includes methods for Bayesian and maximum likelihood inference of tree topologies, branch lengths and model parameters. The Bayesian inference is carried out by a Markov chain Monte Carlo (MCMC) algorithm. A discrete-Gamma variable rate model is included in order to deal with the huge variation in evolutionary rates at different sites in RNA molecules [30]. See Chapter 4 for an introduction to maximum likelihood and Bayesian phylogenetic methods (Sections 4.4.5 and 4.4.7), standard DNA substitution models (Section 4.4.2), and variable rate models (Section 4.4.9). For details of our MCMC sampler see [31] and for details of the substitution models and other programs in the package see the documentation available from the PHASE web-site.

The most recent version of PHASE allows for more than one substitution model to be applied to a data set simultaneously [32]. This is very useful in the context of RNA molecules, where the loops and helices should be described by the most appropriate model in each case. For the results presented here we use a standard DNA substitution model (GTR4) for the RNA loops and a base-pair model (GTR7) for the helices. Each model has its own set of variable rate categories with their own Gamma distribution parameter. The constraint that the total number of substitutions per unit time should equal one is applied to one of the models in order to calibrate the time-scale. The rate of substitutions for the other model is measured relative to this. We do not assume a molecular clock and therefore the trees inferred are unrooted and an outgroup is required in order to place a root.[6]

6.4 An Application: Mammalian Phylogeny

Molecular phylogenetic methods have played an important role in recent important changes in our understanding of mammalian evolution. We now have sequence data from large numbers of species, and the computational methods for analysis of these data sets are improving. One important feature of the mammal tree that is strongly supported by molecular data is that the placental mammals can be divided into four principal groups. This has been shown convincingly by recent studies of large concatenated sets of genes [33, 34, 35]. Using the numbering from [34] these groups are: (I) Afrotheria, containing mammals thought to have originated from Africa, (II) Xenarthra, South American mammals including e.g. armadillos, (III) containing primates, rodents and others, (IV) containing all of the other placental mammals. This classification has only emerged quite recently and includes some surprises. For example, the Afrotherian clade contains many morphologically diverse species that were previously assigned to very distant parts of the mammal tree. It is difficult to find any superficial similarities between many of these species. Also, although most of the mammalian orders have been well established for a long time from morphological similarity and fossil evidence, the early branches in the mammal tree are difficult to resolve using these methods. The evidence offered by molecular data therefore provides useful resolution for the early branches.

The molecular picture described above was obtained using large data sets mostly comprising genes whose DNA is contained in the cell nucleus. Cellular organisms also have a small proportion of their DNA contained in small organelles which exist outside of the cell nucleus, known as mitochondria in animals and chloroplasts in plants. Many taxa have had their entire mitochondrial genomes sequenced, and the mitochondrial DNA therefore provides an

[6] The method of rooting a tree with an outgroup is briefly explained in Section 4.1

important resource for phylogenetic investigations. Studies using mitochondrial DNA have repeatedly contradicted the picture emerging from the above studies (e.g. [36, 37]) and it has been suggested that these results may be artifacts due to the assumption of a homogeneous and stationary substitution model [38]; see Section 4.4.11. In contrast to this, our own studies using large sets of RNA genes from the mitochondrial genome find strong support for the consensus picture emerging [31, 32]. This may be due in some part to our particular choice of genes, as well as the methods used. For example, stability constraints in the RNA helices may make them less susceptible to changes in mutation patterns which can cause non-stationarity in the substitution process. Nevertheless, we believe that our results demonstrate the importance of RNA genes in resolving challenging phylogenetic issues. We show below that using inappropriate substitution models for these genes may result in misleading posterior probabilities and will generally invalidate the statistical support given to a particular phylogenetic hypothesis.

In our most recent study we used a data set comprising the entire complement of RNA genes encoded by the mitochondrial genome of 69 mammals. A small number of non-placental mammals (marsupials and monotremes) are included as an outgroup in order to root the tree of placental mammals. The genes used include the SSU and LSU rRNA as well as all 22 tRNAs. The data set contains 3571 bases in total, consisting of 967 base-pairs and 1637 single sites (full details of the methods and sequences used are provided in [32]). This was a completely unselective set of sequences as it was made up of all mitochondrial sequences publicly available at that time (August 2002). We carried out four independent MCMC runs starting from a random initial tree and each run provided us with 40,000 samples of tree topology, branch lengths and substitution model parameters. The results are summarised in Figure 6.3 which shows a consensus tree from the combined MCMC output from all four runs. This tree was constructed using the majority rule consensus tree method provided by the PHYLIP package [39] which draws a tree containing all sub-trees (*clades*) appearing in more than 50% of samples, as well as the most supported remaining clades which are not contradictory. Although this tree cannot completely capture the information from the MCMC sample, it provides a useful visualisation of the most supported arrangements. Clades supported with less than 100% of the posterior probability have the percentage of posterior probability shown (i.e. the percentage of times they appear in the MCMC output). Mean posterior estimate (MPE) branch lengths are shown on the tree conditional on this topology, i.e. these are the mean branch lengths for every topology identical to the consensus in the MCMC samples.

The consensus tree shows that we find strong support for the four main groups described above. In addition, the resolution appears to be good for later evolutionary events. We find support for all of the established mammalian orders, most of which are strongly supported. It appears that different parts of the RNA molecule provide resolution on different time-scales. In an earlier study [31] we used only data from the RNA helices with the GTR7 base-

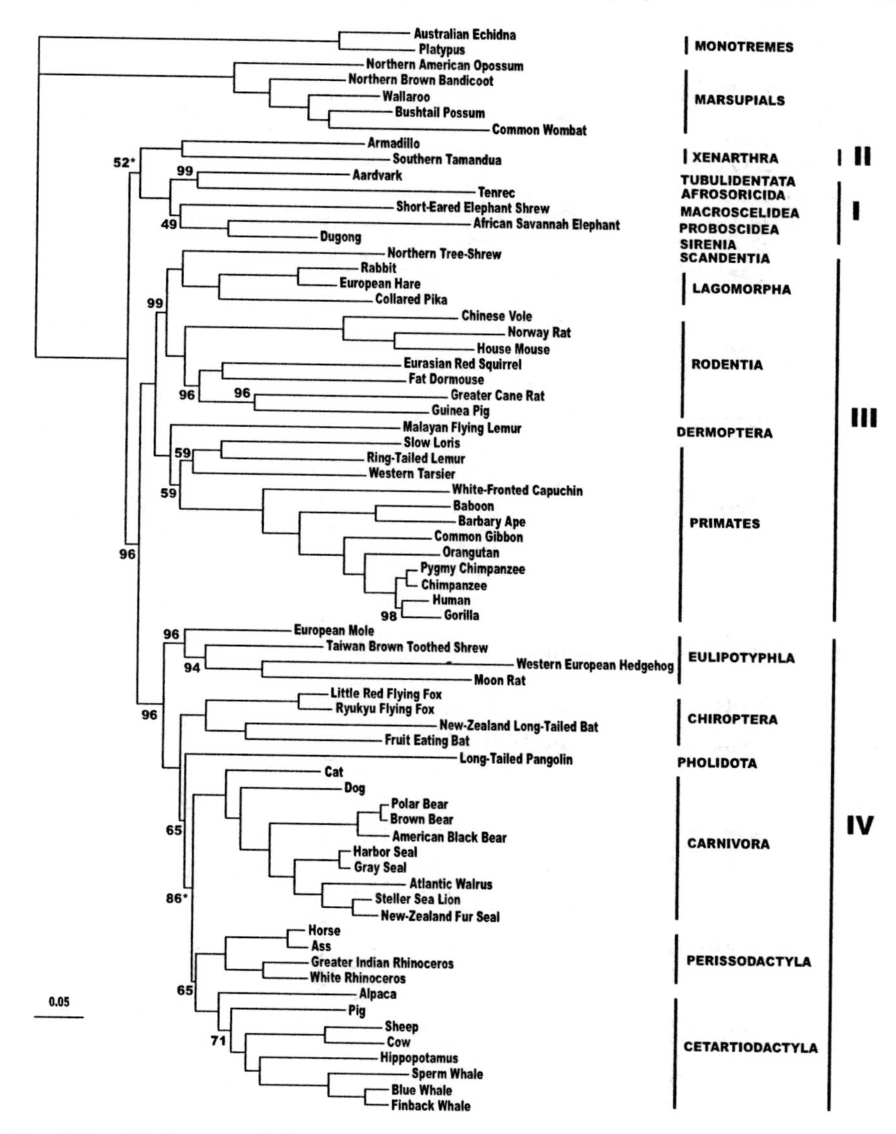

Fig. 6.3. Phylogeny of the mammals inferred from a data set containing all mitochondrial RNA genes. Bayesian posterior probability values are calculated using the PHASE program. Percentages shown are averaged over four independent runs. Internal nodes without percentages are supported with 100% of posterior probability in every run. Percentages marked with an asterix are the most variable with percentages ranging between 5 and 7.5% from the mean over the four runs. The remaining numbers vary by less than 4% over all runs (reprinted from [32] with permission from Elsevier).

pair model. In that study we had good resolution for the early branches in the tree, but many of the later evolutionary events were not well resolved and a number of mammalian orders were found to be paraphyletic (i.e. not compatible with coming exclusively from the same clade). In contrast to this, runs using only the single-stranded RNA loops have very poor resolution for the early branches of the tree. When data from the loops and helices are combined then there is good resolution for early and late evolutionary events.

It is well known that the substitution process in the loops is typically faster than in the helices, since bases in the helices are under selective pressure to maintain stability. However, in our study we found the mean substitution rate to be almost identical in the loops and helices. The reason for this is that we only used parts of loops that could be reliably aligned across all species. Thus we excluded substantial parts of the RNA loops that were most highly variable. The question then remains as to why the helices provide much more information over long time-scales compared with the loops, given that the loops contain almost twice the number of independent features. One answer may be that the alphabet is larger for RNA (7 pairs in GTR7 versus 4 bases in GTR4) and therefore the substitution process contains more memory. Another reason is suggested when we look at the estimated substitution model parameters, shown in Table 6.1. Focusing first on the six canonical base-pairs we see that substitutions requiring only transitions are fastest (i.e. between {AU,GU,GC} or {UA,UG,CG}). This correlates well with the picture described in Section 6.3 and Figure 6.2. We see in particular that double transitions are fastest, suggesting that the one-step substitution process appears to be occurring via a GU/UG intermediate which is never fixed in the population. Substitutions to and from the MM states are not uncommon, although it should be remembered that this is a composite state for all ten unstable pairs and therefore the actual substitution to any particular unstable pair is roughly one tenth of these values. The pattern of substitutions may provide an explanation of why the RNA helices provide resolution over long evolutionary times. We see that changes requiring a double transversion (directly or via a mismatch) will typically be much slower than changes requiring only transitions. It is also true that transitions are typically faster than transversions in the loops, but the difference in the helices is much greater [32]. Therefore, double transversions provide information on much longer time-scales than transitions and will provide useful phylogenetic information over long time-scales.

The rate of substitutions to and from unstable pairs looks higher than might be expected given our arguments about the one-step process dominating under strong selective pressure against mismatches. This problem may in part be due to an unforeseen relationship between the variable rate model and the substitution model used in the helices. Sites with a high substitution rate will tend to be those under weakest selective constraint on conserved structure. Therefore, the proportion of unstable pairs will tend to correlate with the substitution rate and sites with high rates will have more MM states on average. We have observed exactly this pattern in the data set used here

R_{ij}	AU	GU	GC	UA	UG	CG	MM
AU	*	0.2051	0.3682	0.0147	0.0021	0.0006	0.2809
GU	1.5060	*	1.0638	0.0064	0.0029	0.0095	0.1647
GC	0.4954	0.1950	*	0.0009	0.0009	0.0007	0.1463
UA	0.0153	0.0009	0.0007	*	0.1613	0.2774	0.2498
UG	0.0164	0.0031	0.0052	1.2410	*	0.6989	0.2336
CG	0.0009	0.0019	0.0007	0.3880	0.1271	*	0.1793
MM	0.6177	0.0493	0.2391	0.5303	0.0645	0.2721	*

Table 6.1. Mean posterior transition rate estimates for the GTR7 model used for paired sites in the RNA helices (reprinted from [32] with permission from Elsevier).

and this will tend to bias the parameter estimates. For example, the base-pair frequency estimates will tend to be larger than the mean frequency of MM pairs observed in the data [31]. This is because the fastest evolving sites will contribute more information to the frequency estimates, as they provide less correlated samples from the substitution process. As an example one can compare an invariant site with an infinitely rapidly evolving site. The fast site contributes as many samples from the stationary substitution process as there are species in the tree, since there is no memory of the past in any of the samples. By contrast, the invariant site only contributes a single sample for the process. Therefore, the fast site will contribute much more information about the base-pair frequencies and this will tend to increase the MM estimate. The effect on substitution rates is harder to predict but we would expect a similar inflation of the rate to and from these states. These observations suggest that we need to further improve the substitution models in order to fit the data better. We are currently investigating models which assign different parameters to different rate classes in the variable rate model.

It is interesting to ask what happens when a standard 4-state DNA substitution model is applied to data from the RNA helices. Do base-pair models provide us with any advantages over the standard models? We carried out a comparison in [31] using only the helical regions of the mitochondrial RNA and found that the consensus trees obtained by each method were significantly different. It was not obvious which consensus tree was a more accurate representation of the true evolutionary relationship but we did observe that the tree obtained using a standard DNA substitution model tended to find higher posterior probabilities, some of which were for rather dubious arrangements. In Figure 6.4 we plot the number of occurrences of each distinct tree topology (ranked according to posterior probability) for each model. The posterior probability distribution is much more peaked for the DNA model, with the top tree topology having about an order of magnitude greater posterior probability.

We can understand these results by considering what happens if we apply a DNA substitution model to a perfectly base-paired helix (i.e. where all pairs

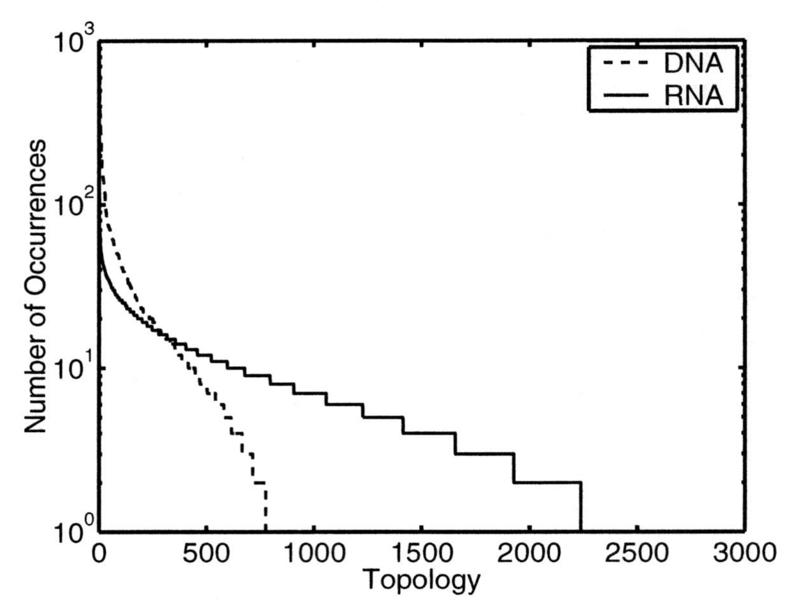

Fig. 6.4. The number of occurrences of each topology is plotted for two MCMC runs using the GTR7 (solid line) and GTR4 (dashed line) substitution models. The topologies are ranked according to the number of occurrences in each case (reprinted from [31] with permission from Oxford University Press).

are Watson–Crick pairs). Let L_1 and L_2 be the likelihood of two different trees given data from one side of the helix. Under a standard DNA substitution model such as the Jukes–Cantor or HKY85 model introduced in Section 4.4.2, the corresponding likelihoods given data from both sides (but treating sites as independent) would be L_1^2 and L_2^2 for each tree respectively.[7] Under a uniform prior the likelihood ratio gives the ratio of posterior probabilities for the two trees. The ratio is L_1/L_2 in the first case and L_1^2/L_2^2 in the second case. So, if one tree is 100 times more likely than another given information from one side of the helix, it will be 10,000 times more likely given information from both. This effect tends to make the posterior probability distribution more peaked than it should be. A similar argument also applies to bootstrap support values, discussed in Section 4.4.6, which will tend to be over-estimated when sequence data are strongly correlated. This suggests that it is dangerous to ignore correlations due to base-pairing and our results in Figure 6.4 show that the effects in real data may be significant.

[7] This assumes symmetries in the frequencies (e.g. $\Pi_C = \Pi_G$ and $\Pi_T = \Pi_A$) that hold if model parameters are estimated from perfectly base-paired data.

6.5 Conclusion

RNA molecules are used extensively in phylogenetic studies. Their strongly conserved secondary structure can be used to improve the alignment of highly diverged sequences and this in turn can improve phylogenetic accuracy. Computational methods can be used to determine the secondary structure from sequence information alone and comparative methods in particular provide an accurate method of structure prediction when a large number of related sequences are available. However, the substitution models used in most phylogenetic studies ignore the strong covariation of base-paired sites. We have implemented a number of substitution models that treat base-paired sites in the RNA helices as a unit of evolution and these are included in the PHASE phylogenetic inference software package. The most recent version allows for an arbitrary number of substitution models to be used simultaneously. This means that we can use models specific to the RNA helices along with standard DNA substitution models applied to unpaired sites in the RNA loops.

Our results on a large data set of mammalian mitochondrial RNA are very promising. This is the first study using mitochondrial DNA and a completely unselective set of species to find support for monophyly of all mammalian orders, and to find support for the same four early branching groups observed in recent studies of much larger data sets mainly comprising nuclear genes. We show that using inappropriate substitution models for the RNA helices will artificially inflate posterior probabilities in a Bayesian analysis and it is therefore important to correctly account for covariation in the helices.

The substitution models used in molecular phylogenetics need to be improved further, as many of the simplifying assumptions used are violated in real data sets. In this study we observed a non-trivial relationship between the variable rate model and the substitution rate matrix in base-pair models, suggesting that these cannot be treated as independent of one another. There may also be differences between the substitution processes in different genes, or different parts of the same gene. Most of the models currently used assume a stationary and homogeneous Markov model of the substitution process, as discussed in Section 4.4.2. These assumptions can be violated in real data sets. Non-stationary and non-homogeneous substitution models have been introduced [40, 41], and are discussed in Section 4.4.11, but these methods are not widely available in phylogenetic inference software and are not appropriate for all types of data. The length of sequences used in phylogenetics studies is sometimes of the order of 10,000 bases and in this case there will be sufficient data to accurately estimate the parameters of quite complex models.

The Bayesian inference methodology is attractive in phylogenetic inference as there is often uncertainty about certain phylogenetic features. Posterior probabilities allow us to quantify the degree of uncertainty in these features. For example, in Figure 6.3 there is no resolution for the relative positioning of the clades (I), (II) and (III,IV) despite the fact that these clades themselves are strongly supported. Bootstrap support values provide an alternative method of determining the confidence in phylogenetic features, but the computational cost of finding the maximum likelihood tree for many bootstrap samples is considerable; see Figure 4.35 on page 134.

Recently there has been some debate about the relative merits of Bayesian posterior probabilities and bootstrap support values (see e.g. [42, 43, 44]). It appears that bootstrap support values are more conservative than posterior probabilities and the relationship between the quantities is often nonlinear. Some see this as evidence that bootstrap proportions are biased, while others see it as a positive aspect of the bootstrap method. Bayesian posterior probabilities use the likelihood ratio in order to score the relative posterior probability of two competing hypotheses. This quantity has been shown to have much higher variance between sites in real data sets than would be expected under the assumed parametric model of the substitution process [45]. It has therefore been argued that this will lead to over-confidence in a hypothesis with higher likelihood. This problem appears to stem from the fact that substitution models are much simpler than the actual evolutionary processes at work. The interpretation of posterior probabilities is unclear when the actual data is produced by a process very different from the class of models considered. It has therefore been argued that bootstrap support values are a better measure of the actual variability observed in the data and provide a more robust estimate of the confidence in the result. Some recent work attempts to reconcile these two very different methods and to produce bootstrap-like quantities from an MCMC algorithm [45]. However, the interpretation and relative merits of both methods remain under debate. Our own work demonstrates that both posterior probabilities and bootstrap support values can be misleading when the substitution model ignores strong inter-site dependencies. We believe that the best way to proceed is to develop increasingly realistic models of the substitution process and that is the focus of our research.

Acknowledgments

This work was supported by the UK Biotechnology and Biological Sciences Research Council. We would like to thank Vivek Gowri-Shankar for useful comments on a preliminary draft.

References

[1] Olsen GJ and Woese CR. *FASEB*, 7:113–123, 1993.
[2] Boucher Y, Nesbo CL, and Doolittle WF. *Curr Op Microbiol*, 4:285–289, 2001.
[3] Woese CR. *Proc Nat Acad Sci USA*, 97:8392–8396, 2000.
[4] Titus TA and Frost DR. *Mol Phylogenet Evol*, 6:49–62, 1996.
[5] Higgs PG. *Quart Rev Biophys*, 33:199–253, 2000.

[6] Cannone JJ, Subramanian S, Schnare MN, Collet JR, D'Souza LM, Du Y, Feng B, Lin N, Madabusi LV, Müller KM, Pande N, Shang Z, Yu N, and Gutell RR. *BMC Bioinformatics*, 3:2, 2002.

[7] Wang Z and Zhang K. In Jing T, Xu Y, and Zhang MQ, editors, *Current Topics in Computational Molecular Biology*, pages 345–363. MIT Press, Cambridge MA, 2002.

[8] Freier SM, Kierzek R, Jaeger JA, Sugimoto N, Caruthers MH, Nielson T, and Turner DH. *Proc Nat Acad Sci USA*, 83:9373–9377, 1986.

[9] Nussinov R and Jacobson AB. *Proc Nat Acad Sci USA*, 77:6309–6313, 1980.

[10] Waterman MS and Smith TF. *Adv Applied Maths*, 7:455–464, 1986.

[11] Zuker M. *Science*, 244:48–52, 1989.

[12] McCaskill JS. *Biopolymers*, 29:1105–1119, 1990.

[13] Higgs PG. *J Chem Soc Faraday Trans*, 91:2531–2540, 1995.

[14] Konings DAM and Gutell RR. *RNA*, 1:559–574, 1995.

[15] Fields DS and Gutell RR. *Folding & Design*, 1:419–430, 1996.

[16] Morgan SR and Higgs PG. *J Chem Phys*, 105:7152–7157, 1996.

[17] Gutell RR, Lee JC, and Cannone JJ. *Curr Op Struct Biol*, 12:302–310, 2002.

[18] Gutell RR, Power A, Hertz GZ, Putz EJ, and Stormo GD. *Nucl Acids Res*, 20:5785–5795, 1992.

[19] Durbin R, Eddy S, Krogh A, and Mitchison G. *Biological Sequence Analysis*. Cambridge University Press, Cambridge UK, 1998.

[20] Page DM and Holmes EC. *Molecular Evolution - A Phylogenetic Approach*. Blackwell Science, Cambridge (UK), 1998.

[21] Kimura M. *Theor Pop Biol*, 7:364–398, 1985.

[22] Stephan W. *Genetics*, 144:419–426, 1996.

[23] Higgs PG. *Genetica*, 102/103:91–101, 1998.

[24] Crow JF and Kimura M. *An Introduction to Population Genetics Theory*. Harper & Row, New York, 1970.

[25] Schöniger M and Von Haeseler A. *Mol Phylogenet Evol*, 3:240–247, 1994.

[26] Muse S. *Genetics*, 139:1429–1439, 1995.

[27] Rzhetsky A. *Genetics*, 141:771–783, 1995.

[28] Savill NJ, Hoyle DC, and Higgs PG. *Genetics*, 157:399–411, 2001.

[29] Tillier ERM and Collins RA. *Genetics*, 148:1993–2002, 1998.

[30] Yang Z. *J Mol Evol*, 39:306–314, 1994.

[31] Jow H, Hudelot C, Rattray M, and Higgs PG. *Mol Biol Evol*, 19:1591–1601, 2002.

[32] Hudelot C, Gowri-Shankar V, Jow H, Rattray M, and Higgs PG. *Mol Phylogenet Evol*, 28:241-252, 2003.

[33] Madsen O, Scally M, Douady CJ, Kao DJ, DeBry RW, Adkins R, Amrine HM, Stanhope MJ, de Jong W, and Springer MS. *Nature*, 409:610–614, 2001.

[34] Murphy WJ, Eizirik E, Johnson WE, Zhang YP, Ryder A, and O'Brien SJ. *Nature*, 409:614–618, 2001.

[35] Murphy WJ, Eizirik E, O'Brien SJ, Madsen O, Scally M, Douady CJ, Teeling E, Ryder OA, Stanhope MJ, de Jong WW, and Springer MS. *Science*, 294:2348–2351, 2001.
[36] Penny D, Hasegawa M, Waddell PJ, and Hendy MD. *Syst Biol*, 48:76–93, 1999.
[37] Arnason U, Adegoke JA, Bodin K, Born EW, BE Yuzine, Gullberg A, Nilsson M, Short VS, Xu X, and Janke A. *Proc Nat Acad Sci USA*, 99:8151–8156, 2002.
[38] Lin Y-H, McLenachan PA, Gore AR, Phillips MJ, Ota R, Hendy MD, and Penny D. *Mol Biol Evol*, 19:2060–2070, 2002.
[39] Felsenstein JP. *Cladistics*, 5:164–166, 1989.
[40] Yang Z and Roberts D. *J Mol Biol*, 14:717–724, 1995.
[41] Galtier N and Gouy M. *J Mol Evol*, 44:632–636, 1998.
[42] Wilcox TP, Zwickl DJ, Heath TA, and Hillis DM. *Mol Phylogenet Evol*, 25:361–371, 2002.
[43] Douady CJ, Delsuc F, Boucher Y, Doolittle WF, and Douzery EJP. *Mol Biol Evol*, 20:248–254, 2003.
[44] Alfaro ME, Zoller S, and Lutzoni F. *Mol Biol Evol*, 20:255–266, 2003.
[45] Waddell PJ, Kishino H, and Ota R. *Genome Informatics Series*, 13:82–92, 2002.

7

Statistical Methods in Microarray Gene Expression Data Analysis

Claus-Dieter Mayer[1] and Chris A. Glasbey[2]

[1] Biomathematics & Statistics Scotland, BioSS Office at the Rowett Research Institute, Aberdeen AB21 9SB, UK, claus@bioss.ac.uk
[2] Biomathematics & Statistics Scotland, King's Buildings, Edinburgh EH9 3JZ, UK, chris@bioss.ac.uk

Summary. Microarrays allow the simultaneous measurement of the expression levels of thousands of genes. This unique data structure has inspired a completely new area of research in statistics and bioinformatics. The objective of the present chapter is to review some of the main statistical tools used in this context. We will mainly focus on low-level preprocessing steps: image analysis, data transformation, normalization, and multiple testing for differential expression. The high-level inference of genetic regulatory interactions from preprocessed microarray data will be covered in Chapters 8 and 9.

7.1 Introduction

Microarrays have been a key element in the biotechnological revolution of recent years. They have enabled life scientists to monitor the expression of thousands of genes simultaneously and thus to obtain snapshots of the state of a complete genome. This development has inspired many new research projects, which promise to give us important information about the molecular biological processes that rule our lives. However, due to both the enormous volume and the unique structure of microarray data, completely new problems of data handling and statistical analysis have to be tackled. It is the second problem, the statistical analysis, that we will be concerned with in this chapter. We will cover some of the main statistical challenges and discuss relevant contributions that have been made to the field so far.

7.1.1 Gene Expression in a Nutshell

To understand microarray measurements and their relevance we will first summarize the relevant biology. In the nucleus of each cell we find strands of DNA, consisting of long chains of the nucleotides C, T, G and A. The four nucleotides are paired in the sense that A forms a weak bond with T, and

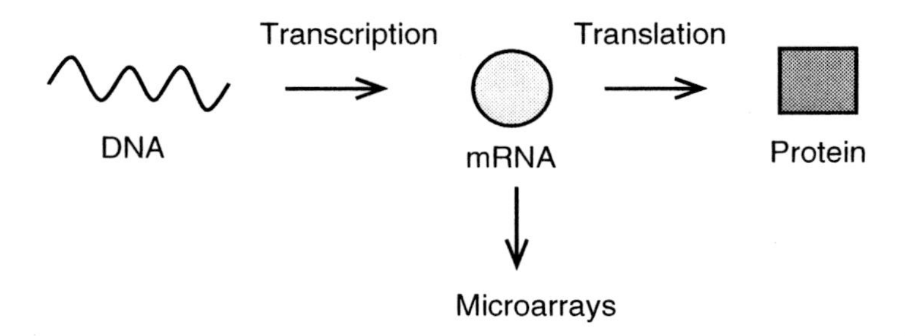

Fig. 7.1. Steps in protein synthesis, and what microarrays measure.

C with G. This is reflected in the structure of DNA: strands are arranged in pairs forming a *double helix*, where the second strand consists of the complementary nucleotides. *Genes* are certain subchains of the DNA that contain important information. Each nucleotide triplet codes for an amino acid, with the 64 possible triplets producing 20 different amino acids. The sequences of these amino acids formed by a gene produce the corresponding *protein*.

Transcription is the first step in *protein synthesis*, i.e. the process by which a gene produces a protein. An enzyme (*RNA polymerase*) uses DNA as a template and makes a complementary strand of short-lived messenger RNA (*mRNA*). The structure of RNA is similar to that of DNA, except that the nucleotide U substitutes T. The second step is *splicing*, where regions that are not coding for proteins are removed from the sequence. *Translation* is the final step by which a protein is produced. Microarrays measure mRNA abundance for each gene. As almost all biological processes are carried out by proteins, a direct measurement of protein level in a cell might seem more relevant. However, this is harder to measure than mRNA, and the amount of mRNA transcribed should correlate with *gene expression*, i.e. the rate at which a gene produces the corresponding protein. Figure 7.1 gives a summary.

7.1.2 Microarray Technologies

The main principle behind all methods for measuring gene expression is to utilize the bonds between the base pairs A/(T or U) and C/G by *hybridizing* samples to a pool of complementary sequences representing the genes of interest. The number of molecules in the target that bind to the probe should reflect gene expression. Although there is occasional confusion in the literature about these two terms, we will follow the recommended nomenclature and refer to the samples as *targets* and the complementary sequences as *probes*.

For single genes such techniques have been available for some time (e.g. Northern blotting). The breakthrough brought about by microarray technology is, however, that it allows us to monitor the expression of thousands of genes simultaneously.

Several microarray technologies have been developed. A very popular one, based on oligonucleotide chips, is produced by the company Affymetrix. On these arrays each gene is represented by a set of 14 to 20 short sequences of DNA, termed *oligonucleotides*. These oligonucleotides are referred to as the *perfect match (PM)* and each of them is paired with a corresponding *mismatch (MM)*, which is identical to the PM-Probe except for one nucleotide in the center of the sequence. The motivation for this approach is that any hybridization that occurs just by chance should affect both probes equally, whereas the correct gene will preferably hybridize to the PM-Probe. By measuring the difference between these two intensities the chance of observing false positives should be reduced.

Sets of pairs of oligonucleotides are synthesized directly onto a chip (*in situ synthesis*) by a light-directed chemical process (*photolithography*). Then, complementary RNA (*cRNA*) is obtained from the sample of interest (after transcription of mRNA to cDNA, which is then back transcribed), fluorescently labelled and hybridized to the array. After scanning, for each gene the set of PM- and MM-values is summarized in a single number. There has been some debate in the literature as to how this should be done (see Irizarry et al. [25] and the references therein).

The other widely used microarray technology is *cDNA-arrays*, in which two samples are usually analyzed simultaneously in a comparative fashion. In this technology, probes of purified DNA are spotted onto a glass slide by a robot. These are usually longer sequences compared with oligonucleotides, often consisting of complete genes. Also, in contrast to oligonucleotide arrays which are usually bought ready-made, many research groups spot their own cDNA-arrays. In this process the choice of the probes is an important problem.

In an experiment, mRNA is extracted from an experimental sample and a reference sample, and both are transcribed into the more stable cDNA. One sample is labelled by a fluorescent dye, usually Cy3 (green), and the other by Cy5 (red). The samples are mixed and the mixture is then hybridized to the array. According to the base pairing rules, the amount of cDNA that is hybridized to a particular spot for each of the two samples should be proportional to the level of expression of this gene in the samples. After hybridization the array is scanned at the wavelength of the two dyes producing two images as shown in Figure 7.2, which can be considered as the data in its rawest form. These particular arrays were scanned at 10μm resolution, resulting in digital images approximately 2000×2000 pixels in size. For presentation purposes these black and white images are usually overlaid and differently colored (again green/red) resulting in the well-known microarray images.

The data for a single sample are often also referred to as a *channel*, so that there are usually two channels in a cDNA microarray experiment, whereas Affymetrix chips yield one-channel data. For each of the two channels the next step is an analysis of the image with an appropriate piece of software (see Section 7.2). The main results of this analysis are an intensity value for each spot and its background, resulting in four values altogether. The standard

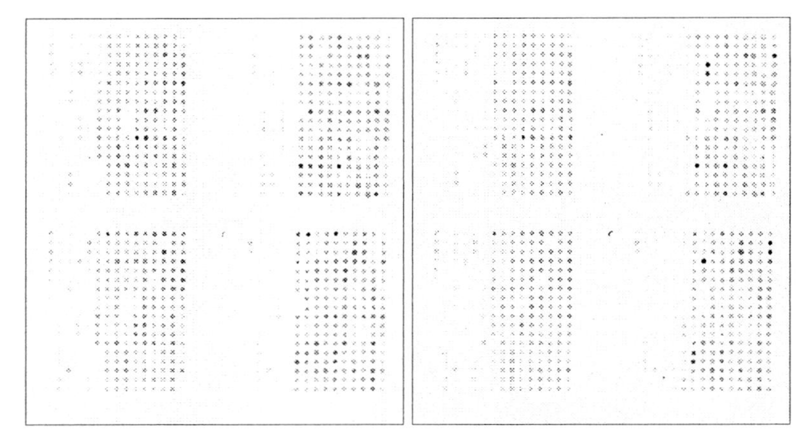

Fig. 7.2. Two channels of an HCMV cDNA microarray, comparing two viral strains.

procedure is to subtract the background intensity from the spot intensity for each of the channels and to then use the ratio of the two as a measure of relative gene expression.

We will focus on those steps in the analysis which use statistical tools. Section 7.2 will deal with the initial image analysis of scanned cDNA-microarray slides, Section 7.3 discusses the transformation of data obtained from the image analysis. In Section 7.4 we will discuss the extremely important problem of normalization, whereas Section 7.5 studies statistical methods to filter out genes which are differentially expressed between different experimental conditions. There is no space here to discuss all the different methods that have been proposed to analyze genes in a multivariate way and find classes or groups of genes or experiments that behave similarly, but the last section gives some references where the reader can find more information on this topic.

7.2 Image Analysis

Image analysis is the first stage in the analysis of microarray data, in order to summarize the information in each spot and to estimate the level of expression of each gene. Computer packages such as *QuantArray* [21], *ScanAlyse* [16], *GenePix* [2], *UCSF Spot* [26] and *NHGRI Image processing software tools* [33] implement a range of methods. Here we consider the basic steps involved in image analysis: image enhancement, gridding and estimation of spot and background intensities. For illustration we will use microarray images from an experiment concerning Human Cytomegalovirus (HCMV). Details about this experiment can be found in [18].

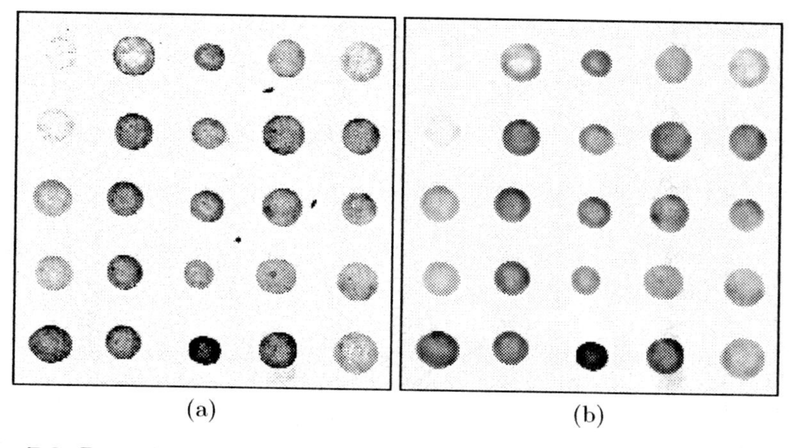

Fig. 7.3. Part of one of the HCMV channels before and after median filtering.

7.2.1 Image Enhancement

Noise can be a problem in scanned microarray images, including both small random specks and trends in background values. Filters are a set of image analysis methods that can be used to reduce noise in images (see, for example, Glasbey and Horgan [19], ch. 3). One of the simplest non-linear filters is the *median filter*. For a filter of size $(2m+1) \times (2m+1)$, the output is

$$z_{i_1,i_2} = \text{median}\,\{y_{i_1+j_1,i_2+j_2} \;:\; j_1,j_2 = -m,\ldots,m\} \qquad \text{for all } i_1,i_2,$$

where y_{i_1,i_2} (or, more succinctly, y_i) denotes the original pixel value in row i_1, column i_2. Figure 7.3 shows a small part of one of the HCMV channels before and after the application of a 5×5 median filter, from which we see that most of the contamination has been removed.

The background of a microarray image is often not uniform over the entire array and needs to be removed or adjusted for. These changes of fluorescent background are usually gradual and smooth across an array, and may be due to many technical reasons. Yang et al. [47] proposed the *top-hat filter* as a way to remove this trend. The trend can be estimated using a *morphological opening* (see, for example, Glasbey and Horgan [19], ch. 5), obtained by first replacing each pixel by the minimum local intensity in a region and then performing a similar operation on the resulting image, using the local maximum. For a region, we use a square of size $(2m+1) \times (2m+1)$ centered on each pixel, where m is a non-negative integer used to specify the size of the top-hat filter. Pixels, z_i, in the opened image will be given by

$$z_i = \max_j \, x_{i+j}, \qquad \text{where } x_k = \min_j \, y_{k+j}, \qquad \text{for } |j_1|,|j_2| \le m,$$

with y again denoting the original pixel values. If the top-hat filter uses a structuring element that is larger than the spots, then only the pixels in the spots will be substantially changed from y_i to z_i. As there is little background trend visible in Figure 7.3, the top-hat filter makes little difference in this case.

7.2.2 Gridding

The next step is to superimpose a lattice on each microarray image, adjusted for location shifts and small rotations. This is termed *gridding*, and can be done either automatically or semi-automatically [26, 39, 47]. Since each element of an array is printed automatically to a defined position, the final probe signals form a regular array. Typically, in a semi-automatic system, a scientist identifies the four corners of each block of spots on a computer display of an array, possibly using orientation markers, termed *landing lights*. Then, the computer interpolates a grid on the assumption that spots are positioned approximately equidistantly. Each software package has its own algorithm. For example, the NHGRI procedure [33] is as follows: 1) detect strong targets, 2) find their centers (e.g., center of mass), 3) regress four-corner coordinates of each subarray from these centers of strong signals. The final grid-overlay precisely segments each target, which enables future processing tasks to concentrate on only one target. Figure 7.4 shows the result of gridding one of the HCMV channels. In this case, each grid square is a 41×41 array of pixels containing the spot approximately at its center, where 41 corresponds to the inter-spot spacing.

7.2.3 Estimators of Intensities

To identify which pixels in each gridded square should be classified as *spot* and which as *background*, computer packages have implemented a range of methods: *QuantArray* [21] applies thresholds to the histogram of pixel values in a target region around a spot, *ScanAlyse* [16] uses a circle of fixed radius, *GenePix* [2] allows the circle radius to vary from spot to spot, and *UCSF Spot* [26] uses histogram information within a circle. Alternatives are to fit a scaled bivariate Gaussian density function to pixel values [39], possibly using a robust fitting method [7], k-means clustering [6], edge detection [30] and seeded region growing [47]. For a review of image segmentation including many more methods, see, for example, Glasbey and Horgan [19], ch. 4. Here, we consider two well-established estimators of spot intensities, those based on discs and on proportions of histogram values, as illustrated in Figure 7.5.

We need to calculate $\bar{y}^{(S)}$, the mean spot intensity, separately for each channel, and $\bar{y}^{(B)}$, the mean background intensity. If the spot center is at pixel location ν, we can use the disc estimator

$$\bar{y}^{(S)}_{\text{DISC}} = \frac{1}{\#} \sum_{\|i-\nu\|<R^{(S)}} y_i \qquad \text{and} \qquad \bar{y}^{(B)}_{\text{DISC}} = \frac{1}{\#} \sum_{\|i-\nu\|>R^{(B)}} y_i, \tag{7.1}$$

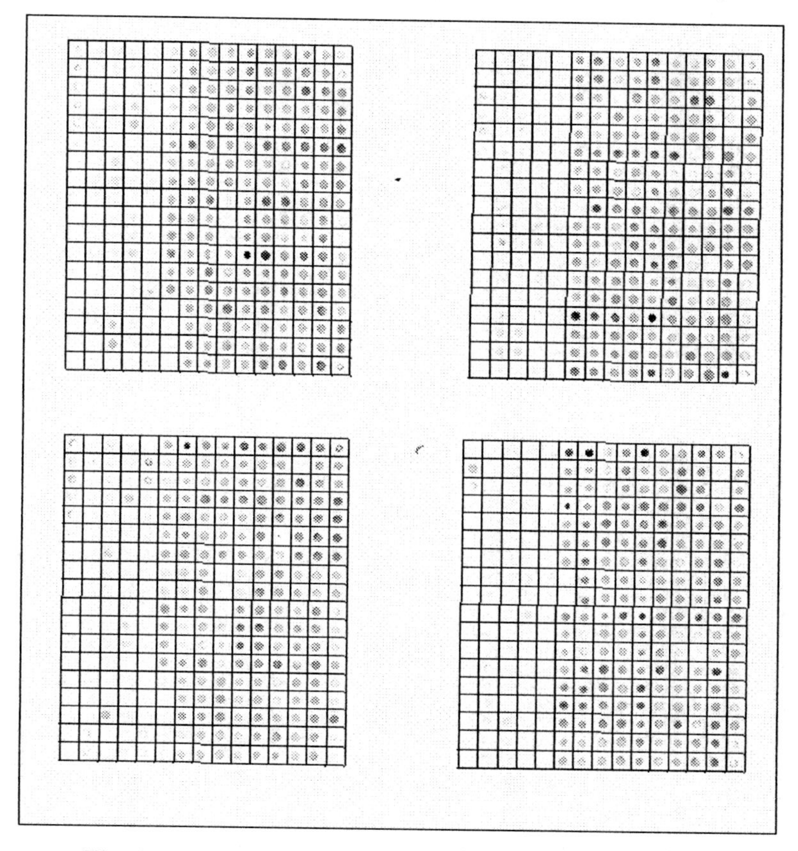

Fig. 7.4. Image of one HCMV channel with grid overlaid.

where # denotes the number of terms in each sum, and we specify radii $R^{(S)}$ and $R^{(B)}$. We may choose ν to maximize $\bar{y}^{(S)}$, using a systematic search. So, $\bar{y}^{(S)}_{\mathrm{DISC}}$ is the average value of those pixels located inside a disc of radius $R^{(S)}$ centred on ν (such as the disc in Figure 7.5(a)), and $\bar{y}^{(B)}_{\mathrm{DISC}}$ is the average pixel value for locations outside a disc of radius $R^{(B)}$ also centred on ν and inside the grid square. We may use constant values for $R^{(S)}$ and $R^{(B)}$, or different values in each grid square.

Alternatively, we can ignore the spatial information and use the proportion estimator. We rank $y_i \quad (i = 1, \ldots, N)$ $(N = 41^2$ in our illustration), for each channel independently, giving $y_{(1)} \leq y_{(2)} \leq \cdots \leq y_{(N)}$,and use

$$\bar{y}^{(S)}_{\mathrm{PROP}} = \frac{1}{\#} \sum_{i=Np^{(S)}}^{N} y_{(i)} \qquad \text{and} \qquad \bar{y}^{(B)}_{\mathrm{PROP}} = \frac{1}{\#} \sum_{i=1}^{Np^{(B)}} y_{(i)}$$

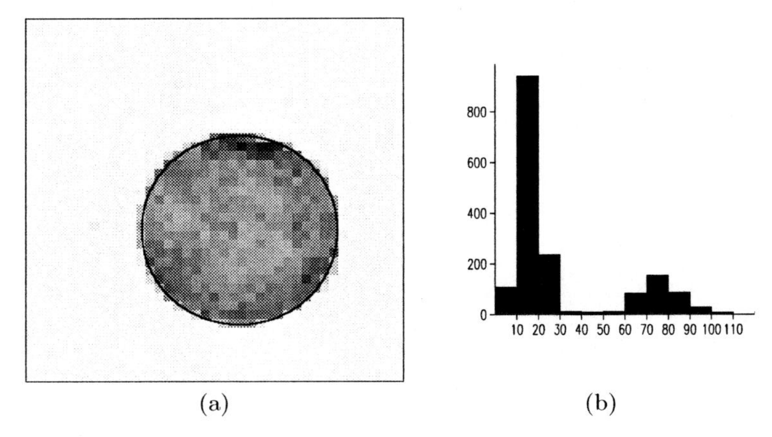

Fig. 7.5. A single spot in HCMV microarray with superimposed disc, and histogram of pixel values on square-root scale.

for specified proportions $p^{(S)}$ and $p^{(B)}$. So, $\bar{y}^{(S)}_{\mathrm{PROP}}$ is the average value of pixels greater than $p^{(S)}\%$ (such as data in the right mode in Figure 7.5(b)) and $\bar{y}^{(B)}_{\mathrm{PROP}}$ is the average of those less than $p^{(B)}\%$. Again, we may fix $p^{(S)}$ and $p^{(B)}$ or use different values in each grid square.

For either disc or proportion estimators, in a two-channel experiment, we then estimate the rate of expression of channel 2 relative to channel 1, denoted c, by either

$$\hat{c} = \frac{\bar{y}_2^{(S)}}{\bar{y}_1^{(S)}} \qquad \text{or} \qquad \hat{c} = \frac{\bar{y}_2^{(S)} - \bar{y}_2^{(B)}}{\bar{y}_1^{(S)} - \bar{y}_1^{(B)}},$$

i.e. without or with background subtraction. However, background subtraction can lead to negative estimates, which we have set to small positive values before log-transforming [8]. Background correction will usually be unnecessary if a top-hat filter has been used in the image enhancement step. Glasbey and Ghazal [18] consider how to select optimal settings for image processing parameters.

7.3 Transformation

A *transformation* of the intensities which result from the image analysis is usually the next step in the data analysis. From a statistical point of view the motivation for such a transformation is to find a scale on which the data can be analyzed by classical methods, i.e. methods for linear models with normally distributed errors (e.g. ANOVA, regression). For this reason the aim of a suitable transformation is that the rescaled data satisfy a model with

1. additive effects

2. normal (or at least symmetric) error distributions
3. homogeneous variances.

It might seem difficult to fulfil all these requirements simultaneously, but fortunately these three properties are not independent of each other. For example, measurement errors are usually the result of a combination of uncontrolled effects. In an additive model the central limit theorem thus implies that these errors (approximately) follow a normal distribution.

Often the mechanism that produced the data can be modelled and the corresponding transformation can be derived from this model (we will come back to this point later). If this is not the case, one can use exploratory methods to retrieve information about the right transformation from the data themselves. Among these the so-called *delta method* can be applied to find a variance-stabilizing transformation. Let X denote a univariate real-valued variable measured in an experiment and assume that its variance σ^2 is a function of the mean μ, i.e. we have

$$\mathrm{Var}(X) = \sigma^2(\mu). \tag{7.2}$$

Let now g be a differentiable function on the real line. If we transform our variable by g, a Taylor-expansion

$$g(X) = g(\mu) + (X - \mu)g'(\mu) + o(|X - \mu|) \tag{7.3}$$

thus yields

$$\mathrm{Var}(g(X)) \approx \sigma^2(\mu)(g'(\mu))^2 \tag{7.4}$$

as a first-order approximation of the variance of the transformed variable. A variance-stabilizing transformation should result in constant right-hand side in the last equation and solving the corresponding differential equation results in

$$g(x) = c_1 \int_0^x \frac{1}{\sigma(y)}\,dy + c_2 \tag{7.5}$$

for some constants c_1 and c_2.

The simplest and possibly most common application of this approach arises if the standard deviation σ is a linear function of the mean. Here the variance-stabilizing function turns out to be the logarithm. The ratio of the standard deviation divided by the mean is also called the *coefficient of variation*, which in this case is constant for the untransformed data. Surprisingly the pioneering paper of Chen et al. [9], which has to be regarded as the starting point of microarray statistics, assumes such a constant coefficient of variation ("a biochemical consequence of the mechanics of transcript production") but does not consider a *log-transformation*. Instead, these authors formulate a model where the original intensities are normally distributed. This leads to a fairly simple decision rule to determine whether a gene is differentially expressed or not based on the red/green-ratio, cf. Section 7.5.1. The skewness of the data and the fact that the intensities are restricted to be positive are further indicators for the need of a log-transformation. For this reason many following papers preferred such a log-transformation to the approach of Chen et al. [9]. Most prominently, several papers by Speed and collaborators propose this transformation and his web page includes the dogma "Always log!" in his section of "Hints and Prejudices" (cf. `http://stat-www.berkeley.edu/users/terry/zarray/Html/log.html`).

Hoyle et al. [22] discuss some other interesting related points. They show that the log-normal distribution not only models the distribution of each spot-intensity fairly well but that it also approximates the overall distribution of all gene expressions measured in the genome of interest and that the corresponding variance of the log-transformed distribution is a biological characteristic of the particular genome. They also argue that the observed spot intensity for the g-th gene X_g is a product of the true mRNA abundance t_g multiplied by a gene-specific error term ε_g, i.e. $X_g = t_g \varepsilon_g$. In the same way in which an additive model is linked to normal distributions by the central limit theorem, a multiplicative model naturally corresponds to lognormal distributions.

Despite all the evidence supporting a log-transformation, there are also some problems involved here. Usually the image analysis software gives a spot intensity and a background intensity for each channel (dye) and the standard method is to subtract the background intensity. For weak spots this will occasionally lead to negative values, where a log-transformation is not applicable. Even if the background-corrected values are positive but very small this can lead to high variability for the log-transformed data.

An interesting paper in this context is the work by Newton et al. [32], who model the untransformed data by Gamma distributions, i.e. a family of densities of the form

$$f_{\vartheta,a}(x) = \frac{\vartheta^a x^{a-1} \exp(-\vartheta x)}{\Gamma(a)} \quad \text{for } x \geq 0, \tag{7.6}$$

where $\vartheta > 0$ is a scale parameter, $a > 0$ models the shape of the distribution and Γ denotes the Gamma function. The mean of such a distribution is $\mu = a/\vartheta$, the standard deviation is given by $\sqrt{a}/\vartheta = \mu/\sqrt{a}$. This implies that this model also assumes a constant coefficient of variation just like the log-normal model and the approach of Chen et al. A log-transformation applied to Gamma distributed data will achieve two of the aforementioned aims, i.e. it will result in additive effects and homogeneous variances, but the assumption of normality will not hold.

Newton et al. assume that the shape parameter is the same for both channels but allow for different scale parameters. They use a hierarchical model in which the two shape parameters themselves are independent observations from a Gamma distribution. Their model leads to an estimate of the form $\frac{R+\nu}{G+\nu}$ for the ratio of the two channels. Here R and G denote the intensities of the red and green channel respectively, and ν is the scale parameter of the prior Gamma distribution, which has to be estimated from the data. The interesting point is that the problem of high variability for the ratio of weak spots can be reduced by adding ν and thus the effect of background correction can be counterbalanced as well.

A more explicit way to deal with inhomogeneous variability across the range of intensities is presented in two related papers by Durbin et al. [14] and Huber et al. [23]. Both papers propose a variance-stabilizing transformation motivated by a model introduced by Rocke and Durbin [35]. For the intensity X_{ig} of gene g measured on channel i ($i = 1, 2$) this model assumes the form

$$X_{ig} = b_i + t_{ig}e^{\eta_{ig}} + \varepsilon_{ig}. \tag{7.7}$$

Here b_i denotes a background intensity level common to all spot intensities on that channel, t_{ig} is the true gene expression of interest, and η_{ig} and ε_{ig} are families of independent mean-zero normal distributions with variances $\sigma^2_{i\eta}$ and $\sigma^2_{i\varepsilon}$. The distribution thus becomes a convolution of a log-normal distribution, which is dominant for large gene expressions t_{ig}, and a normal distribution that models lowly expressed genes. The mean and variance of this distribution are given by

$$\mathcal{E}(X_{ig}) = b_i + t_{ig}e^{\sigma^2_{i\eta}/2} \tag{7.8}$$

and

$$\mathrm{Var}(X_{ig}) = t^2_{ig}e^{\sigma^2_{i\eta}}(e^{\sigma^2_{i\eta}} - 1) + \sigma^2_{i\varepsilon}. \tag{7.9}$$

As the gene expression effect t_{ig} is the only term here which changes with the genes, we see that the variance depends on the mean via a polynomial of degree 2. Using the delta-method and solving the integral in (7.5) Huber et al. showed that the corresponding variance-stabilizing transformation is given by the arsinh function

$$g(x) = \gamma \mathrm{arsinh}(a + bx), \tag{7.10}$$

which is related to the logarithm via

$$\mathrm{arsinh}(x) = \log(x + \sqrt{x^2 + 1}). \tag{7.11}$$

Durbin et al. derive a transformation, which is exactly of the same type up to an unimportant shift. Note that this is a family of transformations, rather than a single transformation, as in the case of the log-transformation. The choice of the specific transformation is based on parameters a and b, which depend on the relative magnitudes of the additive and multiplicative errors and have to be estimated from the data. Having to estimate parameters and lack of comparability of transformations between data sets are both drawbacks of this approach.

In a very recent paper Cui et al. [11] have suggested a generalization of the Rocke and Durbin model in (7.7) for a two-channel experiment, where a second error term is added to both the multiplicative and the additive error, which is gene-dependent but the same for both channels:

$$X_{ig} = b_i + t_{ig}e^{\eta_g + \zeta_{ig}} + \varepsilon_g + \delta_{ig}. \tag{7.12}$$

This modelling approach takes into account the fact that measurements at the same spot will be more correlated. The authors show that many typical features of microarray data can be simulated from this model. As variance-stabilizing transformation they propose the so-called *linlog* function

$$h_d(x) = \begin{cases} \log(d) + x/d & x < d \\ \log(x) + 1 & x \geq d \end{cases}$$

Here d is a parameter that can be chosen or estimated from the data, separately for each channel. This transformation is very similar to the arsinh transformation. It is linear for small intensities and logarithmic for large intensities, but in contrast to the arsinh function these properties hold strictly and not just approximately, which of course causes the function to be less smooth. The authors also suggest the use of a shift of the same size but with a different sign in both channels prior to the transformation, in order to remove possible curvature from the MA plot.

To conclude, we would like to mention that choosing a variance-stabilizing transformation is not the only way to handle heterogeneous variances. An alternative way is to model and/or estimate the variance and incorporate this estimate into the subsequent analysis. One example for this approach is the work of Rudemo et al. [36], where the variability of the log-ratio of the two channels is assumed to decay exponentially with the log-harmonic mean of the two intensities.

7.4 Normalization

Normalisation/calibration has proven to be one of the main problems in the analysis of microarray data. Results from studies ignoring this problem are highly questionable. We will give an overview of how problems can be visualized by explorative analysis. Subsequently, we will also present some of the main remedies that have been proposed for this issue.

7.4.1 Explorative Analysis and Flagging of Data Points

One of the main characteristics of microarray experiments is the vast amount of data they yield. A second feature is that, due to the complex mechanism producing these data, artifacts and freak observations are quite common. Therefore it is extremely important to use good visualization and exploration tools that allow one to get a first overview of the data and to single out observations of poor data quality.

Histograms of log-intensities and log-ratios, which show the empirical distribution of measurements across genes, and scatterplots of the log-intensities of two channels from a cDNA-array or two different one-channel arrays, are

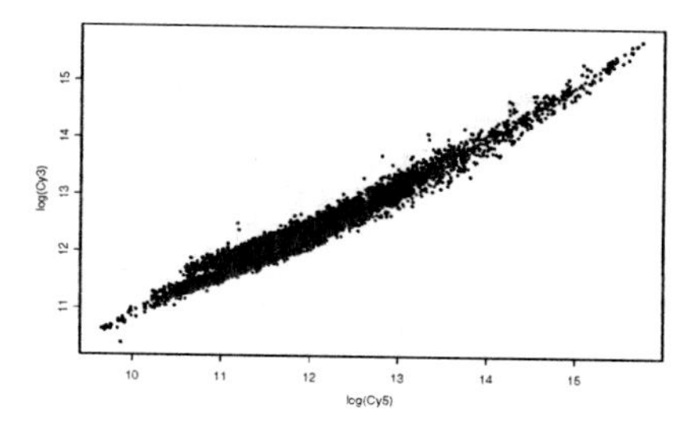

Fig. 7.6. Scatterplot of two log-intensities.

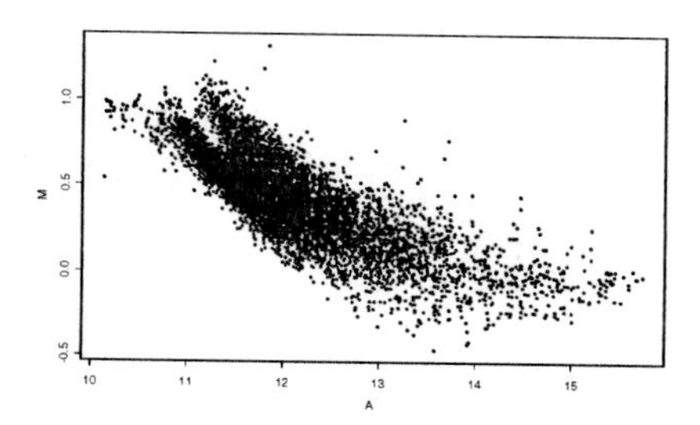

Fig. 7.7. MA-plot of two log-intensities.

the most common visualization tools. Figure 7.6 shows such a plot, where non-differentially expressed genes are expected to lie on the diagonal line with slope 1. Typically, the majority of genes can be expected not to change their expression, so deviations of the data cloud from this diagonal indicate experimental artifacts, which are to be corrected for by the normalization step (see following paragraphs). Terry Speed's group has suggested replacing this plot by a very similar one, which basically is a 45° degree rotation, cf. [46]. In the so-called *MA-plot* the mean log-intensity of the two channels M is plotted against the log-ratio of the two channels A. In Figure 7.7 we see the MA-version of the previous plot. Here the reference line of "no differential expression" is now a horizontal line, which makes it easier to spot deviations. There is also more space in such a plot to display the residuals at all intensity levels, so that a spurious impression of correlation is reduced. Apart from these more psychological reasons there is also a mathematical/statistical argument to prefer the MA-plot: some normalization methods use a regression approach and fit a curve to the plot. In the original plot an arbitrary choice has to be made as to which of the two channels is being treated as an explanatory variable and which one is the response (which can make a substantial difference!), whereas in the MA-plot both channels are treated equally.

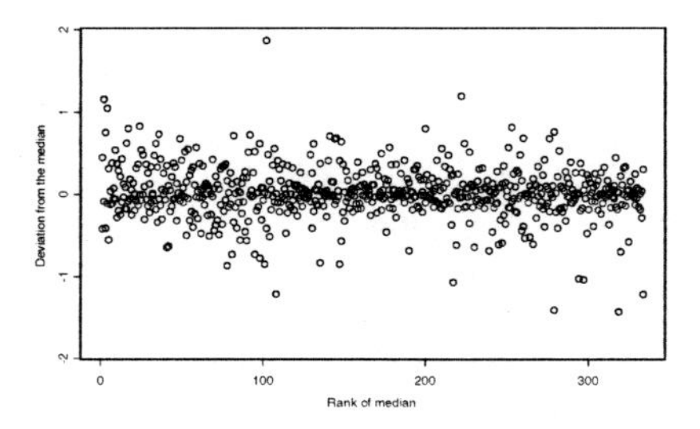

Fig. 7.8. Deviation of replicates from the median.

If there are *technical replicates* within an array, i.e. if genes have been spotted more than once, it is advisable to explore the consistency of measurements for the replicates of the same gene. In Figure 7.8 and Figure 7.9 we show two such plots for an example where genes on a two-channel array were spotted in triplicates (more than three spots per gene are neither common nor necessary). For Figure 7.8 we took minimum, median and maximum of the triplicates of each gene for one channel and displayed the ranks of the median along the x-axis. The y-axis shows differences between the maximum (minimum) and median plotted on the positive (negative) part. It is quite easy to single out questionable spots by eye in this plot. The plot in Figure 7.9 is similar. Here, we plotted the sample mean of the three replicates versus the sample standard deviation. Spots in the upper part of the plot correspond to genes where at least one of the replicates does not coincide with the others. This plot also indicates whether the log-transformation has stabilized the variance successfully. If so, mean and standard deviation should be uncorrelated, whereas trends in this plot indicate that other transformations might be more suitable (cf. the previous section).

Spots which are revealed as questionable by an exploratory analysis are usually *flagged*, i.e. the data spreadsheet has a special column, where a flagging symbol is entered for each spot of poor quality. Typically the image analysis software already does some of this flagging. Some programs have options to flag all genes where the spot-intensity falls below a certain threshold (for example the background intensity for two-channel arrays or the MM-intensity for Affymetrix-arrays). For data handling reasons, it is not advisable to remove flagged genes completely from further analysis as, for example, genes with low intensities are not necessarily artifacts, but might contain the valuable information that the corresponding gene is simply not expressed on this array. Where possible, the flagging status should be taken into account in the data analysis or, at least, it should be checked for all those genes which have been detected as playing an important role in the analysis.

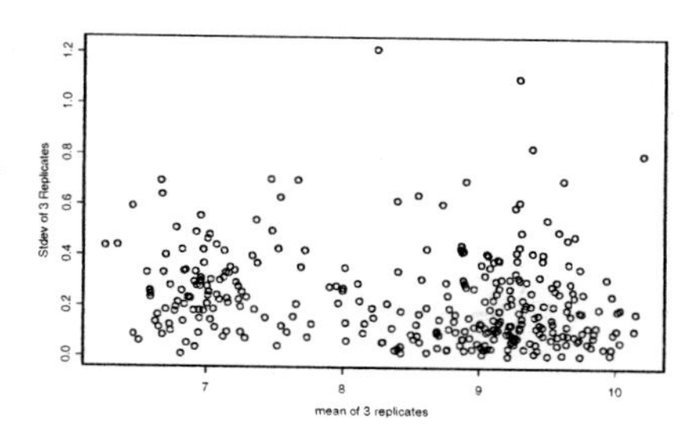

Fig. 7.9. Sample mean of tree replicates plotted against sample standard deviation.

7.4.2 Linear Models and Experimental Design

The exploratory plots introduced in the previous section indicate that the intensities measured on microarrays are not equal to the original mRNA abundance but are disturbed by a series of systematic experimental effects. These include effects depending on the array, dye, spot location, print-tip, intensity level, scanner settings and many more factors. Normalization and calibration is needed to remove these effects from the data and to reveal the true gene expression levels as clearly as possible. One strategy to deal with this problem is to include spots on the array which control for these effects. A typical example of this are so-called *housekeeping genes*. These are positive controls, i.e. genes which are known to be highly expressed at a constant level under different experimental conditions. Negative controls, i.e. genes which are not expected to be expressed at all, are also commonly used. *Spiking* is another control technique. Here spots with synthetic cDNA are included on the array and the samples are "spiked" with a known amount of the corresponding DNA. This should result in a constant spot-intensity. These and other control strategies clearly depend very much on the specific experiment and will not be discussed in detail here. A general problem is that the controls often do not behave as expected and give highly variable results. Although control spots can be a very helpful tool to monitor the experiment and its analysis, a calibration based only on these spots is highly questionable.

The first set of normalization methods we will discuss try to jointly model the treatment effects of interest and the experimental effects that we try to eliminate. This approach has been introduced and described in a series of papers by Gary Churchill's group at the Jackson Laboratory. A typical model for the log-transformed gene expression measured in a cDNA microarray experiment would be

$$X_{ijkg} = \mu + A_i + D_j + T_k + G_g + (AG)_{ig} + (TG)_{kg} + \varepsilon_{ijkg}, \qquad (7.13)$$

cf. Kerr et al. [29]. Here A_i denotes the effect of array i, D_j the effect of dye j, T_k corresponds to treatment k, G_g to gene g and combinations of letters denote interactions of the corresponding effects. The error terms ε_{ijkg} are assumed to be independent and identically distributed with mean 0. Normal distributions are not assumed though. The authors use a bootstrapping technique instead to calculate significances. The parameters of interest in this model are the treatment-gene interactions $(TG)_{kg}$, whereas all other parameters are included for normalization purposes. Naturally factors or interactions can flexibly be removed from or added to model, where the number of degrees of freedom which can be used up is constrained by the number of observations.

Wolfinger et al. [44] and Wernisch et al. [42] proposed to replace fixed effects for the experimental effects in the *Analysis of Variance (ANOVA)* model above by random effects, which leads to a *mixed model*. This means that, for example, the array effects A_i are treated as random variables which are independently identically normally distributed with mean 0 and variance σ_A^2 (similar assumptions are made for other effects in the model). Both papers use the *residual maximum likelihood (REML)* approach to estimate these variance components, which can then be compared to find out which factors and levels of the experiment account for the largest variability in the observations.

One of the nice features of these linear models is that they facilitate the comparison of different experimental designs. For example in a *dye swap* experiment, i.e. a cDNA-microarray experiment where the same two samples are hybridized again on a second array but with interchanged dyes, averaging the log-ratio measurements from the two arrays can eliminate the dye effect from the model. Kerr and Churchill [28] consider more complicated designs, so-called *loop designs*, which are also balanced with respect to the dyes. These designs are proposed as an alternative to the classical *reference design*, where all samples are compared with the same common reference. Figures 7.10 and 7.11 show the difference between a reference and a loop design in the simplest non-trivial case of three samples. For more complicated situations there are many fairly complex possible loop-designs and Kerr and Churchill compare these in terms of *A-optimality*, a criterion which minimizes the average variance of the parameter estimators.

Estimated variance components in a mixed model can be used to choose the number of required replicates at different levels of the experiment as shown by Wernisch et al. [42], who discuss how optimal choices can be made under constraints given by a limit on the total cost of experiments.

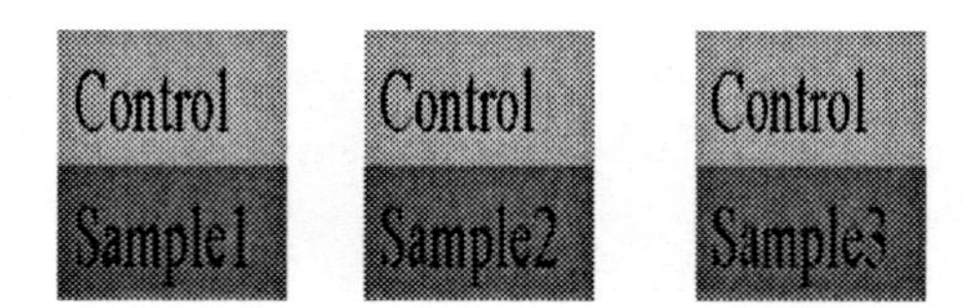

Fig. 7.10. Reference design for three samples.

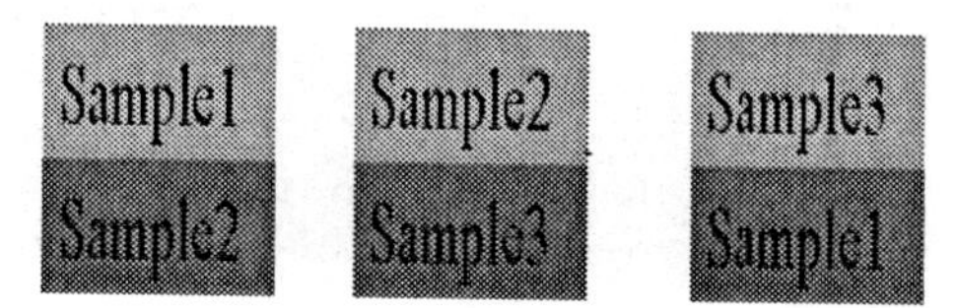

Fig. 7.11. Loop design for three samples.

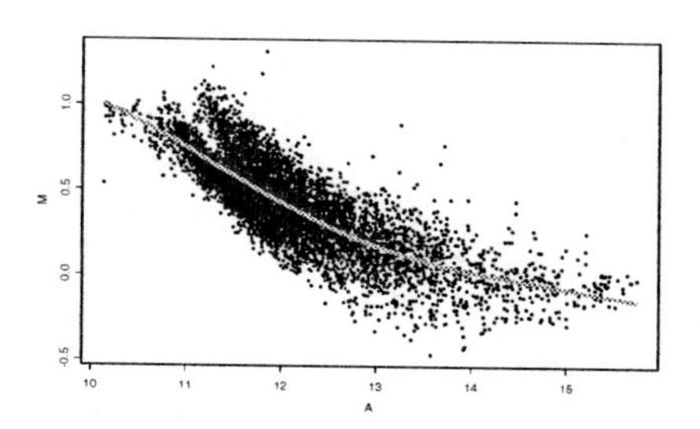

Fig. 7.12. MA-plot with fitted loess curve

7.4.3 Non-linear Methods

Parameter estimation and design optimization in the linear models discussed in the previous section are only meaningful if the underlying model is appropriate. Unfortunately, there is strong evidence that some effects in microarray experiments do not fit into this linear framework. In many two-channel experiments so-called "banana-shapes" occur in the MA-plots indicating that the dye effects can change with the gene-expression level.

Most normalization methods are based on the assumption that the majority of genes will not change their expression across samples and experimental conditions. For small targeted arrays this is a questionable assumption but for larger or whole genome arrays it is certainly reasonable. Under this assumption the majority of points in an MA-plot should scatter around the x-axis once the data have been normalized. The most popular method to achieve this seems to be the *loess (or lowess) normalization*, as discussed in the papers by Yang et al., cf. [46] and [45]. Loess is a robust local regression method that fits a curve to the MA-plot and then uses the residuals from this fit as normalized log-ratio values. The loess regression, as implemented in R, the statistical programming language most widely used for microarray analysis, has one main parameter: the *span*, that defines the percentage of data, which are declared to be in the neighborhood of a point x on the x-axis. Subsequently, a polynomial is fitted to these points by minimizing a weighted sum of squares. The weights are determined by a weight function and decrease for larger distances from x. Figure 7.12 shows a loess fit to the MA-plot of Figure 7.7.

There are several variations of the loess normalization. As each sub-grid of spots on a microarray is spotted by a different print-tip, different calibration might be necessary for each sub-grid. Yang et al. [46] propose to fit loess curves to each of these sub-grids separately in such a case. This approach removes spatial effects within the slide to some extent. A robust regression fit of the M-values against the spatial coordinates is an alternative method for the reduction of spatial effects.

7.4.4 Normalization of One-channel Data

For oligonucleotide arrays there is little variation in the amount of DNA spotted and the same dye is used for all arrays, so that normalization should be less important for this technology. Nevertheless exploratory analysis reveals that there still is some need for calibration, cf. Bolstad et al. [5]. Schadt et al. [37] proposed to find a *rank invariant set of genes*, i.e. a group of genes whose ranked expression values do not differ between the current array and some common baseline array by more than some threshold. The scatterplot of the expression values for this invariant set is then smoothed by a spline function, which represents the relationship between non-differentially expressed genes and is used to normalize the data.

Bolstad et al. [5] study and compare several methods that do not require the choice of a baseline array. One of these is the *quantile normalization*, where the measurements on each array are replaced by their ranks and then back-transformed by a common monotone transformation. According to the comparative study by these authors the quantile normalization seems to be slightly better than the method of Schadt et al. and two generalizations of the loess normalization to more than two channels.

7.5 Differential Expression

A basic question in the analysis of gene expression data is whether a gene changes its expression under different experimental conditions. Depending on the experimental set-up this might mean comparison of the two channels on a cDNA microarray with each other, comparison of the ratios against a common reference across two-channel experiments or comparison of intensities of one-channel experiments performed under different conditions.

7.5.1 One-slide Approaches

In the early days of microarrays, scientists chose an arbitrary fold-change (e.g. 2) as a threshold and defined every gene showing an expression ratio higher than this threshold as differentially expressed. Since the replication of microarray experiments is expensive and was even more expensive some years ago, early attempts to improve this ad hoc decision rule focused on comparing expression values across genes within one array.

The paper by Chen et al. [9] gives one example of this approach. Recall that these authors modelled the original intensities by normal distributions via

$$X_{ig} = \mu_{ig}\varepsilon_{ig}. \tag{7.14}$$

Here i indicates the channels 1,2, g indicates the genes. The error terms ε_{ig} are independently normally distributed with mean 1 and variance c^2, i.e. we have

$$\mathcal{E}(X_{ig}) = \mu_{ig}, \quad \mathrm{Var}(X_{ig}) = \mu_{ig}^2 c^2. \tag{7.15}$$

Under the null-hypothesis

$$H_0 : \{\mu_{1g} = \mu_{2g}\} \tag{7.16}$$

of no differential expression the distribution of the ratio X_{1g}/X_{2g} thus only depends on the unknown coefficient of variation c, which the authors propose to estimate from a set of control genes that are known to be non-differentially expressed. By using the null-distribution of the ratio, the significance of the evidence for differential expression can be calculated for each gene.

Newton et al. [32] propose an alternative method to assess the evidence for differential expression of each gene. As mentioned before, these authors model expression intensities with the Gamma distribution as given in (7.6). Their Bayesian approach leads to a modified ratio estimate of the form $(X_{1g}+\nu)/(X_{2g}+\nu)$, where ν is a hyper-parameter estimated from the data. This ratio estimates a theoretical ratio of the scale parameters ϑ_1 and ϑ_2 of the Gamma distributions. The authors' hierarchical model assumes that the parameters themselves are independently generated from another Gamma distribution for differentially expressed genes, i.e. if $\vartheta_1 \neq \vartheta_2$ holds. Under the null-hypothesis, however, the two parameters are identical and it is thus assumed that the prior distribution only yields one observation. This leads to a mixture model for the prior distribution. By using the EM-algorithm and modelling the mixture parameter by yet another level of prior distributions the authors derive a probability of differential expression given the observed outcome.

Lee et al. [31] also use a mixture approach. They model data from a two-channel experiment, where one channel was not used at all, leading to a one-channel situation. Here the log-intensities are modelled by a mixture of two normal distributions, where the component with lower mean represents background noise measured for non-expressed genes and the other component describes the distribution of "real" expression values across genes. This is similar to the approach in Newton et al. [32]. Maximum-likelihood estimation of the parameters yields an estimated posterior probability for a gene to be differentially expressed.

7.5.2 Using Replicated Experiments

Although the methods mentioned so far can be helpful to summarize data from a single microarray experiment, only a sufficient number of replications can help to decide whether the change in expression of a gene is really significant or not. In the following, we focus on the situation where we have observed transformed and normalized expression quantities x_{ig}, where the first m measurements (for indices $1 \leq i \leq m$) were taken under condition A and a second group of n measurements ($m+1 \leq i \leq m+n$) were observed under condition B. The measurements are assumed to be either log-ratios (or related measurements of differential expressions) in series of two-channel experiments with a common reference or expressions (on an appropriate scale) from one-channel experiments.

Different versions of t-statistics

The most commonly used tool in this situation is the *t-test-statistic*

$$\frac{\bar{x}_{gA} - \bar{x}_{gB}}{SED_g}, \tag{7.17}$$

which relates the difference between the group averages for gene g to the *standard error* of this difference (SED_g). The calculation of this SED has been the topic of major discussions in this context. The classical approach (as implemented in any standard statistical software package) is to base the SED on the pooled sum of squares given by

$$SED^2_{gp} = \frac{m+n}{mn(m+n-2)} \left(\sum_{i=1}^{m} (x_{ig} - \bar{x}_{gA})^2 + \sum_{i=m+1}^{m+n} (x_{ig} - \bar{x}_{gB})^2 \right) \tag{7.18}$$

$$= \frac{m+n}{m+n-2} \left(\frac{m-1}{n} s^2_{gA} + \frac{n-1}{m} s^2_{gB} \right). \tag{7.19}$$

Here s_{gA} and s_{gB} denote the standard error estimates for the group means. This version of the t-statistic assumes that, under the null hypothesis, not only the means of the variables but also the variances (or in general the whole underlying distribution) are equal in both groups. In the case of variance heterogeneity the *Welch-statistic* is an alternative method, which uses

$$SED^2_{gw} = s^2_{gA} + s^2_{gB} \tag{7.20}$$

as an estimate of the standard error of the difference.

It is interesting that most publications have focused on the Welch-version of the t-statistic, cf. the seminal paper of Dudoit et al. [13] or Baldi and Long [4]. If one was truly convinced of the variance stabilizing properties of the preceding transformation the classical t-statistic would seem more appropriate. In this case a further improvement could be achieved by using the sums of squares of *all* genes, i.e. choosing

$$SED^2_p = \frac{1}{G} \sum_{g=1}^{G} SED^2_{gp}, \tag{7.21}$$

where G denotes the number of genes. Clearly this will give a much better estimator of the SED, if the assumption of variance homogeneity holds. This touches upon a general problem with all the SED estimators discussed above: since the sample sizes are usually very small, they are highly variable. In particular small SED estimates can appear by chance resulting in very high t-values even when differences in expression are small.

As a result of their Bayesian approach, Baldi and Long [4] propose to use a modified SED^2 estimate that is given by a linear combination of Welch's SED_{gw}^2 and a hyperparameter σ_0^2, which reflects a prior assumption on the expected variability. An obvious estimate for σ_0^2 would be SED_p^2, yielding an estimator that combines the variability of this particular gene with the average variability of all genes.

Several authors have suggested other modifications of the SED, for example Tusher et al. [41], who add a constant s_0 to SED_{gp} that is chosen such that the correlation between nominator and denominator is minimized.

Resampling methods and non-parametric tests

Usually any test statistic is transformed to a number in the unit interval, the *p-value*, which reflects the probability of obtaining a value at least as extreme as the observed one under the null-hypothesis. For the calculation of the p-value the distribution of the test statistic under the null-hypothesis has to be known. In the case of independently normally distributed variables with equal variances this distribution is a t_{m+n-2}-distribution for the classical t-statistic (using SED_{gp} as the denominator). Under variance heterogeneity only approximations (t-distributions with non-integer degrees of freedom) are available for the Welch-statistic.

For large sample sizes the central limit theorem ensures that the statistic is approximately normally distributed. Thus it is less crucial that the assumption of normally distributed data holds. Unfortunately, the sample size, i.e. the number of slides, is typically very small in microarray experiments, so these asymptotic laws cannot be applied.

If variables are independently identically distributed (*i.i.d.*) under the null hypothesis, *permutation tests* are a solution for this problem. Based on the fact that, under the null-hypothesis, every permutation of the data (*resampled* data set) could have been observed with the same probability, the test-statistic is recalculated for each of the $\binom{m+n}{m}$ possibilities to split up the observed data into the two groups. The p-value is then determined based on this permutation distribution. For larger sample sizes the number of permutations gets very high, so that usually only a subset of all possible permutations are generated in a Monte Carlo simulation.

To control a false positive (type 1 error) rate of $\alpha \in (0, 1)$ a t-statistic with a p-value below α is called *significant*. Under an i.i.d. hypothesis it can be easily shown that permutation tests control this error rate exactly, independent of the underlying distribution. This is no longer true if variables are not identically distributed under the null hypothesis, e.g. if they are allowed to have different variances. Still it can be shown that, provided an appropriate SED estimator is used, permutation versions of the Welch-test have the same asymptotic behavior as the original version of the test using the t-distribution, cf. Janssen [27]. Permutation methods have been widely applied to microarray data, cf. Dudoit et al. [13] or Tusher et al. [41].

A particular class of permutation tests are rank tests, which use only the ranks of the observations within the pooled sample rather than the original data. Rank test are also called nonparametric tests as they do not depend on distributional assumptions. The most common rank statistic is the Wilcoxon-statistic, which is based on the sum of the ranks in each group. The calculation of p-values for rank tests is the same as for permutation tests and again p-values are only accurate under an i.i.d. null-hypothesis.

7.5.3 Multiple Testing

All tests for differential expression discussed so far try to control the false positive rate for one particular gene only. If we apply a test to each of 20,000 genes on an array and a significance level of 5% is chosen, we would thus expect 1000 false positive discoveries even if none of the genes are differentially expressed. This sort of multiple testing problem has some tradition in statistics but it has hardly ever been as relevant as in this context. Finding a multiple testing strategy for microarray data is further complicated by the fact that the measurements for different genes will in general not be independent of each other. The main contributions to this area have been made by Terry Speed's group in Berkeley (cf. [13], [17]) and the Stanford group (cf. [41], [15] and [40]), each following one of two very different approaches to this problem.

The family wise error rate

The first and classical approach is to control the *family wise error rate (FWER)*, i.e. the probability that there are any false positives among the thousands of statements. By definition, this is a rather conservative strategy, which reduces the number of significant findings quite dramatically. The simplest way to control the FWER is the Bonferroni method, where the adjusted significance level is the original one divided by the numbers of observations (or, alternatively, adjusted p-values are given by multiplication with this number).

Dudoit et al. [13] suggest controlling the FWER by using a permutation-based procedure first introduced by Westfall and Young [43]. This is called the *step-down* method because it looks sequentially at the set of ordered observed p-values

$$p_{r_1} \leq p_{r_2} \leq \cdots \leq p_{r_n}, \tag{7.22}$$

where r_j gives the gene for which the j-th smallest p-value occurred. Starting with the smallest, each of these p-values is then replaced by an *adjusted p-value*, which has to be below the chosen FWER (typically 5%) to be called significant. Let $P_1, \ldots, P_G$ denote random variables describing the p-values of genes $1, \ldots, G$. If $\mathbf{H_0}$ denotes the intersection of all null-hypotheses, i.e. no genes are differentially expressed, the steps of this algorithm are:

Step 1: Choose the adjusted smallest p-value as

$$\tilde{p}_{r_1} = P[\min(P_{r_1}, \ldots, P_{r_G}) \leq p_{r_1} \mid \mathbf{H_0}].$$

This means that we compare the smallest observed p-value with the distribution this smallest value has, if there are no differential genes.

Step j: Choose

$$\tilde{p}_{r_j} = \max\left(\tilde{p}_{r_{j-1}} \ , \ P[\min(P_{r_j}, \ldots, P_{r_G}) \leq p_{r_j} \mid \mathbf{H_0}] \right).$$

Again the jth smallest p-value is studied under the distribution of the smallest value among the $G - j + 1$ remaining genes. The maximum ensures that the sequence of adjusted p-values has the same ordering as the original ones.

Although the marginal distribution of each single p-value is known to be uniform under $\mathbf{H_0}$, we know little about the dependence structure, so that the joint distribution of p-values needed above is unknown in general. Again a permutation strategy can be used here, where a simultaneous permutation for all gene allows to estimate the joint distribution (this is only true to some extent: this approach assumes that the dependence structure is the same under the different treatments!). Details of the exact algorithm can be found in Dudoit et al. [13].

The false discovery rate

As mentioned before, FWER-methods tend to be fairly conservative, i.e. they often result in very few significant findings. One reason for this is that trying to avoid *any* false positives is a very cautious strategy. Many scientists probably are happy to accept some false positives provided they have an estimate of how many errors there will be. The *false discovery rate (FDR)* and related approaches address this point of view. The FDR is defined as the expected ratio of rejected true null-hypotheses divided by the total number of rejected hypotheses. (The *positive false discovery rate (pFDR)* is a closely related rate, which is given by the same expected value, but conditional on the null-hypothesis being rejected at least once.) If all hypotheses are true, the FDR is identical to the FWER, but in general they will be different. We refer to the PhD thesis of Storey [40] for a more detailed discussion of the control and estimation of the (p)FDR in a microarray context.

One related application we would like to mention is the *Significance Analysis of Microarray (SAM)* method described by Tusher et al. [41], as this has been implemented in a widely used free software package (cf. `http://www-stat.stanford.edu/~tibs/SAM/index.html`). One feature of this software is that rather than controlling the FDR it gives estimates for the FDR and the number of expected false positives for a user-defined threshold. This is quite different from the classical approach of choosing a certain acceptable rate (say 5%) and then calculating thresholds for test statistics accordingly. In some way this addresses the fact that often microarrays are not so much used to verify hypotheses as to generate them, i.e. to screen for genes that might be differentially expressed.

As before, one of the main problems in estimating the FDR is the unknown dependence structure between the genes and SAM uses a simulation approach that is similar to the one in the Westfall and Young algorithm discussed above.

7.6 Further Reading

So far, we have only considered preprocessing methods, experimental design and the detection of single differentially expressed genes. In some way, these methods do not fully exploit microarray technology, which allows us to have a look at all genes spotted on an array simultaneously. Thus, the true challenge is to correlate the complete observed gene expression pattern with the experimental conditions under which it was observed. From a statistical point of view we are facing a multivariate problem here, where we can either regard each experiment/slide as a unit with G components (G = number of genes) or each gene as a unit for which we observe a vector of K measurements (K = number of slides). Multivariate statistics offer a sometimes confusingly high number data analysis methods and most of these have been applied or adapted to microarray analysis. For example, *principal component analysis (PCA)* , as used in Alter et al. [1] is a classical tool which reduces the dimensionality of the data. By *singular value decomposition (SVD)* of the (empirical) variance-covariance or correlation matrix, PCA yields *eigengenes* (i.e. linear combinations of genes) or *eigenarrays* (linear combinations of slides) that account for the largest variability in the data. Often, these principal components are then used to find groups or *clusters* of arrays or genes in a second step. If prior knowledge is available these groups or classes might already be known. In this case the problem is to allocate observations to the appropriate group. This is a *classification* problem, where typically the classes are modelled probabilistically. Prominent examples are experiments for tumor classification as in Golub et al. [20]. In other cases without any prior knowledge the data are used to find such groupings and a wide range of such *clustering* methods has been proposed for microarray analysis. For an excellent overview on classification and clustering methods for microarrays we refer to the contributions of Dudoit and Fridlyand [12] and Chipman et al. [10] in the recently published book edited by Speed [38], which also covers many other aspects of microarray statistics. A range of other books have been published lately or are about to be published soon, cf. [3] or [34]. A shorter but very comprehensive overview can be found in Huber et al. [24].

References

[1] O. Alter, P. Brown, and D. Botstein. Singular value decomposition for genome-wide expression data processing and modeling. *Proceedings of the National Academy of Sciences of the USA*, 97:10101–6, 2000.

[2] Axon Instruments, Inc. *GenePix 400A User's Guide*. 1999.

[3] P. Baldi and W. Hatfield. *DNA Microarrays and Gene Expression*. Cambridge University Press, 2002.

[4] P. Baldi and A. Long. A Bayesian framework for the analysis of microarray expression data: Regularized t-test and statistical inferences of gene changes. *Bioinformatics*, 17:509–519, 2001.

[5] B. Bolstad, R. A. Irizarry, M. Astrand, and T. Speed. A comparison of normalization methods for high density oligonucleotide array data based on bias and variance. *Bioinformatics*, 19(2):185–193, 2002.

[6] D. Bozinov and J. Rahnenführer. Unsupervised technique for robust target separation and analysis of microarray spots through adaptive pixel clustering. *Bioinformatics*, 18:747–756, 2002.

[7] N. Brändle, H.-Y. Chen, H. Bischof, and H. Lapp. Robust parametric and semi-parametric spot fitting for spot array images. In *ISMB'00 – 8th International Conference on Intelligent Systems for Molecular Biology*, pages 46–56, 2000.

[8] C. S. Brown, P. C. Goodwin, and P. K. Sorger. Image metrics in the statistical analysis of DNA microarray data. *Proceedings of the National Academy of Sciences of the USA*, 98:8944–8949, 2001.

[9] Y. Chen, E. Dougherty, and M. Bittner. Ratio-based decisions and the quantative analysis of cDNA microarray images. *Journal of Biomedical Optics*, 2:364–374, 1997.

[10] H. Chipman, T. Hastie, and R. Tibshirani. Clustering microarray data. In T. Speed, editor, *Statistical Analysis of Gene Expression Microarray Data*, pages 159–200. Chapman & Hall/CRC, 2003.

[11] X. Cui, M. Kerr, and G. Churchill. Transformations for cDNA microarray data. *Statistical Applications in Genetics and Molecular Biology*, 2, 2003.

[12] S. Dudoit and J. Fridlyand. Classification in microarray experiments. In T. Speed, editor, *Statistical Analysis of Gene Expression Microarray Data*, pages 93–158. Chapman & Hall/CRC, 2003.

[13] S. Dudoit, Y. Yang, M. Callow, and T. Speed. Statistical methods for identifying differentially expressed genes in replicated cDNA microarray experiments. Technical Report 578, Statistics Dept, UC Berkeley, 2000.

[14] B. Durbin, J. Hardin, D. Hawkins, and D. Rocke. A variance-stabilizing transformation for gene-expression microarray data. *Bioinformatics*, 18:105–110, 2002.

[15] B. Efron, R. Tibshirani, J. Storey, and V. Tusher. Empirical Bayes analysis of a microarray experiment. *Journal of the American Statistical Association*, 96:1151–1160, 2001.

[16] M. B. Eisen. *ScanAlyse.* 1999. (Available at `http://rana/Stanford.EDU/~software/`)

[17] Y. Ge, S. Dudoit, and T. Speed. Resampling-based multiple testing for microarray data analysis. Technical Report 633, Statistics Dept, UC Berkeley, 2003.

[18] C. A. Glasbey and P. Ghazal. Combinatorial image analysis of DNA microarray features. *Bioinformatics*, 19:194–203, 2003.

[19] C. A. Glasbey and G. W. Horgan. *Image Analysis for the Biological Sciences.* Wiley, Chichester, 1995.

[20] T. Golub, D. Slonim, P. Tamayo, C. Huard, M. Gaasenbeek, J. Mesirov, H. Coller, M. Loh, J. Downing, M. Caligiuri, C. Bloomfield, and E. Lander. Molecular classification of cancer: class discovery and class prediction by gene expression monitoring. *Science*, 286:531–537, 1999.

[21] GSI Luminomics. *QuantArray Analysis Software, Operator's Manual.* 1999.

[22] D. Hoyle, M. Rattray, R. Jupp, and A. Brass. Making sense of microarray data distributions. *Bioinformatics*, 18:576–584, 2002.

[23] W. Huber, A. von Heydebreck, H. Sültmann, A. Proustka, and M. Vingron. Variance stabilization applied to microarray data calibration and to quantification of differential expression. *Bioinformatics*, 18:96–104, 2002.

[24] W. Huber, A. von Heydebreck, and M. Vingron. Analysis of microarray gene expression data. In *Handbook of Statistical Genetics.* Wiley, second edition, 2003.

[25] R. Irizarry, B. Bolstad, F. Collin, L. Cope, B. Hobbs, and T. Speed. Summaries of affymetrix genechip probe level data. *Nucleic Acids Research*, 31:e 15, 2003.

[26] A. N. Jain, T. A. Tokuyasu, A. M. Snijders, R. Segraves, D. G. Albertson, and D. Pinkel. Fully automatic quantification of microarray image data. *Genome Research*, 12:325–332, 2002.

[27] A. Janssen. Studentized permutation tests for non i.i.d. hypotheses and the generalized Behrens–Fisher problem. *Statististics and Probability Letters*, 36:9–21, 1997.

[28] M. Kerr and G. Churchill. Experimental design for gene expression microarrays. *Biostatistics*, 2:183–201, 2001.

[29] M. Kerr, M. Martin, and G. Churchill. Analysis of variance for gene expression microarray data. *Journal of Computational Biology*, 7:819–837, 2000.

[30] J. H. Kim, H. Y. Kim, and Y. S. Lee. A novel method using edge detection for signal extraction from cDNA microarray image analysis. *Experimental and Molecular Medicine*, 33:83–88, 2001.

[31] M. Lee, F. Kuo, G. Whitmore, and J. Sklar. Importance of replication in microarray gene expression studies: Statistical methods and evidence from repetetive cDNA hybridizations. *Proceedings of the National Academy of Sciences of the USA*, 97:9834–9839, 2000.

[32] M. Newton, C. Kendziorski, C. Richmond, F. Blattner, and K. Tsui. On differential variability of expression ratios: Improving statistical inference about gene expression changes from microarray data. *Journal of Computational Biology*, 8:37–52, 2000.

[33] NHGRI. *Image processing software tools.* 2003. (Available at `http://www.nhgri.nih.gov/DIR/LCG/15K/HTML/img_analysis.html`)

[34] G. Parmigiani, E. S. Garrett, R. Irizarry, and S. Zeger, editors. *The Analysis of Gene Expression Data.* Springer, 2003.

[35] D. Rocke and B. Durbin. A model for measurement error for gene expression arrays. *Journal of Computational Biology*, 8:557–569, 2001.

[36] M. Rudemo, T. Lobovkin, P. Moștad, S. Scheidl, S. Nilsson, and P. Lindahl. Variance models for microarray data. Technical report, Mathematical Statistics, Chalmers University of Technology, 2002.

[37] E. Schadt, C. Li, B. Eliss, and W. Wong. Feature extraction and normalization algorithms for high-density oligonucleotide gene expression array data. *Journal of Cellular Biochemistry*, 84:120–125, 2002.

[38] T. Speed, editor. *Statistical Analysis of Gene Expression Microarray Data.* Chapman & Hall/CRC, 2003.

[39] M. Steinfath, W. Wruck, H. Seidel, H. Lehrach, U. Radelof, and J. O'Brien. Automated image analysis for array hybridization experiments. *Bioinformatics*, 17:634–641, 2001.

[40] J. Storey. *False Discovery Rates: Theory and Applications to DNA Microarrays.* PhD thesis, Department of Statistics, Stanford University, 2002.

[41] V. Tusher, R. Tibshirani, and G. Chu. Significance analysis of microarrays applied to the ionizing radiation response. *Proceedings of the National Academy of Sciences of the USA*, 98:5116–5121, 2001.

[42] L. Wernisch, S. Kendall, S. Soneji, A. Wietzorrek, T. Parish, J. Hinds, P. Butcher, and N. Stoker. Analysis of whole-genome microarray replicates using mixed models. *Bioinformatics*, 19:53–61, 2003.

[43] P. Westfall and S. Young. *Resampling-based multiple testing: examples and methods for p-value adjustment.* Wiley series in probability and mathematical statistics. Wiley, 1993.

[44] R. Wolfinger, G. Gibson, E. Wolfinger, L. Bennett, H. Hamadeh, P. Bushel, C. Afshari, and R. Paules. Assessing gene significance from cDNA microarray expression data via mixed models. *Journal of Computational Biology*, 8(6):625–637, 2001.

[45] Y. Yang, S. Dudoit, P. Luu, D. Lin, V. Peng, J. Ngai, and T. Speed. Normalization for cDNA microarray data: a robust composite method addressing single and multiple slide systematic variation. *Nucleic Acids Research*, 30(4):e 15, 2002.

[46] Y. Yang, S. Dudoit, P. Luu, and T. Speed. Normalization for cDNA microarray data. In M. Bittner, Y. Chen, A. Dorsel, and E. Dougherty, editors, *Microarrays: Optical Technologies and Informatics*, volume 4266 of *Proceedings of SPIE*, 2001.

[47] Y. H. Yang, M. J. Buckley, S. Dudoit, and T. P. Speed. Comparison of methods for image analysis on cDNA microarray data. *Journal of Computational and Graphical Statistics*, 11:108–136, 2002.

8

Inferring Genetic Regulatory Networks from Microarray Experiments with Bayesian Networks

Dirk Husmeier

Biomathematics and Statistics Scotland (BioSS)
JCMB, The King's Buildings, Edinburgh EH9 3JZ, UK
dirk@bioss.ac.uk

Summary. Molecular pathways consisting of interacting proteins underlie the major functions of living cells, and a central goal of molecular biology is to understand the regulatory mechanisms of gene transcription and protein synthesis. Several approaches to the reverse engineering of genetic regulatory networks from gene expression data have been explored. At the most refined level of detail is a mathematical description of the biophysical processes in terms of a system of coupled differential equations that describe, for instance, the processes of transcription factor binding, protein and RNA degradation, and diffusion. Besides facing inherent identifiability problems, this approach is usually restricted to very small systems. At the other extreme is the coarse-scale approach of clustering, which provides a computationally cheap way to extract useful information from large-scale expression data sets. However, while clustering indicates which genes are co-regulated and may therefore be involved in related biological processes, it does not lead to a fine resolution of the interaction processes that would indicate, for instance, whether an interaction between two genes is direct or mediated by other genes, or whether a gene is a regulator or regulatee. A promising compromise between these two extremes is the approach of Bayesian networks, which are interpretable and flexible models for representing conditional dependence relations between multiple interacting quantities, and whose probabilistic nature is capable of handling noise inherent in both the biological processes and the microarray experiments. This chapter will first briefly recapitulate the Bayesian network paradigm and the work of Friedman et al. [8], [23], who spearheaded the application of Bayesian networks to gene expression data. Next, the chapter will discuss the shortcomings of *static* Bayesian networks and show how these shortcomings can be overcome with *dynamic* Bayesian networks. Finally, the chapter will address the important question of the reliability of the inference procedure. This inference problem is particularly hard in that interactions between hundreds of genes have to be learned from very sparse data sets, typically containing only a few dozen time points during a cell cycle. The results of a simulation study to test the viability of the Bayesian network paradigm are reported. In this study, gene expression data are simulated from a realistic molecular biological network involving DNAs, mRNAs and proteins, and then regulatory networks are inferred from these data in a reverse engineering approach, using dynamic Bayesian networks and Bayesian learning with Markov chain Monte Carlo. The simulation results are presented as receiver operator characteristics (ROC) curves. This allows an estimation of the proportion of spurious gene interactions incurred for a specified target proportion of recovered true interactions. The findings demonstrate how the network inference performance varies with the training set size, the degree of inadequacy of prior assumptions, the experimental sampling strategy, and the inclusion of further, sequence-based information.

8.1 Introduction

Molecular pathways consisting of interacting proteins underlie the major functions of living cells. A central goal of molecular biology is therefore to understand the regulatory mechanisms of gene transcription and protein synthesis, and the invention of DNA microarrays, which measure the abundance of thousands of mRNA targets simultaneously, has been hailed as an important milestone in this endeavour. Several approaches to the reverse engineering of genetic regulatory networks from gene expression data have been explored, reviewed, for example, in [6] and [5].

At the most refined level of detail is a mathematical description of the biophysical processes in terms of a system of coupled differential equations that describe, for example, the processes of transcription factor binding, diffusion, and RNA degradation; see, for instance, [4]. While such low-level dynamics are critical to a complete understanding of regulatory networks, they require detailed specifications of both the relationship between the interacting entities as well as the parameters of the biochemical reaction, such as reaction rates and diffusion constants. Obviously, this approach is therefore restricted to very small systems. In a recent study, Zak et al. [30] found that a system of ordinary differential equations describing a regulatory network of three genes with their respective mRNA and protein products is not identifiable when only gene expression data are observed, and that rich data, including detailed information on protein–DNA interactions, are needed to ensure identifiability of the parameters that determine the interaction structure.

At the other extreme of the spectrum is the coarse-scale approach of clustering, illustrated in Figure 8.1. Following up on the seminal paper by Eisen et al. [7], several clustering methods have been applied to gene expression data, reviewed, for instance, in [6]. Clustering provides a computationally cheap way to extract useful information out of large-scale expression data sets. The underlying conjecture is that co-expression is indicative of co-regulation, thus clustering may identify genes that have similar functions or are involved in related biological processes. The disadvantage, however, is that clustering only indicates which genes are co-regulated; it does *not* lead to a fine resolution of the interaction processes that indicates, for example, whether an interaction between two genes is direct or mediated by other genes, whether a gene is a regulator or regulatee, and so on. Clustering, in effect, only groups interacting

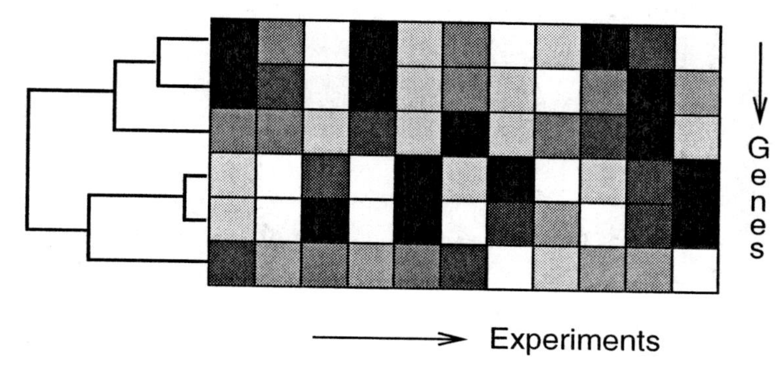

Fig. 8.1. Hierarchical clustering of gene expression data. Rows represent genes, columns represent experimental conditions, and grey levels show the amount of up or down regulation with respect to a control. Genes with similar expression levels across different conditions are grouped together. The algorithm is, in principle, similar to the method of Figure 4.9.

genes together in a monolithic block, where the detailed form of the regulatory interaction patterns is lost; see Figure 8.2 for an illustration.

A promising compromise between these two extremes is the approach of Bayesian networks, introduced in Chapter 2, which were first applied to the problem of reverse engineering genetic networks from microarray expression data in [8], [23], and [12]. Bayesian networks are interpretable and flexible models for representing probabilistic relationships between multiple interacting entities. At a *qualitative* level, the structure of a Bayesian network describes the relationships between these entities in the form of conditional independence relations. At a *quantitative level*, relationships between the interacting entities are described by conditional probability distributions. The probabilistic nature of this approach is capable of handling noise inherent in both the biological processes and the microarray experiments. This makes Bayesian networks superior to Boolean networks ([18], [19]), which are deterministic in nature.

8.2 A Brief Revision of Bayesian Networks

Recall from Section 2.1 that a Bayesian network consists of a set of *nodes* connected by *directed edges*. The nodes represent random variables, while the edges represent conditional dependence relations between these random variables. A Bayesian network defines a factorization of the joint probability of all the nodes into a product of simpler conditional probabilities, by (2.1). In applying this method to the inference of genetic networks, we associate nodes with genes and their expression levels, while edges indicate interactions between the genes. For instance, the network structure of Figure 2.1 suggests

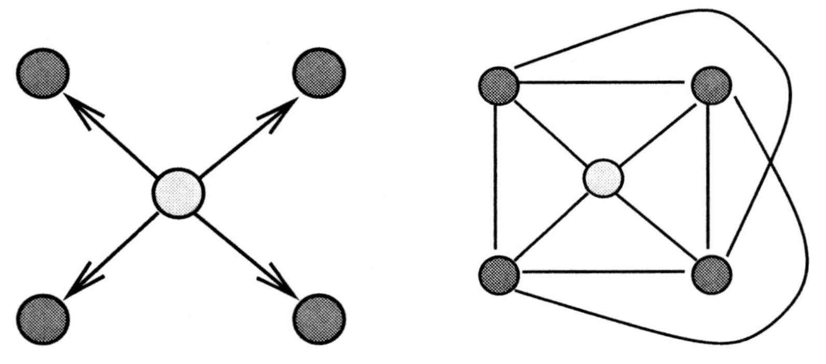

Fig. 8.2. Shortcomings of clustering. The left figure shows a hypothetical gene regulatory network, where the transcription of the centre gene initiates the transcription of four other genes. The right figure shows the outcome of a standard clustering approach. All five genes are grouped together due to their correlated expression, but the detailed form of their interaction remains unknown.

that gene A initiates the transcription cascade, that genes B and C co-regulate gene D, and that gene D mediates the interaction between genes (B, C) and E.

Recall from Section 2.1 that we distinguish between the *model* or *network structure* $\mathcal{M}$, which is the set of edges connecting the nodes, and the *network parameters* $\mathbf{q}$. Given a family $\mathcal{F}$ of (conditional) probability distributions, the latter define the conditional probabilities associated with the edges and determine, for example, whether the influence of one gene on another is of the form of an excitation or inhibition. An illustration can be found in Figure 2.10. Our objective is to learn the network from gene expression data $\mathcal{D}$, resulting from a microarray experiment and an appropriate normalization method, as discussed in Chapter 7. In a nutshell, learning effectively means sampling network structures $\mathcal{M}$ from the posterior probability

$$P(\mathcal{M}|\mathcal{D}) = \frac{1}{Z}P(\mathcal{D}|\mathcal{M})P(\mathcal{M}) \tag{8.1}$$

where $Z = \sum_{\mathcal{M}} P(\mathcal{D}|\mathcal{M})P(\mathcal{M})$ is a normalization factor, $P(\mathcal{M})$ is the prior probability on network structures, and

$$P(\mathcal{D}|\mathcal{M}) = \int P(\mathcal{D}|\mathbf{q}, \mathcal{M})P(\mathbf{q}|\mathcal{M})d\mathbf{q} \tag{8.2}$$

is the marginal likelihood for network structures, which requires the parameters $\mathbf{q}$ to be integrated out; see Section 2.2.1 for a more detailed discussion. If certain regularity conditions, discussed in [14], are satisfied and the data are *complete* (meaning that we do not have any missing values), the integral in (8.2) is analytically tractable. Two function families $\mathcal{F}$ of conditional probability distributions for which this closed-form solution of (8.2) is possible are

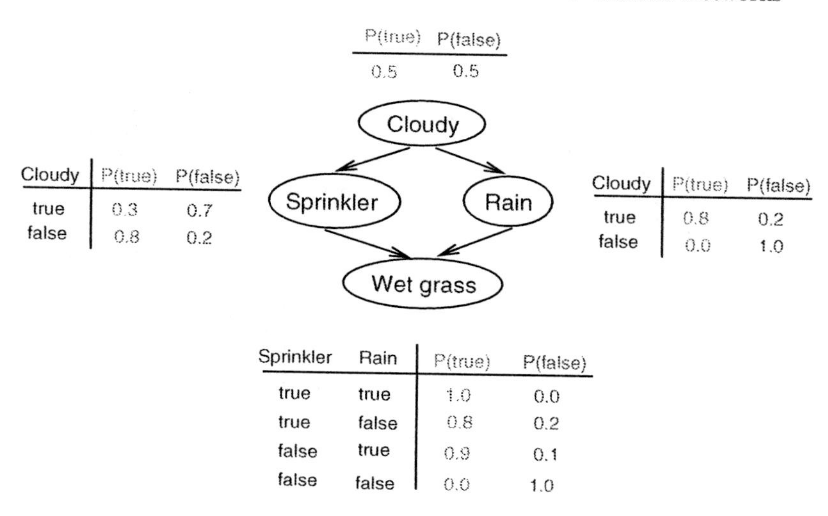

Fig. 8.3. Multinomial conditional probability distribution. A multinomial conditional probability distribution is basically a table that lists the probabilities of discrete events for each combination of the discrete settings of the parents. The figure shows an example for a simple network with binary units that can take on the values TRUE and FALSE (indicating, for example, whether or not the grass is wet, or whether or not a sprinkler is used). In gene expression data, the discretization usually contains three values: underexpressed (−1), not differently expressed (0), and overexpressed (1), depending on whether the expression rate is significantly lower than, similar to, or greater than control, respectively. Adapted from [20], by permission of Cambridge University Press.

the *linear Gaussian* and the *multinomial* distribution. The *multinomial distribution* is illustrated in Figure 8.3 and discussed at length in [14]. It allows us to model a nonlinear regulation scheme, like the one illustrated in Figure 8.4. However, the price to pay is a discretization of the data, as described in the caption of Figure 8.3, and this inevitably incurs a certain information loss. Also, the number of parameters increases exponentially with the number of parents. The *linear Gaussian* model is given by

$$p(x_i|\mathbf{x}_{pa[i]}) = N\left(\mathbf{w}^\dagger \mathbf{x}_{pa[i]}; \sigma\right) \tag{8.3}$$

where $pa[i]$ are the parents of node i, $\mathbf{x}_{pa[i]}$ represents the (column) vector of random variables associated with $pa[i]$, $N(\mu; \sigma)$ denotes a Normal distribution with mean μ and standard deviation σ, $\mathbf{w}$ is a parameter (column) vector, and the superscript $\dagger$ denotes matrix transposition. The linear Gaussian model does not suffer from the information loss caused by discretization, and the number of parameters increases linearly rather than exponentially with the number of parents. The disadvantage, however, is that nonlinear regulation patterns, like the one illustrated in Figure 8.4, can *not* be modelled in this

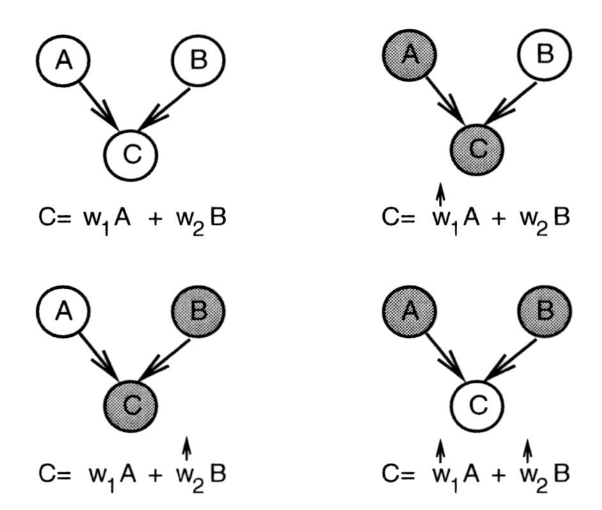

Fig. 8.4. Nonlinear interaction. Gene C is co-regulated by two genes, A and B. The regulation is of an XOR type: gene C is up-regulated, symbolized by a grey shading, if either gene A is up-regulated, but not gene B (top right), or if gene B is up-regulated, but not gene A (bottom, left). Otherwise, gene C is down-regulated, represented by a node without shading (top left, bottom right). This co-regulation pattern is intrinsically nonlinear and can *not* be predicted with the linear Gaussian model (8.3), as indicated in the figure. The positive correlation between genes A and C (top, right) requires a positive weight parameter w_1; the positive correlation between genes B and C (bottom, left) requires a positive weight parameter w_2. With both parameters w_1 and w_2 positive, an upregulation of both genes A and B will lead to a positive weighted sum, $w_1A + w_2B > 0$. Consequently, up-regulation is predicted where, in reality, the gene is down-regulated (bottom, right).

way. For this reason the benchmark studies reported later in Sections 8.8 and 8.9 choose $\mathcal{F}$ to be the family of multinomial conditional probabilities. For a more comprehensive discussion and further details, see [8].

Now, recall from Section 2.2.2 that direct sampling from (8.1) is impossible due to the intractability of the denominator. We therefore have to resort to a Markov chain Monte Carlo (MCMC) simulation, as discussed in Section 2.2.2.

8.3 Learning Local Structures and Subnetworks

Recall from Table 2.1 that the number of possible network structures $\mathcal{M}$ increases super-exponentially with the number of nodes. For a large and informative data set $\mathcal{D}$, the posterior probability $P(\mathcal{M}|\mathcal{D})$ is usually dominated by only a few network structures $\mathcal{M}$, which allows us to reasonably infer the *global* network structure from the data. However, microarray data are usually sparse, meaning that hundreds of gene expression levels are measured for only

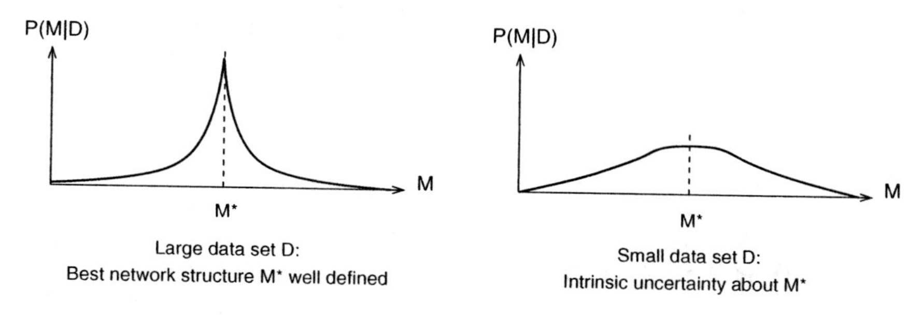

Fig. 8.5. Inference uncertainty. The vertical axis shows the posterior probability $P(\mathcal{M}|\mathcal{D})$, the horizontal axis represents the model structure $\mathcal{M}$. *Left:* When the data set $\mathcal{D}$ is sufficiently large and informative, $P(\mathcal{M}|\mathcal{D})$ has a pronounced maximum at the true network structure $\mathcal{M}^*$. *Right:* For sparse data, the distribution $P(\mathcal{M}|\mathcal{D})$ is diffuse and many different structures have similarly high posterior probability scores.

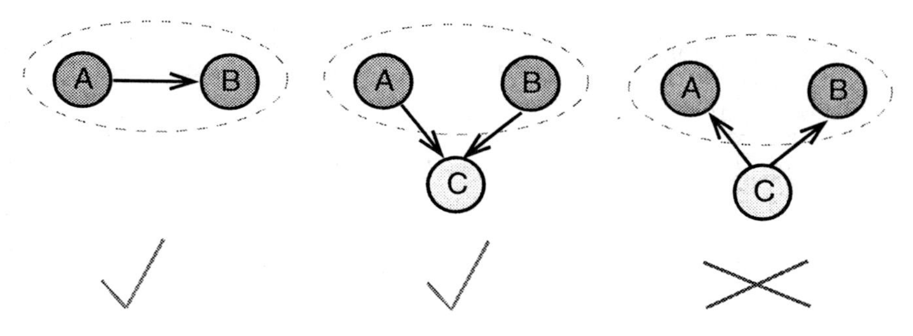

Fig. 8.6. Markov neighbours. Markov neighbours are nodes that are not d-separated by any other measured variable in the domain. This includes parent–child relations (*left*), where one gene regulates another gene, and spouse relations (*middle*), where two genes co-regulate a third gene. In the configuration on the *right*, nodes A and B are d-separated by node C, hence they do *not* satisfy the Markov relation. See Figures 2.7 and 2.8 for a revision of the concept of d-separation.

a few time points or under a small number of different experimental conditions. Consequently, the posterior distribution of the network structure given the data, $P(\mathcal{M}|\mathcal{D})$, is diffuse, and a huge number of different networks are plausible given the data. An illustration is given in Figure 8.5.

Since the vagueness of $P(\mathcal{M}|\mathcal{D})$ does not allow a reasonable inference of the *global* network structure, Friedman et al. [8] suggested focusing on low-dimensional features of the high-scoring networks and then examining the posterior probability of these features given the data. Formally, a feature is a binary indicator variable, which is 1 if the feature is present in the given network structure $\mathcal{M}$, and 0 otherwise:

$$f(\mathcal{M}) = \begin{cases} 1 \text{ if } \mathcal{M} \text{ satisfies the feature} \\ 0 \text{ otherwise} \end{cases} \tag{8.4}$$

Three features applied in [8] and [23] are Markov, order, and separator relations.

Markov relations are illustrated in Figure 8.6. The definition is based on the concepts of *d-separation* and the *Markov blanket*, which were introduced in Section 2.1. Two nodes A and B are Markov neighbours if they are in each other's Markov blanket, that is, if they are not d-separated by any other node. If two variables are in a Markov relation, no other variable in the model mediates the dependence between them. In the context of gene expression analysis, a Markov relation indicates that the two genes are related in some joint biological regulation process or interaction.

Separator relations identify (sets of) nodes that mediate the dependence between other (sets of) nodes. For instance, in Figure 8.6, node C satisfies the separator relation when nodes A and B are *not* in each other's Markov blanket, which holds for the subfigure on the right. In the context of gene expression analysis, a gene that acts as a separator mediates the regulatory interactions between the separated genes.

Order relations indicate that two nodes in the network are connected by a directed path, that is, a path whose edges all have the same direction. Recall from Section 2.2.4 that for complete observation and under the causal Markov assumption, a directed path in a PDAG implies a causal relation. Since gene expression data do not capture processes related to protein activities and post-translational modifications (see Section 8.9, especially Figure 8.15), the condition of complete observability is not satisfied. Consequently, an order relation has to be interpreted as an *indication* rather than a proof that two genes *might* be involved in a causal relation.

The posterior probability of a feature f is given by

$$P(f|\mathcal{D}) = \sum_{M} f(\mathcal{M})P(\mathcal{M}|\mathcal{D}) \tag{8.5}$$

By mapping the *high-dimensional* space of network structures $\mathcal{M}$ into the *low-dimensional* feature space, the posterior probabilities can be assumed to become more informative and less diffuse. In practice, we cannot compute (8.5) directly because the number of possible network structures $\mathcal{M}$ is far too large (see Table 2.1 on page 28). Consequently, we resort again to MCMC, and approximate (8.5) from the MCMC sample $\{\mathcal{M}_1, \ldots, \mathcal{M}_T\}$:

$$P(f|\mathcal{D}) = \frac{1}{T}\sum_{i=1}^{T} f(\mathcal{M}_i) \tag{8.6}$$

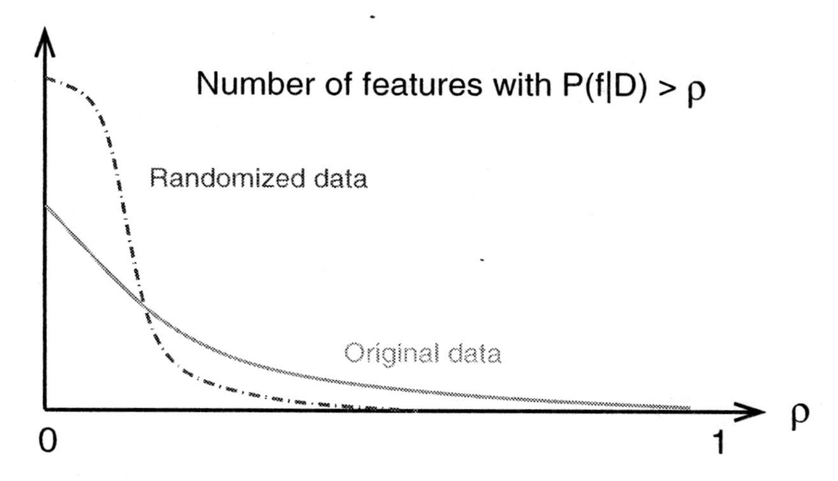

Fig. 8.7. Confidence scores for local features in the yeast cell cycle. The figure illustrates the results obtained in the study of Friedman et al. [8]. The plot shows the number of local features whose posterior probability $P(f|\mathcal{D})$ exceeds a given threshold $\rho \in [0, 1]$. The approximation of $P(f|\mathcal{D})$ in [8] is based on (8.6), but uses a MAP/ bootstrapping approach rather than Bayesian MCMC (consequently, the plotted score is not a proper posterior probability). The solid line shows the results on the yeast data. The dash-dotted line shows the results on the randomized data. The actual graphs in [8] show certain variations and deviations from the plot in the present figure depending on which type of feature (Markov versus order relations) was chosen, and depending on which model for the conditional probabilities was selected (multinomial versus linear-Gaussian). However, the main characteristic of the plots in [8] is captured by the present figure in that the distribution of confidence estimates for the original data has a longer and heavier tail in the high-confidence region.

8.4 Application to the Yeast Cell Cycle

Friedman et al. [8] applied Bayesian networks to the yeast microarray data of Spellman et al. [27], which contain 76 gene expression measurements of the mRNA levels of 6177 genes,[1] taken during six time series under different experimental conditions. Of these 6177 genes, 800 genes showed significant variations over the different cell-cycle stages and were selected for further analysis. In learning from these data, Friedman et al. [8] treated individual gene expression measurements as independent samples. To model the temporal nature of the cellular processes, an additional node was introduced to denote the cell cycle phase, and this node was forced to be the root in all the networks learned. A vague prior[2] $P(\mathcal{M})$ that did not incorporate any biological domain knowledge was used. Instead of the Bayesian approach, expressed

[1] More accurately: open reading frames.

[2] For more details on the prior, see [8], page 605, and [14].

in (8.1) and discussed in Section 1.3, the authors applied a penalized maximum likelihood/ bootstrap procedure akin to the one described in Section 1.2, but with the maximum likelihood estimate replaced by the MAP estimate of (1.16) on page 13. Bootstrapping is computationally expensive,[3] as discussed in Section 1.4. To reduce the computational costs, Friedman et al. [8] applied a heuristic simplification, which they called the *sparse candidate* algorithm. This algorithm identifies a small number of best candidate parents – first based on a local correlation measure, and later iteratively adapted during the search. The search algorithm is restricted to networks in which the parents of a node are chosen from the set of candidate parents of this node. This restriction results in a much smaller search space and, consequently, a considerable reduction in the computational costs.

The confidence for local features is computed from (8.6), where the set of learned network structures, $\{\mathcal{M}_i\}$, is obtained from a bootstrap rather than an MCMC sample – hence the confidence scores obtained in [8] are not proper posterior probabilities (although the actual difference may be small).

To estimate the credibility of the confidence assessment, the authors created a random data set by permuting the order of the experiments independently for each gene. In this randomized data set, genes are independent of each other and one does not expect to find true features. Figure 8.7 illustrates the results found in [8]. Local features in the random data tend to have notably lower confidence scores than those in the true data, and the distribution of confidence scores in the original data has a longer and heavier tail in the high-confidence region than the distribution of confidence scores in the random data. Friedman et al. [8] therefore suggest that local features with high confidence scores are likely to reflect true features of the underlying genetic regulatory network.

8.4.1 Biological Findings

A striking feature that emerged from the application of Bayesian networks to the yeast data is the existence of a few dominant genes. To quantify this notion, Friedman et al. [8] introduced a dominance score,[4]

$$\Psi(X) = \sum_{Y} P(X \to Y|\mathcal{D}) \tag{8.7}$$

[3] Recall that in most other applications, the Bayesian MCMC approach is computationally less expensive than bootstrapping, as discussed, for example, in Section 4.4.7, especially Figure 4.35. In the present situation, however, the computation of the Hastings ratio, discussed in Section 2.2.2 and illustrated in Figure 2.16, is prohibitively expensive.

[4] See [8], page 615, for the exact definition of this dominance score, which deviates slightly from (8.7). Also, recall that the confidence scores in [8] are not proper posterior probabilities, as discussed before.

where $X \rightarrow Y$ represents the feature that gene X is an ancestor of gene Y in a directed path from X to Y. A gene with a high dominance score is indicative of a potential causal source of the cell-cycle process, and only a few genes were found to have a high dominance score. These high-scoring genes are known to be directly involved in initiating or controlling the cell cycle, to play key roles in essential cell functions, or to be involved in DNA repair and transcription initiation. These findings suggest that the analysis can discover true biological features of the cell-cycle process.

When looking at *Markov relations*, the two conditional probability models employed – the *multinomial* and the *linear-Gaussian* distributions – were found to lead to different results. A Markov pair $A \leftrightarrow B$ with a high confidence score $P(A \leftrightarrow B|\mathcal{D})$ under one model did not necessarily have a high confidence score under the other. This lack of agreement is not too surprising: the multinomial model can capture nonlinear dependence relations, which the linear-Gaussian model inevitably misses. On the other hand, the discretization of the data required for the application of the multinomial model may lose information that is available to the linear-Gaussian model. Friedman et al. [8] found that for the multinomial distribution, the analysis discovered several high-scoring Markov pairs that had a low correlation in their expression and were therefore grouped into different clusters with a standard clustering algorithm. These high-scoring Markov pairs included several pairs of genes with similar biological functions,[5] which suggests that Bayesian networks can find biological features that are not amenable to standard clustering methods. However, supporting the inference results with biological findings from the literature has certain intrinsic problems, as discussed later, in Section 8.9.

As demonstrated in Figure 8.2, Bayesian networks may overcome the limitations of conventional clustering techniques by modelling the detailed form of the interactions between the genes. Especially, the identification of *separator relations* allows us to infer which genes mediate the dependence between other genes. For instance, the clustering algorithm applied in [27] groups the five genes CLN2, RNR3, SVS1, SRO4, and RAD51 together in the same cluster. Figure 8.11 shows a high-confidence subnetwork inferred in [8], involving the same genes. It is seen that RNR3, SVS1, SRO4, and RAD51 are separated by their common parent CLN2 and do not have any links between each other. This finding agrees with biological knowledge: CLN2 has a central and early cell cycle control function, whereas there are no known biological relationships between the other genes.

Figure 8.8 shows a subnetwork from a different analysis, reported in [23]. In the inferred high confidence subnetwork, several low-osmolarity response genes

[5] Examples are LAC1 $\leftrightarrow$ YNL300W (LAC1 is a GPI transport protein, and YNL300W is modified by GPI), FAR1 $\leftrightarrow$ ASH1 (both proteins participate in a mating-type switch), and SAG1 $\leftrightarrow$ MF-ALPHA-1 (SAG1 induces the mating process, and MF-ALPHA-1 is an essential protein that participates in the mating process).

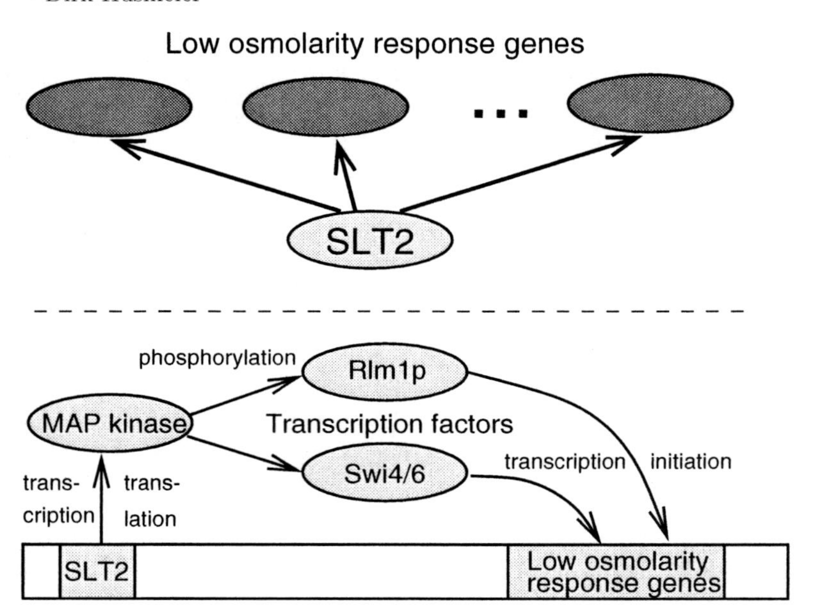

Fig. 8.8. Separator relations. In the analysis of Pe'er et al. [23] gene SLT2 was found to d-separate several low-osmolarity response genes. The top figure shows the subnetwork with the highest posterior probability, which suggests that SLT2 initiates the transcription of several low-osmolarity response genes. The bottom figure shows a network suggested in the biological literature. SLT2 encodes the enzyme MAP kinase, which activates two transcription factors by phosphorylation. The activated transcription factors bind to the promoter regions of several low-osmolarity genes and thereby initiate their transcription. Reprinted from [16], by permission of the Biochemical Society.

are separated by their parent, SLT2. This concurs with biological findings: SLT2 encodes the enzyme MAP kinase, which post-translationally activates two transcription factors, which in turn activate the low-osmolarity response genes.

In both cases, the inference with Bayesian networks has explained away dependencies and has provided an enhanced insight into the underlying molecular architecture of pathways. In Figure 8.8, all separated genes share similar biological functions. This finding can be used to assign novel putative functions to yet unannotated genes: when a previously uncharacterized gene is found to be a child of a given parent node, it may have a function related to that of the other children. Also, note that in both cases, Figures 8.8 and 8.11, the Bayesian network has uncovered intra-cluster structures among correlated genes that are not amenable to standard clustering methods.

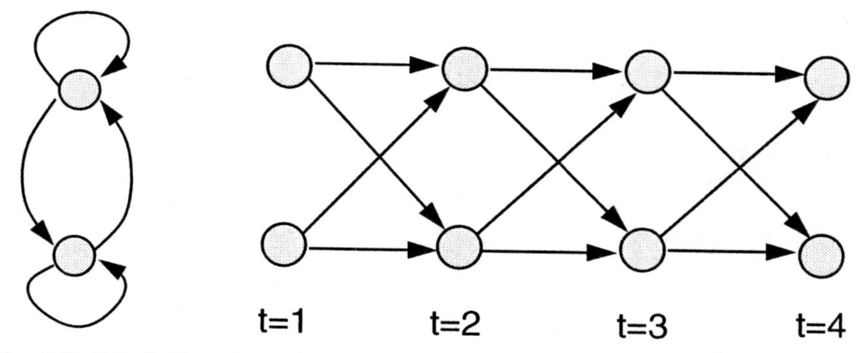

Fig. 8.9. Modelling feedback with dynamic Bayesian networks. *Left:* Recurrent network comprising two genes with feedback that interact with each other. This structure is *not* a Bayesian network. *Right:* Equivalent dynamic Bayesian network obtained by unfolding the recurrent network in time. Note that similar unfolding methods have been applied in the study of recurrent neural networks ([15], page 183). Reprinted from [17], by permission of Oxford University Press.

8.5 Shortcomings of Static Bayesian Networks

The approach outlined above has several limitations. The first obvious restriction results from the problem of *equivalence* classes, discussed in Section 2.2.3. Take, for example, Figure 2.18. All networks have the same skeleton, but differ with respect to the edge directions. Expanding the joint probability $P(A, B, C)$ according to (2.1), however, gives the same factorization for three of the networks irrespective of the edge directions. These networks are therefore *equivalent* and cannot be distinguished on the basis of the data. The consequence is that for a given Bayesian network structure $\mathcal{M}$ sampled from the posterior probability distribution (8.1), we have to identify the whole equivalence class $\mathcal{C}(\mathcal{M})$ to which $\mathcal{M}$ belongs, and then discard all those edge directions which are not unequivocal among all $\mathcal{M}' \in \mathcal{C}(\mathcal{M})$. An example is given in Figure 2.19, where the subfigure on the right shows the equivalence class that corresponds to the Bayesian network on the left. Note that this equivalence loses substantial information about the edge directions and thus about possible causal interactions between the genes.[6] A second, possibly more serious drawback, is given by the acyclicity constraint, which rules out feedback loops like those in the bottom right of Figure 2.10. Since feedback is an essential feature of biological systems, the usefulness of Bayesian networks for modelling genetic regulatory interactions is questionable.

[6] See Section 2.2.4 for a discussion of the relation between edge directions and causal interactions.

8.6 Dynamic Bayesian Networks

Consider Figure 8.9, left, which shows a simple network consisting of two genes. Both genes have feedback loops and interact with each other, ruling out the applicability of DAGs. However, interactions between genes are usually such that the first gene is transcribed and translated into protein, which then has some influence on the transcription of the second gene. This implies that the interaction is not instantaneous, but that its effect happens with a time delay after its cause. The same applies to the feedback loops of genes acting back on themselves. We can therefore *unfold* the recurrent network of Figure 8.9, left, *in time* to obtain the directed, acyclic network of Figure 8.9, right. The latter is again a proper DAG and corresponds to a *dynamic Bayesian network*. For details, see [9] and [21]. Note that similar unfolding methods have been applied in the study of recurrent neural networks ([15], page 183). To avoid an explosion of the model complexity, parameters are tied such that the transition probabilities between time slices $t-1$ and t are the same for all t. The true dynamic process is thus approximated by a homogeneous Markov model. Following [17], and as opposed to [9], intra-slice connections, that is, edges within a time slice, are not allowed because this would correspond to instantaneous interactions. Note that with this restriction, a dynamic Bayesian network avoids the ambiguity of the edge directions, discussed in Section 8.5: reversing an edge corresponds to an effect that precedes its cause, which is impossible. The approach has the further advantage of overcoming one of the computational bottlenecks of the MCMC simulations. Recall that the acceptance probabilities (2.33) of the Metropolis-Hastings sampler depend on the Hastings ratio, that is, the ratio of the proposal probabilities. As illustrated in Figure 2.16, the computation of the Hastings ratio implies an acyclicity check for all networks in the neighbourhood of a given candidate network. For networks with many nodes these neighbourhoods and, consequently, the computational costs become prohibitively large. It is presumably for this reason that a proper MCMC approach was not attempted in [8] and [23], as discussed in Section 8.4. Since the unfolding process of Figure 8.9 automatically guarantees acyclicity, the computation of the Hastings ratio becomes trivial for dynamical Bayesian networks, thereby overcoming this major computational bottleneck.

8.7 Accuracy of Inference

The main challenge for the inference procedure is that interactions between hundreds of genes have to be learned from short time series of typically only about a dozen measurements. The inevitable consequence is that the posterior distribution over network structures becomes diffuse, as discussed earlier in Section 8.3, and illustrated in Figure 8.5, and it is therefore important

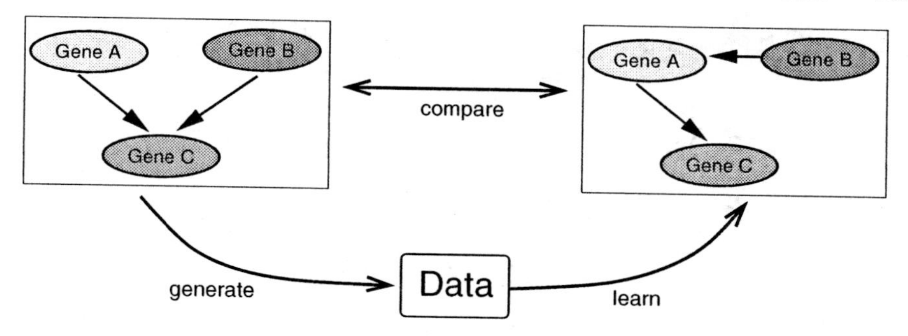

Fig. 8.10. Synthetic simulation study. Synthetic data are generated from a known Bayesian network. Then, new networks are sampled from the posterior distribution with MCMC and compared with the true network. Reprinted from [17], by permission of Oxford University Press.

to somehow quantify how much can be learned from the data in this unfavourable situation. Also, note that the sparseness of the data implies that the prior $P(\mathcal{M})$ has a non-negligible influence on the posterior $P(\mathcal{M}|\mathcal{D})$ (8.1) and should therefore be devised so as to capture known features of biological networks. A reasonable approach, adopted in most applications of Bayesian networks to the reverse engineering of genetic networks, is to impose a limit on the maximum number of edges converging on a node, $FI(\mathcal{M})$, and to set $P(\mathcal{M}) = 0$ if $FI(\mathcal{M}) > \alpha$, for some *a priori* chosen value of α. This prior incorporates our current assumptions about the structure of genetic networks, namely, that the expression of a gene is controlled by a comparatively small number of active regulators, while, on the other hand, regulator genes themselves are unrestricted in the number of genes they may regulate. The practical advantage of this restriction on the maximum "fan-in" is a considerable reduction of the computational complexity, which improves the convergence and mixing properties of the Markov chain in the MCMC simulation. The following two sections will report the results of the benchmark study [17], whose objective was to empirically estimate how much can be learned about genetic regulatory networks from sparse gene expression data. Recall from Section 8.2 that $\mathcal{F}$ is the family of multinomial conditional probabilities.

8.8 Evaluation on Synthetic Data

To evaluate the performance of the inference procedure on sparse data sets, we can proceed as shown in Figure 8.10. Synthetic data, $\mathcal{D}$, are generated from a known Bayesian network, $\mathcal{M}_0$. Then, new networks $\mathcal{M}_i$ are sampled from the posterior distribution $P(\mathcal{M}|\mathcal{D})$. From a comparison between this sample, $\{\mathcal{M}_i\}$, and the true network, $\mathcal{M}_0$, we can estimate the accuracy of the inference procedure. Denote by $P(e_{ik}|\mathcal{D})$ the posterior probabil-

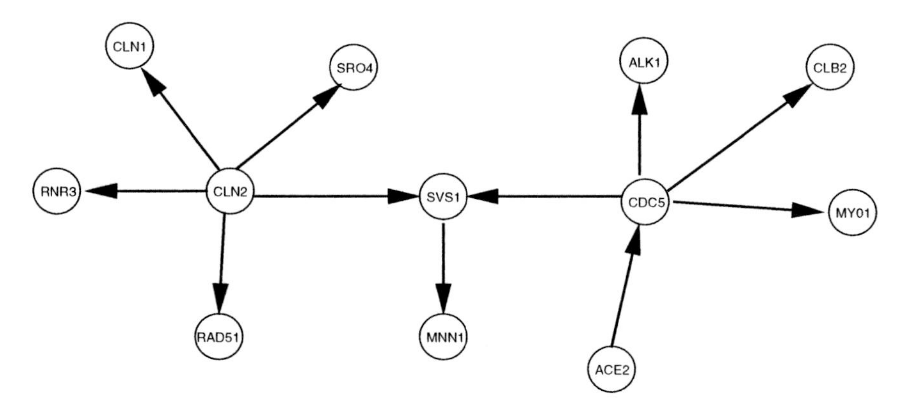

Fig. 8.11. Synthetic genetic network. The structure of the true Bayesian network used in this study is that of a subnetwork of the yeast cell cycle, taken from [8]. 38 unconnected nodes were added, giving a total number of 50 nodes. Reprinted from [17], by permission of Oxford University Press.

ity of an edge e_{ik} between nodes i and k, which is given by the proportion of networks in the MCMC sample $\{\mathcal{M}_i\}$ that contain this edge. Let $\mathcal{E}(\rho) = \{e_{ik} | P(e_{ik}|\mathcal{D}) > \rho\}$ denote the set of all edges whose posterior probability exceeds a given threshold $\rho \in [0, 1]$. From this set we can compute (1) the *sensitivity*, that is, the proportion of recovered true edges, and (2) the complementary *specificity*, that is, the proportion of erroneously recovered spurious edges. To rephrase this: For a given threshold ρ we count the number of true positive (TP), false positive (FP), true negative (TN), and false negative (FN) edges. We then compute the sensitivity = $TP/(TP + FN)$, the specificity = $TN/(TN + FP)$, and the complementary specificity = 1-specificity = $FP/(TN + FP)$. Rather than selecting an arbitrary value for the threshold ρ, we repeat this scoring procedure for several different values of $\rho \in [0, 1]$ and plot the ensuing sensitivity scores against the corresponding complementary specificity scores. This gives the *receiver operator characteristics* (ROC) curves of Figures 8.13 and 8.18. The diagonal dashed line indicates the expected ROC curve for a random predictor. The ROC curve of Figure 8.13, top left, solid line indicates a perfect retrieval of all true edges without a single spurious edge. In general, ROC curves are between these two extremes, with a larger *area under the ROC curve* (AUROC) indicating a better performance. The true network (or, more precisely, the true inter-slice connectivity of the dynamic Bayesian network) is shown in Figure 8.11. Two different conditional probability distributions were associated with the edges. *Simulation 1:* Noisy regulation according to a binomial distribution with the following parameters. Excitation: $P(on|on) = 0.9, P(on|off) = 0.1$; inhibition: $P(on|on) = 0.1, P(on|off) = 0.9$; noisy XOR-style co-regulation: $P(on|on, on) = P(on|off, off) = 0.1$, $P(on|on, off) = P(on|off, on) = 0.9$. *Simulation 2:* Stochastic interaction, where all parameters were chosen at

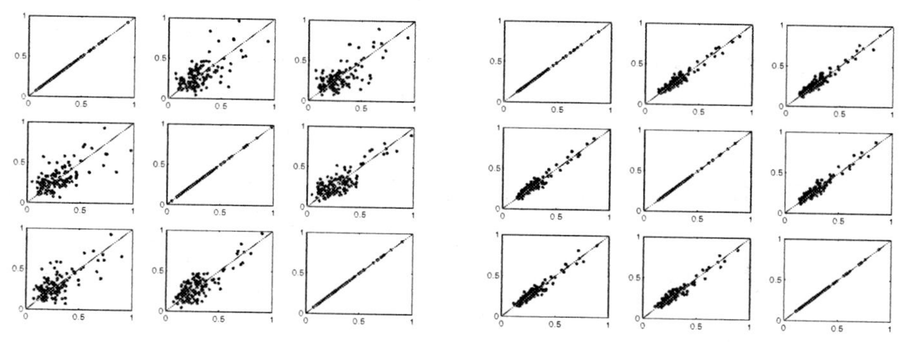

Fig. 8.12. Convergence test for MCMC. The figure shows an application of the MCMC convergence test of Figure 2.17. Each MCMC simulation was repeated three times, using the same training data $\mathcal{D}$, but starting from different random number generator seeds. The posterior probabilities of the edges $P(e_{ik}|\mathcal{D})$ obtained from different simulations are plotted against each other, leading to a 3-by-3 matrix of subfigures, where subfigure (1,1) plots the posterior probability scores obtained from simulation 1 against those of simulation 1 (so the scores obviously lie on a straight line), subfigure (1,2) plots the scores from simulation 1 against those from simulation 2, subfigure (2,1) plots the scores from simulation 2 against those from simulation 1 (hence subfigure (2,1) is the mirror image of subfigure (1,2)), and so on. *Left:* Burn-in = 10,000 steps, sampling phase = 10,000 steps. The agreement between the posterior probabilities obtained from different simulations is poor, which indicates insufficient convergence of the Markov chain. *Right:* Burn-in = 100,000 steps, sampling phase = 100,000 steps. The agreement between the posterior probabilities obtained from different simulations is satisfactory, hence the simulation passes the (necessary) convergence test.

random. The latter simulations were repeated with both a binomial and a trinomial distribution. Since the results were similar, only the results for the trinomial case will be reported here. All simulations were repeated for three different time series of length $N = 100$, $N = 30$, and $N = 7$. In a second series of simulations, 38 redundant unconnected nodes we added to the true network as *confounders*, giving a total of 50 nodes. For each setting, networks were sampled from the posterior distribution $P(\mathcal{M}|\mathcal{D})$ with MCMC. Based on an initial convergence test depicted in Figure 8.12, both the burn-in and sampling phases were chosen to contain 100,000 Metropolis-Hastings steps. All simulations were then repeated three times for different training data $\mathcal{D}$, generated from different random number generators. The results are summarized in Figure 8.13. The ROC curves show which price in terms of erroneously predicted spurious edges has to be paid for a target recovery rate of true edges. For instance, for a training set size of $N = 100$ generated from the noisy regulation network without redundant nodes, all true edges can be recovered without incurring any false spurious edges (Figure 8.13, top left, solid line). With redundant nodes, we can still recover 75% of the true edges at a zero false

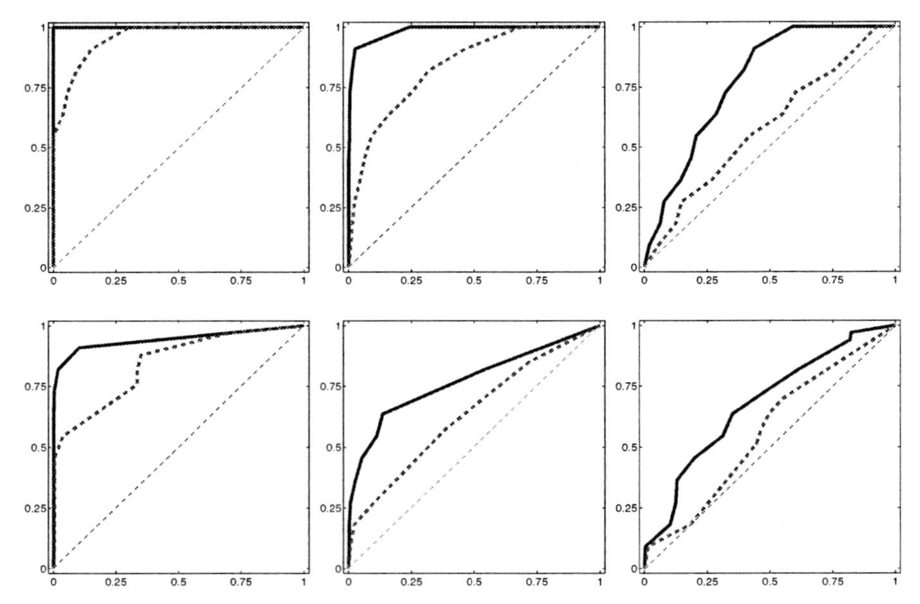

Fig. 8.13. ROC curves for the synthetic data, averaged over three MCMC simulations. The columns correspond to different training set sizes. *Left column:* 100; *middle column:* 30; *right column:* 7. The rows represent different network sizes. *Top row:* Networks without redundant nodes. *Bottom row:* Networks with 38 unconnected nodes (50 nodes in total). In each subfigure the sensitivity (proportion of recovered true edges) is plotted against the complementary specificity (proportion of false edges). The thin, diagonal dashed line is the expected ROC curve of a random predictor. The solid thick line shows the ROC curve for simulation 1 (noisy regulation), the dashed thick line that of simulation 2 (stochastic interaction). The maximum fan-in was set to $\alpha = 2$. Reprinted from [17], by permission of Oxford University Press.

positive rate, while a price of 25% false positives has to be paid if we want to increase the true prediction rate to 90% (Figure 8.13, bottom left, solid line). However, a time series of 100 gene expression measurements is much larger than what is usually available in the laboratory practice, and a realistic experimental situation corresponds much more to Figure 8.13, bottom right. Here, the inference scheme hardly outperforms a random predictor when the true network has stochastic interactions (thick dashed line). This scenario might be over-pessimistic in that real gene interactions are not stochastic, but exist for a reason. However, even for a true network with noisy regulation (solid line), we have to pay a price of 25% spurious edges in order to recover 50% of the true edges, or of 50% spurious edges for a true recovery rate of 75%.

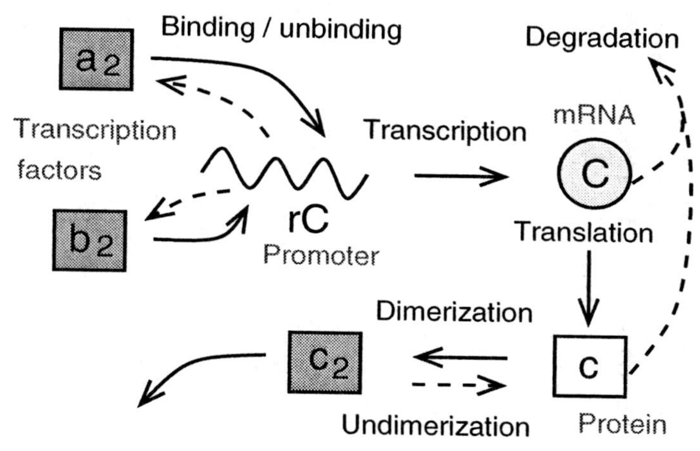

Fig. 8.14. Elementary molecular biological processes. Two transcription factor dimers a_2 and b_2 bind to the *cis* regulatory site rC in the promoter region upstream of a gene, influencing its rate of transcription. The transcribed mRNA C is translated into protein c, which dimerizes into c_2 to form a new active transcription factor that can bind to other *cis* regulatory sites. Reprinted from [17], by permission of Oxford University Press.

8.9 Evaluation on Realistic Data

Synthetic simulations, as discussed in the previous section, are an important tool to obtain an upper bound on the performance of an inference scheme, that is, they indicate how much can at most be learned about gene interactions for a given training set size. A good performance, however, is no guarantee that we will be able to infer this amount of information in practice. First, the conditional probabilities resulting from the true, underlying biological process are different from those associated with the edges of the Bayesian network, which means, we have a mismatch between the real data-generating process and the model used for inference. Second, the true continuous signals are typically sampled at discrete time points, which loses information, especially if the sampling intervals are not matched to the relaxation times of the true biological processes. Third, gene expression ratios are typically discretized, as discussed in Section 8.2, which inevitably adds noise and causes a further loss of information; see Figure 8.16.

In an attempt to achieve a more realistic estimation, several authors have tested their inference methods on real microarray data, testing if *a priori* known gene interactions (reported in the biological literature) could be recovered with their learning algorithms. While this approach addresses the shortcomings mentioned above, it has two inherent problems, resulting from the absence of known gold standards. First, the estimation of the sensitivity is controversial. Having detected an interaction between two genes from microarray expression data with Bayesian networks, authors tend to search

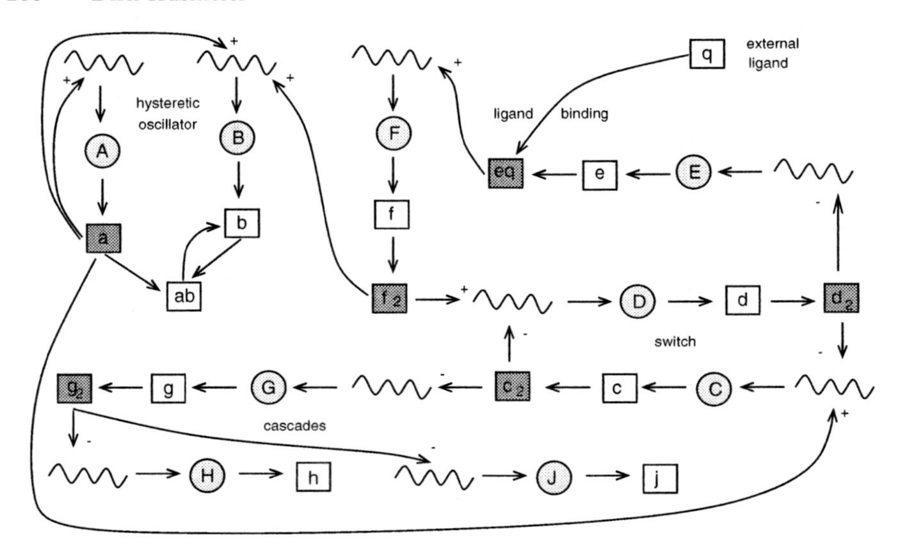

Fig. 8.15. Realistic biological network composed of the elementary processes of Figure 8.14, taken from [29] in a slightly modified form. Oscillating lines represent *cis* regulatory sites in the gene upstream regions (promoters), mRNAs are symbolized by upper case letters in circles, proteins are shown by lower case letters in squares. Shaded squares indicate active transcription factors, where in all but two cases this activation is effected by dimerization, and in one case by ligand binding. The symbols + and − indicate whether a transcription factor acts as an activator or inhibitor. The network contains several subnetworks reported in the biological literature. The subnetwork involving mRNAs A and B is a hysteretic oscillator. A is translated into protein a, which is an active transcription factor that activates the transcription of B. B is translated into protein b, which forms a dimer ab. This dimerization reduces the amount of free transcription factors a, and oscillations result as a consequence of this negative feedback loop. The subnetwork involving mRNAs C and D is a switch: each mRNA is translated into a transcription factor that inhibits the transcription of the other mRNA, thereby switching the competing path "off". Finally, the subnetwork involving mRNA F is triggered by an external ligand, which is needed to form an active transcription factor dimer. Reprinted from [17], by permission of Oxford University Press.

for evidence for this interaction in the biological literature. Often this search involves proteins whose sequences are similar to the ones encoded by genes included in the performed experiment. Besides the fundamental problem that sequence similarity does not necessarily imply similar functions, there is an inherent arbitrariness in deciding on a cut-off value for the similarity score,[7] and it is not clear how independent this selection is from the outcome of the prediction. The second and more serious drawback is the difficulty in estimating the false detection rate. This is because on predicting a gene interaction that

[7] This similarity score is, for instance, given by the E-score of a BLAST [1] search.

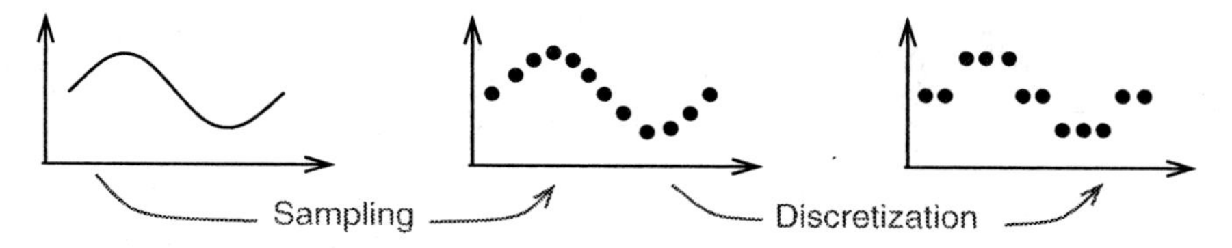

Fig. 8.16. Sampling and discretization. Information contained in the true time dependent mRNA abundance levels is partially lost due to sampling and discretization. Adapted from [26], by permission of Oxford University Press.

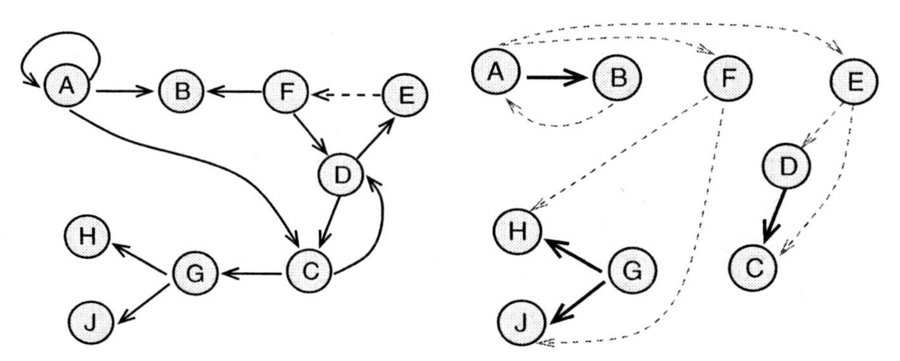

Fig. 8.17. Realistic simulation study. *Left:* Genetic network corresponding to the full molecular biological regulation network of Figure 8.15. Information on protein translation and dimerization is lost, and only mRNA abundance data, obtained from the microarray experiment, are available. The dashed line indicates an interaction that is triggered by the presence of an external ligand. *Right:* Genetic network learned from the sampled and discretized data (see text). Solid arrows show true edges, dashed arrows represent spurious edges. Reprinted from [17], by permission of Oxford University Press.

is not supported by the literature, it is impossible to decide, without further expensive interventions in the form of multiple gene knock-out experiments, whether the algorithm has discovered a new, previously unknown interaction, or whether it has flagged a false edge.

To proceed, the only satisfactory way is a compromise between the above two extremes and to test the performance of an inference scheme on realistic simulated data, for which the true network is known, and the data-generating processes are similar to those found in real biological systems. The study in [17] applied the model regulatory network proposed by Zak et al. [29], which is shown in Figure 8.15 and which contains several structures similar to those in the literature, like a hysteretic oscillator [3], a genetic switch [10], as well as a ligand binding mechanism that influences transcription. The elementary processes are shown in Figure 8.14 and are described by the following system of differential equations, which describe the processes of transcription factor binding, transcription, translation, dimerization, mRNA degradation, and protein degradation:

$$\frac{d}{dt}[a_2.rC] = \lambda^+_{a_2.rC}[a_2][rC] - \lambda^-_{a_2.rC}[a_2.rC]$$
$$\frac{d}{dt}[C] = \lambda_{rC}[rC] + \lambda_{a_2.rC}[a_2.rC] + \lambda_{b_2.rC}[b_2.rC] - \lambda_C[C]$$
$$\frac{d}{dt}[c] = \lambda_{Cc}[C] - \lambda_c[c], \qquad \frac{d}{dt}[c_2] = \lambda^+_{cc}[c]^2 - \lambda^-_{cc}[c_2] \qquad (8.8)$$

Here, the λ_i are kinetic constants, available from the references in [29], t represents time, [.] means concentration, $a_2.rC$ and $b_2.rC$ represent transcription factors a_2 and b_2 bound to the *cis*-regulatory site rC, and the remaining symbols are explained in the caption of Figure 8.15. The system of differential equations (8.8) is taken from chemical kinetics ([2], Chapter 28). Consider, for instance, the formation and decay of a protein dimer: $c + c \leftrightarrow c_2$. The forward reaction (formation) is second order, involving two monomers. Consequently, the time derivative of the dimer concentration, $\frac{d}{dt}[c_2]$, is proportional to the square of the concentration of the monomer, $[c]^2$. The reverse reaction (decay) is first order, and $\frac{d}{dt}[c_2]$ is proportional to the concentration of the dimer, $[c_2]$. Both processes together are described by the second equation in the last row of (8.8). The remaining equations can be explained similarly. The system of differential equations for the whole regulatory network of Figure 8.15 is composed of these elementary equations, with three additional but similar equations for ligand binding, ligand degradation, and heterodimerization ($a, b \leftrightarrow ab$). The resulting set of differential equations is stiff and needs to be integrated numerically with a high-order adaptable step-size method (e.g. Runge–Kutta–Fehlberg). Note that except for a, all transcription factors dimerize before they are active, that each gene has more than one rate of transcription, depending on whether promoters are bound or unbound, and that the presence of different time scales makes it representative of a real biological system and a suitable challenge for the Bayesian network inference algorithm. In contrast to [29], the system was augmented by adding 41 spurious, unconnected genes (giving a total of 50 genes), which were up- and down-regulated at random.

The first experiment followed closely the procedure in [29]. Ligand was injected for 10 minutes at a rate of 10^5 molecules/minute at time 1000 minutes. Then, 12 data points were collected over 4000 minutes in equi-distant intervals, which, as opposed to [29], also had to be discretized, as illustrated in Figure 8.16; recall from Section 8.2 that the need for this discretization is a consequence of using the function family $\mathcal{F}$ of trinomial conditional probabilities. The discretization was based on the following simple procedure: $y \to 1$ if $y - y_{min} > \frac{2(y_{max} - y_{min})}{3}$, $y \to -1$ if $y - y_{min} < \frac{y_{max} - y_{min}}{3}$, and $y \to 0$ otherwise. The learning algorithm for Bayesian networks was applied as described in the previous sections. Three different structure priors were used, with maximum fan-ins of 2, 3, and 4 edges. The resulting ROC curves are shown in the top of Figure 8.18. The areas under the ROC curves are small, and the low slope of the ROC curves at the left-hand side of the complementary specificity interval (the x-axis) implies that even the dominant true edges

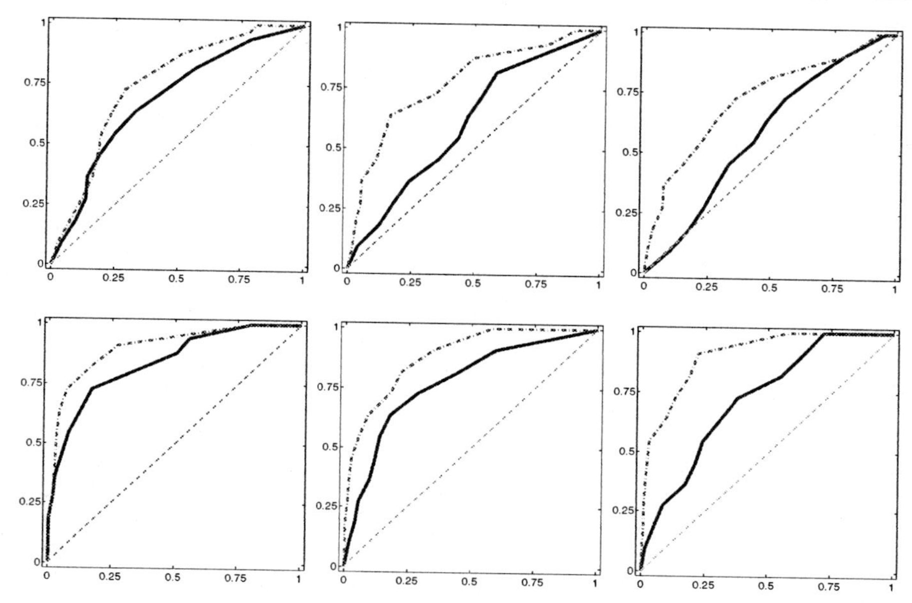

Fig. 8.18. ROC curves for the realistic simulated data, averaged over three MCMC simulations. The rows represent different sampling periods. *Top row:* Sampling over a long time interval of 4000 minutes, which mainly covers the system in equilibrium. *Bottom row:* Restricting the sampling to a short 500-minute time interval immediately after ligand injection, when the system is in a perturbed non-equilibrium state. The columns correspond to different structure priors. *Left column:* maximum fan-in = 2; *middle column:* maximum fan-in = 3; *right column:* maximum fan-in = 4. In each subfigure the sensitivity (proportion of recovered true edges) is plotted against the complementary specificity (proportion of false edges). The thin, diagonal dashed line is the expected ROC curve of a random predictor. The solid line shows the ROC curve obtained from gene expression data alone, while the dash-dotted line shows the ROC curve obtained when including sequence information. Reprinted from [17], by permission of Oxford University Press.

are obscured by a large proportion of spurious edges. This concurs with the findings of Zak et al. [29], who concluded that inferring genetic networks from gene expression data alone was impossible.

The second experiment adopted a sampling strategy different from [29]. An analysis of the mRNA abundance levels reveals regular oscillations when the system is in equilibrium. Such signals are known to have a low information content; consequently, it seems to make better sense to focus on the time immediately after external perturbation, when the system is in disequilibrium. The sampler therefore collected 12 data points over a shorter interval of only 500 minutes immediately after ligand injection, between times 1100 and 1600 minutes. The resulting ROC curves are shown in the bottom of Figure 8.18. The areas under the ROC curves have significantly increased, and the larger slope of the curves in the low-sensitivity range implies that the dominant true edges are obscured by far fewer spurious edges.

Recall that in order to obtain a network from the posterior probability on edges, $P(e_{ik}|\mathcal{D})$, we have to choose a threshold ρ and discard all edges with $P(e_{ik}|\mathcal{D}) < \rho$. Figure 8.17, right, shows, for the most restrictive prior (maximum fan-in = 2), the resulting sub-network of non-spurious genes. The threshold ρ was chosen so as to obtain the same number of edges (namely 11) between non-spurious nodes as in the true network. Four true edges, shown as thick arrows, have been recovered (which was consistent in all three MCMC simulations). The probability of finding at least this number of true edges by chance is given by $p = \sum_{k=4}^{11} \binom{11}{k} \left(\frac{11}{50^2}\right)^k \left(\frac{50^2-11}{50^2}\right)^{(11-k)} \approx 10^{-7}$, which indicates that the inference procedure has captured real structure in the data. However, this structure is only *local* in nature. The *global* network inferred in this way, shown in Figure 8.17, right, shows little resemblance with the true network, depicted in Figure 8.17, left. The ROC curves of Figure 8.18 reveal that the complete set of true edges can only be recovered at a false positive rate of about 75%. Consequently, it is only the most salient local gene interactions that can be inferred from the mRNA abundance data, and the price for this in terms of false positive edges can be obtained from the ROC curves of Figure 8.18. While this number, in absolute terms, is still so large that an experimental verification is indispensable, Figure 8.18 also suggests that the search for new genetic interactions preceded and supported by a Bayesian network analysis is significantly more effective than a search from *tabula rasa*. The amount of improvement can, again, be quantified from the ROC curves. Also, note that the most restrictive prior (maximum fan-in = 2) gave consistently the best results, which is in agreement with the true network structure (Figure 8.17, left). This underlines the obvious fact that, for small data sets, the inclusion of available prior knowledge improves the performance of the inference scheme, and the amount of improvement is quantifiable from the ROC curves.

Given that mRNA abundance levels only convey partial information about a biological regulatory network, it is natural to combine microarray data with genomic and proteomic data. On the genomic side, the identification of certain regulatory sequence elements in the upstream region of a gene [28] can be exploited to predict which transcription factors are most likely to bind to a given promoter, and this sequence-based estimation can be further assisted experimentally with localization assays [24]. When location data or known binding motifs in the sequence indicate that a transcription factor, say a, binds to the promoter of another gene, say rB, the respective edge, $A \to B$ in this case, should be enforced. A straightforward way to incorporate this additional information in the induction was proposed by Hartemink et al. [13]: when genomic location data indicate that particular edges corresponding to transcription factor binding reactions should be present, the model prior is modified such that network structures lacking these suggested edges have probability zero. However, location data are usually noisy, and this intrinsic uncertainty is not allowed for by such rigid constraints. An approach that is more involved was proposed by Segal et al. [25], who modelled both the outcome of localization experiments as well as the occurrence of certain binding motifs in the promoter region probabilistically. The method applied in [17] is pitched between these two extremes. It modifies the model prior in a way similar to [13], but allows for uncertainty in sequence motif identification and location data. Let $y \rightarrow rX$ denote the event that transcription factor y binds to the promoter r upstream of gene X, and let $B[y]$ represent the set of indicated binding regions for y. Then

$$\frac{P(y \rightarrow rX | r \in B[y])}{P(y \rightarrow rX | r \notin B[y])} = \phi \tag{8.9}$$

for some value $\phi > 1$. In words: Equation (8.9) expresses the fact that on identifying a binding region for transcription factor y in the promoter of gene X, this transcription factor is ϕ times as likely to bind to X than in the absence of such an indication. The value of ϕ can be related to the p-value of location data [24] and/or the pattern score for binding motifs [28]. To quantify the amount of improvement in the induction that can be achieved by combining expression and location data, the previous simulations were repeated for a value of $\phi = 2$ under the assumption that complete location data indicating all regulatory sequence elements are available. The resulting ROC curves are shown as dash-dotted lines in Figure 8.18, which, as expected, give a consistent improvement on the earlier results obtained from gene expression data alone. Equation (8.9) is certainly over-simplified. However, the analysis described here and the comparison of the respective ROC curves allows us to give a rough quantitative estimation of the amount of improvement achievable by merging microarray with sequence and location data.

For a comparison of the simulation results reported here with the related simulation studies in [26] and [29], see the discussion in the final section of [17].

8.10 Discussion

The simulation studies described in the previous two sections suggest that in agreement with Section 8.3, local structures of genetic networks can, to a certain extent, be recovered. The results depend on the prior used in the Bayesian inference scheme, with a smaller mismatch between reality and prior assumptions obviously leading to better predictions. The amount of this improvement can be quantified from the ROC curves. The results also depend on the sampling scheme. Interestingly, collecting data of the perturbed system in disequilibrium following ligand injection gives better results than when the system is in equilibrium. This finding may suggest that gene expression measurements should, at best, be taken during the relaxation of a biological system after external intervention.

Note, however, that the *global* network inferred from the data is meaningless. This shortcoming, illustrated in Figure 8.17, is a direct consequence of the fact that for sparse data $\mathcal{D}$, the posterior distribution of network structures, $P(\mathcal{M}|\mathcal{D})$, is diffuse. Consequently, as discussed earlier in Section 8.3, it is essential to sample networks from $P(\mathcal{M}|\mathcal{D})$, rather than search for a single high-scoring network. From such a sample of structures we can identify edges with high posterior probability and use them to identify local features and subnetworks with high posterior support. However, a high posterior probability in itself is no guarantee that the respective edge represents a true genetic interaction, partly as a consequence of the fact that the number of spurious interactions, increasing with the square of the number of nodes, substantially outweighs the number of true interactions. Consequently, detected true features of a genetic network are inevitably obscured by a considerable amount of spurious ones. This should be taken as a cautionary note for those trying to back up detected interactions with circumstantial evidence from the biological literature. In practical applications, one has to find a compromise between the number of true edges one wants to detect, and the price in terms of spurious edges one is prepared to pay. The ROC curves shown in the present work do not offer a universal law from which a practical decision support system for the biologist could easily be derived. They do, however, demonstrate empirically how the sensitivity–specificity score ratios vary with the training set size, the degree of inadequacy of prior assumptions, the experimental sampling strategy, and the inclusion of further, sequence-based information.

As a final remark, note that gene expression data do not contain information on post-transcriptional and post-translational processes. It would therefore be more appropriate to allow for incomplete observations by including hidden nodes in the Bayesian network architecture. Ong et al. [22] described a dynamic Bayesian network with hidden nodes, where the subnetworks pertaining to the hidden nodes incorporated substantial prior knowledge about operons. In general, we would like to *learn* such network structures from (incomplete) data. The practical complication of this approach is that (8.2) has no longer a closed-form solution. In principle we could sample from the joint distribution of model structures *and* their associated parameters with trans-dimensional reversible jump MCMC [11], as discussed in Section 2.3.7, but convergence and mixing of the Markov chain may become prohibitively slow. The next chapter discusses a linear state-space approach (Kalman smoother) to model the influence of unobserved regulators on gene expression levels. While the inherent linearity constraint excludes the modelling of nonlinear gene interactions, like those in Figure 8.4, it allows a part of the inference procedure to be solved analytically – equivalent to the analytic solution of (8.2) – and this renders the overall inference scheme practically viable.

Acknowledgments

The work on this chapter was supported by the Scottish Executive Environmental and Rural Affairs Department (SEERAD). I would like to thank Jill Sales, Marco Grzegorczyk, Florian Markowetz, Lynn Broadfoot, and Philip Smith for their critical feedback on and proofreading of a draft version of this chapter.

References

[1] S. F. Altschul, W. Gish, W. Miller, E. W. Myers, and D. J. Lipman. Basic local alignment search tool. *Journal of Molecular Biology*, 215:403–410, 1990.

[2] P. W. Atkins. *Physical Chemistry*. Oxford University Press, Oxford, 3rd edition, 1986.

[3] N. Barkai and S. Leibler. Circadian clocks limited by noise. *Nature*, 403:267–268, 2000.

[4] T. Chen, H. L. He, and G. M. Church. Modeling gene expression with differential equations. *Pacific Symposium on Biocomputing*, 4:29–40, 1999.

[5] H. De Jong. Modeling and simulation of genetic regulatory systems: A literature review. *Journal of Computational Biology*, 9(1):67–103, 2002.

[6] P. D'haeseleer, S. Liang, and R. Somogyi. Genetic network inference: from co-expression clustering to reverse engineering. *Bioinformatics*, 16(8):707–726, 2000.

[7] M. B. Eisen, P. T. Spellman, P. O. Brown, and D. Botstein. Cluster analysis and display of genome-wide expression patterns. *Proceedings of the National Academy of Sciences of the United States of America*, 95:14863–14868, 1998.

[8] N. Friedman, M. Linial, I. Nachman, and D. Pe'er. Using Bayesian networks to analyze expression data. *Journal of Computational Biology*, 7:601–620, 2000.

[9] N. Friedman, K. Murphy, and S. Russell. Learning the structure of dynamic probabilistic networks. In G. F. Cooper and S. Moral, editors, *Proceedings of the Fourteenth Conference on Uncertainty in Artificial Intelligence (UAI)*, pages 139–147, San Francisco, CA, 1998. Morgan Kaufmann Publishers.

[10] T. S. Gardner, C. R. Cantor, and J. J. Collins. Construction of a genetic toggle switch in *Escherichia coli*. *Nature*, 403:339–342, 2000.

[11] P. Green. Reversible jump Markov chain Monte Carlo computation and Bayesian model determination. *Biometrika*, 82:711–732, 1995.

[12] A. J. Hartemink, D. K. Gifford, T. S. Jaakkola, and R. A. Young. Using graphical models and genomic expression data to statistically validate models of genetic regulatory networks. *Pacific Symposium on Biocomputing*, 6:422–433, 2001.

[13] A. J. Hartemink, D. K. Gifford, T. S. Jaakkola, and R. A. Young. Combining location and expression data for principled discovery of genetic network models. *Pacific Symposium on Biocomputing*, 7:437–449, 2002.

[14] D. Heckerman. A tutorial on learning with Bayesian networks. In M. I. Jordan, editor, *Learning in Graphical Models*, Adaptive Computation and Machine Learning, pages 301–354, Cambridge, MA, 1999. MIT Press.

[15] J. Hertz, A. Krogh, and R. G. Palmer. *Introduction to the Theory of Neural Computation.* Addison Wesley, Redwood City, CA, 1991.

[16] D. Husmeier. Reverse engineering of genetic networks with Bayesian networks. *Biochemical Society Transactions*, 31(6):1516–1518, 2003.

[17] D. Husmeier. Sensitivity and specificity of inferring genetic regulatory interactions from microarray experiments with dynamic Bayesian networks. *Bioinformatics*, 19:2271–2282, 2003.

[18] S. A. Kauffman. Metabolic stability and epigenesis in randomly connected nets. *Journal of Theoretical Biology*, 22:437–467, 1969.

[19] S. A. Kauffman. *The Origins of Order, Self-Organization and Selection in Evolution.* Oxford University Press, 1993.

[20] P. J. Krause. Learning probabilistic networks. *Knowledge Engineering Review*, 13:321–351, 1998.

[21] K. P. Murphy and S. Milan. Modelling gene expression data using dynamic Bayesian networks. Technical report, MIT Artificial Intelligence Laboratory, 1999. http://www.ai.mit.edu/~murphyk/Papers/ismb99.ps.gz.

[22] I. Ong, J. Glasner, and D. Page. Modelling regulatory pathways in *E. coli* from time series expression profiles. *Bioinformatics*, 18(Suppl.1):S241–S248, 2002.

[23] D. Pe'er, A. Regev, G. Elidan, and N. Friedman. Inferring subnetworks from perturbed expression profiles. *Bioinformatics*, 17:S215–S224, 2001.

[24] B. Ren, F. Robert, J. J. Wyrick, O. Aparicio, E. G. Jennings, I. Simon, J. Zeitlinger, J. Schreiber, N. Hannett, E. Kanin, T. L. Volkert, C. J. Wilson, S. P. Bell, and R. A. Young. Genome-wide location and function of DNA binding proteins. *Science*, 290:2306–2309, 2000.

[25] E. Segal, Y. Barash, I. Simon, N. Friedman, and D. Koller. From promoter sequence to expression: a probabilistic framework. *Research in Computational Molecular Biology (RECOMB)*, 6:263–272, 2002.

[26] V. A. Smith, E. D. Jarvis, and A. J. Hartemink. Evaluating functional network inference using simulations of complex biological systems. *Bioinformatics*, 18:S216–S224, 2002. (ISMB02 special issue).

[27] P. Spellman, G. Sherlock, M. Zhang, V. Iyer, K. Anders, M. Eisen, P. Brown, D. Botstein, and B. Futcher. Comprehensive identification of cell cycle-regulated genes of the yeast *Saccharomyces cerevisiae* by microarray hybridization. *Molecular Biology of the Cell*, 9:3273–3297, 1998.

[28] J. Vilo, A. Brazma, I. Jonassen, A. Robinson, and E. Ukkonen. Mining for putative regulatory elements in the yeast genome using gene expression data. In P. E. Bourne, M. Gribskov, R. B. Altman, N. Jensen,

D. Hope, T. Lengauer, J. C. Mitchell, E. Scheeff, C. Smith, S. Strande, and H. Weissig, editors, *Proceedings of the Eighth International Conference on Intelligent Systems for Molecular Biology (ISMB)*, pages 384–394. AAAI, 2000.

[29] D. E. Zak, F. J. Doyle, G. E. Gonye, and J. S. Schwaber. Simulation studies for the identification of genetic networks from cDNA array and regulatory activity data. *Proceedings of the Second International Conference on Systems Biology*, pages 231–238, 2001.

[30] D. E. Zak, F. J. Doyle, and J. S. Schwaber. Local identifiability: when can genetic networks be identified from microarray data? *Proceedings of the Third International Conference on Systems Biology*, pages 236–237, 2002.

9

Modeling Genetic Regulatory Networks using Gene Expression Profiling and State-Space Models

Claudia Rangel[1], John Angus[1], Zoubin Ghahramani[2], and David L. Wild[3]

[1] Claremont Graduate University, 121 E. Tenth St., Claremont, CA 91711, USA
claudia.rangel@cgu.edu john.angus@cgu.edu
[2] Gatsby Computational Neuroscience Unit, University College London, UK
zoubin@gatsby.ucl.ac.uk
[3] Keck Graduate Institute, 535 Watson Drive, Claremont CA 91711, USA
david_wild@kgi.edu

Summary. We describe a Bayesian network approach to infer genetic regulatory interactions from microarray gene expression data. This problem was introduced in Chapter 7 and an alternative Bayesian network approach was presented in Chapter 8. Our approach is based on a linear dynamical system, which renders the inference problem tractable: the E-step of the EM algorithm draws on the well-established Kalman smoothing algorithm. While the intrinsic linearity constraint makes our approach less suitable for modeling non-linear genetic interactions than the approach of Chapter 8, it has two important advantages over the method of Chapter 8. First, our approach works with continuous expression levels, which avoids the information loss inherent in a discretization of these signals. Second, we include hidden states to allow for the effects that cannot be measured in a microarray experiment, for example: the effects of genes that have not been included on the microarray, levels of regulatory proteins, and the effects of mRNA and protein degradation.

9.1 Introduction

The application of high-density DNA microarray technology to gene transcription analyses, introduced in Chapter 7, has been responsible for a real paradigm shift in biology. The majority of research groups now have the ability to measure the expression of a significant proportion of an organism's genome in a single experiment, resulting in an unprecedented volume of data being made available to the scientific community. This has in turn stimulated the development of algorithms to classify and describe the complexity of the transcriptional response of a biological system, but efforts towards developing the analytical tools necessary to exploit this information for revealing interactions between the components of a cellular system are still in their early stages.

The availability of such tools would allow a large-scale systematic approach to pathway reconstruction in organisms of clinical and pharmaceutical relevance (i.e. mouse and human). With present technologies, such an approach is possible only in relatively simple model systems where genome coverage genetic screenings are accessible (i.e. *D. melanogaster*, *C. elegans*). In more complex organisms reconstructing pathways is often a demanding exercise that can involve a large research group for a considerable period of time. The popular use of clustering techniques, reviewed in [9], whilst allowing qualitative inferences about the co-regulation of certain genes to be made, do not provide models of the underlying transcriptional networks which lend themselves to statistical hypothesis testing.

Many of the tools which have been applied in an exploratory way to the problem of reverse engineering genetic regulatory networks from gene expression data have been reviewed in [30] and [27]. These include Boolean networks [1, 15, 26], time-lagged cross-correlation functions [3], differential equation models [14] and linear and non-linear autoregression models [8, 28, 7, 29]. Although these techniques have produced models which appear biologically plausible, based on circumstantial evidence from the biological literature, many have been derived from public domain data with insufficient replication given that these papers attempt to reconstruct the interactions of large numbers (sometimes thousands) of genes from small data sets, with the consequent likelihood of model overfitting. Smith *et al.* [24], Yeung *et al.* [31] and Zak *et al.* [33] have attempted to evaluate reverse engineering techniques by the use of simulated data from *in silico* networks. Zak *et al.* considered linear, log-linear and non-linear (squashing function) regressive models and concluded that these methods were unable to identify the generating network from simulated gene expression data alone, and constituted little more than curve fitting.

Murphy and Mian [18] have shown that many of these published models can be considered special cases of a general class of graphical models known as Dynamic Bayesian Networks (DBNs), discussed in Section 8.6. Bayesian networks, introduced in Chapter 2, have a number of features which make them attractive candidates for modeling gene expression data, such as their ability to handle noisy or missing data, to handle hidden variables such as protein levels which may have an effect on mRNA expression levels, to describe locally interacting processes and the possibility of making causal inferences from the derived models. The application of Bayesian networks to microarray data analysis was first explored experimentally in the pioneering work of Friedman *et al.* [10], who described a technique known as the *sparse candidate algorithm* for learning the network structure directly from fully-observed data; see Section 8.3 for further details. Friedman *et al.* applied this method to the gene expression time series data of Spellman *et al.* [25], as discussed in Section 8.4, and produced networks which again appeared biologically plausible. This work has, nonetheless, some limitations. The time series measurements were considered to be independent and identically distributed (iid), which is clearly not the case (the authors acknowledge this and introduce a root variable to model dependency of expression level on the cell cycle phase). Gene expression measurements were also discretized into a multinomial distribution, with consequent loss of information. However, in an attempt to robustly evaluate the model networks derived, Friedman *et al.* proposed the use of a bootstrapping procedure, based on identifying which model structures where repeatedly inferred with a high probability from repeated random resamplings of the data. Recently, a number of other authors have described Bayesian network models of gene expression data. Although microarray technologies have made it possible to measure time series of the expression level of many genes simultaneously, we cannot hope to measure all possible factors contributing to genetic regulatory interactions, and the ability of Bayesian networks to handle such hidden variables would appear to be one of their main advantages as a modeling tool. However, most published work to date has only considered either static Bayesian networks with fully observed data [20] or static Bayesian networks which model discretized data but incorporate hidden variables [6, 32]. Following Friedman *et al.*, Ong *et al.* [19] have described a dynamic Bayesian network model for *E. coli* which explicitly includes operons as hidden variables, but again uses discretized gene expression measurements. There would, therefore, appear to be a need for a dynamic modeling approach which can both accommodate gene expression measurements as continuous, rather than discrete, variables and which can model unknown factors as hidden variables.

We have applied linear dynamical systems modeling to reverse engineer transcriptional networks from expression profiling data [21, 22]. In order to test the validity of our approach we have applied it both to synthetic (*in silico*) data and real experimental data obtained from a well-established model of T-cell activation in which we have monitored a set of relevant genes across a time series [21, 22]. Linear-Gaussian state-space models (SSM), also known as linear dynamical systems [23] or Kalman filter models [5, 17], are a subclass of dynamic Bayesian networks used for modeling time series data and have been used extensively in many areas of control and signal processing. SSM models have a number of features which make them attractive for modeling gene expression time series data. They assume the existence of a hidden state variable, from which we can make noisy continuous measurements, which evolves with Markovian dynamics. In our application, the noisy measurements are the observed gene expression levels at each time point, and we assume that the hidden variables are modeling effects which cannot be measured in a gene expression profiling experiment, for example: the effects of genes which have not been included on the microarray, levels of regulatory proteins, the effects of mRNA and protein degradation, etc. Our SSM models have produced testable hypotheses, which have the potential for rapid experimental validation.

9.2 State-Space Models (Linear Dynamical Systems)

In linear state-space models, a sequence of $p-$dimensional observation vectors $\{\mathbf{y}_1, ..., \mathbf{y}_T\}$, is modeled by assuming that at each time step $\mathbf{y}_t$ was generated from a $K-$dimensional hidden state variable $\mathbf{x}_t$, and that the sequence $\{\mathbf{x}_t\}$ defines a first-order Markov process. The most basic linear state space model can be described by the following two equations:

$$\mathbf{x}_{t+1} = \mathbf{A}\mathbf{x}_t + \mathbf{w}_t \tag{9.1}$$

$$\mathbf{y}_t = \mathbf{C}\mathbf{x}_t + \mathbf{v}_t \tag{9.2}$$

where $\mathbf{A}$ is the state dynamics matrix, $\mathbf{C}$ is the state to observation matrix and $\{\mathbf{w}_t\}$ and $\{\mathbf{v}_t\}$ are uncorrelated Gaussian white noise sequences, with covariance matrices $\mathbf{Q}$ and $\mathbf{R}$, respectively.

9.2.1 State-Space Model with Inputs

Often, the observations can be divided into a set of input (or exogenous) variables and a set of output (or response) variables. Allowing inputs to both the state and observation equation, the equations describing the linear state space model then become:

$$\mathbf{x}_{t+1} = \mathbf{A}\mathbf{x}_t + \mathbf{B}\mathbf{h}_t + \mathbf{w}_t \tag{9.3}$$

$$\mathbf{y}_t = \mathbf{C}\mathbf{x}_t + \mathbf{D}\mathbf{u}_t + \mathbf{v}_t \tag{9.4}$$

where $\mathbf{h}_t, \mathbf{u}_t$ are the inputs to the state and observation vectors, $\mathbf{A}$ is the state dynamics matrix, $\mathbf{B}$ is the input to state matrix, $\mathbf{C}$ is the state to observation matrix, and $\mathbf{D}$ is the input to observation matrix. A Bayesian network representation of this model is shown in Figure 9.1.

The state and observation noise sequences, $\{\mathbf{w}_t\}$ and $\{\mathbf{v}_t\}$ respectively, are generally taken to be white noise sequences, with $\{\mathbf{w}_t\}$ and $\{\mathbf{v}_t\}$ orthogonal to one another. Here, we make the additional assumption that these noise sequences are Gaussian distributed, and independent of the initial values of $\mathbf{x}$ and $\mathbf{y}$. Note that noise vectors may also be considered hidden variables. The conditional distributions of the states and the observables are given by:

$$P(\mathbf{x}_{t+1}|\mathbf{x}_t, \mathbf{h}_t) \sim N(\mathbf{A}\mathbf{x}_t + \mathbf{B}\mathbf{h}_t, \mathbf{Q}),\ P(\mathbf{y}_t|\mathbf{x}_t, \mathbf{u}_t) \sim N(\mathbf{C}\mathbf{x}_t + \mathbf{D}\mathbf{u}_t, \mathbf{R})$$

where $\mathbf{Q}$ and $\mathbf{R}$ are the state and observation noise covariances respectively, both assumed to be non-singular, and the notation $N(\mathbf{m}, \mathbf{S})$ signifies a multivariate normal distribution with mean $\mathbf{m}$ and covariance matrix $\mathbf{S}$. Hence we have that

$$P(\mathbf{y}_t|\mathbf{x}_t, \mathbf{u}_t) = \frac{\exp\{-\frac{1}{2}(\mathbf{y}_t - \mathbf{C}\mathbf{x}_t - \mathbf{D}\mathbf{u}_t)^{\dagger}\mathbf{R}^{-1}(\mathbf{y}_t - \mathbf{C}\mathbf{x}_t - \mathbf{D}\mathbf{u}_t)\}}{(2\pi)^{p/2}|\mathbf{R}|^{1/2}} \tag{9.5}$$

where the superscript $\dagger$ denotes matrix transposition, and

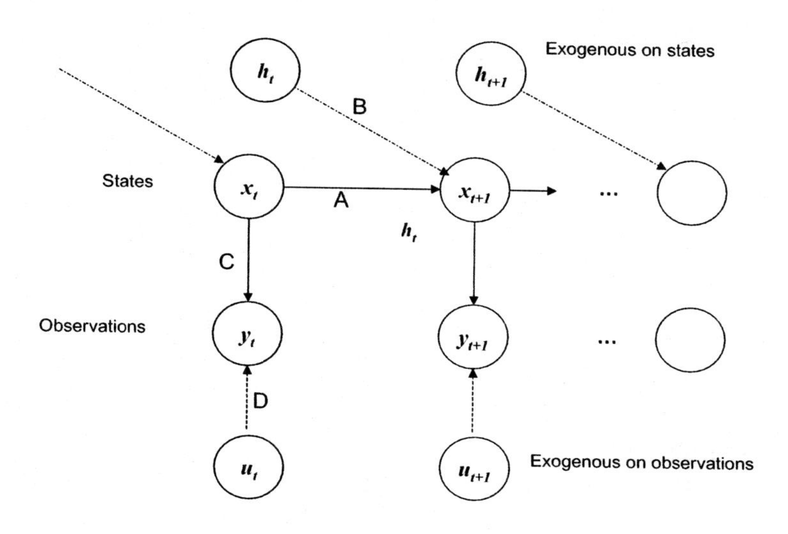

Fig. 9.1. SSM model with inputs.

$$P(\mathbf{x}_{t+1}|\mathbf{x}_t, \mathbf{h}_t) = \frac{\exp\{-\frac{1}{2}(\mathbf{x}_{t+1} - \mathbf{A}\mathbf{x}_t - \mathbf{B}\mathbf{h}_t)^\dagger \mathbf{Q}^{-1}(\mathbf{x}_{t+1} - \mathbf{A}\mathbf{x}_t - \mathbf{B}\mathbf{h}_t)\}}{(2\pi)^{K/2}|\mathbf{Q}|^{1/2}} \tag{9.6}$$

Applying the factorization rule for Bayesian networks (2.1) to the graph of Figure 9.1 gives:

$$P(\{\mathbf{x}_t\}, \{\mathbf{y}_t\}|\{\mathbf{h}_t\}, \{\mathbf{u}_t\}) = P(\mathbf{x}_1) \prod_{t=1}^{T-1} P(\mathbf{x}_{t+1}|\mathbf{x}_t, \mathbf{h}_t) \prod_{t=1}^{T} P(\mathbf{y}_t|\mathbf{x}_t, \mathbf{u}_t) \tag{9.7}$$

Note the similarity of this equation with the corresponding expansion (2.51) for hidden Markov models (HMMs), discussed in Section 2.3.4 and depicted in Figure 2.27. The main difference between HMMs and SSMs is that the hidden states of the former – $\{S_t\}$ in (2.51) – are discrete, whereas the hidden states of the latter – $\{\mathbf{x}_t\}$ in (9.7) – are continuous. We will henceforth simplify the notation by dropping the exogenous input variables $\mathbf{h}_t$ and $\mathbf{u}_t$ from the conditional distributions; it should be understood that these are always given and therefore all distributions over $\mathbf{x}_t$ and $\mathbf{y}_t$ are conditioned on them.

The unknown parameters $\boldsymbol{\theta}$ of the SSM model may be learned from the training data in a maximum likelihood sense by applying the Expectation-Maximization (EM) algorithm, introduced in Section 2.3.3. All we have to do is adapt equations (2.48) and (2.49), which were defined for *discrete* hidden states, to *continuous* hidden states:[4]

$$F(\boldsymbol{\theta}) = \int Q(\mathcal{S}) \log \frac{P(\mathcal{D}, \mathcal{S}|\boldsymbol{\theta})}{Q(\mathcal{S})} d\mathcal{S} \tag{9.8}$$

$$KL[Q, P] = \int Q(\mathcal{S}) \log \frac{Q(\mathcal{S})}{P(\mathcal{S}|\mathcal{D}, \boldsymbol{\theta})} d\mathcal{S} \tag{9.9}$$

where $\mathcal{D} = \{\mathbf{y}_t\}$ are the observations, $\mathcal{S} = \{\mathbf{x}_t\}$ are the hidden states, and $Q(\mathcal{S})$ is an arbitrary distribution on the hidden states. We can now decompose the log-likelihood $L(\boldsymbol{\theta}) = \log P(\mathcal{D}|\boldsymbol{\theta})$ according to (2.50):

$$L(\boldsymbol{\theta}) = F(\boldsymbol{\theta}) + KL[Q, P] \tag{9.10}$$

9.2.2 EM Applied to SSM with Inputs

E-step:

The maximization in the EM algorithm depends on expectations of the log complete likelihood $\log P(\mathcal{D}, \mathcal{S}|\boldsymbol{\theta}) = \log P(\{\mathbf{x}_t\}, \{\mathbf{y}_t\}|\boldsymbol{\theta})$, by (9.8). From (9.5)–(9.7), and assuming $P(\mathbf{x}_1)$ is $N(\boldsymbol{\mu}_1, \mathbf{Q}_1)$, this is given by (modulo a factor of -2)

$$\begin{aligned} &-2 \log P(\{\mathbf{x}_t\}, \{\mathbf{y}_t\}|\boldsymbol{\theta}) = \\ &\sum_{t=1}^{T-1} (\mathbf{x}_{t+1} - \mathbf{A}\mathbf{x}_t - \mathbf{B}\mathbf{h}_t)^\dagger \mathbf{Q}^{-1} (\mathbf{x}_{t+1} - \mathbf{A}\mathbf{x}_t - \mathbf{B}\mathbf{h}_t) \\ &+ \sum_{t=1}^{T} (\mathbf{y}_t - \mathbf{C}\mathbf{x}_t - \mathbf{D}\mathbf{u}_t)^\dagger \mathbf{R}^{-1} (\mathbf{y}_t - \mathbf{C}\mathbf{x}_t - \mathbf{D}\mathbf{u}_t) \\ &+ (\mathbf{x}_1 - \boldsymbol{\mu}_1)^\dagger \mathbf{Q}_1^{-1} (\mathbf{x}_1 - \boldsymbol{\mu}_1) + (T-1) \log |\mathbf{Q}| \\ &+ T \log |\mathbf{R}| + T(p+K) \log(2\pi) + \log |\mathbf{Q}_1| \end{aligned} \tag{9.11}$$

Using the identity $\mathbf{v}^\dagger \boldsymbol{\Sigma} \mathbf{v} = \operatorname{tr}(\boldsymbol{\Sigma} \mathbf{v} \mathbf{v}^\dagger)$ and expanding the quadratic terms above, we see that taking the necessary conditional expectation of (9.11) in the E-step requires computation (for the current values of the parameters) of all terms of the form

$$\hat{\mathbf{x}_t} = \mathcal{E}\left[\mathbf{x}_t | \mathbf{y}_1, \mathbf{y}_2, ..., \mathbf{y}_T\right] \tag{9.12}$$

$$\mathbf{U}_t = \mathcal{E}\left[\mathbf{x}_t \mathbf{x}_t^\dagger | \mathbf{y}_1, \mathbf{y}_2, ..., \mathbf{y}_T\right] \tag{9.13}$$

$$\mathbf{U}_{t+1,t} = \mathcal{E}\left[\mathbf{x}_t \mathbf{x}_{t+1}^\dagger | \mathbf{y}_1, \mathbf{y}_2, ..., \mathbf{y}_T\right] \tag{9.14}$$

These terms can be computed from the Kalman filter and smoother algorithm, which will be discussed below.

[4] Note that in (2.48) and (2.49), $\mathbf{q}$ is used instead of $\boldsymbol{\theta}$.

M-step:

Here, we solve for the parameters $\boldsymbol{\theta} = \{\mathbf{A}, \mathbf{B}, \mathbf{C}, \mathbf{D}, \mathbf{Q}, \mathbf{R}, \mathbf{Q}_1, \boldsymbol{\mu}_1\}$ that maximize the conditional expectation from the E-step, which is equivalent to maximizing F in (9.8):

$$\text{M step}: \quad \boldsymbol{\theta}_{k+1} \leftarrow \arg_{\boldsymbol{\theta}} \max \int P(\mathcal{S}|\mathcal{D}, \boldsymbol{\theta}_k) \log P(\mathcal{S}, \mathcal{D}|\boldsymbol{\theta}) d\mathcal{S} \tag{9.15}$$

where $\mathcal{D} = \{\mathbf{y}_t\}$, and $\mathcal{S} = \{\mathbf{x}_t\}$. Recall from Section 2.3.3 that since F is equal to the log likelihood at the beginning of each M-step, as seen from (9.10), and since the E-step does not change $\boldsymbol{\theta}$, we are guaranteed not to decrease the likelihood after each combined EM-step.

It is clear from (9.11) and (9.15) that the M-step is accomplished by taking the partial derivative of the expected log likelihood with respect to each parameter, setting it to zero, and solving. That is, the parameters from the M-step are found by minimizing the conditional expectation of (9.11), utilizing (9.12)–(9.14). It turns out to be admissible for this problem to find partial derivatives of (9.11) first, set them to 0, and then take the conditional expectation of the resulting equations before solving for the parameter estimates. For instance, if we want to solve for the matrix $\mathbf{C}$ in the M-step, we set the partial derivative of (9.11) equal to zero and solve. Since only the third term in (9.11) depends on $\mathbf{C}$, we only need to compute:

$$\begin{aligned} &\frac{\partial\left[-2\log P(\{\mathbf{x}_t\}, \{\mathbf{y}_t\})\right]}{\partial \mathbf{C}} \\ &= \frac{\partial\left[\sum_{t=1}^{T}(\mathbf{y}_t - \mathbf{C}\mathbf{x}_t - \mathbf{D}\mathbf{u}_t)^{\dagger}\mathbf{R}^{-1}(\mathbf{y}_t - \mathbf{C}\mathbf{x}_t - \mathbf{D}\mathbf{u}_t)\right]}{\partial \mathbf{C}} = 0 \\ &\Longrightarrow \sum_{t=1}^{T} \mathbf{y}_t\mathbf{x}_t^{\dagger} - \mathbf{C}\sum_{t=1}^{T} \mathbf{x}_t\mathbf{x}_t^{\dagger} - \mathbf{D}\sum_{t=1}^{T} \mathbf{u}_t\mathbf{x}_t^{\dagger} = 0 \end{aligned} \tag{9.16}$$

Taking conditional expectations of the terms involving the hidden states, and using the notation (9.12)–(9.14), and then solving for $\mathbf{C}$, the M-step equation for $\mathbf{C}$ becomes:

$$\mathbf{C} = \left(\sum_{t=1}^{T} \mathbf{y}_t\hat{\mathbf{x}}_t^{\dagger} - \mathbf{D}\sum_{t=1}^{T} \mathbf{u}_t\hat{\mathbf{x}}_t^{\dagger}\right)\left(\sum_{t=1}^{T} \mathbf{U}_t\right)^{-1} \tag{9.17}$$

Repeating this recipe for $\mathbf{D}$ yields another equation, and these two equations can be solved simultaneously for $\mathbf{C}$ and $\mathbf{D}$ in closed form. Similarly, these same procedures lead to the computations for the other parameters needed to complete the M-step.

9.2.3 Kalman Smoothing

The Kalman smoother solves the problem of estimating the expectation values (9.12)–(9.14) for a linear-Gaussian state-space model. It consists of two parts:

a forward recursion which uses the observations from $\mathbf{y}_1$ to $\mathbf{y}_t$, known as the Kalman filter, and a backward recursion which uses the observations from $\mathbf{y}_T$ to $\mathbf{y}_{t+1}$. The forward and backward recursions together are also known as the Rauch–Tung–Streibel (RTS) smoother. Treatments of Kalman filtering and smoothing can be found in [5, 17].

To describe the filter-smoother recursions, it is useful to define the quantities $\mathbf{x}_t^r$ and $\mathbf{V}_t^r$, the conditional expectation of the state vector and its error covariance matrix, respectively, given observations $\{\mathbf{y}_1, ..., \mathbf{y}_r\}$:

$$\mathbf{x}_t^r = \mathcal{E}[\mathbf{x}_t|\mathbf{y}_1, \ldots, \mathbf{y}_r] \tag{9.18}$$
$$\mathbf{V}_t^r = \mathrm{Var}[\mathbf{x}_t|\mathbf{y}_1, \ldots, \mathbf{y}_r] \tag{9.19}$$

The Kalman filter consists of the following forward recursions:

$$\mathbf{x}_{t+1}^t = \mathbf{A}\mathbf{x}_t^t + \mathbf{B}\mathbf{h}_t \tag{9.20}$$
$$\mathbf{V}_{t+1}^t = \mathbf{A}\mathbf{V}_t^t\mathbf{A}^\dagger + \mathbf{Q} \tag{9.21}$$
$$\mathbf{K}_t = \mathbf{V}_t^{t-1}\mathbf{C}^\dagger(\mathbf{C}\mathbf{V}_t^{t-1}\mathbf{C}^\dagger + \mathbf{R})^{-1} \tag{9.22}$$
$$\mathbf{x}_t^t = \mathbf{x}_t^{t-1} + \mathbf{K}_t(\mathbf{y}_t - \mathbf{C}\mathbf{x}_t^{t-1} - \mathbf{D}\mathbf{u}_t) \tag{9.23}$$
$$\mathbf{V}_t^t = (\mathbf{I} - \mathbf{K}_t\mathbf{C})\mathbf{V}_t^{t-1} \tag{9.24}$$

where $\mathbf{x}_1^0 = \boldsymbol{\mu}_1$ and $\mathbf{V}_1^0 = \mathbf{Q}_1$ are the prior mean and covariance of the state, which are model parameters. Equations (9.20) and (9.21) describe the forward propagation of the state mean and variance before having accounted for the observation at time $t+1$. The mean evolves according to the known dynamics $\mathbf{A}$ which also affects the variance. In addition the variance also increases by $\mathbf{Q}$, the state noise covariance matrix. The observation $\mathbf{y}_t$ has the effect of shifting the mean by an amount proportional to the prediction error $\mathbf{y}_t - \mathbf{C}\mathbf{x}_t^{t-1} - \mathbf{D}\mathbf{u}_t$, where the proportionality term $\mathbf{K}_t$ is known as the Kalman gain matrix. Observing $\mathbf{y}_t$ also has the effect of reducing the variance of the state estimator.

At the end of the forward recursions we have the values for $\mathbf{x}_T^T$ and $\mathbf{V}_T^T$. We now need to proceed backwards and evaluate the influence of future observations on our estimate of states in the past:

$$\mathbf{K}_{t-1} = \mathbf{V}_{t-1}^{t-1}\mathbf{A}(\mathbf{V}_t^{t-1})^{-1} \tag{9.25}$$
$$\mathbf{x}_{t-1}^T = \mathbf{x}_{t-1}^{t-1} + \mathbf{K}_{t-1}(\mathbf{x}_t^T - \mathbf{A}\mathbf{x}_{t-1}^{t-1} - \mathbf{B}\mathbf{h}_{t-1}) \tag{9.26}$$
$$\mathbf{V}_{t-1}^T = \mathbf{V}_{t-1}^{t-1} + \mathbf{K}_{t-1}(\mathbf{V}_t^T - \mathbf{V}_t^{t-1})\mathbf{K}_{t-1}^\dagger \tag{9.27}$$

where $\mathbf{K}_t$ is a gain matrix with a similar role to the Kalman gain matrix. Again, equation (9.26) shifts the mean by an amount proportional to the prediction error $\mathbf{x}_t^T - \mathbf{A}\mathbf{x}_{t-1}^{t-1} - \mathbf{B}\mathbf{h}_{t-1}$. We can also recursively compute the covariance across two time steps

$$\mathbf{V}_{t,t-1}^T = \mathbf{V}_t^t\mathbf{K}_{t-1}^\dagger + \mathbf{K}_t(\mathbf{V}_{t+1,t}^T - \mathbf{A}\mathbf{V}_t^t)\mathbf{K}_{t-1}^\dagger \tag{9.28}$$

which is initialized with

$$\mathbf{V}_{T,T-1}^{T} = (\mathbf{I} - \mathbf{K}_T\mathbf{C})\mathbf{A}\mathbf{V}_{T-1}^{T-1} \tag{9.29}$$

The expectations (9.12)–(9.14) required for EM can now be readily computed.

9.3 The SSM Model for Gene Expression

To model the effects of the influence of the expression of one gene at a previous time point on another gene and its associated hidden variables, we modified the SSM model with inputs described in the previous section as follows. We let the observations $\mathbf{y}_t = \mathbf{g}_t$, where $\mathbf{g}_t$ is the vector of suitably transformed and normalized[5] gene expression levels at time t, and the inputs $\mathbf{h}_t = \mathbf{g}_t, \mathbf{u}_t = \mathbf{g}_{t-1}$ to give the model shown in Figure 9.2. This model is described by the following equations:

$$\mathbf{x}_{t+1} = \mathbf{A}\mathbf{x}_t + \mathbf{B}\mathbf{g}_t + \mathbf{w}_t \tag{9.30}$$

$$\mathbf{g}_t = \mathbf{C}\mathbf{x}_t + \mathbf{D}\mathbf{g}_{t-1} + \mathbf{v}_t \tag{9.31}$$

Here, matrix $\mathbf{D}$ captures direct gene–gene expression level influences at consecutive time points, matrix $\mathbf{C}$ captures the influence of the hidden variables on gene expression levels at each time point, whilst $\mathbf{CB} + \mathbf{D}$ represents all possible gene-gene interactions at consecutive time points, including those mediated via a hidden state variable.

9.3.1 Structural Properties of the Model

There are basically three important properties to look at in the state-space representation of time series: stability, controllability, and observability. Conditions for stability, observability and controllability of the general model (9.3) and (9.4) can be formulated, but as we will show later, our gene expression model (9.30) and (9.31) can be cast in the framework of the simpler model (9.1) and (9.2), so it is sufficient to address these structural properties for the model (9.1) and (9.2).

For *stability* of the model (9.1) and (9.2), what is required is that the matrix $\mathbf{A}$ have spectral radius less than one. In other words we will require that the eigenvalues of $\mathbf{A}$ be less than one in magnitude (see [2] or [4]). This is denoted $\rho(\mathbf{A}) < 1$.

The model (9.1) and (9.2) is *controllable* if the state vector can be "controlled" to evolve from a given, arbitrary initial state $\mathbf{x}_0$ to a given, arbitrary final state $\mathbf{x}_t$ at a future time by a judicious choice of the inputs $\{\mathbf{w}_t\}$. With the state noise covariance non-singular, it can be shown [4] that the model is

[5] The transformation and normalization of microarray gene expression data is discussed in Sections 7.3 and 7.4.

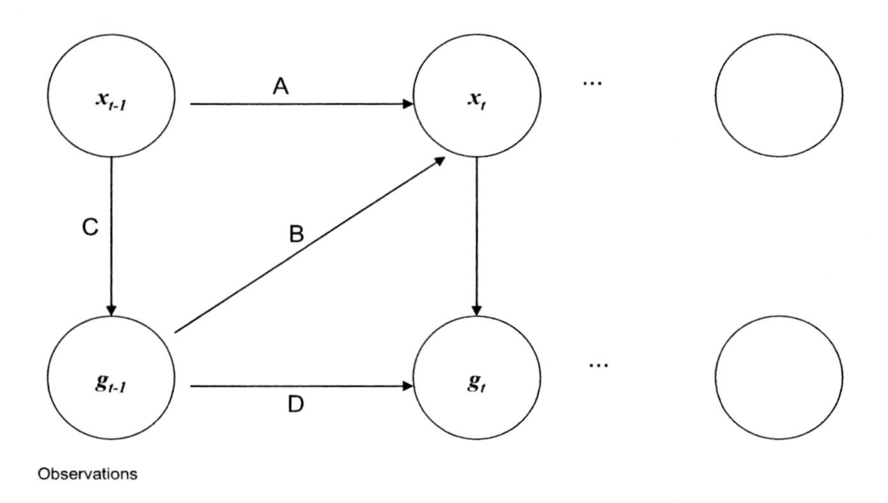

Fig. 9.2. The SSM model for gene expression.

controllable *if and only if* $[\mathbf{I}, \mathbf{A}, \mathbf{A}^2, ..., \mathbf{A}^{K-1}]$ is full rank where $K = \dim(\mathbf{x}_t)$. On the other hand *observability* is associated with the outputs. The state space model is observable if, when the noise vectors are all taken to be 0 vectors, the initial state vector can be reconstructed from a sequence of output observations $\mathbf{y}_t$. From [4], it follows that the state space model (9.1) and (9.2) will be observable *if and only if* $\left[\mathbf{C}^\dagger, \mathbf{A}^\dagger C^\dagger, (\mathbf{A}^2)^\dagger \mathbf{C}^\dagger, ..., (\mathbf{A}^{K-1})^\dagger \mathbf{C}^\dagger\right]$ has full rank for $K = \dim\ (\mathbf{x}_t)$.

A state space model that is both controllable and observable is minimal in the sense that its state vector has the smallest possible dimension. This minimality condition turns out to be important in determining what parameters in the model (9.30) and (9.31) can be estimated unambiguously. This leads to the concept of *identifiability*.

9.3.2 Identifiability and Stability Issues

Consider an observable random vector or matrix $\mathbf{Y}$ defined having probability distribution $P_\theta \in \{P_\phi : \boldsymbol{\phi} \in \Theta\}$ where the parameter space Θ is an open subset of the n-dimensional Euclidean space. We say that this model is *identifiable* if the family $\{P_\phi : \boldsymbol{\phi} \in \Theta\}$ has the property that $P_\theta \equiv P_\phi$ if and only if $\boldsymbol{\theta} = \boldsymbol{\phi} \in \Theta$. It is conventional in this parametric setting to say that in this case, the parameter vector $\boldsymbol{\theta}$ is identifiable. It is easy to see why this property is important, for without it, it would be possible for different values of the parameters $\boldsymbol{\theta}$ to give rise to identically distributed observables, making the statistical problem of estimating $\boldsymbol{\theta}$ ill-posed.

The identifiability problem has been studied extensively for the simple linear dynamic system model (9.1) and (9.2). Taking the model to be stable, and defining the unknown parameters to be the composite of $\mathbf{A}, \mathbf{C}, \mathbf{Q}, \mathbf{R}$, it is known that without any restrictions on the parameters, this model is not identifiable (see, for example [13]). In fact, it is easily seen that by a coordinate transformation of the state variable $\widetilde{\mathbf{x}}_t = \mathbf{T}\mathbf{x}_t$ with $\mathbf{T}$ a nonsingular matrix, the model

$$\widetilde{\mathbf{x}}_{t+1} = \mathbf{T}\mathbf{A}\mathbf{T}^{-1}\widetilde{\mathbf{x}}_t + \mathbf{T}\mathbf{w}_t \tag{9.32}$$

$$\mathbf{y}_t = \mathbf{C}\mathbf{T}^{-1}\widetilde{\mathbf{x}}_t + \mathbf{v}_t \tag{9.33}$$

gives rise to a sequence of observations $\{\mathbf{y}_t, t = 1, 2, ..., T\}$ that has the same joint distribution as the sequence of observables from the model (9.1) and (9.2). Therefore, in the model (9.1) and (9.2), if we write the parameter in the form

$$\boldsymbol{\theta} = [\mathbf{A}, \mathbf{C}, \mathbf{Q}, \mathbf{R}] \tag{9.34}$$

it follows that for a fixed value of $\boldsymbol{\theta}$, each parameter in the set

$$\left\{\boldsymbol{\theta}_T : \boldsymbol{\theta}_T = \left[\mathbf{T}\mathbf{A}\mathbf{T}^{-1}, \mathbf{C}\mathbf{T}^{-1}, \mathbf{T}\mathbf{Q}\mathbf{T}^{\dagger}, \mathbf{R}\right], \det(\mathbf{T}) \neq 0\right\} \tag{9.35}$$

gives rise to an observation sequence $\{\mathbf{y}_t, t = 1, 2, ..., T\}$ having the same joint distribution as the one generated by $\boldsymbol{\theta}$. When the model (9.1) and (9.2) is both controllable and observable, (9.35) in fact defines the only variations on a given parameter $\boldsymbol{\theta}$ that can lead to observation sequences $\{\mathbf{y}_t\}$ all having the same joint distribution as the one emanating from $\boldsymbol{\theta}$ [13].

It turns out that by restricting the structure of the matrices $\mathbf{A}, \mathbf{C}$, the model (9.1) and (9.2) can be rendered identifiable. See, for example, [13] and [16]. However, restricting to one of these identifiable forms is unnecessary if interest is focused on certain subparameters, or functions of subparameters of $\boldsymbol{\theta}$.

This motivates a concept of *extended identifiability*. We shall say that $\boldsymbol{\vartheta}$ is a subparameter of $\boldsymbol{\theta}$ if $\boldsymbol{\vartheta}$ is a function of $\boldsymbol{\theta}$, and we will write $\boldsymbol{\vartheta} \equiv \boldsymbol{\vartheta}(\boldsymbol{\theta})$ to denote this. For example, defining the parameter $\boldsymbol{\theta}$ as in (9.34), $\boldsymbol{\vartheta} = \mathbf{A}$ is a subparameter. We shall say that the subparameter $\boldsymbol{\vartheta}(\boldsymbol{\theta})$ is identifiable in the extended sense if $P_{\theta} \equiv P_{\phi}$ implies that $\boldsymbol{\vartheta}(\boldsymbol{\theta}) = \boldsymbol{\vartheta}(\boldsymbol{\phi})$ for any $\boldsymbol{\theta} \in \Theta$, $\boldsymbol{\phi} \in \Theta$.

In the gene expression model (9.30) and (9.31), the use of lagged observables as inputs presents no theoretical or practical problems for estimating the state $\mathbf{x}_t$ based on the observations $\{\mathbf{y}_1, \mathbf{y}_2, ..., \mathbf{y}_t\}$, when $\mathbf{A}, \mathbf{B}, \mathbf{C}, \mathbf{D}, \mathbf{Q}, \mathbf{R}$ are known, as the Kalman filter theory allows having the inputs $\mathbf{u}_t$ and $\mathbf{h}_t$ be measurable functions of $\{\mathbf{y}_1, \mathbf{y}_2, ..., \mathbf{y}_t\}$. However, this approach does alter the treatment of both identifiability and stability. To study this model in these regards, it is helpful to transform it to the more conventional state-space form (9.1) and (9.2) for which these properties have been well studied.

Define a new state vector to be $\widetilde{\mathbf{x}}_t^\dagger = \left(\mathbf{x}_t^\dagger, \mathbf{g}_t^\dagger\right)^\dagger$. Then the gene expression model (9.30) and (9.31) can be rewritten in a new state space form with a noiseless observation equation as

$$\widetilde{\mathbf{x}}_{t+1} = \mathbf{A}_0 \widetilde{\mathbf{x}}_t + \widetilde{\mathbf{w}}_t \tag{9.36}$$

$$\mathbf{g}_t = \mathbf{H} \widetilde{\mathbf{x}}_t \tag{9.37}$$

where the matrices $\mathbf{A}_0$ and $\mathbf{H}$ are given by

$$\mathbf{A}_0 = \begin{pmatrix} \mathbf{A} & \mathbf{B} \\ \mathbf{CA} & \mathbf{CB} + \mathbf{D} \end{pmatrix}, \ \mathbf{H} = \begin{pmatrix} \mathbf{0} \ \mathbf{I} \end{pmatrix} \tag{9.38}$$

and the white noise term in the state equation and its variance matrix become

$$\widetilde{\mathbf{w}}_t = \begin{pmatrix} \mathbf{w}_t \\ \mathbf{C}\mathbf{w}_t + \mathbf{v}_{t+1} \end{pmatrix}, \ \widetilde{\mathbf{Q}} = \begin{pmatrix} \mathbf{Q} & \mathbf{Q}\mathbf{C}^\dagger \\ \mathbf{CQ} & \mathbf{CQC}^\dagger + \mathbf{R} \end{pmatrix} \tag{9.39}$$

Notice here that the variance matrix $\widetilde{\mathbf{Q}}$ above remains non-singular (since both $\mathbf{Q}$ and $\mathbf{R}$ are assumed non-singular). It is now easy to resolve the issue of stability for (9.30) and (9.31) in terms of this model. The model (9.30), (9.31) will be stable if and only if the matrix $\mathbf{A}_0$ in (9.38) has spectral radius less than 1. Moreover, we will have controllability and observability if and only if the matrices

$$[\mathbf{I}, \mathbf{A}_0, \mathbf{A}_0^2, ..., \mathbf{A}_0^{\mathbf{K}_0 - 1}] \tag{9.40}$$

$$\left[\mathbf{H}^\dagger, \mathbf{A}_0^\dagger \mathbf{H}^\dagger, (\mathbf{A}_0^2)^\dagger \mathbf{H}^\dagger, ..., (\mathbf{A}_0^{\mathbf{K}_0 - 1})^\dagger \mathbf{H}^\dagger\right] \tag{9.41}$$

have full rank, where now $\mathbf{K}_0$ is the row dimension of $\mathbf{A}_0$.

Now, in terms of identifiability, it is easy to see that not all coordinate transformations of the state vector in this model (9.36), (9.37) will lead to identically distributed observations. This is because of the constraint on the form of $\mathbf{H}$ which fixes the coordinate system for $\mathbf{g}_t$. However, arbitrary transformations of the portion of the state vector corresponding to $\mathbf{x}_t$ will lead to indistinguishable observations. In fact, let the modified state vector

$$\overline{\mathbf{x}}_t = \begin{pmatrix} \mathbf{T} & \mathbf{O} \\ \mathbf{O} & \mathbf{I} \end{pmatrix} \widetilde{\mathbf{x}}_t \tag{9.42}$$

be defined with $\mathbf{T}$ a non-singular square matrix conforming with $\mathbf{x}_t$. Then for fixed values of $\mathbf{A}, \mathbf{B}, \mathbf{C}, \mathbf{D}, \mathbf{Q}, \mathbf{R}$, the state space model

$$\overline{\mathbf{x}}_{t+1} = \mathbf{A}_{0,T} \overline{\mathbf{x}}_t + \overline{\mathbf{w}}_t, \ \mathbf{A}_{0,T} = \begin{pmatrix} \mathbf{TAT}^{-1} & \mathbf{TB} \\ \mathbf{CAT}^{-1} & \mathbf{CB} + \mathbf{D} \end{pmatrix} \tag{9.43}$$

$$\mathbf{g}_t = \mathbf{H}\overline{\mathbf{x}}_t \tag{9.44}$$

with white noise (and its corresponding variance matrix) given by

$$\overline{\mathbf{w}}_t = \begin{pmatrix} \mathbf{T} & \mathbf{O} \\ \mathbf{O} & \mathbf{I} \end{pmatrix} \widetilde{\mathbf{w}}_t, \; \overline{\mathbf{Q}} = \begin{pmatrix} \mathbf{TQT}^\dagger & \mathbf{TQC}^\dagger \\ \mathbf{CQT}^\dagger & \mathbf{CQC}^\dagger + \mathbf{R} \end{pmatrix}$$

will generate observations that are identically distributed with those of (9.36), (9.37). Here it is easily seen that, when the model (9.36), (9.37) is both controllable and observable, then we have that, for example, $\mathbf{CB} + \mathbf{D}$, is identifiable in the extended sense. Also, when $\mathbf{A}$ is non singular, $\mathbf{CB}$ is invariant to the choice of the arbitrary non-singular matrix $\mathbf{T}$ in (9.42), since it can be computed from elements of $\mathbf{A}_{0,T}$ in (9.43) by $\mathbf{CB} = \mathbf{CAT}^{-1}(\mathbf{TAT}^{-1})^{-1}\mathbf{TB}$, and therefore $\mathbf{D}$ is also identifiable in the extended sense.

Thus, we define the admissible set for the parameters $\mathbf{A}, \mathbf{B}, \mathbf{C}, \mathbf{D}, \mathbf{Q}, \mathbf{R}$ to be such that $\rho(\mathbf{A}_0) < 1$, and that both (9.40) and (9.41) are full rank.

9.4 Model Selection by Bootstrapping

9.4.1 Objectives

The size of the search space (i.e. the space of all gene–gene interaction networks) increases super-exponentially with the number of parameters of the model. Following Friedman *et al.* [10] we have developed a bootstrap procedure to identify "high probability" gene-gene interaction networks which are shared by a significant number of sub-models built from randomly resampled data sets. In our procedure we use bootstrap methods to find confidence intervals for the parameters defining the gene-gene interaction networks (i.e. the elements of $\mathbf{CB} + \mathbf{D}$) so we can eliminate those that are not significantly different from zero. Thresholding the elements of the matrix $\mathbf{CB} + \mathbf{D}$ using these confidence levels we can obtain a connectivity matrix which describes all gene-gene interactions over successive time points.

9.4.2 The Bootstrap Procedure

Recall the SSM model defined by the two equations (9.30) and (9.31). Estimated parameters for this model $[\hat{\mathbf{A}}, \hat{\mathbf{B}}, \hat{\mathbf{C}}, \hat{\mathbf{D}}]$, as well as estimates of the covariances $\hat{\mathbf{Q}}, \hat{\mathbf{R}}$, are computed using the EM algorithm (with straightforward modifications for more than one replicate) as described above.

The key idea in the bootstrap procedure, introduced in Chapter 1, especially Section 1.2 and Figure 1.5, is to resample with replacement the replicates within the original data. By resampling from the replicates N_B times (where the value N_B is a large number, say 200 or 300) we can estimate, among other things, the sampling distributions of the estimators of the elements of $\mathbf{CB}+\mathbf{D}$, which is the identifiable gene-gene interaction matrix in the gene-expression model (9.30) and (9.31). In general once we have estimates of these distributions, we can make statistical inferences about those underlying parameters (in particular, confidence intervals and hypothesis tests).

Each "technical" replicate represents a reproduction of the same experiment under the same circumstances and assumptions. Hence replicates are assumed to be independent and identically distributed with unknown (multivariate) cumulative probability distribution F_0. That is, the ith replicate consists of a time series $\mathbf{Y}_i = \left(\mathbf{y}_1^i, \mathbf{y}_2^i, ..., \mathbf{y}_T^i\right)$ with each $\mathbf{y}_t^i$ a p-dimensional vector (one component for each gene). Thus, the collection $\mathcal{D} = \{\mathbf{Y}_1, \mathbf{Y}_2, ..., \mathbf{Y}_N\}$ can be viewed as a sequence of N iid random matrices, each with cumulative distribution F_0. Under this assumption, a *bootstrap sample* $\mathcal{D}^* = \{\mathbf{Y}_1^*, \mathbf{Y}_2^*, ..., \mathbf{Y}_N^*\}$ is obtained by selecting at random with replacement, N elements from $\mathcal{D} = \{\mathbf{Y}_1, \mathbf{Y}_2, ..., \mathbf{Y}_N\}$.

Following is the bootstrap procedure for the model (9.30) and (9.31) with data collected as described above. Let us denote a generic element of the matrix $\mathbf{CB} + \mathbf{D}$ by $\boldsymbol{\theta}$. The following steps lead to a bootstrap confidence interval for $\boldsymbol{\theta}$ using the percentile method.

1. Calculate estimates for the unknown matrices $\mathbf{A}, \mathbf{B}, \mathbf{C}, \mathbf{D}$ from the full data set with replicates using the EM algorithm. From the estimates $\hat{\mathbf{B}}, \hat{\mathbf{C}}, \hat{\mathbf{D}}$, compute $\widehat{\boldsymbol{\theta}}$, the estimate of the given element of $\mathbf{CB} + \mathbf{D}$.
2. Generate N_B independent bootstrap samples $\mathcal{D}_1^*, \mathcal{D}_2^*, ..., \mathcal{D}_{N_B}^*$ from the original data.
3. For each bootstrap sample compute bootstrap replicates of the parameters. This is done using the EM algorithm on each bootstrap sample $\mathcal{D}_i^*, i = 1, 2, ..., N_B$. This yields bootstrap estimates of the parameters
$$\{\hat{\mathbf{A}}_1^*, \hat{\mathbf{B}}_1^*, \hat{\mathbf{C}}_1^*, \hat{\mathbf{D}}_1^*\}, \{\hat{\mathbf{A}}_2^*, \hat{\mathbf{B}}_2^*, \hat{\mathbf{C}}_2^*, \hat{\mathbf{D}}_2^*\}, ..., \{\hat{\mathbf{A}}_{N_B}^*, \hat{\mathbf{B}}_{N_B}^*, \hat{\mathbf{C}}_{N_B}^*, \hat{\mathbf{D}}_{N_B}^*\}.$$
4. From $\{\hat{\mathbf{B}}_1^*, \hat{\mathbf{C}}_1^*, \hat{\mathbf{D}}_1^*\}$, $\{\hat{\mathbf{B}}_2^*, \hat{\mathbf{C}}_2^*, \hat{\mathbf{D}}_2^*\}$, ..., $\{\hat{\mathbf{B}}_{N_B}^*, \hat{\mathbf{C}}_{N_B}^*, \hat{\mathbf{D}}_{N_B}^*\}$, compute the corresponding bootstrap estimates of the parameter of interest, leading to $\widehat{\boldsymbol{\theta}}_1^*, \widehat{\boldsymbol{\theta}}_2^*, ..., \widehat{\boldsymbol{\theta}}_{N_B}^*$. For the given parameter $\boldsymbol{\theta}$, estimate the distribution of $\widehat{\boldsymbol{\theta}} - \boldsymbol{\theta}$ by the empirical distribution of the values
$$\left\{\widehat{\boldsymbol{\theta}}_j^* - \widehat{\boldsymbol{\theta}} : j = 1, 2, ..., N_B\right\}.$$
Using quantiles of this latter empirical distribution to approximate corresponding quantiles of the distribution of $\widehat{\boldsymbol{\theta}} - \boldsymbol{\theta}$, compute an estimated confidence interval on the parameter $\boldsymbol{\theta}$.
5. Test the null hypothesis that the selected parameter is 0 by rejecting the null hypothesis if the confidence interval computed in step 4 does not contain the value 0.
6. Repeat steps 4 and 5 for each element of $\mathbf{CB} + \mathbf{D}$.

9.5 Experiments with Simulated Data

To evaluate our method to reverse engineer gene regulatory networks using data collected from cDNA microarray experiments, we simulate a microarray experiment *in silico*, generating a synthetic data set using our gene expression model. Synthetic data are generated from an initial network defined by the connectivity matrix in the matrix $\mathbf{CB} + \mathbf{D}$. The idea is to determine if we are able to recover the same network using the SSM model and bootstrap procedure described earlier and also to estimate the size of the data set needed by the method to reconstruct the underlying network.

9.5.1 Model Definition

We generate simulated data from the model (9.30) and (9.31). The covariance matrices $\mathbf{Q}, \mathbf{R}$ add some Gaussian noise to the simulated data and are defined to be diagonal with $\mathbf{Q}$ taken to be the identity matrix. Simulated data are generated from a model that is stable, controllable and observable.

9.5.2 Reconstructing the Original Network

An SSM model is trained on the simulated data to estimate the model parameters. Then a bootstrap analysis as described in Section 9.4.2 is performed to estimate the distributions of the parameter estimates and compute confidence intervals on elements of $\mathbf{CB} + \mathbf{D}$. Based on those confidence bounds some elements in this matrix are set to zero. We formulate this as a simple decision problem with two hypotheses as described in step 5 in Section 9.4.2:

$$
\begin{aligned}
H_0 &: (\mathbf{CB} + \mathbf{D})_{i,j} = 0 \qquad (\textit{no connection}) \\
&\quad vs \\
H_1 &: (\mathbf{CB} + \mathbf{D})_{i,j} \neq 0 \qquad (\textit{connection})
\end{aligned}
$$

where H_0 is rejected when 0 is not within the confidence interval. Thresholding the $\hat{\mathbf{C}}\hat{\mathbf{B}} + \hat{\mathbf{D}}$ matrix using this criterion produces a connectivity matrix or directed graph where the diagonal elements represent self–self interactions at consecutive time steps. A number of experiments were performed using different numbers of nodes and the results are described in the next section.

9.5.3 Results

The following are the results for 3 and 39 nodes (genes). Whilst 3 nodes were selected for simplicity, the 39-node network was taken from results obtained using the real experimental data described in Section 9.6. We are interested in determining what would be the appropriate sample size in terms of replicates as well as time points to correctly reconstruct the underlying network. However, we will emphasize the case with 40 or 50 replicates and 10 time points

Table 9.1. True and estimated parameter values for different numbers of replicates.

	Rep.					
True	10	20	30	40	50	60
-0.35	-0.3634	-0.4342	-0.4212	-0.3921	-0.3818	-0.3548
0.51	0.6571	0.3647	0.7463	0.6010	0.8022	0.7706
0.51	0.2491	0.4503	0.4662	0.4437	0.4109	0.3751
0	-0.0087	-0.0051	-0.0056	-0.0048	-0.0049	-0.0028
0.25	0.1422	0.1929	0.2254	0.2461	0.2506	0.2461
0	0.0028	0.0014	0.0006	0.0014	0.0031	0.0002
0.14	0.1450	0.2215	0.2269	0.1882	0.1723	0.1348
0.35	0.2412	0.5519	0.1609	0.2855	0.0192	0.0419
0.635	0.9647	0.7168	0.6927	0.7227	0.7573	0.8004

since this is approximately the size of the real experimental data set described in Section 9.6. Due to dimensional complexity, results will be presented differently as the number of nodes increases.

Network evaluation – 3 × 3 matrix example

Table 9.1 shows the parameter estimates for 6 different sample ("technical replicate") sizes from the initial fit of the SSM model. In all cases the number of time points is 10.

The first column represents the vectorized form of the 3 × 3 matrix $\mathbf{CB}+\mathbf{D}$. The columns following are the parameter estimates for sample sizes of $10, 20, ..., 60$. We can see that 40 samples are certainly enough for a "good" estimate of the model parameters in terms of magnitude and sign. Hence, we can choose that sample size and run the bootstrap experiment on this example with 10 time points and 40 replicates.

The results after thresholding based on the confidence bounds are presented in the form of a connectivity matrix. For this example with 3 nodes all connections except for (3,2) (the 8th element of the matrix) were recovered at a 90% confidence level on each connection. Figure 9.3 shows the upper and lower bounds calculated based on the 5th and 95th quantiles from 100 bootstrap samples (top plot) and the 20th and 80th quantiles (bottom plot). Note that with a 60% confidence level the original structure is finally recovered. This can been seen in the plot: based on the test that rejects H_0 whenever zero is not between the upper and lower confidence bounds, those elements that were not originally zero all result in a rejection of H_0, while elements that were originally zero result in tests where H_0 could not be rejected.

It is important to point out that the 8th element corresponding to connection $(3, 2)$ shows a high standard error compared with others (a standard error of about 0.4949 as opposed to others of the order of magnitude of 0.0038).

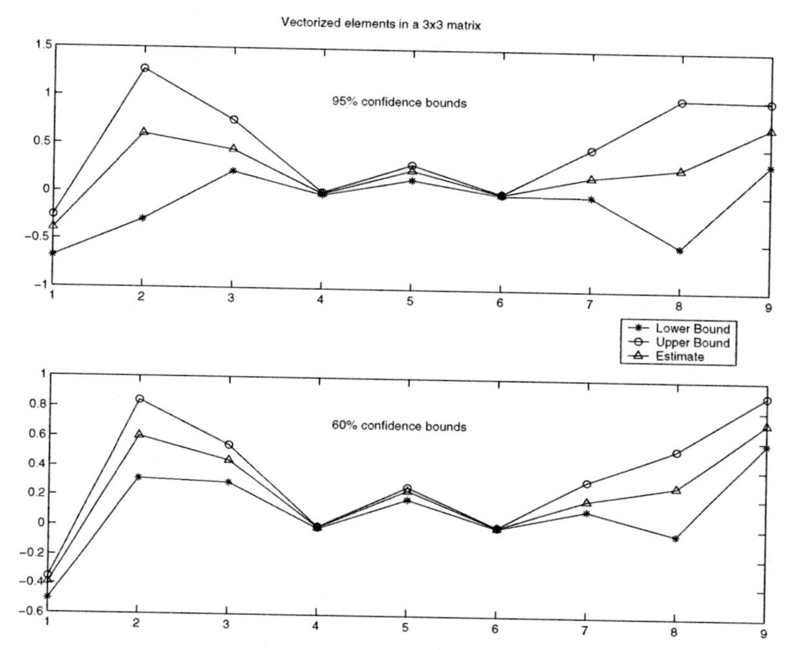

Fig. 9.3. Bootstrap results with 90% and 60% confidence levels.
Note that the first 3 points are the elements in the first row and the next 3 are the elements in the second row and so on.

Network evaluation – 39 × 39 sparse matrix example

The results for the 39 × 39 node simulation are presented using ROC (Receiver Operating Characteristics) plots. These curves are obtained by computing the hit and false alarm rates for different thresholds (i.e. the confidence level placed on testing individual connections). The hit rate or *sensitivity* is the true positive fraction, $TP/(TP + FN)$, and the false alarm rate or complimentary *specificity* is the false positive fraction, $FP/(FP+TN)$, from the number of true/false positives and negatives, where:

TP = number of actual connections that are declared connections
FP = number of non-connections that are declared connected
FN = number of actual connections that are declared not connected
TN = number of non-connections that are declared not connected.

The problem can be stated based on a hypothesis testing problem where the ROC is a plot (for varying thresholds) of $P(\text{reject } H_0|H_1) = TP/(TP+FN)$ versus $P(\text{reject } H_0|H_0) = FP/(FP+TN)$ where H_0 and H_1 are defined as in Section 9.5.2. The plot runs as $P(\text{reject } H_0|H_0)$ varies between 0 and 1. These are all computed based on a comparison of the estimated graph with the true

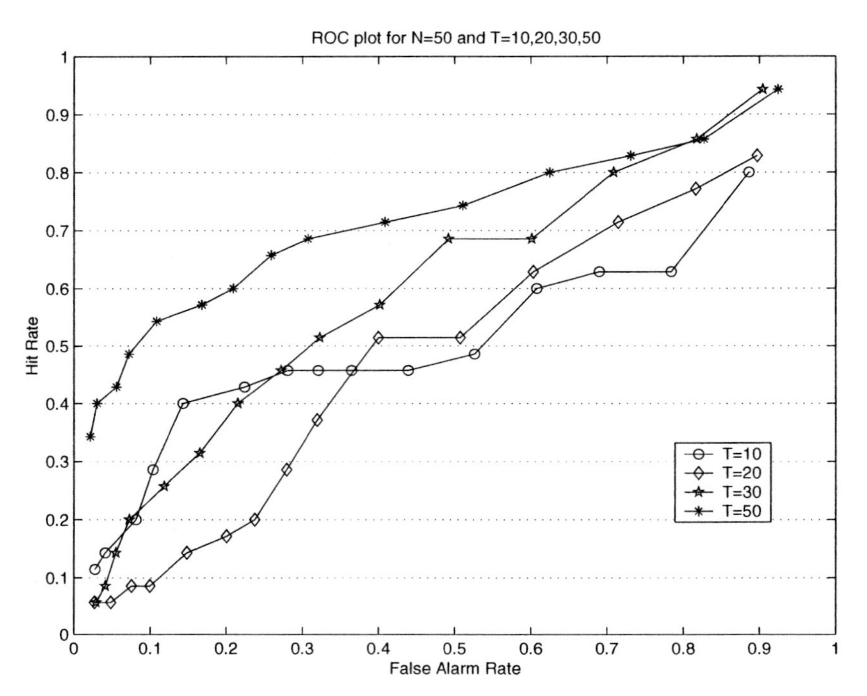

Fig. 9.4. ROC plot for 39×39 graph with 50 replicates and different time series lengths.

or actual graph. So, for a given number of time points T and a given number of replicates N, the process for generating the graph is simulated for many different values of 2α (where $1 - 2\alpha$ is the nominal confidence level used on each connection for testing H_0) ranging between 0 and 1 giving us one ROC curve. This process is repeated for different combinations of T and N, each combination generating another ROC curve. In the ROC plots shown here points in each curve represent the rate values computed based on different thresholds (nominal confidence levels). A total of 15 points are plotted for confidence levels in the sequence $\{99, 98, 96, 94, 90, 85, 80, 75, 70, 60, 50, 40, 30, 20, 10\}\%$. On the ROC curve, the "hit" axis represents the fraction of the total actual connections in the network that are correctly identified. The "false alarm" axis represents one minus the fraction of non-connections that are correctly identified.

We generated a sparse 39×39 matrix which had $c = 35$ actual connections and $n - c = 1486$ non-connections. Simulations were performed with different sample sizes N and different numbers of time points T to generate three ROC plots. Figure 9.4 shows the case for 50 replicates and different time series lengths. We see that longer sequences are advantageous, especially once T reaches 50. We can also compare the results we obtain for different time series lengths whilst fixing the confidence level threshold on individual connections to some value, say 80%. For this threshold, with sequences of length 20 we get that 20% of the true connections are recovered correctly while 76% of the non-connections are recovered correctly. With sequences of length 50 these numbers go up to 60% and 80% respectively.

We also examined the effect of increasing the number of replicates to 100. This is shown in Figure 9.5. As would be expected results are generally better.

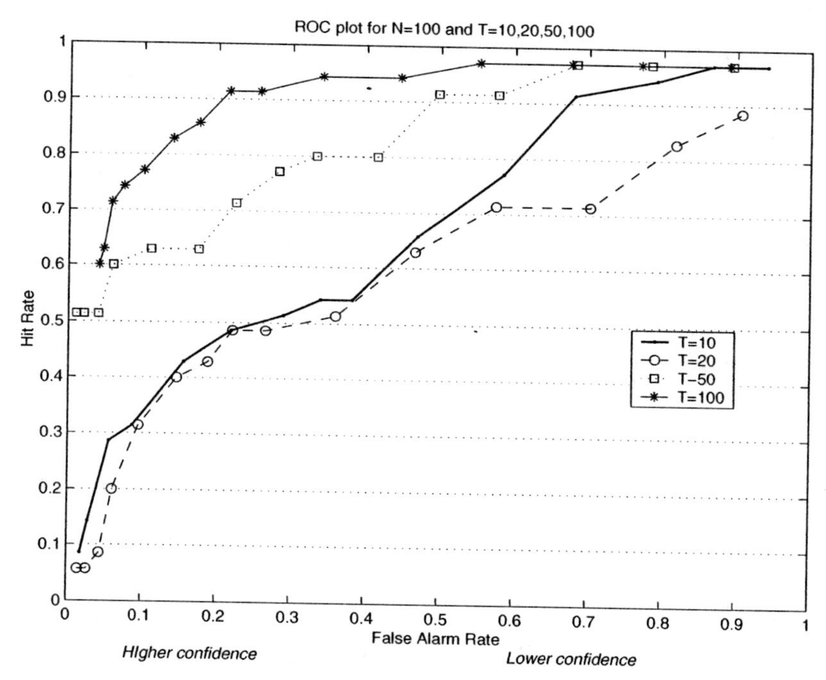

Fig. 9.5. ROC plot for 100 replicates and different time series lengths.

For $N = 100$ and $T = 100$, thresholding again at a confidence level of 80% results in 86% true connections and 82% non-connections recovered, a clear improvement on the results for $N = 50$ and $T = 50$. A more conservative confidence threshold of 99% results in the first point on the ROC curve corresponding to $T = 100$, i.e. $(0.05, 0.6)$. This indicates that one can recover 60% of true connections along with 95% of non-connections.

The last simulation experiment fixes the time series length to $T = 10$ (corresponding to our experimental data) and varies the number of replicates. This is shown in Figure 9.6.

This last set of simulations shows that an increase in performance can be obtained by increasing the number of replicates. The size of the experimental gene expression data described below is approximately $N = 50$ and $T = 10$.

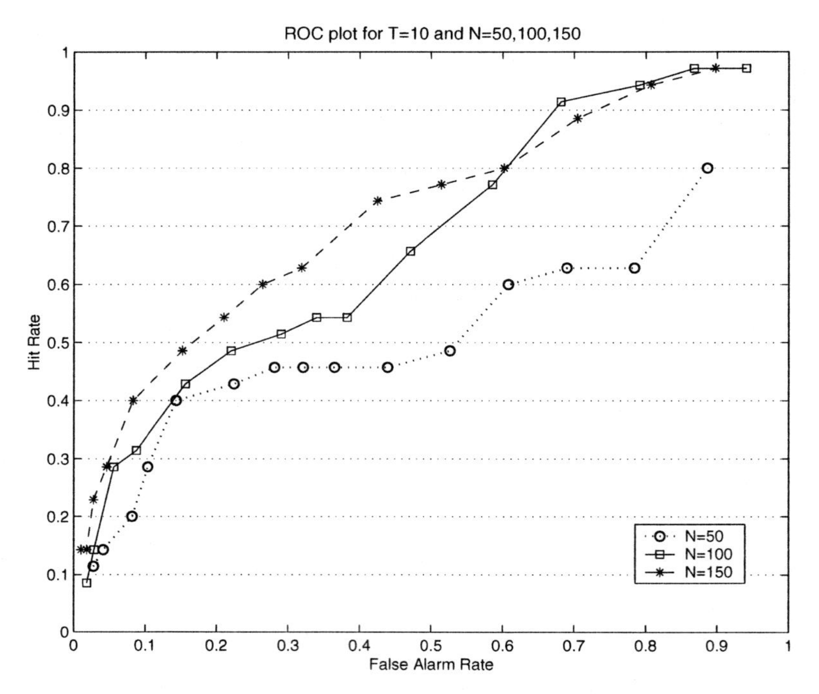

Fig. 9.6. 39-node ROC plot for different number of replicates and $T = 10$.

9.6 Results from Experimental Data

Care must be taken in extrapolating these simulation results to experiments with actual gene expression data. First of all, while the simulations were idealized in that the data were actually generated from a linear dynamical system, in real gene expression data one would expect to see nonlinearities, more or less noise, and possibly many hidden variables. Finally, the confidence threshold chosen should depend on the relative costs one would associate with falsely positive connections versus missed connections, and on the assumed sparsity of the graph. Clearly, if it is desired to have a high percentage of overall correctness in the graph that is identified, then it is advisable to set the confidence level high on testing individual connections in a large, sparsely connected graph. However, in the limit of claiming that nothing is connected we would get a high percentage correct score but an uninteresting hypothesis.

Figure 9.7 shows results obtained from an experimental data set obtained from a well-established model of T-cell activation in which we have monitored a set of relevant genes across a time series. Details of this work are published elsewhere [21]. The data set comprises 58 genes, 44 replicates (comprising two independent experiments of 34 and 10 "technical" replicates respectively) and 10 time points. Following the bootstrap procedure described above, the confidence level on individual connections was set to 99.66%. At this confi-

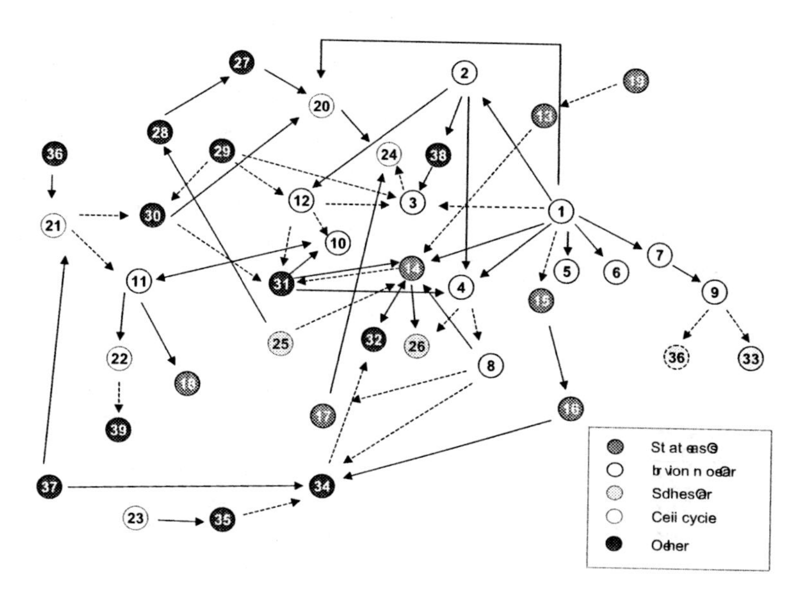

Fig. 9.7. Directed graph representing the elements of the CB + D matrix. The main functional categories involved in T lymphocyte response (cytokines, proliferation and apoptosis) are marked in different shades. Numbers refer to genes in Table 9.2. Positive coefficients of the **CB + D** matrix are represented by solid arrows; negative coefficients are represented by dotted arrows. Reprinted from [21], by permission of Oxford University Press.

dence level we obtain a directed graph comprising 39 connected nodes with 76 connections. From a strictly topological point of view FYN-binding protein (FYB, gene 1) occupies a crucial position in the graph since it has the highest number of outward connections. Interestingly, the majority of the genes that are directly related to inflammation response are directly connected to or located in close proximity of FYB. The topology of the graph and the functional grouping fit well with the fact that this gene is an important adaptor molecule in the T-cell receptor signalling machinery and is, therefore, very high in the hierarchy of events downstream of cell activation. This model has yielded plausible biological hypotheses concerning the role of FYB and Interleukin-2 in T-cell activation, which have the potential for experimental validation [21].

9.7 Conclusions

Despite the linear assumptions inherent in state-space models, the results presented above indicate that they are a useful tool for investigating gene transcriptional networks. The bootstrap procedure we have described provides a

Table 9.2. Gene numbers and descriptions for the graph shown in Figure 9.7.

Number	Gene description
1	FYN-binding protein (FYB-120/130)
2	interleukin 3 receptor, alpha (low affinity)
3	CD69 antigen (p60, early T-cell activation antigen)
4	TNF receptor-associated factor 5
5	interleukin 4 receptor
6	GATA-binding protein 3
7	interleukin 2 receptor, γ (severe combined immunodeficiency)
8	interferon (alpha, beta and omega) receptor 1
9	chemokine (C-X3-C) receptor 1
10	zinc finger protein, subfamily 1A, 1 (Ikaros)
11	interleukin 16 (lymphocyte chemoattractant factor)
12	nuclear factor of kappa light polypeptide gene enhancer in B-cell
13	jun B proto-oncogene
14	caspase 8, apoptosis-related cysteine protease
15	clusterin (complement lysis inhibitor, SP-40,40, sulfated glycoprotein 2
16	apoptosis inhibitor 2
17	caspase 4, apoptosis-related cysteine protease
18	caspase 7, apoptosis-related cysteine protease
19	survival of motor neuron 1, telomeric
20	cyclin A2
21	cell division cycle 2 (cdc2)
22	proliferating cell nuclear antigen
23	cyclin-dependent kinase 4
24	retinoblastoma-like 2 (p130)
25	catenin (cadherin-associated protein), beta 1 (88kD)
26	integrin, alpha M (complement component receptor 3 α)
27	phosphodiesterase 4B, cAMP-specific
28	SKI-interacting protein
29	inhibitor of DNA binding 3, dominant negative
30	myeloperoxidase
31	myeloid cell leukemia sequence 1 (BCL2-related)
32	colony stimulating factor 2 receptor, α
33	CBF1 interacting corepressor
34	cytqochrome P450, subfamily XIX (aromatization of androgens)
35	mitogen-activated protein kinase 9
36	early growth response 1
37	jun D proto-oncogene
38	quinone oxidoreductase homolog
39	Ribosomal protein S6 Kinase

robust statistical approach to identifying "high probability" sub-models with a given level of statistical confidence. Application of the method to experimental microarray gene expression data has yielded plausible biological hypotheses which have the potential for rapid experimental validation.

Future work will include investigating Bayesian approaches to model selection using Markov chain Monte Carlo (MCMC) methods, as introduced in Section 2.2.2, and applied in Chapter 8. Recall from the discussion in Section 4.4.7 and Figure 4.35, that this may lead to a considerable reduction in the computational costs. This approach will also allow us to examine the robustness of the inferences with respect to choices in the prior distribution over parameters, and to study different choices for the hierarchical prior over parameters. One attraction of this approach is that it is possible to incorporate priors in the form of known connections supported by the literature, including constraints with regard to the sign of the interaction (i.e. negative–repression or positive–promotion). An alternative approach will explore the use of variational Bayesian methods, which were briefly discussed in Section 2.3.6. The theory of variational Bayesian learning has been successfully applied to learning non-trivial SSM model structures in other application domains [11, 12], which suggests that it will provide good solutions in the case of modeling gene expression data. Our initial experiments with linear dynamics also pave the way for future work on models with realistic nonlinear dynamics.

Acknowledgments

The authors would like to thank Francesco Falciani (University of Birmingham, formerly Lorantis Ltd, UK) for the microarray data described in Section 9.6 and Figure 9.7, and Brian Champion (Lorantis Ltd) for his enthusiastic support of the project. Part of this work is based on C.R.'s PhD dissertation for Claremont Graduate University and part was previously published in [22]. C.R. acknowledges support from the Keck Graduate Institute of Applied Life Sciences.

References

[1] T. Akutsu, S. Miyano, and S. Kuhara. Identification of genetic networks from a small number of gene expression patterns under the boolean network model. *Pac. Symp. Biocomput.*, pages 17–28, 1999.

[2] M. Aoki. *State Space Modeling of Time Series.* Springer-Verlag, New York, 1987.

[3] A. Arkin, P. Shen, and J. Ross. A test case of correlation metric construction of a reaction pathway from measurements. *Science*, 277:1275–1279, 1997.

[4] P. Brockwell and R. Davis. *Time Series: Theory and Methods.* Springer-Verlag, New York, 1996.
[5] R. G. Brown and P. Y. Hwang. *Introduction to Random Signals and Applied Kalman Filtering.* John Wiley and Sons, New York, 1997.
[6] G. Cooper and E. Herskovits. A Bayesian method for the induction of probabilistic networks from data. *Machine Learning*, 9:309–347, 1992.
[7] T. G. Dewey and D. J. Galas. Generalized dynamical models of gene expression and gene classification. *Funt. Int. Genomics*, 1:269–278, 2000.
[8] P. D'Haeseleer, X. Wen, S. Fuhrman, and R. Somogyi. Linear modeling of mRNA expression levels during CNS development and injury. *Pacific Symposium for Biocomputing*, 3:41–52, 1999.
[9] J. Dopazo, E. Zanders, I. Dragoni, G. Amphlett, and F. Falciani. Methods and approaches in the analysis of gene expression data. *Journal of Immunological Methods*, 250:93–112, 2001.
[10] N. Friedman, M. Linial, I. Nachman, and D. Pe'er. Using Bayesian networks to analyze expression data. *J. Comput. Biol.*, 7:601–620, 2000.
[11] Z. Ghahramani and M. Beal. Variational inference for Bayesian mixture of factor analysers. *Advances in Neural Information Processing Systems*, 12:449–455, 2000.
[12] Z. Ghahramani and M. Beal. Propagation algorithms for variational Bayesian learning. *Advances in Neural Information processing Systems*, 13, 2001.
[13] E. Hannan and M. Deistler. *The Statistical Theory of Linear Systems.* John Wiley, New York, 1988.
[14] B. Kholodenko, A. Kiyatkin, F. Bruggeman, E. Sontag, H. Westerhoff, and J. Hoek. Untangling the wires: a strategy to trace functional interactions in signaling and gene networks. *Proc. Natl. Acad. Sci.*, 99:12841–12846, 2002.
[15] S. Liang, S. Fuhrman, and R. Somogyi. Identification of genetic networks from a small number of gene expression patterns under the boolean network model. *Pac. Symp. Biocomput.*, pages 18–29, 1998.
[16] L. Ljung. *System Identifiability*, 2nd ed. Prentice Hall, New Jersey, 1999.
[17] R. J. Meinhold and N. D. Singpurwalla. Understanding the Kalman Filter. *The American Statistician*, 37(2):123–127, 1983.
[18] K. Murphy and S. Mian. Modelling gene expression data using dynamic Bayesian networks. *Proc. Intelligent Systems for Molecular Biology*, August 1999.
[19] I. Ong, J. Glasner, and D. Page. Modelling regulatory pathways in *E. coli* from time series expression profiles. *Bioinformatics*, 18(1):S241–S248, 2002.
[20] D. Pe'er, A. Regev, G. Elidan, and N. Friedman. Inferring subnetworks from perturbed expression profiles. *Proc. 9th International Conference on Intelligent Systems for Molecular Biology (ISMB)*, 2001.
[21] C. Rangel, J. Angus, Z. Ghahramani, M. Lioumi, E.A. Sotheran, A. Gaiba, D. L. Wild, and F. Falciani. Modeling T-cell activation us-

ing gene expression profiling and state space models. *Bioinformatics*, 20 (9): 1316-1372, 2004.

[22] C. Rangel, D. L. Wild, F. Falciani, Z. Ghahramani, and A. Gaiba. Modelling biological responses using gene expression profiling and linear dynamical systems. In *Proceedings of the 2nd International Conference on Systems Biology*, pages 248–256. Omipress, Madison, WI, 2001.

[23] S. Roweis and Z. Ghahramani. A unifying review of linear Gaussian models. *Neural Computation*, 11:305–345, 1999.

[24] V. Smith, E. Jarvis, and A. Hartemink. Evaluating functional network influence using simulations of complex biological systems. *Bioinformatics*, 18(1):S216–S224, 2002.

[25] P. Spellman, G. Sherlock, M. Zhang, V. Iyer, K. Anders, M. Eisen, P. Brown, D. Botstein, and B. Futcher. Comprehensive identification of cell cycle-regulated genes of the yeast *Saccharomyces cerevisiae* by microarray hybridization. *Mol. Biol. Cell.*, 9:3273–3297, 1998.

[26] R. Thomas. Boolean formalization of genetic control circuits. *J. Theor. Biol.*, 42(3):563–586, 1973.

[27] E. van Someren, L.F. Wessels, E. Backer, and M. Reinders. Genetic network modeling. *Pharmacogenomics*, 3:507–525, 2002.

[28] E. van Someren, L.F. Wessels, and M. Reinders. Linear modeling of genetic networks from experimental data. *Proc. 9th International Conference on Intelligent Systems for Molecular Biology (ISMB)*, 8:355–366, 2000.

[29] D. Weaver, C. Workman, and G. Stormo. Modeling regulatory networks with weight matrices. *Pacific Symposium for Biocomputing*, 4:112–123, 1999.

[30] L. Wessels, E. van Someren, and M. Reinders. A comparison of genetic network models. *Pacific Symposium for Biocomputing*, 6:508–519, 2001.

[31] M. Yeung, J. Tegner, and J. Collins. Reverse engineering gene networks using singular value decomposition and robust regression. *Proc. Natl. Acad. Sci.*, 99:6163–6168, 2002.

[32] C. Yoo, V. Thorsson, and G. Cooper. Discovery of causal relationships in a gene-regulation pathway from a mixture of experimental and observational DNA microarray data. *Pac. Symp. Biocomput.*, pages 422–433, 2002.

[33] D. Zak, F. Doyle, G. Gonye, and J. Schwaber. Simulation studies for the identification of genetic networks from cDNA array and regulatory activity data. In *Proceedings of the 2nd International Conference on Systems Biology*, pages 231–238. Omipress, Madison, WI, 2001.

Part III

Medical Informatics

10

An Anthology of Probabilistic Models for Medical Informatics

Richard Dybowski[1] and Stephen Roberts[2]

[1] InferSpace, 143 Village Way, Pinner HA5 5AA, UK.
richard@inferspace.com
[2] University of Oxford, Department of Engineering Science, Parks Road, Oxford OX1 3PJ, UK.
sjrob@robots.ox.ac.uk

Summary. We present a collection of examples that illustrate how probabilistic models can be applied within medical informatics, along with the relevant statistical theory.

We begin by listing the desirable features of a clinical probability model and then proceed to look at a wide range of techniques that can be used for model development. These include logistic regression, neural networks, Bayesian networks, class probability trees, and hidden Markov models.

Because of the growing interest in applying Bayesian techniques to probabilistic models, we have emphasized the Bayesian approach throughout the chapter.

10.1 Probabilities in Medicine

Two fundamental activities of medicine are diagnosis (disease identification) and prognosis (forecasting patient outcome). It is possible to express both diagnosis and prognosis probabilistically; for example, statement ξ in conditional probability $p(\xi|clinical\ observations)$ can refer to the presence of a particular disease or to a patient's survival whilst in hospital. In this chapter, we will illustrate various approaches that have been used in practice to estimate this type of probability. The use of probabilistic models for detection in biomedical data is discussed in the final section.

We have not attempted an exhaustive review of the literature. Instead, we have compiled an "anthology" that illustrates a number of examples, which we have combined with relevant theory.

10.2 Desiderata for Probability Models

There are several features that we would like to see in a probability model:

- *High accuracy.* Clearly, we would like the estimate of a class conditional probability provided by a model to be as close as possible to the correct value for that conditional probability.
- *High discrimination.* The misclassification rate (or, better still, the misclassification cost) exhibited by a probability model should be as low as possible.
- *Accessible interpretation.* Instead of existing as a "black box", the model should provide a set of input-output relationships that are comprehensible to the intended user. There are several advantages to having an interpretable model. One advantage is that the model may provide a previously unknown but useful input-output summary: an educational role. Another advantage is that an input-output summary can be compared with known facts. This may disclose an error in the model: a diagnostic role.
- *Short construction time.* The time taken to construct a model should be as short as possible. This is advantageous if the model has to be updated with new data on a regular basis.
- *Short running time.* Once a probability model is built, the time taken to compute a result from the model should be as short as possible, particularly for real-time applications.
- *Robust to missing data.* Missing data are a reality for many clinical data sets; therefore, it should be possible to build a probability model from an incomplete data set, and it should also be possible to apply the probability model to a new but incomplete feature vector.
- *Ability to incorporate pre-existing knowledge.* Inclusion of background knowledge can aid model development and make the interpretation of a model more accessible.

In the following sections, where appropriate, we will highlight the extent to which the above desiderata are fulfilled by the techniques under discussion.

10.3 Bayesian Statistics

The two ideologies of statistics are the Bayesian approach and the classical or frequentist approach [e.g., 7].

The aim of both Bayesian and classical statistics is to estimate the parameters $\boldsymbol{\phi}$ of a joint probability distribution $p(\mathbf{x}|\boldsymbol{\phi})$ from which a set of observed data $\mathcal{D}$ were sampled. In classical statistics, this is usually done by estimating the parameters $\hat{\boldsymbol{\phi}}$ that maximize the likelihood $p(\mathcal{D}|\boldsymbol{\phi})$: the *maximum likelihood approach* [e.g., 5]. Once obtained, the *maximum likelihood estimate* (MLE) $\hat{\boldsymbol{\phi}}$ provides the estimated distribution $p(\mathbf{x}|\hat{\boldsymbol{\phi}})$ from which inferences can be made.

In the classical approach, which is discussed in more detail in Chapter 1, Section 1.2, uncertainty in the estimate $\hat{\boldsymbol{\phi}}$ is traditionally quantified using a 95% confidence interval; however, this is *not* to be interpreted as a 95% chance of ϕ residing within the interval; the correct interpretation of the classical confidence interval is given in Section 1.2. Furthermore, the classical confidence interval is either based on an asymptotic behaviour of maximum likelihood estimates, which does not hold for small-sized samples, or else bootstrapping is used. The latter approach, which is described in Section 1.2, and illustrated in Figure 1.5, usually suffers from exorbitant computational costs (see the caption of Figure 4.35 on for a discussion).

Bayesian statistics, introduced in more detail in Section 1.3, provides an alternative framework with which to consider parameter uncertainty. Instead of striving for a point estimate of ϕ (the classical approach), a Bayesian considers a probability distribution for ϕ, with $p(\phi|\mathcal{D})$ expressing the uncertainty in ϕ given $\mathcal{D}$. If $p(\phi)$ is the assumed distribution of ϕ prior to observing $\mathcal{D}$, *Bayes' theorem*

$$p(\phi|\mathcal{D}) \propto p(\phi)p(\mathcal{D}|\phi) \tag{10.1}$$

represents how a Bayesian's belief in ϕ has changed on observing $\mathcal{D}$ (*Bayesian updating*). Relationship (10.1) holds irrespective of the sample size, and a natural interpretation can be given to the 95% confidence interval based on $p(\phi|\mathcal{D})$ (the *credible interval*). If a single estimate of ϕ is required, the mode of $p(\phi|\mathcal{D})$, the *maximum a posteriori* (MAP), can be quoted.

Although the MAP for ϕ is expected to differ from its MLE because of the influence of the prior $p(\phi)$ in (10.1), this influence decreases as the size of $\mathcal{D}$ increases, which causes the MAP to converge toward the MLE. Increasing the size of $\mathcal{D}$ also decreases the variance of $p(\phi|\mathcal{D})$ and, thus, the uncertainty in ϕ. If there is no preferred shape for the prior distribution $p(\phi)$, a flat (*uninformative*) prior can be used, which makes all possible values of ϕ equally likely.[3] In this case, the MAP and MLE will coincide, even when sample sizes are small; Section 1.4 for a more comprehensive discussion.

10.3.1 Parameter Averaging and Model Averaging

Suppose that we have a model $\mathcal{M}$ that enables us to determine the probability that $y = 1$ when a vector of features $\mathbf{x}$ is given.[4] We can write this probability as $p(y = 1|\mathbf{x}, \boldsymbol{\theta})$, where $\boldsymbol{\theta}$ is a vector of model parameters. Suppose also that $\mathcal{D}$ is a set of exemplars sampled from the same distribution that provided $\mathbf{x}$. The classical approach to using $p(y = 1|\mathbf{x}, \boldsymbol{\theta}, \mathcal{M})$ is to first obtain the MLE $\hat{\boldsymbol{\theta}}$ from $\mathcal{D}$ and then use $\hat{\boldsymbol{\theta}}$ for the parameters of the model; in other words, predictions are based on $p(y = 1|\mathbf{x}, \hat{\boldsymbol{\theta}}, \mathcal{M})$. The Bayesian approach, on the other hand, is to regard all the possible values of $\boldsymbol{\theta}$, and to average over these possibilities according to their posterior distribution $p(\boldsymbol{\theta}|\mathcal{D}, \mathcal{M})$:

$$p(y = 1|\mathbf{x}, \mathcal{M}, \mathcal{D}) = \int_{\boldsymbol{\theta}} p(y = 1|\mathbf{x}, \boldsymbol{\theta}, \mathcal{M})p(\boldsymbol{\theta}|\mathcal{D}, \mathcal{M})\mathrm{d}\boldsymbol{\theta}. \tag{10.2}$$

[3] There are challenges with using priors. Kass and Wasserman [80] and Irony and Singpurwalla [65] provide discussions on this topic. See also Section 11.3.2

[4] y denotes a class label.

Equation (10.2) fully accounts for parameter uncertainty.

Of course, in addition to being uncertain about $\boldsymbol{\theta}$ for a given $\mathcal{M}$, we can also be uncertain about $\mathcal{M}$; however, in the Bayesian framework, we can deal with model uncertainty in an analogous way to how parameter uncertainty was handled. In other words, if $p(\mathcal{M}|\mathcal{D})$ is the posterior distribution over the set of all possible models, we can take account of the model uncertainty by averaging over these models:

$$p(y=1|\mathbf{x},\mathcal{D}) = \sum_{\mathcal{M}} p(y=1|\mathbf{x},\mathcal{M},\mathcal{D})p(\mathcal{M}|\mathcal{D}). \tag{10.3}$$

Thus, both model and parameter uncertainty can be accounted for by using Equation (10.3) in combination with (10.2).[5]

Because of the advantages of the Bayesian paradigm, we will emphasize its use throughout this chapter.

10.3.2 Computations

With maximum-likelihood estimation, most of the computational effort is concerned with the optimization of likelihood $p(\mathcal{D}|\boldsymbol{\theta})$ as a function of $\boldsymbol{\theta}$. In contrast, Bayesian inference requires integration over multidimensional spaces, such as the integration required for Equation (10.2).

A practical problem with Bayesian inference is determining an integration such as (10.2) for realistically complex posterior distributions $p(\boldsymbol{\theta}|\mathcal{D})$. For most practical problems, a solution will not be available analytically. In some cases, the required integration can be achieved satisfactorily through the use of simplifying assumptions or approximations; if not, computational tools are required.

A computational tool that simplifies the Bayesian analysis of even the most complex data is *Markov chain Monte Carlo* (MCMC) [e.g., 50]. This technique was introduced by physicists in 1953 [103, 57], and its adoption by the statistical community has been supported by the advances in computing technology that have taken place since the early 1980s. Basically, MCMC provides a mechanism for generating observations from an arbitrarily complex probability distribution, such as the posterior distribution associated with a Bayesian analysis.

To illustrate the use of MCMC, consider Equation (10.2). This equation can be approximated as

$$p(y=1|\mathbf{x},\mathcal{M},\mathcal{D}) \approx \frac{1}{L}\sum_{i=1}^{L} p(y=1|\mathbf{x},\boldsymbol{\theta}_i,\mathcal{M}),$$

where $\{\boldsymbol{\theta}_1,\ldots,\boldsymbol{\theta}_L\}$ represents a random sample from the posterior distribution $p(\boldsymbol{\theta}|\mathcal{D})$. MCMC can generate this sample, as discussed in Section 2.2.2.

[5] The computation of the marginal likelihood $p(\mathcal{D}|\mathcal{M})$, on which the posterior $p(\mathcal{M}|\mathcal{D})$ depends via $p(\mathcal{D}|\mathcal{M}) \propto p(\mathcal{D}|\mathcal{M})p(\mathcal{M})$, is discussed in Section 2.2.1.

10.4 Logistic Regression

In a regression analysis of y regressed on $\mathbf{x}$, we design a function (*regression function*) $f(\mathbf{x}, \boldsymbol{\theta})$ such that

$$\widehat{\mathcal{E}}(Y|\mathbf{x}; \boldsymbol{\theta}) = f(\mathbf{x}, \boldsymbol{\theta}), \tag{10.4}$$

where $\boldsymbol{\theta}$ is a vector of model parameters. In the classic approach, this is done by estimating the parameter vector $\hat{\boldsymbol{\theta}}$ that maximizes the likelihood function $p(\mathcal{D}|\boldsymbol{\theta})$ with respect to a given data set $\mathcal{D}$.

If Y is binary-valued for a two-class classification problem, (10.4) can be replaced by

$$\widehat{p}(y = 1|\mathbf{x}; \boldsymbol{\theta}) = f(\mathbf{x}, \boldsymbol{\theta}), \tag{10.5}$$

in which case the regression function provides a probability model.

In medical informatics, the most common approach to deriving (10.5) is to use *logistic regression* [63, 26, 81, 55]. A main-effects logistic regression model with regression coefficients $\boldsymbol{\beta}$ has the form

$$\widehat{p}(y = 1|\mathbf{x}; \boldsymbol{\beta}) = \ell\left(\beta_0 + \sum_i \beta_i x_i\right), \tag{10.6}$$

where ℓ is the logistic function: $\ell(\xi) = \exp(\xi)/(1 + \exp(\xi))$. Because of the exponential nature of ℓ, the MLE of $\boldsymbol{\beta}$ cannot be determined analytically; instead it is obtained iteratively, typically using an iterative weighted least-squares procedure [35].

Example 1. The primary role of intensive care units (ICUs) is to monitor and stabilize the vital functions of patients with life-threatening conditions. To aid ICU nurses and intensivists with this work, *scoring systems* have been developed to express the overall state of an ICU patient as a numerical value.

At first, the scoring systems were additive models $\sum_{i=1}^{M} \alpha_i(x_i)$, where function $\alpha_i(\cdot)$ gave the number of points associated with attribute value x_i [85, 82, 48]. The selection of attributes and functions were determined subjectively through panels of experts. Lemeshow et al. [92] replaced the use of subjective additive models with logistic regression, where the response variable is a defined outcome (e.g., alive whilst in hospital). This approach is used in the probabilistic scoring systems APACHE III [84], SAPS II [47], and MPM II [91]. A comparison of scoring systems has shown that those derived by logistic regression perform similarly to each other but are better than those obtained subjectively [22].

Prognostic logistic regression models have been used in various ways for intensive-care medicine. These include the stratification of patients for therapeutic drug trials [83] and the comparison of ICUs [67]. ◁

Sometimes, the linear functional form of a main-effects logistic regression model does not provide an adequate model, and multiplicative interaction terms have to be included; for example,

$$\widehat{p}(y=1|\mathbf{x};\boldsymbol{\beta}) = \ell\left(\beta_0 + \sum_i \beta_i x_i + \sum_{i<j} \beta_{ij} x_i x_j + \sum_{i<j<k} \beta_{ijk} x_i x_j x_k\right). \quad (10.7)$$

Example 2. Hosmer and Lemeshow [63] describe a logistic regression analysis of low birth-weight data, birth weight less than 2500 g being the binary response variable Y. The candidate explanatory variables included mother's age (X_1), weight at last menstrual period less than 110 lb (X_2), black skinned (X_3), neither white or black skinned (X_4), smoked during pregnancy (X_5), history of premature labour (X_6), history of hypertension (X_7), and uterine irritability present (X_8). The main-effects model with the sum

$$\begin{aligned} -1.217 &- 0.046X_1 + 0.842X_2 + 1.073X_3 + 0.815X_4 \\ &+ 0.807X_5 + 1.282X_6 + 1.435X_7 + 0.658X_8 \end{aligned}$$

had a log-likelihood of -98.78; however, the addition of two multiplicative interaction terms

$$\begin{aligned} -0.512 &- 0.084X_1 - 1.730X_2 + 1.083X_3 + 0.760X_4 \\ &+ 1.153X_5 + 1.232X_6 + 1.359X_7 + 0.728X_8 \\ &+ 0.147X_1X_2 - 1.407X_5X_2 \end{aligned}$$

improved the fit, the log-likelihood increasing to -96.01. $\triangleleft$

In addition to including interaction terms, it may also be necessary to transform some of the variables in order to improve the fit of a logistic regression model to data. A classic approach is the Box–Cox method [15]. Other possible problems that need to be considered are the presence of collinearity and overly influential observations [e.g., 63, 26, 55].

10.5 Bayesian Logistic Regression

There are two problems with the classic approach to logistic regression given above. Firstly, there is the assumption that variables Y and $\mathbf{X}$ are related by a single model with a pre-specified structure $\mathcal{M}$, but this does not take account of the fact that we are uncertain about $\mathcal{M}$. Secondly, for a given choice of $\mathcal{M}$, we are, in truth, uncertain about the vector $\boldsymbol{\beta}$ of parameter values associated with $\mathcal{M}$, yet the maximum-likelihood approach imposes a single set of parameter values on $\mathcal{M}$. In principle, these two criticisms can be addressed by regarding logistic regression within the framework of Bayesian statistics.

In the Bayesian framework, we express the uncertainty in parameter vector $\boldsymbol{\beta}$ for a given model $\mathcal{M}$ by the posterior probability distribution $p(\boldsymbol{\beta}|\mathcal{M},\mathcal{D})$, where $\mathcal{D}$ is the observed data; therefore, we have

$$p(y=1|\mathbf{x},\mathcal{M},\mathcal{D}) = \int_{\boldsymbol{\beta}} p(y=1|\mathbf{x},\boldsymbol{\beta},\mathcal{M})p(\boldsymbol{\beta}|\mathcal{M},\mathcal{D})\mathrm{d}\boldsymbol{\beta}. \tag{10.8}$$

where

$$p(y=1|\mathbf{x},\boldsymbol{\beta},\mathcal{M}) = \left\{1+\exp\left[-\boldsymbol{\beta}^{\mathsf{T}}\mathbf{x}\right]\right\}^{-1}. \tag{10.9}$$

A common Bayesian assumption is that the posterior distribution $p(\boldsymbol{\beta}|M,\mathcal{D})$ is Gaussian, but, with $p(y=1|\mathbf{x},\boldsymbol{\beta},\mathcal{M})$ defined by (10.8), the resulting integral in (10.8) cannot be solved analytically. However, Spiegelhalter and Lauritzen [149] derived the approximation

$$\int_{\theta}(1+\exp[-\theta])^{-1}p(\theta|\nu,\sigma^2)\mathrm{d}\theta \approx (1+\exp[-c\nu])^{-1}, \tag{10.10}$$

where $\theta \sim Normal(\nu,\sigma^2)$ and c is equal to $(1+\xi^2\sigma^2)^{-1/2}$ for an appropriate value of ξ. This was done via the approximation

$$(1+\exp[-\theta])^{-1} \approx \Phi(\xi\theta), \tag{10.11}$$

where Φ is the probit function [31].

If ξ^2 is set equal to $\pi/8$, as suggested by MacKay [99], then, from (10.9) and (10.10), we obtain the *Spiegelhalter–Lauritzen–MacKay (SLM) approximation*

$$p(y=1|\mathbf{x},\mathcal{M},\mathcal{D}) \approx \left\{1+\exp\left[-\boldsymbol{\beta}_{\mathrm{MP}}^{\mathsf{T}}\mathbf{x}\Big/\sqrt{1+\frac{\pi\mathsf{Var}(\boldsymbol{\beta}^{\mathsf{T}}\mathbf{x}|\mathbf{x},\mathcal{M},\mathcal{D})}{8}}\right]\right\}^{-1}, \tag{10.12}$$

where $\boldsymbol{\beta}_{\mathrm{MP}}$ is the mode of $p(\boldsymbol{\beta}|\mathcal{M},\mathcal{D})$, and $\mathsf{Var}(\boldsymbol{\beta}^{\mathsf{T}}\mathbf{x}|\mathbf{x},\mathcal{M},\mathcal{D})$ is the variance of the posterior distribution $p(\boldsymbol{\beta}^{\mathsf{T}}\mathbf{x}|\mathbf{x},\mathcal{M},\mathcal{D})$. Bishop [13] discusses the error in ignoring the square root in (10.12).

There is, however, still the uncertainty in the choice for model $\mathcal{M}$. This uncertainty can be dealt with by averaging over all possible models:

$$p(y=1|\mathbf{x},\mathcal{D}) = \sum_{\mathcal{M}} p(y=1|\mathbf{x},\mathcal{M},\mathcal{D})p(\mathcal{M}|\mathcal{D}), \tag{10.13}$$

where $p(\mathcal{M}|\mathcal{D})$ is the posterior probability for model $\mathcal{M}$. On substituting (10.8) into (10.13), we have the general expression for *Bayesian model-averaged logistic regression*:

$$p(y=1|\mathbf{x},\mathcal{D}) = \sum_{\mathcal{M}}\int_{\boldsymbol{\beta}} p(y=1|\mathbf{x},\boldsymbol{\beta},\mathcal{M})p(\boldsymbol{\beta}|\mathcal{M},\mathcal{D})\mathrm{d}\boldsymbol{\beta}\,p(\mathcal{M}|\mathcal{D}). \tag{10.14}$$

The SLM approximation provides an estimate of $p(y = 1|\mathbf{x}, \mathcal{M}, \mathcal{D})$ for (10.13), but, in order to perform model-averaging, we also need the posterior model probability $p(\mathcal{M}|\mathcal{D})$. In Section **??**, we discuss the GLIB S-Plus function for estimating this probability, but first we consider the evaluation of the mode and variance required for (10.12).

10.5.1 Gibbs Sampling and GLIB

One route to estimating the mode and variance for (10.12) is to use the *evidence framework* scheme proposed by MacKay [100] and recommended by Bishop [13]; however, the approximations required to satisfy this scheme sometimes make it unreliable. Section 2.3.2 discusses the evidence framework and its disadvantages. An alternative approach is to obtained estimates of the regression coefficients via Gibbs sampling.

Gibbs sampling, illustrated in Figure 5.23, provides a Markov chain simulation of a random walk in the space of $\boldsymbol{\beta}$, which converges to a stationary distribution that equals the joint distribution $p(\boldsymbol{\beta}|\mathcal{M}, \mathcal{D})$ [50]; however, in practice, the convergence is only approximate. In addition to providing an estimate of the mode $\boldsymbol{\beta}_{\text{MP}}$ for (10.12), the stationary distribution also provides an estimate of the variance of $\boldsymbol{\beta}^{\mathsf{T}}\mathbf{x}$ via the estimated covariance for $\boldsymbol{\beta}$. The freeware BUGS package provides a convenient environment in which to conduct Gibbs sampling (Chapter 2).

GLIB

Bayesian model averaging can be performed using the freeware GLIB package [124], which is designed for use within S-Plus. For a given set of models $\mathcal{M}_0, \mathcal{M}_1, \ldots \mathcal{M}_K$ (where $\mathcal{M}_0$ is the null (intercept-only) model), GLIB can estimate the model posterior probabilities $p(\mathcal{M}_k|\mathcal{D})$ for each model in (10.13) through the use of Bayes factors. The *Bayes factor* $B_{i,j}$ associated with models $\mathcal{M}_i$ and $\mathcal{M}_j$ is defined as

$$B_{i,j} = p(\mathcal{D}|\mathcal{M}_i)/p(\mathcal{D}|\mathcal{M}_j). \tag{10.15}$$

Raftery [122] showed that application of the Laplace approximation to the integral in the expression

$$p(\mathcal{D}|\mathcal{M}_k) = \int_{\boldsymbol{\beta}} p(\mathcal{D}|\boldsymbol{\beta}, \mathcal{M}_k)p(\boldsymbol{\beta}|\mathcal{M}_k)\mathrm{d}\boldsymbol{\beta} \tag{10.16}$$

gives an approximation for $\ln B_{k,0}$ that can be calculated using quantities readily provided by regression packages such as GLIM. This enables $p(\mathcal{M}_k|\mathcal{D})$ to be determined through the relationship

$$p(\mathcal{M}_k|\mathcal{D}) = \alpha_k B_{k,0} \Big/ \sum_{r=0}^{K} \alpha_r B_{r,0} \ , \tag{10.17}$$

where $\alpha_k = p(\mathcal{M}_k)/p(\mathcal{M}_0)$. The prior distribution $p(\boldsymbol{\beta}|\mathcal{M}_k)$ in (10.16) is defined by three hyperparameters: ν_1, ψ, and ϕ [78]. GLIB fixes ν_1 and ψ to 1, and ϕ is set to 1.65 by default, because Raftery [122] found these values to be reasonable.

If the number of candidate models is very large, the total time taken by GLIB to compute $p(\mathcal{M}_k|\mathcal{D})$ for each model can be lengthy. In such a situation, a pragmatic approach is to use the `bic.logit` S-Plus function [125]. This uses an approximation for $\ln B_{k,0}$ [123] based on the Bayesian Information Criterion described in Section 2.3.2. Although this approximation is less accurate than that used by GLIB for $\ln B_{k,0}$, `bic.logit` can filter out a large number of candidate models by implementing the following model-selection criteria [121]:

- **First criterion for model selection**
  If a model is far less likely a posteriori than the most likely model, it should be excluded. Therefore, exclude $\mathcal{M}_k$ if

$$p(\mathcal{M}_k|\mathcal{D}) < 0.05p(\mathcal{M}_\star|\mathcal{D}), \tag{10.18}$$

  where $\mathcal{M}_\star$ is the model with maximum $p(\mathcal{M}|\mathcal{D})$. This inequality is equivalent to

$$2\ln B_{k,0} < 2\ln B_{\star,0} - 5.99 \tag{10.19}$$

  if $p(\mathcal{M}_k) = p(\mathcal{M}_\star)$ for all k.
- **Second criterion for model selection (Occam's Window)**
  Exclude any model that receives less support from the data than a simpler model that is nested within it. Therefore, exclude $\mathcal{M}_k$ if there exists $\mathcal{M}_j$ nested within it for which

$$p(\mathcal{M}_j|\mathcal{D}) > p(\mathcal{M}_k|\mathcal{D}). \tag{10.20}$$

  This inequality is equivalent to

$$2\ln B_{j,0} > 2\ln B_{k,0}. \tag{10.21}$$

Example 3. Raftery and Richardson [124] illustrate the use of GLIB for model selection. They used data from a case–control study (379 cases; 475 controls) of risk factors associated with breast cancer. There were 16 possible logistic regression models resulting from the dichotomous inclusion of the following four variables: *alc*, the number of alcoholic drinks per week; *alc*0, whether a person was a drinker or nondrinker; *tfat*, total number of grams of fat consumed per week; and *tsat*, total number of grams of saturated fat consumed per week. In addition, all the models included the classical risk factors associated with breast cancer; namely, age, menopausal status, age at menarche, parity, familial breast cancer, history of benign breast disease, age at end of schooling, and Quetelet's index.

Application of the two model-selection criteria described above resulted in five models (Table 10.1). Model selection was robust to changes in the value of ϕ, the prior variance of the regression parameters. In this example, the regression coefficients estimated under the different models do not vary much; however, Raftery and Richardson point out that this lack of variation across models is not a general occurrence, and inclusion of interaction terms could substantially vary the regression coefficients. $\triangleleft$

Table 10.1. The models selected by Raftery and Richardson [124] using GLIB. The table includes the posterior model probabilities obtained with three values for ϕ. Reprinted from [124] pp. 343 and 345, by courtesy of Marcel Dekker Inc.

	Posterior model probabilities			Regression coefficients			
Model ID	$\phi = 1.00$	$\phi = 1.65$	$\phi = 5.00$	*alc*0	*alc*	*tfat*	*tsat*
3	0.08	0.13	0.31	0.734	–	–	–
7	0.04	0.04	0.03	–	0.038	0.0017	–
8	0.06	0.06	0.05	–	0.039	–	0.0052
9	0.33	0.31	0.25	0.691	–	0.0017	–
10	0.49	0.46	0.37	0.704	–	–	0.0051

10.5.2 Hierarchical Models

A criticism of the Bayesian paradigm is that prior information is rarely rich enough to exactly define a prior distribution, and the uncertainty of priors should be included in a Bayesian model. A *hierarchical Bayesian model* does this by decomposing the prior distribution of the parameters of a model into several conditional levels of distributions. Uncertainty at any level is incorporated into additional prior distributions, thereby creating a hierarchy.

Example 4. An example of hierarchical logistic regression is provided by Clyde et al. [24]. We have created a simplified version for instructional purposes.

For our hierarchical model, we assume that each of the N patients $(y_i, \mathbf{x}_i)$ $(i = 1, \ldots, N)$ in a data set $\mathcal{D}$ has a separate logistic model. The parameters for each model, $(\beta_{i0}, \ldots, \beta_{i|\mathbf{x}|})^{\mathsf{T}} = \boldsymbol{\beta}_i$, are assumed to come from a normal distribution defined by the *hyperparameters* mean μ and variance τ^{-1}, which represents the distribution of the population of the patients. Finally, we use noninformative *hyperpriors* for μ and τ^{-1}. Thus, we have the following hierarchical model:

$$\begin{aligned}
y_i &\sim Bernoulli(p(y_i = 1|\mathbf{x}_i, \boldsymbol{\beta}_i)) \\
\text{logit}[p(y_i = 1|\mathbf{x}_i, \boldsymbol{\beta}_i)] &= \boldsymbol{\beta}_i^{\mathsf{T}}\mathbf{x}_i \\
\boldsymbol{\beta}_{ij} &\sim Normal(\mu, \tau^{-1}) \\
\mu &\sim Normal(0, 10^6) \\
\tau &\sim Gamma(10^{-3}, 10^{-3})
\end{aligned}$$

Gibbs sampling under this model will generate an approximate sample from the posterior distribution $p(\boldsymbol{\beta}_1, \ldots, \boldsymbol{\beta}_N, \mu, \tau|\mathcal{D})$. $\triangleleft$

10.6 Neural Networks

10.6.1 Multi-Layer Perceptrons

Multi-layer perceptrons (MLPs) are the neural networks most commonly encountered in medical research [e.g., 39, 32].[6] A one-hidden-layer MLP with logistic activation functions and a single output node o can be represented by

$$\widehat{p}(y = 1|\mathbf{x}; \mathbf{w}) = \ell\left(w_{(1\to o)} + \sum_h w_{(h\to o)}\ell\left(w_{(1\to h)} + \sum_x w_{(x\to h)}x\right)\right), \tag{10.22}$$

where ℓ is the logistic function (i.e., $\ell(\xi) = \exp(\xi)/(1 + \exp(\xi))$), Σ_h sums over all the hidden nodes, Σ_x sums over all the input nodes, and $w_{(i\to j)} \in \mathbf{w}$ is the *weight* on the connection from node i to node j. Weights $w_{(1\to o)}$ and $w_{(1\to h)}$ are *biases*. From (10.6), it is seen that (10.22) can be regarded as a nonlinear extension of logistic regression consisting of nested logistic models (Chapter 3).

In the standard approach to training an MLP, the MLE of the parameters (weights) $\mathbf{w}$ is found with respect to the negative log likelihood $-\log p(D|\mathbf{w})$ using an optimization procedure. This is often done using the conjugate-gradient or BFGS quasi-Newton algorithm [13, pp. 247–290]. The convention in the neural-network community is to refer to $-\log p(D|\mathbf{w})$ as an *error function* $E(\mathbf{w})$. For probabilistic classification MLPs, the cross-entropy error function $E_{ce}(\mathbf{w})$ should be used, which has $p(D|\mathbf{w})$ identical to that used in logistic regression. Furthermore, in order to prevent overfitting, the error function is augmented with a *regularization term*, which penalizes the creation of large curvatures by the MLP (Section 3.5.1). The most commonly used regularization term is the *weight decay* term:

$$E(\mathbf{w}) = E_{ce}(\mathbf{w}) + \frac{\nu}{2}\sum_{w_i \in \mathbf{w}} w_i^2, \tag{10.23}$$

[6] Chapter 3 provides a short tutorial on MLPs.

where ν is the *regularization constant.* The optimal value for ν has to be determined by trial and error; however, in the Bayesian approach to neural networks (Section 10.7), it can be obtained in a principled manner.

Given the potential of MLPs to model arbitrarily complex functions, and the potentially complex nature of clinical data, interest in the application of MLPs to medical problems increased during the 1990s.

Example 5. The PAPNET computer system [14, 87] was developed to aid the screening of cervico-vaginal smears, a task normally performed manually by technicians. The motivation for developing PAPNET was to reduce misclassification rates [157] and increase sample throughput.

The input to PAPNET is a digitized image of a smear consisting of about 50,000 to 250,000 cells; the output is an abnormality score for each cell and cluster in the smear. Two MLPs are used: one identifies abnormal cells; the other locates abnormal clusters. PAPNET does not provide a final diagnosis; instead, the 64 highest scoring cells and the 64 highest scoring clusters are recorded for the attention of a cytologist.

The published results on the efficacy of PAPNET are varied. For example, Jenny et al. [71] reported that a false negative rate of 5.7% in conventional screening was reduced to 0.4% by PAPNET. In contrast, the PRISMATIC project [119] found the true positive rate for PAPNET-assisted screening (82%) to be similar to that found for conventional screening (83%). However, the same study showed a significantly better true negative rate (77%) for PAPNET-assisted screening than for conventional screening (42%). The total mean time for screening and reporting for conventional screening was 104 min per smear, and for PAPNET-assisted screening it was 39 min.

As a result of a study by Koss et al. [88], the Food and Drug Administration of the United States approved PAPNET as a quality control instrument [87]. $\triangleleft$

10.6.2 Radial-Basis-Function Neural Networks

Equation (10.22) for an MLP can be rewritten as

$$\widehat{p}(y=1|\mathbf{x};\mathbf{w}) = \ell\left(w_{(1\to o)} + \sum_{h} w_{(h\to o)} g_h(\mathbf{x})\right); \tag{10.24}$$

thus, the associated MLP can be regarded as a two-stage structure. In the first stage, there is a projection of $\mathbf{x}$ to an H-dimensional vector $[g_1(\mathbf{x})\cdots g_H(\mathbf{x})]^\mathsf{T}$, where H is the number of hidden nodes in (10.22). The logistic function ℓ is then applied to this vector in the second stage.

A *radial-basis-function network* (RBFNN) for probabilistic classification has a similar form to (10.24),

$$\widehat{p}(y=1|\mathbf{x};\mathbf{w}) = \ell\left(w_0 + \sum_{m=1}^{M} w_m \phi_h(\mathbf{x})\right), \tag{10.25}$$

but *radial basis functions* (RBFs) have replaced the hidden nodes of the MLP.

Unlike an MLP, an RBFNN is constructed in two distinctive steps. First, RBFs $\phi_1, \ldots, \phi_M$ are defined, and, once defined, the parameters of the RBFs are fixed. In the second step, $\phi_1(\mathbf{x}) \ldots \phi_M(\mathbf{x})$ are treated as covariates, and logistic regression is used to estimate the regression coefficients (weights) $w_0, w_1, \ldots, w_M$. When a single output node is used (i.e., the two-class case), the coefficients can be obtained using the usual iterated weighted least squares algorithm of logistic regression [106], which will converge to a single maximum likelihood [4]. The situation for softmax regression (i.e., the multi-class case) is more complicated. Here, Nabney [106] suggests several approaches, including exact determination of a Hessian matrix.

Example 6. Goodacre et al. [52] developed a RBFNN with 2283 inputs (wave numbers from high-dimensional Raman spectra) to discriminate between common infectious agents associated with urinary tract infection. Although the performance of the RBFNN was similar to that of an MLP built with the same inputs, the time required to train the RBFNN was only 2 min, far less than the 30-hour training time required for the MLP. ◁

10.6.3 "Probabilistic Neural Networks"

Kernel density estimation is a nonparametric method for estimating probability distributions [145]. Suppose we have a data set $\mathcal{D}$ consisting of n exemplars, n_k of which are associated with class k. Let $\mathcal{D}^{\{k\}}$ be the subset of $\mathcal{D}$ containing these n_k exemplars. A symmetric *kernel function* $K(\mathbf{x} - \mathbf{x}_i)$ is centered on each $\mathbf{x}_i$ in $\mathcal{D}^{\{k\}}$, and the average of these kernel functions provides an estimate of the class-conditional probability distribution $p(\mathbf{x}|k)$:[7]

$$\widehat{p}(\mathbf{x}|k) = \frac{1}{n_k} \sum_{\mathbf{x}_i \in \mathcal{D}^{\{k\}}} K(\mathbf{x} - \mathbf{x}_i) \ .$$

Consequently, from Bayes' theorem and the estimate $\widehat{p}(k) = n_k/n$, we have

$$\begin{aligned} \widehat{p}(k|\mathbf{x}) &= \frac{\widehat{p}(k)\widehat{p}(\mathbf{x}|k)}{\sum_{k'} \widehat{p}(k')\widehat{p}(\mathbf{x}|k')} \\ &= \frac{\sum_{\mathbf{x}_i \in \mathcal{D}^{\{k\}}} K(\mathbf{x} - \mathbf{x}_i)}{\sum_{k'} \sum_{\mathbf{x}_i \in \mathcal{D}^{\{k'\}}} K(\mathbf{x} - \mathbf{x}_i)} \ . \end{aligned} \tag{10.26}$$

Confusingly, expression (10.26) has been called a *probabilistic neural network* even though there is no apparent biological motivation for doing this.

[7] If $K(\mathbf{x} - \mathbf{x}_i)$ integrates to one then the same is true for $\widehat{p}(\mathbf{x}|k)$.

10.6.4 Missing Data

General responses to the occurrence of missing data are to exclude incomplete exemplars or fill in missing parts with estimates (*imputation*). Unfortunately, imputation is often done in an ad hoc manner; for example, using the unconditional mean or median of the observed values of a variable. When unjustified, these methods can give rise to biased models [49].

There are theoretically sound approaches to the problem of missing data, but the choice of method depends on the type of inference to be made and the assumed missing-data mechanism. A common situation is when a Bayesian- or likelihood-based estimate is required, and the missing-data mechanism is assumed to be ignorable. According to Schafer [142], a mechanism is *ignorable*[8] when (a) the probability that an observation is missing may depend on the observed values $\mathcal{D}_{obs}$ but not on the missing values $\mathcal{D}_{mis}$ (*missing at random* [139]), and (b) the parameters of the missing-data mechanism are distinct from the parameters of the data model $\boldsymbol{\theta}$ (*distinction of parameters*). When ignorability holds, and a data model $p(\mathbf{x}_{obs}, \mathbf{x}_{mis}|\boldsymbol{\theta})$ is assumed, the EM algorithm can be used to impute the missing values by switching iteratively between a current estimate of the parameter $\hat{\boldsymbol{\theta}}$ and a current estimate of the complete data set $(\mathcal{D}_{obs}, \widehat{\mathcal{D}}_{mis})$. The completed data set obtained on convergence can be used to fit a regression model.

A problem with fitting a regression model to a completed data set $(\mathcal{D}_{obs}, \widehat{\mathcal{D}}_{mis})$ is that the resulting model does not convey the uncertainty of the imputations $\widehat{\mathcal{D}}_{imp}$. This can be overcome by assigning a number of imputations $\widehat{\mathcal{D}}_{imp}^{[1]}, \ldots, \widehat{\mathcal{D}}_{imp}^{[\varsigma]}$ to an incomplete data set, fitting a model to each completed data set $(\mathcal{D}_{obs}, \widehat{\mathcal{D}}_{imp}^{[1]}), \ldots, (\mathcal{D}_{obs}, \widehat{\mathcal{D}}_{imp}^{[\varsigma]})$, and averaging over the models (*multiple imputation*) [140, 95]. The spread of the outputs from the models indicates the extent of the uncertainty in the imputations. A standard method for producing multiply-imputed data sets is *data augmentation* [153].

Of course, the existence of a missing-data mechanism implies that a new feature vector could be incomplete. For real-time applications, imputing the new feature vector by a time-consuming iterative technique would be unacceptable; however, there are alternatives:

- Where appropriate, domain heuristics (*cold-deck imputation*) can be adopted, such as the assumption of clinical normality [e.g., 85]
- Sometimes *nearest-neighbour hot-deck imputation* is effective, in which those attribute values contained in the nearest complete case are used [e.g., 94].
- If only a small number η of explanatory variables are prone to incompleteness, 2^{η} regression models could be developed to cover each possible eventuality [e.g., 143].

---

[8] Note that some authors equate "ignorability" to "missing at random" whereas others equate it to "distinction of parameters".

In the context of missing data, there is a virtue in using RBFNNs with Gaussian basis functions if the explanatory variables are continuous. Suppose that

$$\widehat{p}(C_k|\mathbf{x}) = \frac{\sum_{j=1}^{M} w_{kj} G(\mathbf{x}|\boldsymbol{\mu}^{(j)}, \boldsymbol{\Sigma}^{(j)}) p(j)}{\sum_{j=1}^{M} G(\mathbf{x}|\boldsymbol{\mu}^{(j)}, \boldsymbol{\Sigma}^{(j)}) p(j)},$$

is a trained RBFNN with M Gaussian basis functions $G(\mathbf{x}|\boldsymbol{\mu}^{(j)}, \boldsymbol{\Sigma}^{(j)})$, where w_{kj} is the weight from the jth basis function to the node outputting $\widehat{p}(C_k|\mathbf{x})$. Because of a property of multivariate Gaussian distributions, $\widehat{p}(C_k|\mathbf{x}_{obs})$ can be determined for any $\mathbf{x}_{obs} \subseteq \mathbf{x}$ using the existing set of RBFNN parameters w_{kj}, $\boldsymbol{\mu}^{(j)}$, $\boldsymbol{\Sigma}^{(j)}$, and $p(j)$ [156, 49, 38].

10.7 Bayesian Neural Techniques

Adoption of the Bayesian framework by the neural-network community has extended the statistical interpretation of neural networks [e.g., 13, 129] with consequent benefits [e.g., 13, 117]. In fact, Penny et al. [117] have described this development as "second-generation neural computing".

There are several benefits to be had from applying the Bayesian approach to neural networks. These include principled methods for implementing regularization [e.g., 13], variable subset selection (e.g., Chapter 12), and the calculation of error bars [e.g., 41].

When an MLP is trained using the conventional MLE approach, the posterior class-conditional probability $p(y = 1|\mathbf{x}, \mathcal{D})$ is given by

$$p(y = 1|\mathbf{x}, \mathcal{D}) = p(y = 1|\mathbf{x}, \hat{\mathbf{w}}), \tag{10.27}$$

where $\hat{\mathbf{w}}$ is the MLE of weight vector $\mathbf{w}$. A weakness with (10.27) is that it does not take into account the uncertainty associated with $\hat{\mathbf{w}}$; instead, $\hat{\mathbf{w}}$ is treated as if it was the "true" version of $\mathbf{w}$. But, in reality, an infinite number of $\mathbf{w}$ are consistent with $\mathcal{D}$; therefore, a more sensible approach is to take into account all possible $\mathbf{w}$ by integrating over $\mathbf{w}$ space:

$$p(y = 1|\mathbf{x}, \mathcal{D}) = \int_{\mathbf{w}} p(y = 1|\mathbf{x}, \mathbf{w}) p(\mathbf{w}|\mathcal{D}) d\mathbf{w}. \tag{10.28}$$

Integrating out unknown parameters in this manner is a characteristic strategy of the Bayesian framework (Section 10.3.1).

10.7.1 Moderated Output

The single output of a probabilistic MLP can be written as $\ell(r(\mathbf{x}, \mathbf{w}))$, where ℓ is the sigmoidal function of the output node, and $r(\mathbf{x}, \mathbf{w})$ is the input to this node.

An alternative to (10.28) is obtained by using $r(\mathbf{x}, \mathbf{w})$ in place of $\mathbf{w}$:

$$p(y=1|\mathbf{x},\mathcal{D}) = \int_r p(y=1|r)p(r|\mathbf{x},\mathcal{D})\mathrm{d}r \tag{10.29}$$

$$= \int_r \ell(r)p(r|\mathbf{x},\mathcal{D})\mathrm{d}r$$

$$\approx \ell\left[\left(1+\frac{\pi\sigma_r^2(\mathbf{x})}{8}\right)^{-1/2} r(\mathbf{x},\mathbf{w}_{\mathrm{MP}})\right] \quad \text{by (10.12)}, \tag{10.30}$$

where $\sigma_r^2(\mathbf{x})$ is the variance of r. This is given by

$$\sigma_r^2(\mathbf{x}) = \mathbf{h}^{\mathsf{T}}(\mathbf{x})\mathbf{A}^{-1}\mathbf{h}(\mathbf{x}),$$

where element $h_i(\mathbf{x})$ of $\mathbf{h}(\mathbf{x})$ is the partial derivative $\partial r(\mathbf{x},\mathbf{w})/\partial w_i$ at $\mathbf{w}_{\mathrm{MP}}$, and $\mathbf{A}$ is a Hessian matrix, with matrix element $A_{i,j}$ equal to $\partial^2 E(\mathbf{w})/\partial w_i \partial w_j$ at $\mathbf{w}_{\mathrm{MP}}$.

The right-hand side of (10.30) is sometimes referred to as the *moderated output* to distinguish it from the unmoderated output $\ell[r(\mathbf{x},\mathbf{w}_{\mathrm{MP}})]$.

10.7.2 Hyperparameters

The integral of (10.28) contains the posterior probability distribution $p(\mathbf{w}|\mathcal{D})$. This distribution is related to the prior distribution $p(\mathbf{w})$ by Bayes' theorem,

$$p(\mathbf{w}|\mathcal{D}) = p(\mathcal{D}|\mathbf{w})p(\mathbf{w})/p(\mathcal{D}). \tag{10.31}$$

If we assume that the prior is Gaussian,

$$w_i \sim Normal(0, \alpha^{-1}), \tag{10.32}$$

where α is the *hyperparameter*, it follows that $p(\mathbf{w}|\mathcal{D})$ and $p(r|\mathbf{x},\mathcal{D})$ are Gaussian and influenced by α [13]. To take account of the uncertainty in this hyperparameter, we take the Bayesian step of integrating over α as well as r (cf. (10.29)):

$$p(y=1|\mathbf{x},\mathcal{D}) = \int_r p(y=1|r)\int_\alpha p(r|\mathbf{x},\alpha,\mathcal{D})p(\alpha|\mathcal{D})\mathrm{d}\alpha\mathrm{d}r \tag{10.33}$$

$$\approx \int_r p(y=1|r)p(r|\mathbf{x},\alpha_{\mathrm{MP}},\mathcal{D})\mathrm{d}r \tag{10.34}$$

if $p(\alpha|\mathcal{D})$ is sharply peaked at its mode α_{MP}. Comparison of (10.29) with (10.34) suggests that we can replace $r(\mathbf{x},\mathbf{w}_{\mathrm{MP}})$ in the moderated output (10.30) with $r(\mathbf{x},\alpha_{\mathrm{MP}},\mathbf{w}_{\mathrm{MP}})$. But how do we estimate α_{MP} and $\mathbf{w}_{\mathrm{MP}}$?

Both α_{MP} and $\mathbf{w}_{\mathrm{MP}}$ can be determined through the so-called *evidence framework* [e.g., 13].[9] [10] This is done by iterating between the following two steps until convergence is reached:

---

[9] The likelihood $p(\mathcal{D}|\xi)$, where ξ is a statement, is sometimes called the *evidence* for ξ.

[10] Strictly speaking, the evidence-framework approach is not a full Bayesian approach because it does not integrate out the hyperparameters. It is, in fact, a *type-II maximum-likelihood method*.

1. optimize $\mathbf{w}$ for a given α using a standard MLE procedure;
2. re-estimate α using

$$\alpha := \sum_{i=1}^{|\mathbf{w}|} \frac{\lambda_i}{\lambda_i + \alpha} \Big/ \sum_{i=1}^{|\mathbf{w}|} w_i^2 ,$$

where λ_i is an eigenvalue of the Hessian matrix $\mathbf{A} - \alpha\mathbf{I}$.

If $\log p(\mathbf{w}|\mathcal{D})$ is regarded as the total (i.e., regularized) error $E(\mathbf{w})$ [e.g., 117] then from (10.31) and (10.32) (and ignoring the constant term) we have

$$\begin{aligned} E(\mathbf{w}) &= -\log p(\mathcal{D}|\mathbf{w}) - \log p(\mathbf{w}) \\ &= E_{ce}(\mathbf{w}) + \frac{\alpha}{2} \sum_{w_i \in \mathbf{w}} w_i^2, \end{aligned}$$

thus hyperparameter α is acting as the regularization constant ν in (10.23). But the fact that we can determine α_{MP} means that the Bayesian framework has provided us with a principled approach to regularization.

10.7.3 Committees

Suppose that we make the assumption that most of the density of the posterior $p(\mathbf{w}|\mathcal{D})$ is concentrated in non-overlapping regions of $\mathbf{w}$-space that are associated with the maxima of $p(\mathbf{w}|\mathcal{D})$. If $\mathcal{Q}_1, \ldots, \mathcal{Q}_T$ are the regions then

$$p(\mathbf{w}|\mathcal{D}) \approx \sum_{i=1}^{T} p(\mathbf{w}|\mathcal{Q}_i, \mathcal{D}) p(\mathcal{Q}_i|\mathcal{D}); \tag{10.35}$$

consequently, from (10.28), we can write

$$\begin{aligned} p(y=1|\mathbf{x}, \mathcal{D}) &\approx \sum_{i=1}^{T} p(\mathcal{Q}_i|\mathcal{D}) \int_{\mathbf{w} \in \mathcal{Q}_i} p(y=1|\mathbf{x}, \mathbf{w}) p(\mathbf{w}|\mathcal{Q}_i, \mathcal{D}) d\mathbf{w} \\ &= \sum_{i=1}^{T} p(\mathcal{Q}_i|\mathcal{D}) p(y=1|\mathbf{x}, \mathcal{Q}_i, \mathcal{D}). \end{aligned} \tag{10.36}$$

The collection of T models in (10.36) are said to constitute a *committee of networks.*[11]

[11] Regions $\mathcal{Q}_1, \ldots, \mathcal{Q}_T$ are expected to be associated with the minima of an error function $E(\mathbf{w})$. This leads to the maximum-likelihood version of a committee-based prediction,

$$\widehat{p}(y=1|\mathbf{x}) = \frac{1}{T} \sum_{i=1}^{T} p(y=1|\mathbf{x}, \hat{\mathbf{w}}_i),$$

where $\hat{\mathbf{w}}_i$ is the ith local maximum encountered whilst training using random restarts.

An analogous approach can be made using $r(\mathbf{x}, \mathbf{w})$ in place of $\mathbf{w}$. This uses the assumption that, for the posterior $p(r|\mathbf{x}, \mathcal{D})$,

$$p(r|\mathbf{x}, \mathcal{D}) \approx \sum_{i=1}^{T} p(r|\mathbf{x}, \mathcal{R}_i, \mathcal{D}) p(\mathcal{R}_i|\mathcal{D}), \tag{10.37}$$

where $\mathcal{R}_i$ is the region for r corresponding to $\mathcal{Q}_i$ (i.e., $\mathcal{R}_i = \{r(\mathbf{x}, \mathbf{w})|\mathbf{w} \in \mathcal{Q}_i\}$). Substituting (10.37) in (10.29) gives

$$\begin{aligned} p(y=1|\mathbf{x}, \mathcal{D}) &\approx \sum_{i=1}^{T} p(\mathcal{R}_i|\mathcal{D}) \int_{r \in \mathcal{R}_i} p(y=1|r) p(r|\mathbf{x}, \mathcal{R}_i, \mathcal{D}) \mathrm{d}r \\ &= \sum_{i=1}^{T} p(\mathcal{R}_i|\mathcal{D}) \int_{r \in \mathcal{R}_i} \ell(r) p(r|\mathbf{x}, \mathcal{R}_i, \mathcal{D}) \mathrm{d}r \\ &\approx \sum_{i=1}^{T} p(\mathcal{R}_i|\mathcal{D}) \ell \left[\left(1 + \frac{\pi \sigma_r^2(\mathbf{x}; \mathcal{R}_i)}{8} \right)^{-1/2} r(\mathbf{x}, \mathbf{w}_{\mathrm{MP}}; \mathcal{R}_i) \right]. \end{aligned} \tag{10.38}$$

Expression (10.38) provides a moderated output from a committee of networks.

Example 7. Penny et al. [117] used a committee of 10 MLPs, with a moderated output, trained according to the evidence framework. The data consisted of two input features, x_1 and x_2, related to arm tremor. The class labels indicated whether the features were measured from patients with Parkinson's disease and multiple sclerosis or from normal subjects.

Figure 10.1(a) is a plot of $\max p(y|\mathbf{x}, \mathcal{D})$ as a function of x_1 and x_2 obtained from the moderated committee. Dark grey corresponds to $\max p(y|\mathbf{x}, \mathcal{D}) = 0.5$ and white corresponds to $\max p(y|\mathbf{x}, \mathcal{D}) = 1$. Figure 10.1(b) is the plot obtained when one of the MLPs of the committee was trained on the same data using an unmoderated output. It is seen that the single MLP incorrectly gave a high probability in the lower-right region of the input space where data density is relatively low. In contrast, the moderated committee decreased the probability to reflect the greater uncertainty in this region. $\triangleleft$

10.7.4 Full Bayesian Models

Marginal integrals, which appear throughout this discussion of Bayesian neural techniques, may be solved *approximately* in a variety of ways. Sections 10.7.2 and 10.7.3 detail approaches referred to as the *evidence* method [99] in which the joint integration over both parameters $\mathbf{w}$ and hyperparameters α is achieved by making a Gaussian approximation to $p(\mathcal{D}|\mathbf{w}, \alpha)$ and assuming that the distribution over α is very sharply peaked at its *most probable* value

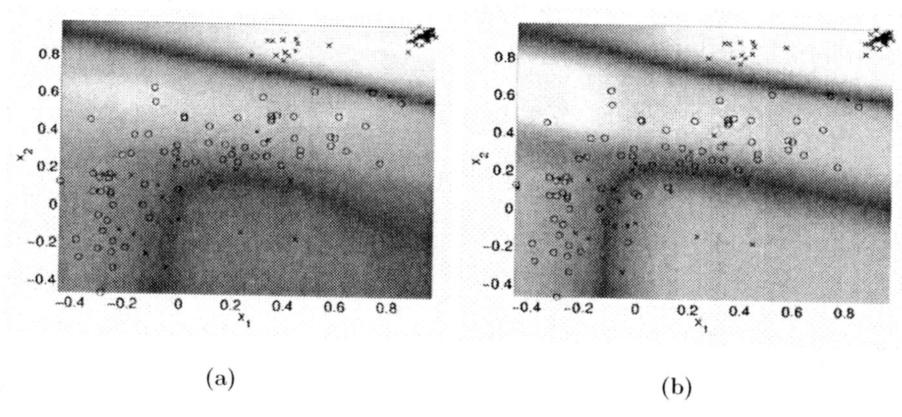

Fig. 10.1. Plots of $\max p(y|\mathbf{x}, \mathcal{D})$ versus features x_1 and x_2 from arm-tremor data when (a) $p(y|\mathbf{x}, \mathcal{D})$ is derived from a moderated committee and (b) $p(y|\mathbf{x}, \mathcal{D})$ is derived from a single unmoderated MLP. Value of $\max p(y|\mathbf{x}, \mathcal{D})$ varies from 0.5 (dark grey) to 1 (white). Data consists of patients ($\times$) and normal subjects ($\circ$). Reprinted from [117] by courtesy of Springer-Verlag.

$p(\alpha|\mathcal{D}) \approx \delta(\alpha - \alpha_{\mathrm{MP}})$. These simplifications, as we have seen, allow for an analytic evaluation of the marginal integral of interest, namely

$$p(y|\mathbf{x}, \mathcal{D}) = \int_{\mathbf{w}} \int_{\alpha} p(y|\mathbf{x}, \mathbf{w}) p(\mathbf{w}|\alpha, \mathcal{D}) p(\alpha|\mathcal{D}) \mathrm{d}\mathbf{w} \mathrm{d}\alpha. \tag{10.39}$$

Such approximations are only forced upon us by the general non-analytic nature of the above equation if we require closed-form solutions. If, however, we may work with a (arbitrarily large) number of *samples* drawn from $p(y|\mathbf{x}, \mathcal{D})$ then we may avoid such approximations and use a sampling strategy.

Sampling approaches are very well known in statistical inference, and a variety of efficient methods have been developed. By far the commonest approaches are the *Markov chain Monte Carlo* (MCMC) methods. Equation (10.39) may be re-written as

$$p(y|\mathbf{x}, \mathcal{D}) = \int_{\mathbf{w}} \int_{\alpha} p(y|\mathbf{x}, \mathbf{w}) p(\mathbf{w}, \alpha|\mathcal{D}) \mathrm{d}\mathbf{w} \mathrm{d}\alpha. \tag{10.40}$$

Hence we may re-formulate our problem of inference as one of sampling from the distribution of $p(\mathbf{w}, \alpha|\mathcal{D})$. The simplest approach is arguably the *Metropolis* method in which samples $\mathbf{w}', \alpha'$ are drawn from *proposal distributions* based on the current $\mathbf{w}, \alpha$ and accepted with a probability

$$Pr(\text{accept}) = \min\left(1, \frac{p(\mathbf{w}', \alpha'|\mathcal{D})}{p(\mathbf{w}, \alpha|\mathcal{D})}\right). \tag{10.41}$$

Neal [108] considers much more efficient approaches to such sampling; namely, *hybrid*. Sampling from the joint distribution $p(\mathbf{w}, \alpha|\mathcal{D})$ is an inefficient scheme, and most sample-based approaches to neural network inference [108, 64] make use of *Gibbs sampling*. In the first step, the hyperparameters α are held fixed and $\mathbf{w}$ is sampled from $p(\mathbf{w}|\alpha, \mathcal{D})$; in the second step, the hyperparameters are sampled from $p(\alpha|\mathbf{w}, \mathcal{D})$. The latter may be re-written as [64]

$$p(\alpha|\mathbf{w}, \mathcal{D}) = \frac{p(\mathbf{w}|\alpha)p(\alpha)}{p(\mathbf{w})} \tag{10.42}$$

in which $p(\mathbf{w})$ and $p(\alpha)$ are the prior distributions over parameters and hyperparameters, respectively. This sampling stage can be made very efficient if these priors are chosen to be of conjugate form to the posteriors.

Husmeier et al. [64] consider such MCMC approaches to neural network evaluation and detail the performance of the method compared with the evidence scheme. They show that, in a biomedical problem of tremor assessment, comparable or superior results are obtained. One key feature of the neural networks discussed by Husmeier et al. [64] and Neal [108] is in the use of hyperparameters that govern the scale of distributions over different groups of parameters. This naturally leads to the concept of *Automatic Relevance Determination* (ARD), which may be used to "prune" away components of a neural network that do not significantly contribute to the desired inference. This has the desirable effect of automatically regulating the complexity of the neural network.

10.8 The Naïve Bayes Model

From Bayes' theorem, the conditional class probability $p(y = i|\mathbf{x})$ is related to the likelihood $p(\mathbf{x}|y = i)$ by

$$p(y = i|\mathbf{x}) = \frac{p(y = i)p(\mathbf{x}|y = i)}{\sum_k p(y = k)p(\mathbf{x}|y = k)}. \tag{10.43}$$

If we make the strong assumption that the elements of $\mathbf{x}$ are independent of each other when y is given then (10.43) simplifies to the so-called naïve Bayes model [155]:

$$p(y = i|\mathbf{x}) = \frac{p(y = i)\prod_{x \in \mathbf{x}} p(x|y = i)}{\sum_k p(y = k)\prod_{x \in \mathbf{x}} p(x|y = k)}. \tag{10.44}$$

In spite of the strong assumption employed by this model, it can be surprisingly effective even when the assumption does not hold [36, 43, 96].

When deciding which of two classes is more likely, (10.44) can be further simplified to the log-odds version

$$\log\left[\frac{p(y = i|\mathbf{x})}{p(y = j|\mathbf{x})}\right] = \log\left[\frac{p(y = i)}{p(y = j)}\right] + \sum_{x \in \mathbf{x}} \log\left[\frac{p(x|y = i)}{p(x|y = j)}\right]. \tag{10.45}$$

Example 8. de Dombal et al. [33] developed a decision support system for the analysis of acute abdominal pain, which was based on the log-odds form of the the naïve Bayes model.

The efficacy of the system was tested using a multi-centre study [1]. According to this study, initial diagnostic accuracy rose from 45.6% to 65.3%. In addition, negative laparotomies fell from 313 cases to 174 cases a year, and perforation rates among appendicitis patient fell from 23% to 11%. $\triangleleft$

10.9 Bayesian Networks

Probabilistic graphical models are a subset of probabilistic models that provide a parsimonious representation of a joint probability distribution $p(X_1, \ldots, X_n)$. This is done using a graphical representation in which the nodes of a graph represent random variables $X_1, \ldots, X_n$, and the edges represent direct probabilistic dependencies. Graphical models are partitioned into two types: directed graphs called *Bayesian networks*[12] and undirected graphs called *Markov nets* or *Markov random fields*. When Bayesian networks are applied to dynamic problems, such as the modelling of signals, they are often referred to as *dynamic probabilistic networks* or *dynamic Bayesian networks* (see Section 8.6 and Figure 8.9. A number of probabilistic models can be represented as graphical models, including näive Bayes models, Gaussian mixtures, hidden Markov models, and Kalman filters. The Bayesian network corresponding to the näive Bayes model of Section 10.8 is shown in Figure 10.2.

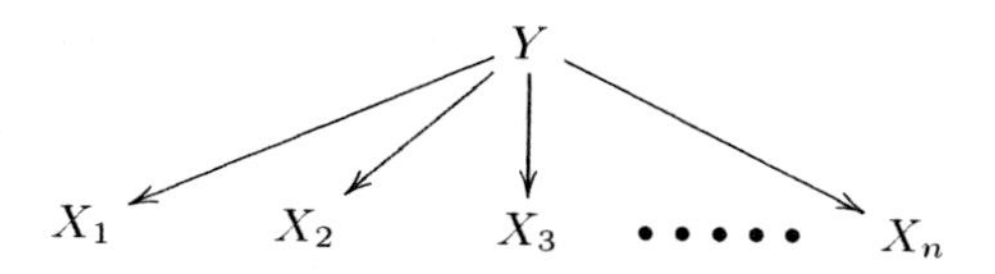

Fig. 10.2. The graphical representation of a näive Bayes model.

Despite the name, Bayesian networks do not necessarily imply a commitment to the Bayesian paradigm. Rather, they are so called because they use Bayes' theorem for probabilistic inference.

A *Bayesian network* (BN) [30, 74, 72] $\mathcal{B}$ for a set of variables $\mathbf{X} = \{X_{v_1}, \ldots, X_{|\mathbf{V}|}\}$ is a pair of mathematical constructs $(\mathcal{G}, \boldsymbol{\theta})$. The first construct, the qualitative component $\mathcal{G} = (\mathbf{V}, \mathbf{E})$, is a directed acyclic graph (DAG) consisting of (i) nodes (vertices) $\mathbf{V}$ in one-to-one correspondence with

[12] The term "Bayesian network" has a number of synonyms, which include *Bayes net*, *Bayesian belief network*, *belief network*, *causal network*, and *probabilistic network*.

the variables $\mathbf{X}$ (with X_u denoting the variable associated with node, or set of nodes, u) and (ii) directed links (edges) $\mathbf{E}$ that connect the nodes. The second construct, the quantitative component $\boldsymbol{\theta} = \{\boldsymbol{\theta}_{v_1}, \ldots, \boldsymbol{\theta}_{v_{|\mathbf{V}|}}\}$, is a set of parameter values that specify all the conditional probability distributions for the nodes of $\mathcal{B}$, where $\boldsymbol{\theta}_v$ defines the conditional probability $p(X_v|X_{\text{pa}(v)})$ of node v given its parents pa(v) in $\mathcal{G}$.[13] For a parentless node v, $p(X_v|X_{\text{pa}(v)})$ is equal to $p(X_v)$. Conditional probability $p(X_v|X_{\text{pa}(v)})$ can be defined by various means, including tables, MLPs (Section 10.6.1), and class probability trees (Section 10.10).

Bayesian network $\mathcal{B}$ models a joint probability distribution $p(\mathbf{X})$ over $\mathbf{X}$, the model depicting the probabilistic dependencies and independencies amongst the variables concerned (Figure 10.3).

The Markov properties of DAGs [111, 158] enable the joint probability distribution $p(X_{\mathbf{V}})$ to be factorized as follows:

$$p(X_{\mathbf{V}}) = p(X_{v_1}, \ldots, X_{v_n}) = \prod_{i=1}^{n} p(X_{v_i}|X_{\text{pa}(v_i)}), \qquad (10.46)$$

thus the global probability $p(X_{\mathbf{V}})$ can be decomposed into a collection of local probabilities. The form of each factor $p(X_{v_i}|X_{\text{pa}(v_i)})$ in (10.46) is specified by $\mathcal{G}$, and the values for $p(X_{v_i}|X_{\text{pa}(v_i)})$ are specified by $\boldsymbol{\theta}$. The advantages of this decomposition are (i) complex systems can be visualized as being composed of simpler models (subgraphs), which facilitates system construction and comprehension, and (ii) because fewer parameters are required for simpler models, parameters can be learnt from less data.

Bayesian networks are pictorial, and clinicians find this computational formalism intuitive and appealing [61, 62, 97, 98]. These networks can provide insight into the way various factors and mechanisms interact to influence the outcome of a disease in a patient. The applicability of BNs to medicine has been investigated in a number of areas, including bone-marrow transplantation [150], intensive care [9], electromyography [2], clinical microbiology [90], and oncology [46].

10.9.1 Probabilistic Inference over BNs

The main use of a BN is to infer probability distributions for the associated variables given a set of observations. More formally, suppose we have the above BN $\mathcal{B}$, and we observe values $\mathbf{w}$ (the *evidence*) for variables $\mathbf{W} \subset \mathbf{X}$. Various techniques have been developed to determine $p(X_i|\mathbf{w})$ for each $X_i \in \mathbf{X} \setminus \mathbf{W}$.[14]

[13] It is more precise to state that the quantitative component consists of (a) a family of (conditional) probability distributions and (b) their parameters $\boldsymbol{\theta}$. Since (a) is usually given and fixed, one usually, in practice, only thinks in terms of $\mathcal{G}$ and $\boldsymbol{\theta}$.

[14] If no observations are made (i.e., $\mathbf{w} = \emptyset$), the estimates are the prior probability distributions $p(X_i)$ for each $X_i \in \mathbf{X}$.

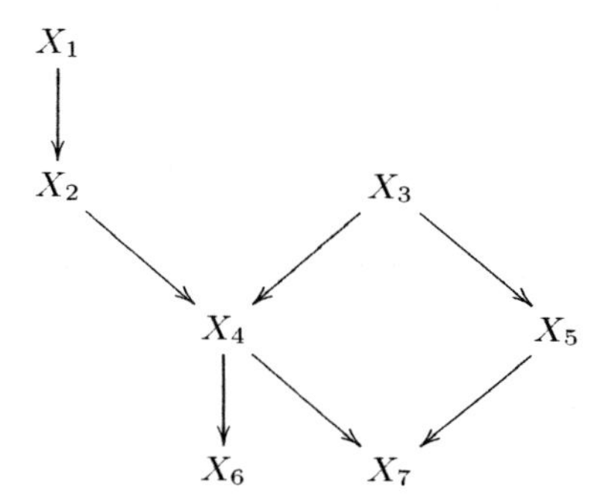

Fig. 10.3. The DAG for a hypothetical BN. The dependencies and independencies can be determined from the graphical structure through application of the *d-separation rules* [112]. For example, from this DAG, we have that the probability of X_4 is independent of the value of X_1 if the value of X_2 is given. The rules also imply that X_4 is independent of X_5 if X_3 is given. The notion of d-separation is extensively discussed in Section 2.1.1 and illustrated in Figures 2.7, 2.8, and 2.9.

In theory, this enables diagnoses and prognoses to be performed when $\mathbf{w}$ is a set of observations such as symptoms, test results, and patient demographics.

The algorithm most commonly used for this purpose is the message-passing (evidence-propagation) algorithm developed by Jensen et al. [73], in which a multiply-connected DAG is replaced by a singly-connected junction tree.[15] However, some exact inference algorithms have been designed for specific types of BNs. For example, the *Quick Medical Reference* (QMR) model consists of an upper layer of disease nodes and a lower layer of symptom nodes [144]. If it is assumed that each disease has an independent chance of causing symptoms, noisy-OR nodes can be used for the symptoms. A problem with the QMR-type network is that the cliques obtained after triangulation can be too large for the junction-tree algorithm to be used for real-time applications; on the other hand, the *quickscore algorithm* [59] is more efficient because it exploits special properties of the noisy-OR node. The variational approach has also been applied to the QMR model [66].

The most commonly-used version of the junction-tree algorithm requires that x_v is discrete for each $v \in \boldsymbol{V}$ (i.e., probabilities $p(x_v|x_{\mathrm{pa}(v)})$ are stored

[15] In order to implement the junction-tree algorithm, a junction tree is formed from a DAG as follows. First, the DAG is *moralized* by adding undirected edges between parents not already joined (*married*). Second, all the directed edges of the moralized graph are made undirected (the *moral graph*). Third, sufficient undirected edges are added to the moral graph to ensure that there are no cycles greater than 3 (*triangulation*). Finally, a tree (the *junction tree*) is formed from the triangulated graph. The nodes of the junction tree correspond to the *cliques* of the triangulated graph, and the edges of the tree correspond to the boundaries between the cliques.

as *conditional probability tables* for each v). But what if some v in $\boldsymbol{V}$ take on continuous values? The usual response to this situation is to discretize the variables in some manner, but this results in an approximation to the continuous case. It is possible to create BNs with continuous-valued nodes, the most common distribution for such variables being the Gaussian. Versions of the junction-tree algorithm can be used when all the nodes are Gaussian (*Gaussian networks*) or when Gaussian nodes have discrete-valued parent nodes but not vice versa (*conditional Gaussian networks*) [141, 89, 29, 93]. When there are discrete nodes with Gaussian parents, *approximate inference* has to be used. A variety of techniques have been proposed for approximate inference. These can be either stochastic, such as *Gibbs sampling*, or deterministic, such as *variational methods* (Section 2.3.6) and *loopy belief propagation* [105].

Another reason for using approximate methods, even when all the nodes are discrete-valued, is that the time taken for the junction-tree algorithm increases with (a) the number of nodes, (b) the number of possible values for the nodes, and (c) the size of the largest clique; consequently, for some BNs, the time required for exact inference is impractical. In this situation, approximate methods must be used instead. An example is the application of a variational technique to the *Promedas* BN [77], which attempts to model the many sub-domains associated with anaemia.

Example 9. In 1989, Beinlich et al. [9] developed a BN (the ALARM system) to diagnose problems with anesthetic-ventilator management in intensive-care units. The BN consisted of 37 nodes associated with such events as hypovolemia and pulmonary embolism. It is one of the demonstration networks available with the Hugin and Hugin Lite packages. ◁

Example 10. The 20-node CHILD BN [148] was developed in conjunction with the Great Ormond Street Hospital for Sick Children, London. The hospital is a major referral centre for neonates with congenital heart disease in South-East England, and the intention was to use the BN to support the diagnosis of cyanosis (the "blue-baby" syndrome).

The structure and all the probabilities required for the network were obtained from domain experts. This was done through the use of Heckerman's similarity-networks technique [58]. This involves asking the expert to provide a network that will differentiate between a pair of diseases that are regarded as being difficult to distinguish. This process is repeated for each such disease pair, and the resulting sub-networks are combined (Section 10.9.4). ◁

Example 11. MammoNet is a BN for the interpretation of mammograms [76]. It consists of five patient-history features (e.g., age at menarch), two physical findings (e.g., presence of pain), and 15 mammographic features (e.g., calcification-cluster shape).

The design of the BN (structure and probabilities) was developed from peer-reviewed articles and expert opinion. When tested with a test set consisting of 77 cases, the network had an ROC-curve area of 0.881. At a probability threshold of 0.15, the BN exhibited a true positive rate of 0.92 and a true negative rate of 0.885. ◁

10.9.2 Sigmoidal Belief Networks

Neural networks can be treated as probabilistic graphical models by regarding the activation functions as providing probabilities at the hidden nodes. For example, for the hth hidden node of the MLP defined by (10.22), we can write

$$\widehat{p}(h = 1|\mathbf{x}; \mathbf{w}) = \ell\left(w_{(1\to h)} + \sum_x w_{(x\to h)}x\right).$$

Treating an MLP as a BN produces the concept of a *sigmoidal belief network* [107]. The advantages of this interpretation include a principled approach to handling missing data for neural-type models. Unfortunately, because of the high fan-ins to the hidden nodes, exact inference is generally not feasible. Because of this problem, Jordan et al. [75] advocated the use of variational approximation for sigmoidal belief networks.

10.9.3 Construction of BNs: Probabilities

One can attempt to elicit the required probabilities $\boldsymbol{\theta}$ of a BN from a domain expert; however, obtaining consistent and accurate values from experts is generally difficult. Conversion of qualitative probabilistic terms into point-valued probabilities is prone to variation [11], and although several aids for assessing probabilities from people (such as the probability wheel) are available [147], the assessment of subjective probabilities is nevertheless a time-consuming task (though recent work has suggested some ingenious techniques for reducing the burden [37, 126]). An alternative approach is to adjust approximate subjective probabilities with complete or incomplete data by means of Bayesian updating (10.1).

Let $\{\varphi_1, \ldots, \varphi_r\}$ be the set of possible values for X_v, and let ρ be a possible value for pa(v). When data $\mathcal{D}$ are complete, and certain assumptions are adopted [149], vector $\boldsymbol{\theta}^{v,\rho}$, equal to

$$\left(p(X_v = \varphi_1|X_{\mathrm{pa}(v)} = \rho)\cdots p(X_v = \varphi_r|X_{\mathrm{pa}(v)} = \rho)\right),$$

can be updated,

$$p(\boldsymbol{\theta}^{v,\rho}|\mathcal{D}) \propto p(\boldsymbol{\theta}^{v,\rho})p(\mathcal{D}|\boldsymbol{\theta}^{v,\rho}), \tag{10.47}$$

using a Dirichlet distribution for the prior $p(\boldsymbol{\theta}^{v,\rho})$. After updating $\boldsymbol{\theta}^{v,\rho}$, a point-valued probability from $p(X_v|X_{\mathrm{pa}(v)} = \rho)$ can be based on the mode of $p(\boldsymbol{\theta}^{v,\rho}|\mathcal{D})$.

Relationship (10.47) can be extended to accommodate incomplete data by means of the EM algorithm (Section 2.3.3 and Figure 2.22.); however, a Gaussian approximation is used for this purpose [79] since the exact Bayesian approach is not tractable in practice [149].

10.9.4 Construction of BNs: Structures

BNs can be built entirely from background knowledge, or induced entirely from data, or constructed from a combination of knowledge and data.

The standard approach to constructing BNs has been to elicit knowledge about $\mathcal{G}$ (and possibly $\boldsymbol{\theta}$) from a domain expert [102]. In the *Pathfinder* approach to knowledge acquisition [58], a domain expert is presented with pairs of diseases, d_1 and d_2, and he is asked to state which manifestations are relevant to the discrimination of d_1 and d_2. The idea is to select disease pairs that are often difficult for non-experts to distinguish. A virtue of this approach is that it enables the construction of a Bayesian network to be decomposed into a set of simpler networks representing subproblems familiar to the expert. This results in a set of local DAGs, and the graph-theoretic union of these DAGs produces a single global DAG.

Given the problems that can occur with knowledge acquisition, there has been a growing interest in constructing Bayesian networks from available data [20, 60]. This alternative approach can lead to improved efficiency in network construction and model accuracy.

The number of directed acyclic graphs (DAGs) that can be constructed from a set of nodes $\mathbf{V}$ grows super-exponentially with $|\mathbf{V}|$ (see Table 2.1); thus, an exhaustive comparison of all possible structures is generally infeasible. Consequently, various search heuristics have been proposed that are able to induce DAGs from data [60], such as the K2 algorithm [27].

A simple heuristic search algorithm is *greedy search*, in which the search space is the set of all possible DAGs having $\mathbf{V}$ as the node set. If the current position in this search space is $\mathcal{G}_{cur}$, the set $\boldsymbol{\Delta}\mathbf{E}(\mathcal{G}_{cur})$ of all possible DAGs that are obtainable from $\mathcal{G}_{cur}$ by adding, deleting or reversing a directed edge is constructed. Let $\mathcal{G}^*$ be the element of $\boldsymbol{\Delta}\mathbf{E}(\mathcal{G}_{cur}) \cup \{\mathcal{G}_{cur}\}$ for which $score(\mathcal{G})$ is maximal with respect to a given scoring function such as the Bayesian information criterion (see Section 2.3.2). If $\mathcal{G}^* = \mathcal{G}_{cur}$ then the search terminates; otherwise, $\mathcal{G}^*$ becomes the next position in search space.

If data are incomplete, one can combine greedy search with the EM algorithm by performing the EM algorithm for each candidate DAG in $\boldsymbol{\Delta}\mathbf{E}(\mathcal{G}_{cur})$, but this is computationally expensive, particularly when random restarts are used to reduce the chance of an EM run converging to a local optimum. A less expensive approach is the *structural EM algorithm* [42] (see also Section 2.3.6 and Section 4.4.5.) in which the search for the best structure takes place within the EM procedure.

10.9.5 Missing Data

As remarked in Sections 10.9.3 and 10.9.4, the EM algorithm can be used to induce probabilities and structures from incomplete training sets, but the assumptions underlying use of the EM algorithm (Section 10.6.4) must be borne in mind.

Because a BN can update the probabilities of its variables with respect to whichever nodes are instantiated, it is able to handle incomplete evidence intrinsically.

10.10 Class-Probability Trees

Tree-structured classifiers (*classification trees*) provide a hierarchical approach to modelling the distribution of a set of class-labelled exemplars $\mathcal{D}$ in the feature space $\Omega[\mathbf{X}]$ of $\mathbf{X}$. Each node ν of a classification tree T is associated with a region $R(\nu, T) \subseteq \Omega[\mathbf{X}]$ that results from a recursive partitioning of $\Omega[\mathbf{X}]$ according to the distribution of $\mathcal{D}$ within $\Omega[\mathbf{X}]$.

Starting at the root node of a classification tree, a new case $\mathbf{x} \notin \mathcal{D}$ is passed down the tree until a leaf node is reached. The decision rule associated with each non-leaf node selects the branch down which $\mathbf{x}$ is passed. If $\mathbf{x}$ reaches leaf node ν_i, and k is the most frequent class in region $R(\nu_i, T)$, then $\mathbf{x}$ is assigned to class k. If $\widehat{p}_{\nu_i,k}$ is the relative frequency $n_{\nu_i,k}/n_{\nu_i}$ of k in $R(\nu_i, T)$ then $\widehat{p}_{\nu_i,k}$ provides an estimate of the conditional class probability $p(k|\mathbf{x})$, whereupon T becomes a *class-probability tree.*

A tree is grown by recursively partitioning feature space $\Omega[\mathbf{X}]$ with respect to $\mathcal{D}$. At each step of the recursive process, there exists a tree T_1, and, for each leaf ν_i of the tree, there is the possibility of selecting a variable X from $\mathbf{X}$, and partitioning (or *splitting*) $R(\nu_i, T_1)$ with respect to X. When a particular partition has been selected, say, $R(\nu_i, T_1)$ into regions R_1 and R_2, two branches are grown from ν_i. The leaf of one branch corresponds to R_1, and the leaf of the other to R_2. These two leaves become leaf nodes ν_j and ν_k for a larger tree T_2, with $R_1 = R(\nu_j, T_2)$ and $R_2 = R(\nu_k, T_2)$.

The most common approach to tree construction is to define a measure of class heterogeneity associated with a node, and choose the split that most reduces the average heterogeneity across the child nodes resulting from the split. A common measure of class heterogeneity at a node is the Gini index $\sum_{k=1}^{K} \widehat{p}_{\nu,k}(1 - \widehat{p}_{\nu,k})$. This is used by the CART tree-induction algorithm [17].

An alternative approach to tree construction is to choose the split that gives the maximum reduction in deviance. The deviance of a tree is defined as

$$D = \sum_{\nu} D_\nu,$$

where D_ν is the contribution by leaf node ν to the deviance:

$$D_\nu = -2 \sum_{k=1}^{K} n_{\nu,k} \log \widehat{p}_{\nu,k}.$$

It follows that, if node s is split into nodes t and u, the reduction in deviance is given by

$$D_s - D_t - D_y = 2\sum_{k=1}^{K}\left[n_{t,k}\log\frac{n_{t,k}n_s}{n_{s,k}n_t} + n_{u,k}\log\frac{n_{u,k}n_s}{n_{s,k}n_u}\right]$$

Once a tree is grown, it is *pruned* to prevent overfitting to the training set. The standard method is to use *cost-complexity pruning* [17]. In the context of deviance, the cost-complexity measure for rooted subtree T is

$$D_\alpha(T) = D(T) + \alpha|T|,$$

where $|T|$ is the number of leaf nodes in T. Parameter α governs the tradeoff between tree size $|T|$ and the goodness of fit $D(T)$ to the data. For any specified α, cost-complexity pruning determines the subtree T_α that minimizes $D_\alpha(T)$. The optimal α, and thus T_α, over a range of α values can be found by using a validation set or cross-validation.

Example 12. Tree induction using deviance-based splits was applied to the low birth-weight data analyzed in Example 2. Optimal pruning was estimated by 10-fold cross-validation with respect to deviance. The attributes selected by the induction were the number of premature labours experienced by the mother (*ptl*), the weight of the mother in pounds at the last menstrual period (*lwt*), and the age of the mother in years (*age*) (Figure 10.4). $\triangleleft$

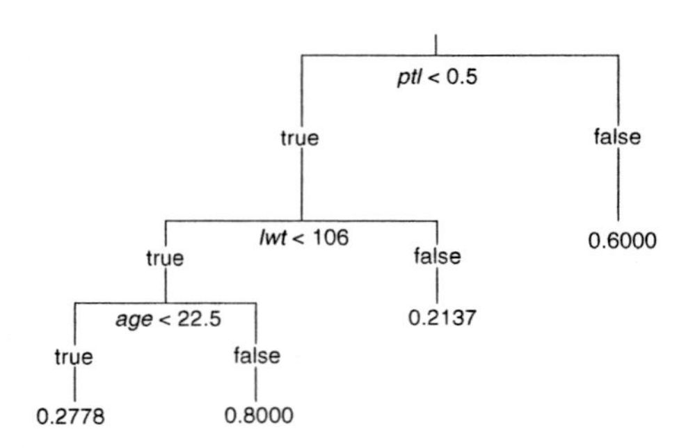

Fig. 10.4. Tree induced from low birth-weight data. The numbers at the leaf nodes are estimates of the conditional probabilities $p(\textit{low birth weight}|\textit{ptl}, \textit{lwt}, \textit{age})$ based on the relative frequencies at the leaf nodes.

10.10.1 Missing Data

One of the attractions of using tree-based models is the ease with which missing values can be handled.

Several approaches to incomplete data have been proposed [17, 129, 56]:

- If the predictors are categorical, create a new category called "missing".

- Use surrogate splits [17]. A *surrogate split* $\tilde{s}_i$ for node t is the split on variable X_i that most accurately predicts the action of the best split $s^\star$ at node t. If a training set is incomplete, the best split $s^\star$ on variable X_j is computed using all the cases that contain a value for X_j. If a new case has a missing value so that $s^\star$ is not defined for that case then, among all the non-missing variables in that case, find the one, X_k, for which $\tilde{s}_k$ has the highest measure of predictive accuracy associated with $s^\star$, and use $\tilde{s}_k$ in place of $s^\star$.
- Estimate the probability of a case at node t going down the left and right branches of t, the probability being conditioned on the attributes used in the earlier splits encountered in the tree.

10.10.2 Bayesian Tree Induction

In the previous section, a single optimal tree T_α was used for the estimation of conditional class probabilities, $p(y = 1|\mathbf{x}, T_\alpha, \mathbf{\Phi}_{T_\alpha})$; where $\mathbf{\Phi}_T$ is a matrix of the class probabilities at the leaf nodes; however, this does not take account of the fact that there is uncertainty in selecting T_α rather than some other tree. The Bayesian response to this uncertainty is to average over all possible trees.[16]

For each possible recursive partitioning of feature space $\Omega[\mathbf{X}]$ with respect to a data set $\mathcal{D}$, there is a corresponding tree $(T, \mathbf{\Phi}_T)$. If $\mathbf{T}$ is the set of all possible trees obtained by each possible recursive partitioning, the Bayesian approach to tree uncertainty is to use

$$p(y = 1|\mathbf{x}, \mathcal{D}) = \sum_{(T,\mathbf{\Phi}_T)\in\mathbf{T}} p(y = 1|\mathbf{x}, T, \mathbf{\Phi}_T)p(T, \mathbf{\Phi}_T|\mathcal{D}). \tag{10.48}$$

A problem with implementing (10.48) is that, for real-world problems, the size of $\mathbf{T}$ is vast. Because of this, Buntine [18, 19] replaced $\mathbf{T}$ in (10.48) with a small set of trees having high posterior probabilities.

Buntine [18] suggested a variety of prior distributions $p(T)$ for trees. These include the following:

- a uniform distribution for all trees (i.e., $p(T)$ is constant);
- a slight preference for simpler trees,

$$p(T) \propto \omega^{|nodes(T)|}, \quad \text{where} \quad \omega < 1;$$

- a prior based on an information-theoretic coding of the complexity of trees [130, 159].

For the posterior

$$p(T, \mathbf{\Phi}_T|\mathcal{D}) = p(T|\mathcal{D})p(\mathbf{\Phi}_T|T, \mathcal{D}),$$

[16] Although theoretically different, the application of "bagging" [16] to tree induction is stylistically related, and it can perform very well as a non-Bayesian variant.

Buntine [18] used

$$p(T|\mathcal{D}) \propto p(T) \prod_{l \in leaves(T)} \frac{Beta_K(n_{1,l} + \alpha_1, \ldots, n_{1,K} + \alpha_K)}{Beta_K(\alpha_1, \ldots, \alpha_K)}, \quad (10.49)$$

$$p(\mathbf{\Phi}_T|T, \mathcal{D}) \propto \prod_{l \in leaves(T)} \frac{1}{Beta_K(\alpha_1, \ldots, \alpha_K)} \prod_{k=1}^{K} p(y = k|\mathbf{x}, T, \mathbf{\Phi}_T)^{n_{k,l}+\alpha-1},$$

where

$$Beta_K(\alpha_1, \ldots, \alpha_K) = \frac{\prod_{i=1}^{K} \Gamma(\alpha_i)}{\Gamma(\sum_{i=1}^{K} \alpha_i)},$$

and he used a version of (10.49) to probabilistically select candidate splits during tree growth.

The simplest approach to pruning is to use the tree with the maximum posterior probability, but this approach is sensitive to the choice of prior. Instead, Buntine [18] used *Bayesian tree smoothing* within the determination of $p(y = 1|\mathbf{x}, \mathcal{D})$. In the standard approach, an example is dropped down a tree until it reaches a leaf node, and the class probabilities associated with that leaf node are returned. The smoothing approach also averages the class-probability vectors encountered along the way from the root node to the leaf node [6].

Another refinement implemented by Buntine [18] was the concept of *option trees*. Option trees are a compact way of storing and growing many thousands of trees together by making note of shared subtrees. In the standard approach to trees, each interior node is associated with a single test, with subtrees rooted at the outcomes of the test. In place of a single test, an option tree has several optional tests, each with their respective subtrees. Only one optional test is chosen from each set of options.

Example 13. Buntine [19] compared three approaches to inducing class-probability trees from a data set of 145 hepatitis patients ($n = 75$ for the training set and $n = 70$ for the test set): CART, Bayesian smoothing, and option trees grown with two-level lookahead. The data set consisted of 20 attributes, including the class label, which recorded whether a patient lived or died. The results are shown in Table 10.2. ◁

10.11 Probabilistic Models for Detection

Analysis of biomedical data has a long history, and it is only relatively recently that probabilistic models *per se* have been used. In the main, such data analysis problems fall into one of three categories. Firstly, given data $\mathcal{D}$, the goal is in the detection of some component of interest, secondly the use of the data in a decision making process, and finally the conditioning of the

Table 10.2. Comparison of CART, Bayesian smoothing, and option trees for the induction of tree-type models from a hepatitis data set [19] (reprinted with permission).

	Time taken (s)			
Method	Training	Testing	Error rate (± std. dev.)	Brier score
CART	4.2	0.1	19.8 ± 3.7	0.35
Bayesian smoothing	1.5	0.1	23.1 ± 4.9	0.32
Option trees	131.0	23.1	18.8 ± 3.6	0.26

data, such as filtering or noise removal. If we consider the act of *detection* of some component within a data stream as tantamount to making the *decision* "is the component present" then we can see that the first and last of the categories above are in fact fundamentally the same process. In this section, we briefly review the traditional approaches to these problems and consider the impact probabilistic modelling has had.

10.11.1 Data Conditioning

We consider as a suitable starting point the use of simple data conditioning approaches, and take classical linear filtering as a good example. The basis of such filtering is well covered in standard texts (for a biomedical perspective, see [e.g., 25]) and will not be covered in detail here. Suffice to say, any digital linear filter can be represented parametrically via a set of coefficients, $\mathbf{a}$ say, which code the filter kernel. These coefficients may be defined by a desired spatial or temporal spectral response, for example, or they may be obtained and adapted based upon the data. The latter, as it requires estimation and inference, is the area in which probabilistic models have had their major impact (see [109] for a comprehensive review of probabilistic methods in signal processing). We consider, as case studies, applications to signal *autoregressive* filtering.

The autoregressive (AR) filter is, in fact, a generative model for the observed data. We consider a time-indexed stream of data $\mathcal{D} = \{x_1, \ldots, x_t, \ldots, x_T\}$. The AR process models the observed data as a linear combination of other (observed) data, normally from the same sequence and from "past" observations and an additive (white) noise process, η. Hence, for a qth order AR model,

$$x_t = \sum_{i=1}^{q} a_i x_{t-i} + \eta_t. \tag{10.50}$$

This is equivalent to modelling the spectral properties of the data as the result of passing a white noise process (flat spectrum) through a resonance filter. This basic model has found much favour in the biomedical community especially for electroencephalogram (EEG) analysis [25, 68, 110]. Traditional methods for estimation of the parameters rely on least-squares optimization. The major problem with such non-probabilistic approaches lies in the fact that no measure of *uncertainty* over the parameters is inferred and hence any further processing (such as the use of the parameters for decision making or classification purposes, e.g. as in [69]) is conditioned on the parameters assuming they are known with absolute precision. If the target variable of interest (i.e. to be inferred) is denoted y, the data $\mathcal{D}$ and the parameters of the AR model $\mathbf{w}$ (i.e. the set of coefficients, a_i, along with the parameters governing the statistics of the noise η) then traditional approaches evaluate the most-probable $\mathbf{w}^*|\mathcal{D}$, followed by $y|\mathbf{w}^*$. This is in sharp contrast to probabilistic approaches in which we wish to infer $p(y|\mathcal{D})$. In a probabilistic setting we achieve this by marginalization, i.e.

$$p(y|\mathcal{D}) = \int_{\mathbf{w}} p(y|\mathbf{w})p(\mathbf{w}|\mathcal{D})d\mathbf{w}. \tag{10.51}$$

This means that the intrinsic uncertainty in the parameters, described by $p(\mathbf{w}|\mathcal{D})$, is taken into account during subsequent computation. This is depicted in the graphical model of Figure 10.5. In [51] the AR model is put into a fully

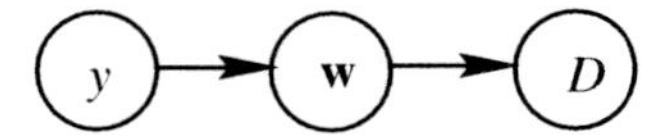

Fig. 10.5. Graphical model for simple AR model. The joint density is given as $p(y, w, \mathcal{D}) = p(\mathcal{D}|w)p(w|y)p(y)$. After some simple manipulation this leads to the marginal of interest in Equation (10.51).

probabilistic framework and applied to speech analysis. A similar model was developed in [115] and applied to EEG analysis. In [114] a Bayesian approach is taken to the multi-dimensional AR (MAR) model with application to EEG data once more. In [151] a fully probabilistic MAR approach is applied to EEG data.

Allowing the set of parameters to become time-varying (i.e., an adaptive AR model) gives rise naturally to the *Kalman–Bucy* filter. This is often discussed as a recursive least squares adaptive filter, but it is more clearly understood in fully probabilistic terms. Early discussions in this vein include the key work of [70] with applications to EEG detailed in [146] and more recently in a Bayesian setting in [118]. Consider a time evolving extension of Equation (10.50),

$$x_t = \sum_{i=1}^{q} a_{i,t}\, x_{t-i} + \eta_t. \tag{10.52}$$

As data becomes available in a causal fashion, the inference problem is to form $p(\mathbf{a}_t|\mathcal{D}_t)$, where $\mathcal{D}_t \stackrel{\text{def}}{=} \{x_1, x_2, ..., x_{t-1}, x_t\}$ and $\mathbf{a} \stackrel{\text{def}}{=} \{a_1, ..., a_q\}$. By noting that $\mathcal{D}_t = \{\mathcal{D}_{t-1}, x_t\}$ we may write via Bayes' theorem

$$p(\mathbf{a}_t|\mathcal{D}_t) = \frac{p(x_t|\mathbf{a}_t, \mathcal{D}_{t-1})p(\mathbf{a}_t|\mathcal{D}_{t-1})}{p(x_t|\mathcal{D}_{t-1})} \tag{10.53}$$

This has the form of a sequential update equation, which may be implemented in a computationally efficient manner. In [21], a Bayesian approach is taken to multi-variate adaptive AR (MAR) models and applied to a variety of biomedical data to great effect.

Few applications of full probabilistic data conditioning (or feature extraction) are found in medical image processing, mainly due to the computational costs involved. Typical solution procedures in this field involve the traditional approach of inferring features from the image, followed by conditioning on those features [e.g., 160] in which parameters from a Markov Random Field are evaluated to perform magnetic resonance image (MRI) analysis. Exceptions to this are discussed in [45, 44, 53]. The blossoming field of magnetic resonance imaging and functional MRI (fMRI) has produced most recent work in the area of applied probabilistic models [e.g., 116].

Recent work in the area of independent component anaylsis (ICA) [133] has been applied in biomedical data analysis and pitched in the framework of probabilistic models. ICA has been applied to problems of both biomedical signal and image processing. The basis of ICA lies in the generative model (see Figure 10.6) for the observed data $\mathbf{x}$ as a linear combination (mixture) of a set of unknown canonical sources, $\mathbf{s}$, and some additive (white) noise process, $\boldsymbol{\eta}$,

$$\mathbf{x} = \mathbf{A}\mathbf{s} + \boldsymbol{\eta} \tag{10.54}$$

in which $\mathbf{A}$ is the mixing process matrix. ICA may be regarded as a model

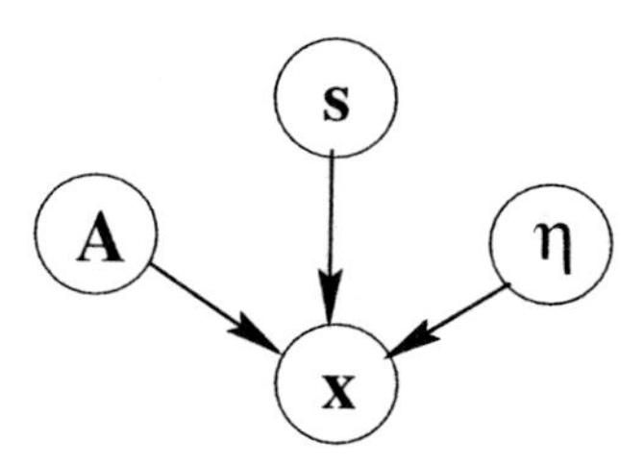

Fig. 10.6. Simple graphical model for ICA in which the observed data, $\mathbf{x}$ is conditionally generated via an unknown mixing matrix, $\mathbf{A}$, a set of unknown sources, $\mathbf{s}$ and a noise process with unknown statistics, η.

of mixing of a set of unknown (and desired) data streams (typical of signal processing applications), or as a method of breaking an observed data set into feature or basis functions (more typical for image processing). Probabilistic models for ICA have come to the fore recently [86, 104, 23] as, although computationally demanding, they offer considerable flexibility. In the *blind source separation* problem, only the observations, $\mathbf{x}$, are available, and the inference of $\mathbf{A}, \mathbf{s}$ and the statistics of $\boldsymbol{\eta}$ is ill-posed. ICA makes the tacit assumption that the desired sources are maximally independent; that is to say, their mutual information is minimal. This is a sufficient condition to make solutions to Equation (10.54) well-posed. With a generative model for the ICA process and, importantly, an explicit density model for the sources, $p(\mathbf{s})$, the goal of ICA is succinctly re-cast as the minimization, under the model, of the mutual information between the sources. This may be achieved by minimizing the Kullback-Leibler (KL) divergence [28] between the joint density and the product of the source marginal densities, i.e.

$$KL[p(\mathbf{s})|| \prod_i p_i(s_i)] = \int_{\mathbf{s}} p(\mathbf{s}) \log \left(\frac{p(\mathbf{s})}{\prod_i p_i(s_i)} \right) d\mathbf{s}. \tag{10.55}$$

This minimization is shown to be equivalent to the maximization of the probability of the data under the model [133]. Several probabilistic approaches have been taken in the literature, from approximate Bayes techniques [136, 86] to sampling methods [133] and *variational learning* approaches [104, 23].

Example 14. As a simple example of ICA operation in a biomedical context we consider the multiple-channel recording of EEG in Figure 10.7. Note the presence of similar signal components in all channels. As we may look at ICA as a fully probabilistic model so we may consider the changes in model evidence as we allow for different priors. In particular, in the context of biomedical signals such as EEG, we may consider positivity priors on the mixing process – justified by the arguments of electrical current addition. Figure 10.8(a) shows the inferred sources with no positivity priors (i.e., the elements of both $\mathbf{A}$ and $\mathbf{s}$ lie in $\mathbb{R}$). Model evidence supports three reconstructed sources. In the case of a positivity prior $\mathbf{A} \in \mathbb{R}_+$, on the other hand, the model evidence is higher than the previous case but only supports two sources, as shown in plot (b) of the same figure. $\triangleleft$

Although fully probabilistic approaches to the ICA inference problem are available, computational pragmatism has meant that the majority of biomedical applications of ICA utilize non-probabilistic approaches with probabilistic methods being used, for example, to infer the number of proposed sources (see, Beckmann et al. [e.g., 8], which exploits probabilistic dimensionality inference methods using PCA to apply to an ICA decomposition of fMRI data).

10.11.2 Detection, Segmentation and Decisions

The basis of probabilistic decision theory lies in the inference of posterior probabilities over the items of interest, be they signal waveforms, image objects, diagnostic outcomes or class decisions. The inference of such probabilities has been undertaken using a variety of approaches in the literature, with neural networks being very popular [40](see Chapter 3 and Section 10.6). The use of classification methods assumes, in general, the availability of a labelled training data set; that is to say, the analysis is performed in a *supervised* manner.

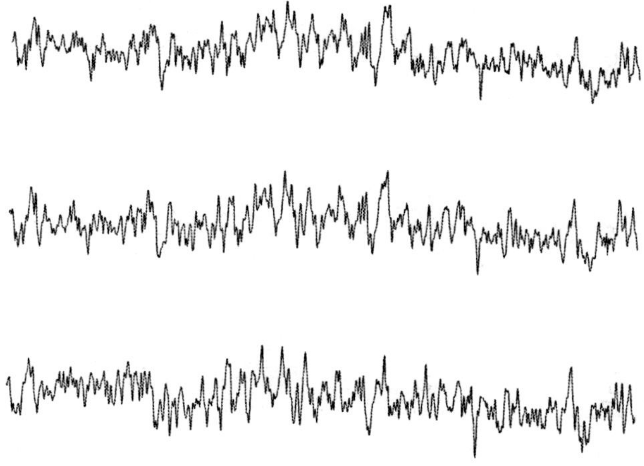

Fig. 10.7. Three recorded channels of EEG. This fragment represents 10 s of data at 128 Hz.

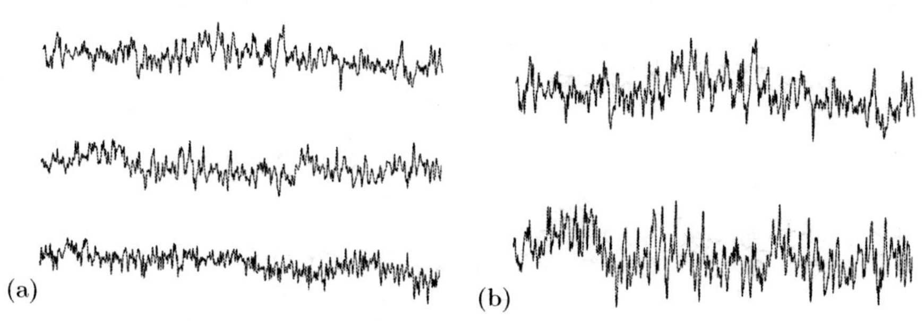

Fig. 10.8. EEG records decomposed into (a) three sources and (b) only two when positivity priors are put over the elements of **A**. The model evidence supports case (b).

In many situations, however, such labels may not exist, and the goal of the analysis is to perform *unsupervised* segmentation or *clustering* of the data. The breaking of data into regions or sets that are self-similar in some sense has been extensively applied to biomedical data [25].

We now turn our attention to three areas: cluster analysis, hidden Markov models, and novelty detection.

10.11.3 Cluster Analysis

We consider a generative model based such that x is generated from one of a simple set of models, indexed by $k = 1, \ldots, K$, one of which is chosen at any instant via an indicator variable, I. The simple graphical model for this is shown in Figure 10.9.

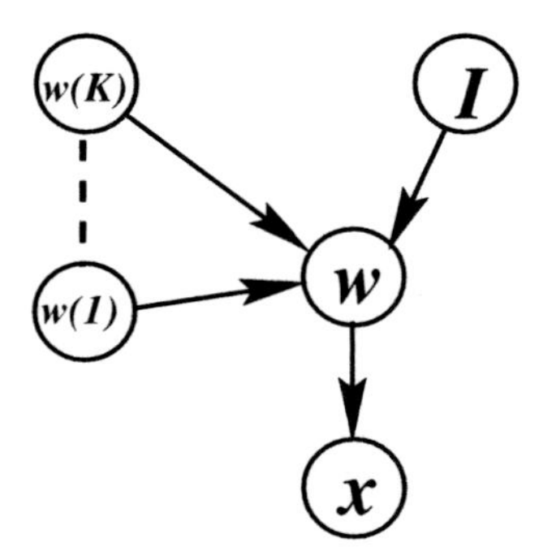

Fig. 10.9. Simple mixture model. Data x is generated by one of a set of K (parametric) models, with internal parameters $w(k)$ chosen from the mixture set via the indicator variable I.

The generative likelihood of datum x under the model is hence,

$$p(x) = \sum_{k=1}^{K} p(I = k)p(x|w(k)). \tag{10.56}$$

For computational and mathematical convenience most work on such mixture models takes each parametric model in the set to be a Gaussian (normal). Indeed this *Mixture of Gaussians* (MoG) model has been extensively used in biomedical data analysis. The model parameters (the set of $w(k)$ and the set of priors $p(I = k)$) may be simplest inferred using a *maximum likelihood* (ML) framework. This gives rise to the well-known Expectation-Maximization (EM) algorithm [34]. This has the typical problems of overfitting associated with all ML approaches and the inherent lack of a principled mechanism for model-order selection; that is, the inference of an appropriate K. Full Bayes implementations of the MoG are analytically cumbersome, but recent approximations based on *variational Bayes learning* and *reversible jump* Markov chain Monte Carlo (MCMC) have proved valuable [3, 134, 128]. The use of such fully probabilistic models has not made a profound impact as yet in the biomedical field. In [134] a reversible-jump MCMC approach was used to segment epileptic signals and detect tumours in MRI images. In [138] quadratic approximations (see, for example, [10]) were used to provide model selection in the unsupervised segmentation of physiological signals.

As case examples of such partitioning approaches, we consider the use of probabilistic Mixture of Gaussians models in biomedical image and signal segmentation.

Example 15. The first example result we show is that of an 8-channel EEG recording from an epileptic subject. A total of 8 hours of data was recorded at 128 Hz. A third-order AR model (see Section 10.11.1) was applied and a Gaussian mixture model fitted. Figure 10.10 shows the resultant log model evidence and model posteriors for varying numbers of clusters, K. Note that a $K = 2$ model is preferred. Figure 10.11 shows 4 s segments of EEG that have highest probability of class membership. We note that one of these (right-hand plot) clearly shows the characteristic 3-Hz "spike and wave" activity of an epileptic seizure. $\triangleleft$

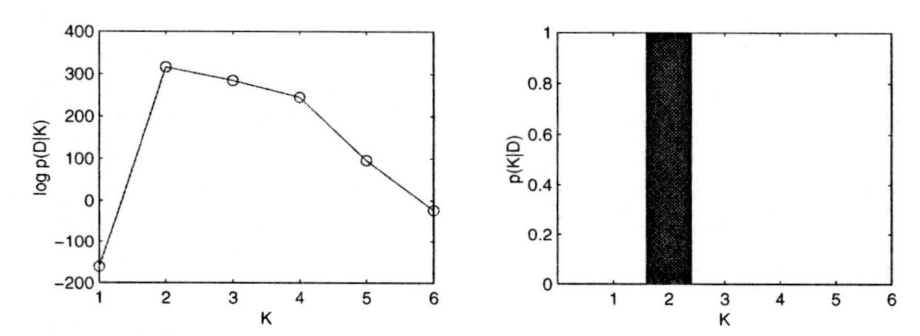

Fig. 10.10. Log evidence (left) and model posteriors for epileptic EEG data.

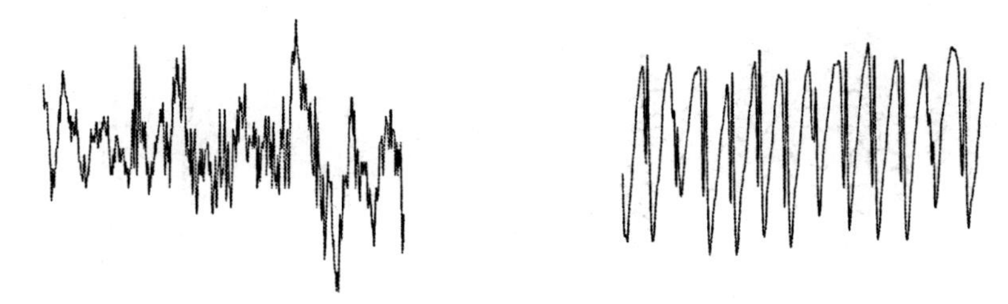

Fig. 10.11. Sections of EEG (4 s each) with maximal class posteriors. The right-hand plot is seizure activity.

The same mixture model approach may be easily applied to medical image segmentation, as the following example shows.

Example 16. Figure 10.12 shows right T2 (left) and proton density (right) magnetic resonance brain images. The grey levels of these two images form a simple two-dimensional space that we can model as generated by a mixture of Gaussians with unknown number. It is found (see [138]) that a $K = 5$ model is optimal. Figure 10.13 shows the posteriors over each of these five clusters (white corresponds to $p = 1$, black to $p = 0$) along with a grey-level coding of the resultant cluster indicator labels. We see that, even without the benefit of spatial models, or any explicit models of brain structure, a simple mixture model segments the image into a set of physiologically meaningful components, including tumours present in the image (bottom left component in the figure). $\triangleleft$

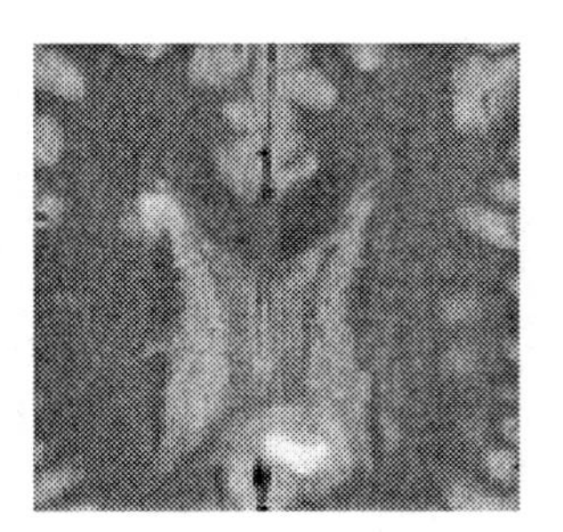

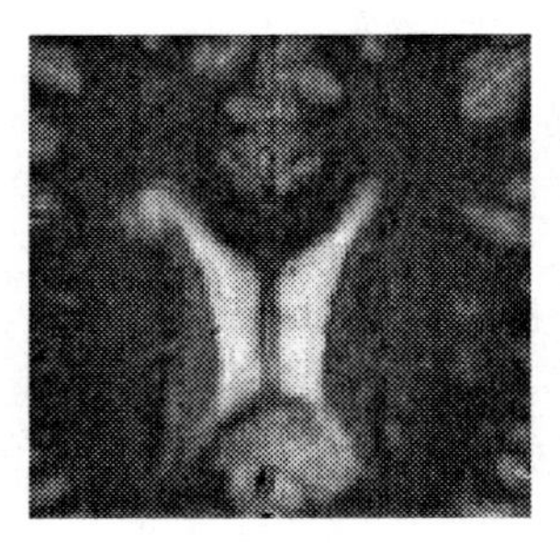

Fig. 10.12. T2 (left) and proton density (right) MR images.

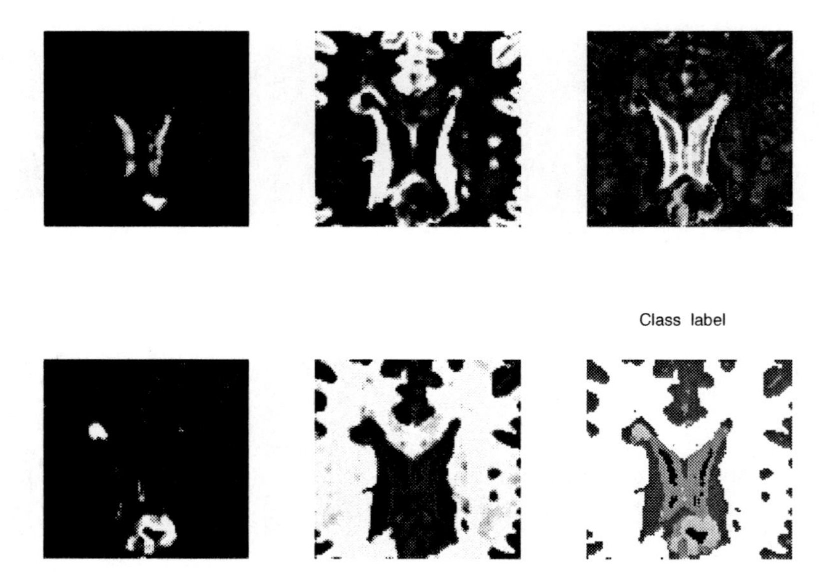

Fig. 10.13. Posterior probabilities of cluster membership. Bottom right shows the resultant class labelling of the MR image. Note the detection of tumours in the 4th cluster posterior (bottom left).

10.11.4 Hidden Markov Models

Hidden Markov models (HHMs) are well-established models with a wide range of applications. The two main components of the HMM are its hidden state sequence, S_t, which encodes state changes in the data, and a set of observation models, which model the within-state dynamics (spatial or temporal) of the data. Each state is associated with an observation model, which generates (from the model's perspective) the observed data, Y_t [120]. The graphical model for a standard HMM is shown in Figure 10.14.

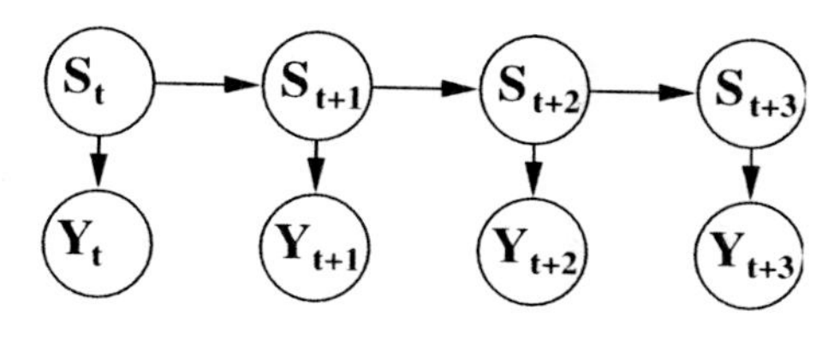

Fig. 10.14. A graphical model representation for the standard Hidden Markov Model. The set of hidden (latent) states S_t form a sequence which evolves under a first-order Markov process. Each state generates an observation, Y_t, according to its observation model.

The HMM has K discrete hidden states, S_i, $i \in [1, K]$, with the state at a given time t being q_t. From each S_i, there is a probability a_{ij} of making the transition to S_j in the next time step:

$$a_{ij} = p(q_{t+1} = S_j | q_t = S_i). \qquad (10.57)$$

These probabilities form the transition matrix $\mathbf{A}$.

Observations are taken at time t, and are denoted Y_t. These follow some observation model $b_j(Y_t)$, defined as:

$$b_j(Y_t) = p(Y_t | q_t = S_j). \qquad (10.58)$$

Due to the Markov property of the graph, the joint density over all states and observations is reduced into a product over neighbouring pairs, i.e.

$$p(\mathbf{S}, \mathbf{Y}) = \prod_{t=1}^{T} p(Y_t|S_t)p(S_t|S_{t-1})p(S_0), \qquad (10.59)$$

where the $p(S_0)$ term is a prior on the starting state of the chain. Computationally efficient message-passing approaches may be developed for solutions to inference in HMMs [120, 112], and, in the fully probabilistic framework, variational learning or sampling may be utilized [131, 101]. These fully Bayesian approaches have been shown to significantly improve performance in a biomedical setting [152].

Example 17. As an example of the use of the HMM in biomedical signal processing, we look at state changes in sections of EEG, recorded over the primary motor cortex, corresponding to imagined finger movements [118]; EEG is known to synchronize and desynchronize with such imagined movements. Figure 10.15 shows a section of EEG along with state paths from a HMM with an autoregressive (AR) observation model (upper path of each block) and a simple two-component Gaussian mixture model operating on the AR coefficients (lower path). We see that the HMM provides a considerably improved detection of areas of synchronized, rhythmic, EEG. As the AR observations model allows for the subsequent projection of the states into the spectral domain, we may look at the prototypical spectra associated with each state. This is shown in Figure 10.16. Note the clear 10 Hz activity associated with the second state, corresponding to the motor cortex "mu" rhythm. The vertical dashed lines indicate the time stamp of computer cues and is not used in the analysis. ◁

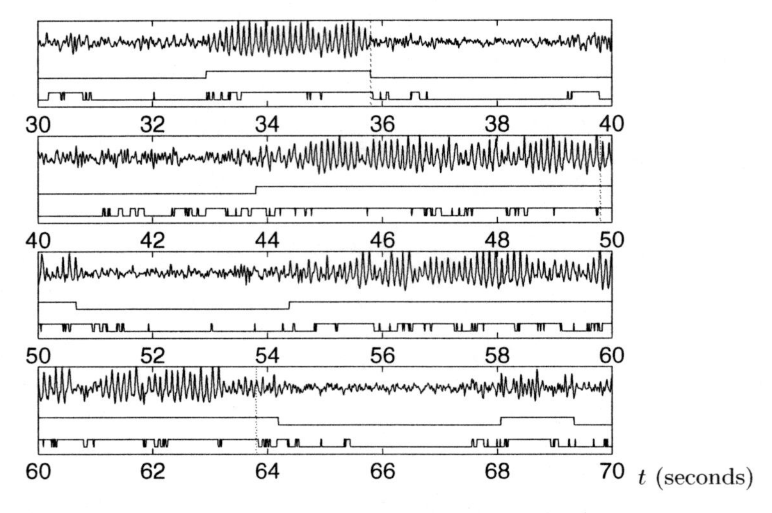

Fig. 10.15. EEG from an imagined movement experiment (top trace in each block). An AR observation model HMM gives an excellent state transition sequence (middle trace) compared with that of a Gaussian mixture model (lower trace).

The fact that HMMs may be cast in the framework of generic graphical (probabilistic) models also means that the observation model may be of arbitrary complexity. Indeed, it is an elegant quality of such an approach that the observed variables, within a Markov state, may be rigorously modelled as generated via another, nested, probabilistic model. Such nested "hierarchies" of probabilistic models enable the formation, for example, of hidden-Markov ICA models [113]. These were shown to be useful in the evaluation of state

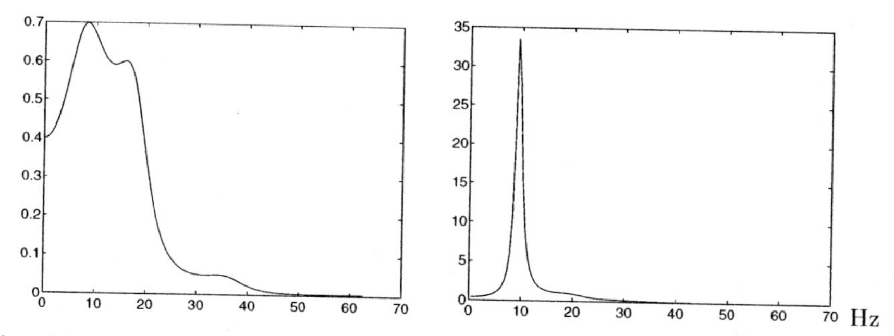

Fig. 10.16. Prototypical power spectra associated with each HMM state. Note that state 2 (right) shows clear association with 10 Hz "mu" activity over the motor cortex.

changes in biomedical signals in which the observed data were linearly mixed (a good model for many electro-physiological signals).

The generic framework of HMMs may be extended to include multiple-state chains that interact in their state-spaces. Such models are usually referred to as *Coupled Hidden Markov Models* (CHMMs), and they have found use in the development of interaction models for different biomedical signals [127]. The advantage of such models lies in the fact that interactions between different sources of information (for example, respiration and EEG or ECG and fMRI responses) may be modelled as interactions between state sequences rather than requiring explicit observation interaction models. Figure 10.17 shows the graphical model for CHMM with two state chains and first-order Markov interactions between all states.

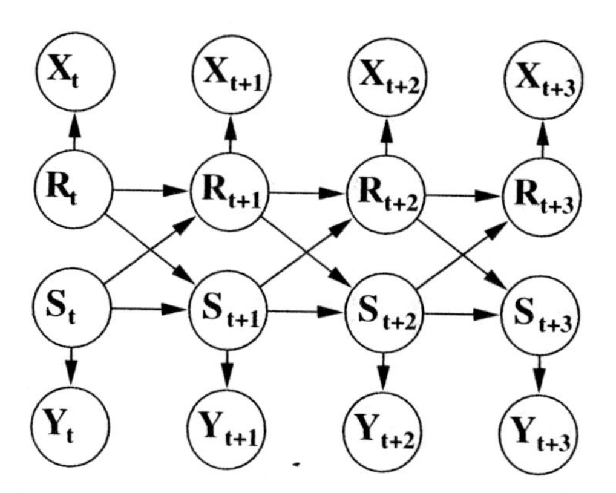

Fig. 10.17. A graphical model representation for a Coupled Hidden Markov Model (CHMM). The set of hidden (latent) states R_t and S_t form sequences which co-evolve under a first-order Markov process. Each state generates an observation, X_t and Y_t, according to its observation model.

10.11.5 Novelty Detection

One of the key problems in biomedical data processing lies in the fact that, whilst copious data from the non-patient population may be acquired, the amount of equivalent patient data may be small. This gives rise to *unbalanced* data sets which, without care, can lead to erroneous or biased results. The key concept of *novelty* or abnormality detection lies in exploiting the large quantities of non-patient data to build a rich model of "normality" against which abnormal results may be screened [135, 12]. Novelty detection approaches have taken two main strands. The first lies in the inference of a model for the normal-data probability density function, $p_N(x)$ say. When an unseen datum, u, is screened it is deemed novel if $p_N(u) < \theta$, where θ is a pre-defined threshold. The latter may be assessed using cross-validation arguments or by balancing the false positive detection rate and the resultant threshold used to screen, for example, EEG abnormalities and breast cancers in X-ray mammograms [135, 12, 154]. The second approach utilizes *extreme value theory* [54] in which the (limit-form) distribution for the extremal (tail) points in any distribution may be inferred. If the model for "normal" data is of Gaussian mixture form (which it may always be chosen to be) then the extreme value distributions are analytic and may be used with ease to detect outlying data. This approach was used for abnormal EEG detection and tumour determination in MRI images [137, 132].

Acknowledgments

We would like to thank Wray Buntine and Peter Weller for their careful reading and constructive comments on an earlier draft of this chapter.

We are grateful to Will Penny and Springer-Verlag for allowing us to reproduce Figure 10.1 from Penny et al. [117], and we are grateful to Adrian Raftery, Sylvia Richardson, and Marcel Dekker Inc. for permission to use the data in Table 10.1, which was taken from Raftery and Richardson [124].

References

[1] I.D Adams, M. Chan, P.C. Clifford, W.M. Cooke, V. Dallos, F.T. de Dombal, M.H. Edwards, D.M. Hancock, D.J. Hewett, N. McIntyre, P.G. Somerville, D.J. Spiegelhalter, J. Wellwood, and D.H. Wilson. Computer-aided diagnosis of acute abdominal pain: a multi-centre study. *British Medical Journal*, 292:800–804, 1986.

[2] S. Andreassen, A. Rosenfalck, B. Falck, K.G. Olesen, and S.K. Andersen. Evaluation of the diagnostic performance of the expert EMG assistant MUNIN. *Electroencephalography and Clinical Neurophysiology*, 101:129–144, 1996.

[3] H. Attias. Inferring parameters and structure of latent variable models by variational Bayes. In *Proceedings of the Fifteenth Conference on Uncertainty in Artificial Intelligence*, 1999.
[4] P. Auer, M. Herbster, and M.K. Warmuth. Exponentially many local minima for single neurons. In D.S. Touretzky, M.C. Mozer, and M.E. Hasselmo, editors, *Advances in Neural Information Processing Systems*, volume 8, pages 316–322. MIT Press, Cambridge, MA, 1996.
[5] A. Azzalini. *Statistical Inference – Based on the Likelihood.* Chapman & Hall, London, 1996.
[6] L.R. Bahl, P.F. Brown, P.V. de Souza and R.L. Mercer. A tree-based language model for natural language speech recognition. *IEEE Transactions on Acoustics, Speech and Signal Processing*, 37(7):1001–1008, 1989.
[7] V. Barnett. *Comparative Statistical Inference.* Wiley, Chichester, 2nd edition, 1982.
[8] C. Beckmann, J.A. Noble, and S. Smith. Investigating the intrinsic dimensionality of FMRI data for ICA. In *Seventh Int. Conf. on Functional Mapping of the Human Brain*, Brighton, UK, 2001.
[9] I.A. Beinlich, H.J. Suermondt, R.M. Chavez, and G.F. Cooper. The ALARM monitoring system: a case study with two probabilistic inference techniques for belief networks. In J. Hunter, J. Cookson, and J. Wyatt, editors, *Proceedings of the 2nd European Conference on Artificial Intelligence in Medicine*, pages 247–256, Berlin, 1989. Springer-Verlag.
[10] J.M. Bernardo and A.F.M. Smith. *Bayesian Theory.* John Wiley, 1994.
[11] R. Beyth-Marom. How probable is probable? A numerical translation of verbal probability expressions. *Journal of Forecasting*, 1:257–269, 1982.
[12] C.M. Bishop. Novelty Detection and Neural Network Validation. *IEE Proc. Vis. Image Signal Processing*, 141:217–222, 1994.
[13] C.M. Bishop. *Neural Networks for Pattern Recognition.* Clarendon Press, Oxford, 1995.
[14] M.E. Boon and L.P. Kok. Using artifical neural networks to screen cervical smears: how new technology enhances health care. In R. Dybowski and V. Gant, editors, *Clinical Applications of Artificial Neural Networks*, chapter 3. Cambridge University Press, Cambridge, 2001.
[15] G.E.P. Box and D.R. Cox. An analysis of transformations (with discussion). *Journal of the Royal Statistical Society*, B26:211–252, 1964.
[16] L. Breiman. Bagging predictors. *Machine Learning*, 24:123–140, 1996.
[17] L. Breiman, J.H. Friedman, R.A. Olshen, and C.J. Stone. *Classification and Regression Trees.* Chapman & Hall, New York, 1984.
[18] W. Buntine. *A Theory of Learning Classification Rules.* PhD dissertation, School of Computing Science, University of Technology, Sydney, February 1990.
[19] W. Buntine. Learning classification trees. *Statistics and Computing*, 2: 63–72, 1991.

[20] W.L. Buntine. A guide to the literature on learning probabilistic networks from data. *IEEE Transactions on Knowledge and Data Engineering*, 8:195–210, 1996.

[21] M. Cassidy and W. Penny. Bayesian nonstationary autoregressive models for biomedical signal analysis. *IEEE Transactions on Biomedical Engineering*, 49(10):1142–1152, 2002.

[22] X. Castella, A. Artigas, J. Bion, A. Kari, and The European/North American Severity Study Group. A comparison of severity of illness scoring systems for intensive care unit patients: Results of a multicenter, multinational study. *Critical Care Medicine*, 23:1327–1332, 1995.

[23] R. Choudrey and S. Roberts. Variational mixture of Bayesian independent component analysers. *Neural Computation*, 15(1), 2003.

[24] M. Clyde, P. Müller, and G. Parmigiani. Inference and design strategies for a hierarchical logistic regression model. In D.A. Berry and D.K. Stangl, editors, *Bayesian Biostatistics*, chapter 11. Marcel Dekker, New York, 1999.

[25] A. Cohen. *Biomedical Signal Processing.* CRC Press, Boca Raton, FL, 1986.

[26] D. Collett. *Modelling Binary Data.* Chapman & Hall, London, 1991.

[27] G.F Cooper and E. Herskovits. A Bayesian method for the induction of probabilistic networks from data. *Machine Learning*, 9:309–347, 1992.

[28] T. Cover and J. Thomas. *Elements of Information Theory.* Wiley, New York, 1991.

[29] R.G. Cowell. Advanced inference in Bayesian networks. In M.I. Jordan, editor, *Learning in Graphical Models*, pages 27–49. MIT Press, Cambridge, MA, 1999.

[30] R.G. Cowell, A.P. Dawid, S.L. Lauritzen, and D.J. Spiegelhalter. *Probabilistic Networks and Expert Systems.* Springer, New York, 1999.

[31] D.R. Cox and E.J. Snell. *Analysis of Binary Data.* Chapman & Hall, London, 2nd edition, 1989.

[32] S.S. Cross. Artifical neural networks in laboratory medicine. In R. Dybowski and V. Gant, editors, *Clinical Applications of Artificial Neural Networks*, chapter 2. Cambridge University Press, Cambridge, 2001.

[33] F.T. de Dombal, D.J. Leaper, J.R. Staniland, A.P. McCann, and J.C. Horrocks. Computer-aided diagnosis of acute abdominal pain. *British Medical Journal*, 2:9–13, 1972.

[34] A.P. Dempster, N.M. Laird, and D.B. Rubin. Maximum likelihood from incomplete data via the EM algorithm. *J. Roy. Stat. Soc.*, 39(1):1–38, 1977.

[35] A.J. Dobson. *An Introduction to Generalized Linear Models.* Chapman & Hall, London, 1990.

[36] P. Domingos and M.J. Pazzani. On the optimality of the simple Bayesian classifier under zero-one loss. *Machine Learning*, 29(2–3):103–130, 1997.

[37] M.J. Druzdel and L.C. van der Gaag. Elicitation of probabilities for belief networks: Combining qualitative and quantitative information.

In P. Besnard and S. Hanks, editors, *Proceedings of the 11th Annual Conference on Uncertainty in Artificial Intelligence*, pages 141–148, San Francisco, CA, 1995. Morgan Kaufman.

[38] R. Dybowski. Classification of incomplete feature vectors by radial basis function networks. *Pattern Recognition Letters*, 19:1257–1264, 1998.

[39] R. Dybowski and V. Gant. Artificial neural networks in pathology and medical laboratories. *Lancet*, 346:1203–1207, 1995.

[40] R. Dybowski and V. Gant, editors. *Clinical applications of artificial neural networks*. Cambridge University Press, 2001.

[41] R. Dybowski and S.J. Roberts. Confidence intervals and prediction intervals for feedforward neural networks. In R. Dybowski and V. Gant, editors, *Clinical Applications of Artificial Neural Networks*, pages 298–326. Cambridge University Press, Cambridge, 2001.

[42] N. Friedman. The Bayesian structural EM algorithm. In G.F. Cooper and S. Moral, editors, *Proceedings of the 14th Conference on Uncertainty in Artificial Intelligence*, pages 129–138, San Francisco, CA, 1998. Morgan Kaufmann.

[43] N. Friedman, D. Geiger, and M. Goldszmidt. Bayesian network classifiers. *Machine Learning*, 29:131–163, 1997.

[44] K.J. Friston, D.E. Glaser, R.N.A. Henson, S. Kiebel, C. Phillips, and J. Ashburner. Classical and Bayesian inference in neuroimaging: Applications. *Neuroimaging*, 16:484–512, 2002.

[45] K.J. Friston, W. Penny, C. Phillips, S. Kiebel, G. Hinton, and J. Ashburner. Classical and Bayesian inference in neuroimaging: Theory. *Neuroimaging*, 16:465–483, 2002.

[46] L.C. van der Gaag, S. Renooij, C.L.M. Witteman, B.M.P. Aleman, and B.G. Taal. Probabilities for a probabilistic network: a case study in oesophageal cancer. *Artificial Intelligence in Medicine*, 25(2):123–148, 2002.

[47] J.-R. Le Gall, S. Lemeshow, and F. Saulnier. A new Simplified Acute Physiology Score (SAPS II) based on a European/North American multicenter study. *Journal of the American Medical Association*, 270(24): 2957–2963, 1993.

[48] J.-R. Le Gall, P. Loirat, A. Alperovitch, P. Glaser, C. Granthil, D. Mathieu, P. Mercier, R. Thomas, and D. Villers. A simplified acute physiology score for ICU patients. *Critical Care Medicine*, 12:975–977, 1984.

[49] Z. Ghahramani and M.I. Jordan. Supervised learning from incomplete data via an EM approach. In J.D. Cowan, G.T. Tesauro, and J. Alspector, editors, *Advances in Neural Information Processing Systems*, volume 6, pages 120–127. Morgan Kaufman, San Mateo, CA, 1994.

[50] W.R. Gilks, S. Richardson, and D.J. Spiegelhalter, editors. *Markov Chain Monte Carlo in Practice*. Chapman & Hall, London, 1996.

[51] S. Godshill and P. Rayner. Statistical reconstruction and analysis of autoregressive signals in impulsive noise. *IEEE Transactions on Speech & Audio Processing*, 6(4):352–372, July 1998.

[52] R. Goodacre, E.M. Timmins, R. Burton, N. Kaderbhai, A.M. Woodward, D.B. Kell, and P.J. Rooney. Rapid identification of urinary tract infection bacteria using hyperspectral whole-organism fingerprinting and artificial neural networks. *Microbiology*, 144(5):1157–1170, 1998.

[53] C. Gössl, D.P. Auer, and L. Fahrmeir. Bayesian spatio-temporal inference in functional magnetic resonance imaging. *Biometrics*, 57(2), 2001.

[54] E.J. Gumbel. *Statistics of Extremes.* Columbia University Press, New York, 1958.

[55] F.E. Harrell. *Regression Modeling Strategies.* Springer, New York, 2001.

[56] T. Hastie, R. Tibshirani, and J. Friedman. *The Elements of Statistical Learning: Data Mining, Inference and Prediction.* Springer, New York, 2001.

[57] W.K. Hastings. Monte Carlo sampling methods using Markov chains and their applications. *Biometrika*, 57:97–109, 1970.

[58] D. Heckerman. *Probabilistic Similarity Networks.* MIT Press, Cambridge, MA, 1990.

[59] D. Heckerman. A tractable inference algorithm for diagnosing multiple diseases. In M. Henrion, R. Shachter, L. Kanal, and J. Lemmer, editors, *Uncertainty in Artificial Intelligence 5*, pages 163–171. North-Holland, New York, 1990.

[60] D. Heckerman. A tutorial on learning with Bayesian networks. In M.I. Jordan, editor, *Learning in Graphical Models*, pages 301–354. MIT Press, Cambridge, MA, 1999.

[61] D. Heckerman, E. Horvitz, and B. Nathwani. Towards normative experts systems: part I – the Pathfinder project. *Methods of Information in Medicine*, 31:90–105, 1992.

[62] D. Heckerman and B. Nathwani. Towards normative experts systems: part II – probability-based representations for efficient knowledge acquisition and inference. *Methods of Information in Medicine*, 31:106–116, 1992.

[63] D.W. Hosmer and S. Lemeshow. *Applied Logistic Regression.* Wiley, New York, 1989.

[64] D. Husmeier, W.D. Penny, and S.J. Roberts. An empirical evaluation of Bayesian sampling with hybrid Monte Carlo for training neural network classifiers. *Neural Networks*, 12:677–705, 1999.

[65] T.Z. Irony and N.D. Singpurwalla. Non-informative priors do not exist: A dialogue with Jose M. Bernardo. *Journal of Statistical Planning and Inference*, 65(1):159–189, 1997.

[66] T. Jaakkola and M.I. Jordan. Variational probabilistic inference and the QMR-DT network. *Journal of Artificial Intelligence Research*, 10: 291–322, 1999.

[67] S. Jacobs, R.W.S. Chang, B. Lee, and B. Lee. Audit of intensive care: A 30-month experience using the APACHE II severity of disease classification system. *Intensive Care Medicine*, 14:567–574, 1988.

[68] B.H. Jansen, J.R. Bourne, and J.W. Ward. Autoregressive estimation of short segment spectra for computerized EEG analysis. *IEEE Trans. on Biomed. Eng*, 28:630–638, 1981.

[69] B.H. Jansen, J.R. Bourne, and J.W. Ward. Identification and labeling of EEG graphic elements using autoregressive spectral estimates. *Comput. Biol. Med.*, 12:97–106, 1982.

[70] A.H. Jazwinski. *Stochastic Processes and Filtering Theory.* Academic Press, 1970.

[71] J. Jenny, I. Isenegger, M.E. Boon, and O.A.N Husain. Consistency of a double PAPNET scan of cervical smears. *Acta Cytologia*, 41:82–87, 1997.

[72] F.V. Jensen. *Bayesian Networks and Decision Graphs.* Springer, New York, 2001.

[73] F.V. Jensen, K.G. Olesen, and S.K. Andersen. An algebra of Bayesian belief universes for knowledge-based systems. *Networks*, 20:637–659, 1990.

[74] M.I. Jordan, editor. *Learning in Graphical Models.* MIT Press, Cambridge, MA, 1999.

[75] M.I. Jordan, Z. Ghahramani, T. Jaakkola, and L.K. Saul. An introdusction to variational methods for graphical models. In M.I. Jordan, editor, *Learning in Graphical Models*, pages 105–161. MIT Press, Cambridge, MA, 1999.

[76] C.E. Kahn, L.M. Roberts, K.A. Shaffer, and P. Haddawy. Construction of a Bayesian network for mammographic diagnosis of breast cancer. *Computers in Biology and Medicine*, 27:19–29, 1997.

[77] H.J. Kappen, W. Wiegerinck, E.W.M.T ter Braak, W.J.P.P ter Burg, M.J. Nijman, Y.L. O, and J.P. Neijt. Approximate inference for medical diagnosis. *Pattern Recognition Letters*, 20:1231–1239, 1999.

[78] R.E. Kass and A.E. Raftery. Bayes factors. Technical Report 254, Department of Statistics, University of Washington, Washington, March 1993. [Technical Report 571, Department of Statistics, Carnegie-Mellon University.]

[79] R.E. Kass and A.E. Raftery. Bayes factors and model uncertainty. *Journal of the American Statistical Association*, 90:773–795, 1995.

[80] R.E. Kass and L. Wasserman. The selection of prior distributions by formal rules. *Journal of the American Statistical Association*, 91(435): 1343–1370, 1996.

[81] D.G. Kleinbaum. *Logistic Regression.* Springer, New York, 1994.

[82] W.A. Knaus, E.A. Draper, D.P. Wagner, and J.E. Zimmerman. APACHE II: A severity of disease classification system. *Critical Care Medicine*, 13:818–829, 1985.

[83] W.A. Knaus, F.E. Harrell, C.J. Fisher, D.P. Wagner, S.M. Opal, J.C. Sadoff, E.A. Draper, C.A. Walawander, K.Conboy, and T.H. Grasela. The clinical evaluation of new drugs for sepsis: A prospective study

design based on survival analysis. *Jouranl of the American Medical Association*, 270(10):1233–1241, 1993.

[84] W.A. Knaus, D.P. Wagner, E.A. Draper, J.E. Zimmerman, M. Bergner, P.G. Bastos, C.A. Sirio, D.J. Murphy, T. Lotring, A. Damiano, and F.E. Harrell. The APACHE III prognostic system: Risk prediction of hospital mortality for critically ill hospitalized patients. *Chest*, 10(6):1619–1635, 1991.

[85] W.A. Knaus, J.E. Zimmerman, D.P. Wagner, E.A. Draper, and D.E. Lawrence. APACHE - Acute Physiology and Chronic Health Evaluation: A physiologically based classification system. *Critical Care Medicine*, 9: 591–597, 1981.

[86] K. Knuth. A Bayesian approach to source separation. In J.-F. Cardoso, C. Jutten, and P. Loubaton, editors, *Proceedings of the First International Workshop on Independent Component Analysis and Signal Separation: ICA-99*, pages 283–288, 1999.

[87] L.G. Koss. The application of PAPNET to diagnostic cytology. In P.J.G. Lisboa, E.C. Ifeachor, and P.S. Szczepaniak, editors, *Artificial Neural Networks in Biomedicine*, chapter 4. Springer, London, 2000.

[88] L.G. Koss, M.E. Sherman, M.B. Cohen, A.R. Anes, T.M. Darragh, L.B. Lemos, B.J. McClellan, and D.L. Rosenthal. Significant reduction in the rate of false-negative cervical smears with neural-network based technology (PAPNET testing system). *Human Pathology*, 28:1196–1203, 1997.

[89] S.L. Lauritzen. Propagation of probabilities, means and variances in mixed graphical association models. *Journal of the American Statistical Association*, 87:1098–1108, 1992.

[90] L. Leibovici, M. Fishman, H.C. Schønheyder, C. Riekehr, B. Kristensen, I. Shraga, and S. Andreassen. A causal probabilistic network for optimal treatment of bacterial infections. *IEEE Transactions on Knowledge and Data Engineering*, 12(4):517–528, 2000.

[91] S. Lemeshow, D. Teres, J. Klar, J.S. Avrunin, S.H. Gehlbach, and J. Rapoport. Mortality probability models (MPM II) based on an international cohort of intensive care unit patients. *Journal of the American Medical Association*, 270(20):2479–2485, 1993.

[92] S. Lemeshow, D. Teres, H. Pastides, J.S. Avrunin, and J.S. Steingrub. A method for predicting survival and mortality of ICU patients using objectively derived weights. *Critical Care Medicine*, 13:519–525, 1985.

[93] U. Lerner, E. Segal, and D. Koller. Exact inference in networks with discrete children of continuous parents. In J. Breese and D. Koller, editors, *Proceedings of the 17th Conference on Uncertainty in Artificial Intelligence*, pages 129–138, San Francisco, CA, 2001. Morgan Kaufmann.

[94] R.J.A. Little and D.B. Rubin. *Statistical Analysis with Missing Data*. Wiley, New York, 1987.

[95] D. Lowe and A.R. Webb. Exploiting prior knowledge in network optimization: an illustration from medical prognosis. *Network: Computation in Neural Systems*, 1:299–323, 1990.

[96] P.J.F. Lucas. Expert knowledge and its role in learning Bayesian networks in medicine: an appraisal. In S. Quaglini, P. Barahona, and S. Andreassen, editors, *Proceedings of Artificial Intelligence in Medicine in Europe 2001 (Lecture Notes in Artificial Intelligence No. 2101)*, pages 156–166, Berlin, 2001. Springer-Verlag.

[97] P.J.F. Lucas, H. Boot, and B.G. Taal. Computer-based decision-support in the management of primary gastric non-Hodgkin lymphoma. *Methods of Information in Medicine*, 37:206–219, 1998.

[98] P.J.F. Lucas, N.G. de Bruijn, K. Schurink, and I.M. Hoepelman. A probabilistic and decision-theoretic approach to the management of infectious disease at the ICU. *Artificial Intelligence in Medicine*, 19(3): 251–279, 2000.

[99] D.J.C. MacKay. The evidence framework applied to classification networks. *Neural Computation*, 4(5):720–736, 1992.

[100] D.J.C. MacKay. A practical Bayesian framework for back-propagation networks. *Neural Computation*, 4(3):448–472, 1992.

[101] D.J.C. MacKay. Ensemble learning for Hidden Markov Models. Technical report, Cavendish Laboratory, University of Cambridge, 1998.

[102] S.M. Mahoney and K.B. Laskey. Network engineering for complex belief networks. In E. Horvitz and F.V. Jensen, editors, *Proceedings of the 12th Conference on Uncertainty in Artificial Intelligence*, pages 389–396, San Francisco, CA, 1999. Morgan Kaufman.

[103] N. Metropolis, A.W. Rosenbluth, M.N. Rosenbluth, A.H. Teller, and E. Teller. Equation of state calculations by fast computing machines. *Journal of Chemical Physics*, 21:1087–1092, 1953.

[104] J. Miskin and D. MacKay. Ensemble learning for blind source separation. In S. Roberts and R. Everson, editors, *Independent Component Analysis: Principles and Practice*, chapter 8. Cambridge University Press, 2001.

[105] K.P. Murphy, Y. Weiss, and M.I. Jordan. Loopy belief propagation for approximation inference: An empirical study. In K.B. Laskey and H. Prade, editors, *Proceedings of the 15th Conference on Uncertainty in Artificial Intelligence*, pages 467–475, San Francisco, CA, 1999. Morgan Kaufman.

[106] I.T. Nabney. Efficient training of RBF networks for classification. In *Proceedings of the Ninth International Conference on Artificial Neural Networks (ICANN99)*, pages 210–215, London, 1999. IEE.

[107] R. Neal. Connectionist learning in belief networks. *Artificial Intelligence*, 56:71–113, 1992.

[108] R.M. Neal. *Bayesian Learning for Neural Networks.* Lecture Notes in Statistics Series No. 118. Springer, Berlin, 1996.

[109] J.J.K. O' Ruanaidth and W.J. Fitzgerald. *Numerical Bayesian Methods Applied to Signal Processing.* Springer, 1996.

[110] J. Pardey, S. Roberts, and L. Tarassenko. A Review of Parametric Modelling Techniques for EEG Analysis. *Med. Eng. Phys*, 18(1):2–11, 1996.

[111] J. Pearl. A constraint-propagation approach to probabilistic reasoning. In L.N. Kanal and J.F. Lemmer, editors, *Uncertainty in Artificial Intelligence*, pages 357–370. North-Holland, Amsterdam, 1986.

[112] J. Pearl. *Probabilistic Reasoning in Intelligent Systems: Networks of Plausible Reasoning.* Morgan Kaufmann, San Mateo, CA, 1988.

[113] W. Penny, R. Everson, and S. Roberts. Hidden Markov independent components analysis. In M. Girolami, editor, *Advances in Independent Components Analysis*, Springer, 2000.

[114] W. Penny and S. Roberts. Bayesian multivariate autoregressive models with structured priors. *IEE Proceedings on Vision, Image and Signal processing*, 149(1):33–41, 2002.

[115] W. Penny and S. Roberts. Variational Bayes for generalised autoregressive models. *IEEE Transactions on Signal Processing*, 50(9):2245–2257, 2002.

[116] W.D. Penny and K.J. Friston. Mixtures of general linear models for functional neuroimaging. *IEEE Transactions on Medical Imaging*, 2003.

[117] W.D. Penny, D. Husmeier, and S.J. Roberts. The Bayesian paradigm: Second generation neural computing. In P.J.G. Lisboa, E.C. Ifeachor, and P.S. Szczepaniak, editors, *Artificial Neural Networks in Biomedicine*, chapter 1. Springer, London, 2000.

[118] W.D. Penny and S.J. Roberts. Dynamic models for nonstationary signal segmentation. *Computers and Biomedical Research*, 32(6):483–502, 1999.

[119] PRISMATIC project management team. Assessment of automated primary screening on PAPNET of cervical smears in the PRISMATIC trial. *The Lancet*, 353:1381–1385, 1999.

[120] M Rabiner. A tutorial on hidden Markov models and selected applications in speech recongnition. *Proceedings of the IEEE*, 77(2):257–286, 1977.

[121] A.E. Raftery. Model selection and accounting for model uncertainty in graphical models using Occam's Window. Technical Report 213, Department of Statistics, University of Washington, Washington, August 1992.

[122] A.E. Raftery. Approximate Bayes factors and accounting for model uncertainty in generalized linear models. Technical Report 255, Department of Statistics, University of Washington, Washington, August 1993.

[123] A.E. Raftery. Bayesian model selection in social research (with discussion by Andrew Gelman, Donald B. Rubin and Robert M. Hauser).

In P.V. Marsden, editor, *Sociological Methodology 1995*, pages 111–196. Blackwells, Oxford, 1995.

[124] A.E. Raftery and S. Richardson. Model selection for generalized linear models via GLIB: Application to nutrition and breast cancer. In D.A. Berry and D.K. Stangl, editors, *Bayesian Biostatistics*, chapter 12. Marcel Dekker, New York, 1999.

[125] A.E. Raftery and C. Volinsky, 1999. *Bayesian Model Averaging Home Page* [WWW]. Available from: http://www.research.att.com/ volinsky/bma.html [Accessed 9 July 1999].

[126] S. Renooij. *Qualitative Approaches to Quantifying Probabilistic Networks.* PhD dissertation, Institute of Information and Computing Sciences, University of Utrecht, March 2001.

[127] I. Rezek and S. Roberts. A Comparison of Bayesian and Maximum Likelihood Learning of Coupled Hidden Markov Models. *IEE Proceedings – Science, Technology & Measurement*, 147(6):345–350, November 2000.

[128] S. Richardson and P.J. Green. On Bayesian analysis of mixtures with an unknown number of components. *Journal of the Royal Statistical Society (Series B)*, 59(4):731–758, 1997.

[129] B.D. Ripley. *Pattern Recognition and Neural Networks.* Cambridge University Press, Cambridge, 1996.

[130] J. Rissanen. Stochastic compexity (with discussion). *Journal of the Royal Statistical Society, Series B*, 49:223–239, 253–265, 1987.

[131] C.P. Robert, G. Celeux, and J. Diebolt. Bayesian estimation of hidden Markov chains: a stochastic implementation. *Statist. Prob. Letters*, 16: 77–83, 1993.

[132] S. Roberts. Extreme Value Statistics for Novelty Detection in Biomedical Signal Processing. *IEE Proceedings – Science, Technology & Measurement*, 147(6):363–367, November 2000.

[133] S. Roberts and R. Everson. *Independent Component Analysis: principles and practice.* Cambridge University Press, 2001.

[134] S. Roberts, C. Holmes, and D. Denison. Minimum entropy data partitioning using Reversible Jump Markov Chain Monte Carlo. *IEEE Transactions on Pattern Analysis and Machine Intelligence*, 23(6), June 2001.

[135] S. Roberts and L. Tarassenko. A probabilistic resource allocating network for novelty detection. *Neural Computation*, 6:270–284, 1994.

[136] S.J. Roberts. Independent component analysis: source assessment and separation, a Bayesian approach. *IEE Proceedings, Vision, Image & Signal Processing*, 145(3):149–154, 1998.

[137] S.J. Roberts. Novelty detection using extreme value statistics. *IEE Proceedings on Vision, Image & Signal Processing*, 146(3):124–129, June 1999.

[138] S.J. Roberts, D. Husmeier, I. Rezek, and W. Penny. Bayesian approaches to Gaussian mixture modelling. *IEEE Transaction on Pattern Analysis and Machine Intelligence*, 20(11):1133–1142, 1998.

[139] D.B. Rubin. Inference and missing data. *Biometrika*, 63:581–592, 1976.

[140] D.B. Rubin. *Multiple Imputation for Nonresponse in Surveys.* John Wiley, New York, 1987.

[141] R. Sachter and C. Kenley. Gaussian influence diagrams. *Management Science*, 35:527–550, 1989.

[142] J.L. Schafer. *Analysis of Incomplete Multivariate Data.* Chapman & Hall, London, 1997.

[143] P.K. Sharp and R.J. Solly. Dealing with missing values in neural network-based diagnostic systems. *Neural Computing and Applications*, 3:73–77, 1995.

[144] M. Shwe, B. Middleton, D. Heckerman, M. Henrion, E.J. Horvitz, and H. Lehmann. Probabilistic diagnosis using a reformulation of the INTERNIST-1 / QMR knowledge base I: The probabilistic model and inference algorithms. *Methods of Information in Medicine*, 30:241–255, 1991.

[145] B.W. Silverman. *Density Estimation for Statistics and Data Analysis.* Chapman & Hall, London, 1986.

[146] D.W. Skagen. Estimation of running frequency spectra using a Kalman filter algorithm. *Journal of Biomedical Engineering*, 10:275–279, 1988.

[147] C.S. Spetzler and C.-A Staël von Holstein. Probability encoding in decision analysis. *Management Science*, 22:340–352, 1975.

[148] D.J. Spiegelhalter and R.G. Cowell. Learning in probabilistic expert systems. In J.M Bernardo, J.O. Berger, A.P. Dawid, and A.F.M. Smith, editors, *Bayesian Statistics 4*, pages 447–465. Clarendon Press, Oxford, 1992.

[149] D.J. Spiegelhalter and S.L. Lauritzen. Sequential updating of conditional probabilities on directed graphical structures. *Networks*, 20:579–605, 1990.

[150] H.J. Suermondt and M.D. Amylon. Probabilistic prediction of the outcome of bone-marrow transplantation. In L.C. Kingsland, editor, *Proceedings of the 13th Symposium on Computer Applications in Medical Care*, pages 208–212, Washington, DC, 1989. IEEE Computer Society Press.

[151] P. Sykacek and S. Roberts. Bayesian time series classification. In *NIPS 2001.* MIT Press, 2001.

[152] P. Sykacek and S. Roberts. Bayesian time series classification. In *Proceedings of Neural Information Processing Systems (NIPS)*, December 2001.

[153] M.A. Tanner and W.H. Wong. The calculation of posterior distributions by data augmentation (with discussion). *Journal of the American Statistical Association*, 82:528–550, 1987.

[154] L. Tarassenko, P. Hayton, N. Cerneaz, and M. Brady. Novelty detection for the detection of masses in mammograms. In *Proceedings of the Fourth IEE International Conference on Artificial Neural Networks*, pages 442–447. IEE, June 1995.

[155] D.M. Titterington, G.D. Murray, L.S. Murray, D.J. Spiegelhalter, A.M. Skene, J.D.F. Habbema, and G.J. Gelpke. Comparison of discrimination techniques applied to a complex data-set of head-injured patients (with discussion). *Journal of the Royal Statistical Society, Series A*, 144:145–175, 1981.

[156] V. Tresp, S. Ahamad, and R. Neuneier. Training neural networks with deficient data. In J.D. Cowan, G. Tesauro, and J. Alspector, editors, *Neural Information Processing Systems*, volume 6, pages 128–135. Morgan Kaufmann, 1994.

[157] Y. van der Graaf, G.P. Vooijs, H.L.J. Gaillard, and D.M.D. Go. Screening errors in cervical cytology smears. *Acta Cytologia*, 31:434–438, 1987.

[158] T. Verma and J. Pearl. Causal networks: Semantics and expressiveness. In R.D. Shachter, T.S. Levitt, L.N. Kanal, and J.F. Lemmer, editors, *Uncertainty in Artificial Intelligence 4*, pages 69–76. North-Holland, Amsterdam, 1990.

[159] C. Wallace and J. Patrick. Coding decision trees. *Machine Learning*, 11 (1):7–22, 1993.

[160] Y. Zhang, M. Brady, and S. Smith. Segmentation of brain MR images through a hidden Markov random field model and the expectation maximization algorithm. *IEEE Transactions on Medical Imaging*, 20 (1):45–57, 2001.

11

Bayesian Analysis of Population Pharmacokinetic/Pharmacodynamic Models

David J. Lunn

Imperial College School of Medicine, London, UK,
d.lunn@ic.ac.uk

Summary. This chapter discusses Bayesian models of groups of individuals who may have taken several drug doses at various times throughout the course of a clinical trial. The Bayesian approach helps the derivation of predictive distributions that contribute to the optimisation of treatments for different target populations.

11.1 Introduction

Pharmacokinetics (PK) can be defined as the study of the time course of drugs and their metabolites within the body. In contrast, pharmacodynamics (PD) is concerned with relating drug effect to either dosage regimen or some relevant drug concentration in the body. While PD is by far the more clinically relevant, PK is generally easier to measure and better understood, and is thus seen as an important intermediate.

Put very simply, when we take/receive a single dose of any drug, the amount (or concentration) of that drug within our bloodstream and bodily tissues begins to increase as the drug is "absorbed" into and distributed throughout our bodies. As the drug is transported around the body, typically via the blood, it will come across various "eliminating" organs, such as the liver, where the drug may be broken down into other compounds (metabolites), and the kidneys, which may filter unchanged drug and/or its metabolites into our urine for excretion. Since the administered dose is finite, absorption (or, more generally, "input") must eventually either cease completely or drop to a level such that the amount of drug leaving the body per unit time is greater than that entering it, at which point the total amount of drug within the body begins a steady decline back towards zero.

Pharmacokinetic models, whether empirical or based on real physiology, aim to accurately characterize the three fundamental processes mentioned above: absorption (or input), distribution, and elimination. They are typically constructed by considering the body as a collection of "compartments" between which drug transfer may or may not occur. This leads to a system of ordinary differential equations parameterized by compartmental volumes and drug transfer rates. Often this system of equations can be solved analytically but the solution is usually non-linear (as a function of model parameters) and potentially very complex.

Regarding pharmacodynamics, different drugs work in different ways, clearly, but all drugs need to "bind" to specific "receptors" within the body in order to produce their desired "effect". Although the mechanism by which this effect is brought about may be quite complex, it is natural to think that the magnitude of the effect will be closely related to the extent of binding, i.e., the number of "occupied" receptors, which will largely be determined by the amount of drug in the vicinity of those receptors. PK models that can predict the time course of drug within this specific vicinity are thus invaluable tools for scientifically linking PK and PD observations together.

Population PK/PD models are concerned with groups of individuals who may have each taken not one but many single doses at various times throughout the course of a clinical trial. The general aim is to determine the central tendency of the concentration–time profile and/or the effect–concentration relationship and quantify the variability in system parameters remaining after controlling for relevant covariates. Use of the Bayesian approach greatly facilitates the subsequent derivation of predictive distributions for clinically relevant (but arbitrarily complex) quantities, which when combined with a suitable "utility" or "loss" function provide a formal and coherent means of optimizing treatments for different target populations [23], for example.

The stochastic elements of population PK/PD models are typically quite straightforward and easily handled by existing general purpose software. However, the complexity of patients' dosing histories coupled with the fact that each dose itself typically requires a complex and non-linear model means that the deterministic component presents some special challenges, regarding mainly model specification but also MCMC sampling and efficiency. This chapter, as well as providing details of the various types of model available, discusses these problems in detail and describes efforts that have been made to alleviate them. Parameterization issues, such as model identifiability and interpretability, are a central theme.

11.2 Deterministic Models

11.2.1 Pharmacokinetics

Empirical models

Perhaps the simplest scenario is when a single dose of drug is administered as an intravenous (IV) bolus and the data comprise measurements of drug concentration in the blood. Since the entire dose is injected as quickly as possible into venous blood, we do not have to worry about modelling the input process; we simply make use of the fact that we know exactly how much drug is in the system just after time zero (0_+, say) and that only disposition (distribution + elimination) occurs thereafter. Figure 11.1 shows genuine measured blood concentrations plotted on a logarithmic scale against time following an IV bolus of some anonymous drug. The logarithmic scale reveals two distinct (approximately) linear portions, which suggests that a bi-exponential model on the natural scale will provide a good fit to the data:

$$C(t) = L_1 \mathrm{e}^{-\lambda_1 t} + L_2 \mathrm{e}^{-\lambda_2 t} \tag{11.1}$$

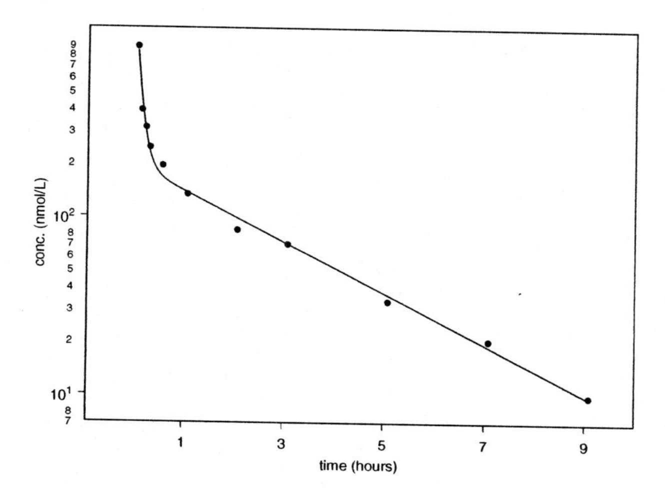

Fig. 11.1. Observed pharmacokinetic profile on logarithmic scale: • measured drug concentration; — fitted bi-exponential (see (11.1)).

where $C(.)$ denotes concentration, t denotes time, and L_1, L_2, λ_1 and λ_2 are unknown parameters. Since $C(0_+) = Dose/V$, where V is the *apparent* volume into which the dose is initially distributed (unknown), it is natural to reparameterize via $L_1 = q \times Dose/V$ and $L_2 = (1 - q) \times Dose/V$, where now q and V replace L_1 and L_2 as unknown parameters and *Dose* is, of course, known. Generally speaking, empirical models for IV boluses all have a similar form, i.e., a sum of exponentials:

$$C(t) = \frac{Dose}{V} \sum_{i=1}^{d} q_i \times \exp(-\lambda_i t), \quad \sum_{i=1}^{d} q_i = 1 \tag{11.2}$$

where d is chosen according to the apparent number of linear phases on a logarithmic plot of the data.

Often it is reasonable to assume that the underlying system is "linear", in the sense that concentrations/amounts of drug within the body, at any time, are directly proportional to the dose received. This provides us with a straightforward way of extending the above model to handle situations where the input process is more complex. We may perceive any input process as comprising a sequence of infinitesimal bolus doses. Let s be a dummy variable representing time and let $R(s)$ denote the rate of absorption/input at time s. Then, within each time interval $(s, s + \mathrm{d}s)$ an amount $R(s)\mathrm{d}s$ enters the system. If that system is linear then the overall response to this sequence of boluses can be obtained by summing the responses to each individual bolus:

$$C(t) = \int_{s=0}^{t} C_\delta(t - s)R(s)\mathrm{d}s \tag{11.3}$$

where $C_\delta(.)$ is known as the *unit impulse dose response* and is given by (11.2) with $Dose = 1$. The two most common choices of input process are *zero-order* and *first-*

order. Zero-order input is where the whole dose is "absorbed" at a constant rate until there is none remaining, at which point the rate of input drops, suddenly, to zero:

$$R(t) = \begin{cases} \frac{Dose}{TI} & 0 < t \leq TI \\ 0 & \text{otherwise} \end{cases}$$

where TI is the duration of input and may either be known, such as in the case of an IV infusion, or unknown. With first-order input, $R(t)$ is assumed to be proportional to $A_0(t)$, the amount of unabsorbed drug remaining at time t: $R(t) = k_a A_0(t)$, where k_a is referred to as the (first-order) absorption rate constant and is typically an unknown parameter. From this assumption we have that $\frac{dA_0}{dt} = -k_a A_0$ and so $R(t) = k_a \times Dose \times e^{-k_a t}$. Both of these forms for $R(.)$ are "compatible" with the general form for bolus responses given in (11.2), in terms of enabling the integration in (11.3), and so closed forms for zero- and first-order models are readily available.

It is worth noting at this point that typically we are modelling drug concentrations in blood, but not all drug necessarily enters the systemic circulation. For example, if a drug is taken orally then a significant proportion of each dose may pass straight through the gut, unabsorbed, and be excreted faecally. Further, that which *is* absorbed will (typically) be absorbed into the hepatic portal vein and must consequently pass through the liver, an eliminating organ, before entering the general circulation. We thus introduce the concept of *bioavailability*, which is the proportion, denoted by F, of the total dose that actually enters the site where measurements are to be made. The impact of this on our modelling equations is that, where appropriate, we must simply replace $Dose$ by $F \times Dose$. However, note that we cannot then estimate both V and F as they generally only appear in the $\frac{F \times Dose}{V}$ term at the beginning of the model – only their ratio is *identifiable*. Another notable consequence of a drug being taken orally, say, is that it may take an appreciable amount of time before any of the drug appears in the blood, because, for example, if the drug is administered in solid form then before any absorption can take place it must first disintegrate and dissolve, as only drug in solution is available for absorption. For this reason, it is sometimes desirable to incorporate an initial "lag-time" ($TLAG$, say) into the input process, e.g.,

$$R(t) = \begin{cases} 0 & 0 < t \leq TLAG \\ k_a.Dose.\exp\{-k_a(t - TLAG)\} & t > TLAG \end{cases}$$

Although still an empirical approach it is possible to re-cast the above models in a setting with some, albeit tenuous, physiologic interpretability. For a drug exhibiting d exponential phases of disposition according to a plot of the PK profile, a d-compartment model can equivalently be constructed. (Although the human body comprises hundreds of separate organs and tissues, we can group together into "compartments" those that have similar levels of perfusion: blood flow divided by the product of the tissue volume and a measure of the drug's solubility in that tissue.) For example, the bi-exponential given in (11.1) can be obtained from the system depicted in Figure 11.2. Here every tissue and organ within the body is assumed to exhibit one of two distinct types of PK behaviour (with respect to the drug in question). Tissues that are so well perfused by the blood that the concentration of drug within them is the same as (or similar to) that in the blood itself are "lumped" together, along with the blood, into a single homogeneous compartment known as

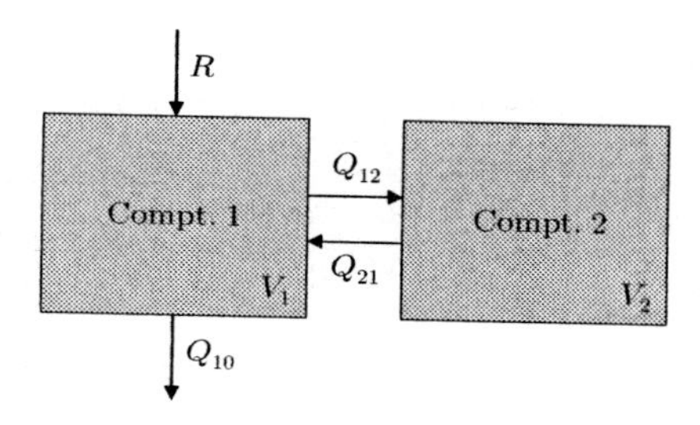

Fig. 11.2. Two-compartment pharmacokinetic model with standard input and disposition.

"the central compartment" or "Compartment 1". Less well-perfused tissues, such as fat, say, collectively comprise "Compartment 2" or "the peripheral compartment". In the figure, V_1 and V_2 denote the apparent volumes (in litres) of Compartments 1 and 2 respectively, and the $Q_{..}$ parameters each represent the "flow-rate" (in litres per hour) of whatever transport mechanism carries the drug in the indicated direction. We assume that the transport mechanism between Compartments 1 and 2 is such that drug flows *through* the peripheral compartment rather than into and out of it separately, and so $Q_{12} = Q_{21} = Q$, say. Q_{10} represents the "flow" of the elimination process and is generally referred to as *clearance* (CL): it is the volume of blood that is *cleared* of drug per unit time. Since the eliminating organs are typically very well perfused, we usually assume that elimination takes place only from the central compartment. Similarly, since we typically take our PK measurements from the blood and that is where the drug usually first appears, it is normal to assume that the input process $R(.)$ inputs drug directly into Compartment 1.

By mass balance, the rate of change of drug in any compartment is given by "rate in" minus "rate out". Intuitively, the rate of drug transfer from one place to another is given by the flow-rate of the transporting medium multiplied by the concentration of drug within that medium, which here we assume is given by the concentration of drug in the compartment from whence it originated:

$$\frac{\mathrm{d}A_1}{\mathrm{d}t} = R(t) - CL.C_1 - Q.C_1 + Q.C_2 \tag{11.4}$$

$$\frac{\mathrm{d}A_2}{\mathrm{d}t} = Q.C_1 - Q.C_2 \tag{11.5}$$

where $A_1(t)$, $C_1(t)$, $A_2(t)$ and $C_2(t)$ denote amounts and concentrations of drug within Compartments 1 and 2 respectively ($A_1 = C_1V_1$, $A_2 = C_2V_2$). (Note that re-expressing the right-hand sides of (11.4) and (11.5) in terms of amounts rather than concentrations reveals all disposition processes to be first-order.) Excepting the input process, (11.4) and (11.5) are linear and can be solved easily using the method of Laplace transforms [17]. Arguably the simplest way of obtaining a full model in closed form is thus to solve (11.4) and (11.5) for a unit impulse dose, i.e., $R(t) = 0$, $A_1(0_+) = 1$, $A_2(0) = 0$, and subsequently evaluate the convolution in (11.3), assuming $R(.)$ is of a suitable form. Solving for a unit impulse dose gives (11.1) with

$$\lambda_1 = \frac{1}{2}\left\{\left(\frac{CL}{V_1} + \frac{Q}{V_1} + \frac{Q}{V_2}\right) + \sqrt{\left(\frac{CL}{V_1} + \frac{Q}{V_1} + \frac{Q}{V_2}\right)^2 - 4 \times \frac{CL}{V_1}.\frac{Q}{V_2}}\right\}$$

$$\lambda_2 = \frac{CL}{V_1} + \frac{Q}{V_1} + \frac{Q}{V_2} - \lambda_1$$

$$q = \frac{\lambda_1 - Q/V_2}{\lambda_1 - \lambda_2}$$

It is worth noting at this point that the model is *far* from linear in its parameters, CL, Q, V_1 and V_2. Indeed, only the most trivial of all PK models can be fully linearized, and so special considerations are required when it comes to analysis (see Section 11.3.4). It is straightforward to see how we can expand on the above ideas to construct, and analyze, more (or even less) complex systems. However, the parameters of such systems, e.g., flow-rates and volumes, do not generally have a directly meaningful physiological interpretation. This is partly because there are no explicit assumptions regarding which tissues/organs constitute each compartment, but is also due to an overly simplistic view of the way in which drug moves around the body. Having said that, it stands to reason that (for some drugs at least) we should expect, and can indeed observe, intuitive correlations between compartmental parameters and measured covariates, such as between clearance (CL) and indicators of hepatic or renal function, or between volume parameters and body weight, say. Thus, such models provide an excellent basis for prediction, in terms of informing about the design of future clinical trials and/or allowing dosage regimens to be tailored to suit individual patients, for instance. In the following subsection we look at a more mechanistic, and thus more directly interpretable, class of models where each compartment comprises a specific set of tissues and the systemic circulation is modelled explicitly. The complexity of such models is such that we have only recently, with today's computational possibilities, been able to entertain the idea of their use within a Bayesian context.[1]

Physiologically-based models

The choice of structure of physiologically-based pharmacokinetic (PBPK) models [3] is not data driven; instead, it is based on biological information regarding the route and nature of drug entry, the various processes of elimination, and the physical/chemical characteristics of the compound under investigation. The *key* differences between such models and their empirical counterparts, however, are that the actual way in which the drug moves around the body, via the blood, is modelled directly, and that the assumed constituents of each compartment can be stated explicitly; the physical connections between compartments are thus understood. Thus, all system parameters are theoretically measurable; that is, they represent real physiological quantities, such as tissue volumes and rates of blood-flow through particular organs.

PBPK models are often seen in a toxicological context [1, 2] where they are used with a view to better understanding the relationship between environmental exposure to "toxic" substances and the onset of adverse health effects (caused, presumably, by high concentrations of toxin in target tissues). Here, (human) data are

[1] See Chapter 1.

typically quite scarce; therefore, models whose parameters can be measured to some extent are particularly useful. From a pharmaceutical perspective, one important role of PBPK models might be to facilitate prediction of the "first dose into man" for a new drug. From pre-clinical animal data and knowledge of how human physiology compares with that of other mammals, we can guess the values of relevant human parameters and thus predict concentrations throughout the body for a given dose. An understanding of the difference between "safe" and toxic concentrations of the drug will then lead us to a (conservative) first dose. Figure 11.3 shows an ex-

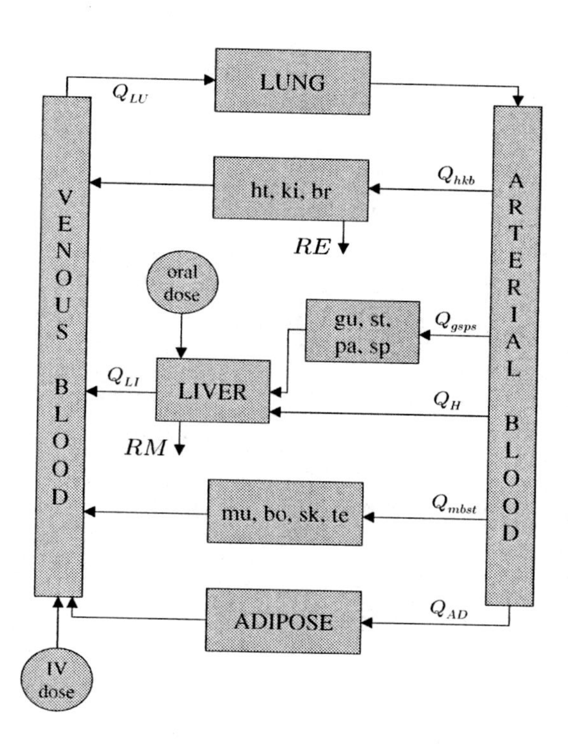

Fig. 11.3. Physiologically based pharmacokinetic model. Abbreviated compartment names are elucidated as follows: "ht, ki, br" – heart, kidneys and brain; "gu, st, pa, sp" – gut, stomach, pancreas and spleen; and "mu, bo, sk, te" – muscle, bone, skin and testes. Note that orally administered drug is generally absorbed across the gut wall into the hepatic portal vein. In order to separate any drug that is being absorbed thus from that which is *recirculating* into the hepatic portal vein, via the tissues of the gut, we tend to assume that, as far as the model is concerned, oral absorption processes input drug directly into the "LIVER" compartment, as shown, rather than the "gu, st, pa, sp" compartment.

ample of a PBPK model that is intended to be largely self-explanatory. The system can be described mathematically via:

$$\frac{dA_{LU}}{dt} = Q_{LU} \times (C_{VEN} - C_{LU}/Kp_{LU}) \quad (11.6)$$

$$\frac{dA_{hkb}}{dt} = Q_{hkb} \times (C_{ART} - C_{hkb}/Kp_{hkb}) - RE(t) \quad (11.7)$$

$$\frac{dA_{gsps}}{dt} = Q_{gsps} \times (C_{ART} - C_{gsps}/Kp_{gsps}) \quad (11.8)$$

$$\frac{dA_{LI}}{dt} = Q_H.C_{ART} + Q_{gsps}.C_{gsps}/Kp_{gsps} + RA(t) - Q_{LI}.C_{LI}/Kp_{LI} - RM(t) \quad (11.9)$$

$$\frac{dA_{mbst}}{dt} = Q_{mbst} \times (C_{ART} - C_{mbst}/Kp_{mbst}) \quad (11.10)$$

$$\frac{dA_{AD}}{dt} = Q_{AD} \times (C_{ART} - C_{AD}/Kp_{AD}) \quad (11.11)$$

$$\frac{dA_{ART}}{dt} = Q_{LU}.C_{LU}/Kp_{LU} - CO.C_{ART} \quad (11.12)$$

$$\frac{dA_{VEN}}{dt} = Q_{hkb}.C_{hkb}/Kp_{hkb} + Q_{LI}.C_{LI}/Kp_{LI} + Q_{mbst}.C_{mbst}/Kp_{mbst} + Q_{AD}.C_{AD}/Kp_{AD} + RI(t) - Q_{LU}.C_{VEN} \quad (11.13)$$

Here, $A_.$ and $C_.$ again represent amounts and concentrations of drug in the indicated compartments, and $Q_.$ and $Kp_.$ denote rates of blood flow and tissue-to-blood partition coefficients, respectively, the latter being equal, by definition, to the ratio of drug concentration in the relevant tissue to that in the blood at equilibrium. The subscripts used for each compartment are defined as follows: LU – lung; hkb – heart, kidneys and brain; $gsps$ – gut, stomach, pancreas and spleen; LI – liver; $mbst$ – muscle, bone, skin and testes; AD – adipose; ART – arterial blood; and VEN – venous blood. (Note that CO is the total cardiac output and that $Q_{LU} = CO$ since all blood must flow through the lungs to be oxygenated; we must also have, for mass balance, that $CO = Q_{hkb} + Q_{gsps} + Q_H + Q_{mbst} + Q_{AD}$, where Q_H represents the liver's *arterial* blood supply and is given by $Q_{LI} - Q_{gsps}$.) Again, the rate of change of drug in each compartment is given by "rate in" minus "rate out". Except for the rate of oral absorption $RA(t)$, the rate of intravenous infusion $RI(t)$, the rate of renal extraction $RE(t)$, and the rate of metabolism in the liver $RM(t)$, all rates are given by blood flows multiplied by the concentrations within those flows. Exit concentrations, however, are typically specified as the relevant tissue concentration divided by the tissue-to-blood partition coefficient – C_{VEN} cannot be used as this corresponds to *combined* (and mixed) venous blood from all compartments (except the lungs).

Standard sub-models for renal extraction and metabolism are given by the first-order equations:

$$RE(t) = CL_R \times C_{hkb}; \quad RM(t) = CL_H \times C_{LI}$$

where CL_H and CL_R denote hepatic and renal clearances, respectively (CL_R represents the combined effects of glomerular filtration and active secretion). In cases where doses are high enough that the liver may, at times, be saturated with drug, in the sense that it has to work at its maximum rate regardless of the concentration, this can be acknowledged by the specification of a non-linear, Michaelis–Menten process ([8], pp. 271–277):

$$RM(t) = \frac{V_{max} \times C_{LI}}{k_m + C_{LI}} \tag{11.14}$$

where V_{max} and k_m are the maximum rate of metabolism and the concentration of drug at which exactly half the maximum rate occurs, respectively. If the drug is broken down via multiple metabolic pathways then a corresponding number of such processes can be added together. In many cases, particularly in toxicological settings, it is the metabolites themselves that are of primary interest, and so $RM(t)$ forms the basis for modelling their kinetics, since it represents their "rate of appearance" within the body.

In general, in all but the simplest of cases, it is not practicable to attempt to solve systems of PBPK equations, such as (11.6)–(11.13), analytically. Instead we need to make use of an appropriate numerical integration routine, which, although increasing analysis time, will, if implemented robustly within a suitable environment, afford the analyst great modelling flexibility, since extremely complex systems can be specified straightforwardly at the differential level. (Note that the fact that the saturable metabolic process in (11.14) is non-linear is then of little consequence.) We may also use such an approach in order to deal with more basic (or empirical) systems that are non-linear, in the PK sense, because their parameters are time-varying.

11.2.2 Pharmacodynamics

The nature of pharmacodynamic measurements depends very much on the drug in question. The goal is to measure efficacy but this is often only observable as the relief of various symptoms, the number and measurability of which vary depending on the condition to be treated. For example, the efficacy of a drug designed to lower a patient's heart-rate can be measured easily and directly on a continuous scale, whereas hayfever (allergic rhinitis) relief, for instance, might best be measured by the patient subjectively rating, on a *categorical* scale, the severity of *each* of his/her symptoms, e.g., sneezing, runny nose, itchy eyes [15]. In short, PD data types, and hence PD model types, are diverse, and so it is difficult to discuss them in any generality. Instead, here we present a few examples that, hopefully, will reflect the essence of PD modelling. We first note, however, that with a good understanding of the drug's mode of action and access to techniques for measuring relevant biomarkers (biological variables related to efficacy), very powerful (but usually very drug-specific) multi-compartment mechanistic models relating concentrations to clinical effects can be constructed – such models will typically best be expressed as a system of ordinary differential equations, to be solved numerically.

Arguably the commonest choice of PD model, for responses on a continuous scale at least, is the "E-max" model. Here it is assumed that a quantum of effect is produced for each molecule of drug that binds to a receptor. Since the number of receptors is finite the "effect site" can become saturated with drug, at which point a maximal effect, E_{max}, is produced. This process is essentially the same as the Michaelis-Menten process mentioned above (see (11.14)), where receptors now play the role previously played by molecules of metabolic enzyme, and so we obtain essentially the same equation:

$$E = \frac{E_{max} \times C_e}{C_{50} + C_e}$$

where E denotes drug effect,[2] C_e is the concentration of drug at the effect site, and C_{50} is the concentration at which 50% of the maximum effect ($E_{max}/2$) is produced. In order that such a model may be "linked" directly to the pharmacokinetics, the PK model must be able to predict concentrations within the vicinity of the effect site, that is, $C_e(.)$. For this reason, a separate "effect compartment" may be required. There exists a simple extension of the E-max model in which C_{50} and both occurrences of C_e are raised to the power γ, an unknown "slope" parameter; this is referred to either as the "Hill equation" or as the "sigmoid E-max model".

In cases where efficacy measures are binary, such as in anaesthesiology (the patient is either asleep or not), we would typically want to assume observations to be distributed according to a Bernoulli distribution with probability parameter π, and then construct a deterministic model to relate π to concentrations at the effect site. One possibility here would be to use the Hill equation with $E_{max} = 1$, i.e., π (or$1 - \pi$) $= C_e^\gamma/(C_{50}^\gamma + C_e^\gamma)$. Another approach, commonly used throughout statistics, would be to specify a linear form for the logistic transform of π (or $1-\pi$), e.g., $\text{logit}(\pi) = z_0 + z_1 C_e$, where z_0 and z_1 are unknown parameters. The advantage of the second type of model, although it is entirely empirical, is that it is easily extended to accommodate explanatory variables other than C_e (via coefficients z_2, z_3, etc.). Also, the logistic approach can be adapted straightforwardly to provide a model for the cumulative probabilities associated with ordered categorical data, such as pain scores from analgesic trials or the hayfever symptom ratings alluded to above [15].

Our final example is of an "indirect response" model. Such a model can be useful for modelling the dynamics of drugs that are designed to inhibit natural physiological processes. As an example, we consider the drug warfarin, which is used to treat thrombophlebitis and pulmonary embolism as it inhibits blood clotting-factor activity (measured via the clotting time of appropriately treated blood samples). Here we let E denote clotting factor activity, and we assume the normal rates of clotting factor synthesis and degradation to be zero-order (with rate constant k_{syn}) and first-order (with rate constant k_{deg}), respectively (such a combination of processes leads to constant levels of clotting factor at steady-state). Warfarin inhibits synthesis and so the following model is appropriate:

$$\frac{\mathrm{d}E}{\mathrm{d}t} = k_{syn}\left(1 - \frac{C_e^\gamma}{C_{50}^\gamma + C_e^\gamma}\right) - k_{deg}E$$

where C_e, in this example, is the concentration of warfarin in the blood. (Note that the above model cannot be expressed in closed form.)

11.3 Stochastic Model

11.3.1 Structure

Here we describe a typical Bayesian population PK/PD model. We begin with the PK aspects and subsequently link these to the pharmacodynamics. Suppose we have a number (n_i) of PK measurements made on each of K individuals, who are indexed

[2] Throughout this chapter, E will denote drug effect and not an error function.

by i. Denote the jth measurement for individual i by y_{ij} and the associated time by t_{ij}. Further, denote the p-dimensional vector of (unknown) PK parameters for individual i by $\boldsymbol{\theta}_i$ and the variance of the residual errors (e.g., observed minus modelled concentrations) by σ^2. At the first of three stages in our statistical model we typically assume

$$p(y_{ij}|\boldsymbol{\theta}_i, \sigma^2) \propto \mathrm{N}(C(\boldsymbol{\theta}_i; t_{ij}; \mathbf{D}_i), \sigma^2) I(y_{ij} \in (l_{ij}, u_{ij})),\ i = 1, ..., K,\ j = 1, ..., n_i \tag{11.15}$$

where, throughout, $p(A|B)$ denotes the conditional probability distribution of A given B. Here the y_{ij} are either concentrations or log-concentrations depending on whether normality or log-normality is the more appropriate assumption for the data. The deterministic PK model for the relevant compartment $C(.)$, which is a function of individual-specific parameters $\boldsymbol{\theta}_i$, time t_{ij}, and individual i's dosing history $\mathbf{D}_i$, is defined on the same scale. The $I(.)$ term in (11.15) above is an indicator function that equals one if $y_{ij} \in (l_{ij}, u_{ij})$ and zero otherwise. This is used for handling censored data; that is to say, measured concentrations that fall below a critical value known as the "limit of detection" (LOD). Such measurements are deemed insufficiently accurate and are thus not reported. The missing data are treated as unknown parameters and assigned distributions that give no support to values outside the known lower and upper bounds l_{ij} and u_{ij}, e.g., $l_{ij} = 0$, $u_{ij} = \mathrm{LOD}$. For non-censored data, i.e., observed values, l_{ij} and u_{ij} are given by $-\infty$ and $+\infty$ respectively.

At the second stage of the model we make distributional assumptions regarding the individual-specific PK parameter vectors $\boldsymbol{\theta}_i$:

$$p(\boldsymbol{\theta}_i|\boldsymbol{\mu}, \boldsymbol{\Omega}) = \mathrm{MVN}_p(\mathbf{Z}_i\boldsymbol{\mu}, \boldsymbol{\Omega}), \quad i = 1, ..., K \tag{11.16}$$

where $\mathrm{MVN}_p(.,.)$ denotes a p-dimensional multivariate normal distribution, $\mathbf{Z}_i$ is a $p \times q$ covariate-effect design matrix for individual i, $\boldsymbol{\mu}$ is a vector of q fixed effect parameters, i.e., intercepts and gradients, which represent the population mean pharmacokinetics, and $\boldsymbol{\Omega}$ is a $p \times p$ variance-covariance matrix that represents the inter-individual variability of PK parameters. In order to make this assumption robust, we first need to ensure that the PK model $C(.)$ is parameterized in terms of quantities for which any value on the whole real line is physically feasible (so that a normality assumption for each $\boldsymbol{\theta}_i$ makes sense); for example, the natural logarithm of clearance (CL). We also need to ensure that the model is *identifiable* by choosing a parameterization such that all vectors in $\mathbb{R}^p$ give rise to *distinct* PK profiles. These issues are discussed fully in Section 11.3.3. (Note that it is not necessary to restrict the covariate model to a linear form, i.e., $\mathcal{E}[\boldsymbol{\theta}_i|\boldsymbol{\mu}, \boldsymbol{\Omega}] = \mathbf{Z}_i\boldsymbol{\mu}$. We do so here for ease of exposition and because it leads to a closed-form full conditional distribution for $\boldsymbol{\mu}$; however, *any* functional form is generally permissible.)

The third stage of our statistical model comprises the prior specification, in which prior distributions are assigned to σ^2, $\boldsymbol{\mu}$ and $\boldsymbol{\Omega}$:

$$p(\sigma^2) = \mathrm{IG}(a, b); \quad p(\boldsymbol{\mu}) = \mathrm{MVN}_q(\boldsymbol{\eta}, \mathbf{H}); \quad p(\boldsymbol{\Omega}) = \mathrm{IW}(\mathbf{S}, \varrho) \tag{11.17}$$

where $\mathrm{IG}(.,.)$ and $\mathrm{IW}(.,.)$ denote inverse-gamma and inverse-Wishart distributions respectively. As this is the final stage of the model, the values of a, b, $\boldsymbol{\eta}$, $\mathbf{H}$, $\mathbf{S}$ and ϱ must be stated explicitly. A discussion of appropriate values for these *hyperparameters* is given in the following subsection (11.3.2).

In cases where there are no PD data, interest is focused on inference about σ^2, $\boldsymbol{\mu}$ and $\boldsymbol{\Omega}$. However, when drug effect *has* been measured, the pharmacokinetics are more of an intermediate interest, and it is the PK model's ability to predict concentrations in some (hypothetical) "effect compartment" that becomes important. The main objective is then to use these concentrations (as a primary predictor) to construct a realistic model for drug effect that will allow the relationship between efficacy and various covariates, including dosage regimen, to be explored.

Suppose we have n_i' effect measurements for individual i, indexed by j' (i.e., $j' = 1, ..., n_i'$). Denote these by $e_{ij'}$ and the times at which they were taken by $\tau_{ij'}$. At the first stage of the statistical model, we assume that each $e_{ij'}$ is a realization from some appropriate distribution $\mathcal{D}(.)$, which is parameterized in terms of a deterministic PD model and some additional distributional parameters $\boldsymbol{\zeta}$ (e.g., variance). The PD model, $E(.)$, is a function of an individual-specific $r \times 1$ vector of PD parameters $\boldsymbol{\phi}_i$ and the pharmacokinetics at time $\tau_{ij'}$,[3] which are determined by $\boldsymbol{\theta}_i$, $\tau_{ij'}$ and $\mathbf{D}_i$:

$$p(e_{ij'}|\boldsymbol{\phi}_i, \boldsymbol{\theta}_i, \boldsymbol{\zeta}) = \mathcal{D}(E(\boldsymbol{\phi}_i; \boldsymbol{\theta}_i; \tau_{ij'}; \mathbf{D}_i), \boldsymbol{\zeta}), \quad i = 1, ..., K, \; j' = 1, ..., n_i' \qquad (11.18)$$

Typically the PK model is compartmental and can predict concentrations in the vicinity of where the drug's effect takes place. In such cases, we usually assume that the dynamics depend upon the kinetics only through these "effect compartment" concentrations, $C_e(.)$:

$$E(\boldsymbol{\phi}_i; \boldsymbol{\theta}_i; \tau_{ij'}; \mathbf{D}_i) = h(\boldsymbol{\phi}_i; C_e(\boldsymbol{\theta}_i; \tau_{ij'}; \mathbf{D}_i))$$

which simplifies the model expression. A simple example of a PK-PD "link model" is, for an efficacy measure on a continuous scale:

$$p(e_{ij'}|\boldsymbol{\phi}_i, \boldsymbol{\theta}_i, \boldsymbol{\zeta}) = \mathrm{N}(h(\boldsymbol{\phi}_i; C_e), \sigma_e^2)$$

where σ_e^2 denotes the residual error variance for the PD data, and $h(.)$ is given by the classic E-max formula:

$$h = \frac{E_{max} \times C_e}{C_{50} + C_e} = \frac{\mathrm{e}^{\phi_{i1}} C_e}{\mathrm{e}^{\phi_{i2}} + C_e}, \text{ say.}$$

If the deterministic PD model is parameterized appropriately, bearing in mind the same issues regarding robustness as were raised for the PK model, then second- and third-stage assumptions analogous to those made for the pharmacokinetics may be specified:

$$p(\boldsymbol{\phi}_i|\boldsymbol{\psi}, \boldsymbol{\Sigma}) = \mathrm{MVN}_r(\mathbf{W}_i\boldsymbol{\psi}, \boldsymbol{\Sigma}), \quad i = 1, ..., K \qquad (11.19)$$

$$p(\boldsymbol{\zeta}) = \mathcal{D}_{\boldsymbol{\zeta}}(\boldsymbol{\xi}); \quad p(\boldsymbol{\psi}) = \mathrm{MVN}_s(\boldsymbol{\chi}, \mathbf{X}); \quad p(\boldsymbol{\Sigma}) = \mathrm{IW}(\mathbf{U}, v) \qquad (11.20)$$

Here $\mathbf{W}_i$ is an $r \times s$ covariate-effect design matrix, $\boldsymbol{\psi}$ is a vector of s fixed-effect parameters, and $\boldsymbol{\Sigma}$ is the $r \times r$ inter-individual variance-covariance matrix for PD parameters. In addition, $\mathcal{D}_{\boldsymbol{\zeta}}(.)$ denotes an appropriate prior for the distributional parameters contained in $\boldsymbol{\zeta}$, e.g., inverse-gamma for the case where $\boldsymbol{\zeta}$ represents a residual variance term, and $\boldsymbol{\xi}$, $\boldsymbol{\chi}$, $\mathbf{X}$, $\mathbf{U}$ and v are hyperparameters that should be assigned fixed values (see below).

[3] Actually, in general, the dynamics may depend on the entire (recent) history of the PK system, but, for the sake of simplicity, such models are not discussed here.

11.3.2 Priors

The distributional forms of priors have traditionally been chosen for mathematical convenience, that is, so that closed form posteriors/full conditionals may be derived analytically. For example, an inverse-gamma prior is typically specified for σ^2 since that is the form of the normal density assumed for each y_{ij} when it is considered as a function of σ^2 (thus all terms involving σ^2 have an inverse-gamma form, which leads to an inverse-gamma full conditional). With the availability nowadays of several reliable methods for sampling from non-standard distributions, however [18, 10, 9, 20], it is worthwhile giving a little more thought towards one's choice of priors. Here, for the sake of simplicity, and also because our model is somewhat generic, we have adopted the traditional approach, but, for specific problems, prior uncertainty regarding σ^2, say, might be better expressed via, for example, a log-normal or uniform distribution [19]. The choice of $a = b = 0.001$ in (11.17) has become somewhat of a standard throughout (applied) Bayesian statistics for "objective" (minimally informative) analyses. While this specification gives rise to a diffuse prior, with a variance for $1/\sigma^2$ of 1000, the location ($\mathrm{E}[1/\sigma^2] = 1$) is quite arbitrary – alternative combinations of a and b can provide equally vague specifications but with more appropriate means. Regarding the specification of more informative priors, we need to match our choice of a and b with whatever expression of prior beliefs seems most natural. In many cases this will be in terms of quantiles for the standard deviation σ (rather than for σ^2 or $1/\sigma^2$) and so experimentation with different values of a and b within a suitable simulation package may be required.

The multivariate normal prior given for $\boldsymbol{\mu}$ in (11.17) is a natural choice and is much easier to specify. Most applied scientists are comfortable with normal distributions and can therefore translate their prior uncertainties into appropriately sized variance terms. For a minimally informative specification, we typically write $\mathbf{H} = \varepsilon^{-1}\mathbf{I}_q$, where $\mathbf{I}_q$ is the $q \times q$ identity matrix and $\varepsilon^{-1} \gg 0$, e.g., 100^2. Generally speaking, the value of $\boldsymbol{\eta}$ is set equal to some prior point estimate for $\boldsymbol{\mu}$. Elements of $\boldsymbol{\eta}$ that correspond to gradient parameters are typically set equal to zero, to reflect an indifferent prior opinion as to the existence of covariate effects, and elements corresponding to intercepts are consequently set equal to prior guesses for the population mean values of each PK parameter.

Our prior for $\boldsymbol{\Omega}$ in (11.17) constitutes a rare example of when compatibility between prior and likelihood is (almost) a practical necessity. If we wish to formulate the model in terms of an entire inter-individual variance-covariance matrix, rather than just the variance terms along with an assumption of independence, then the Wishart/inverse-Wishart is the only closed form distribution that naturally imposes the appropriate constraints: symmetric positive-definiteness. If an informative prior is required then, since the distribution is multidimensional and quite complex, experimentation with different values of ϱ and $\mathbf{S}$ within a software package that is capable of simulating from Wisharts, such as WinBUGS [21, 14], is advisable. However, we rarely wish to be informative about covariance matrices; therefore, we typically set ϱ equal to p (the dimension of the matrix) to obtain the vaguest possible proper prior. The prior mean for $\boldsymbol{\Omega}^{-1}$ is $\varrho\mathbf{S}^{-1}$; therefore, a sensible choice for $\mathbf{S}$ is $\varrho\boldsymbol{\Omega}_0$ where $\boldsymbol{\Omega}_0$ is some prior point estimate for $\boldsymbol{\Omega}$.

The above discussion of priors for the population model's PK component is clearly also applicable to the PD component and so the hyperparameters in (11.20) may be chosen in a similar way.

11.3.3 Parameterization Issues

In order for our assumption of multivariate normality in (11.16) to always make sense, we should ensure that the deterministic PK model is parameterized in terms of quantities for which any real value is physically feasible. Most "natural" PK parameters, such as flow rates and compartmental volumes, are defined on the positive real line; therefore, a logarithmic transform is usually appropriate. However, we cannot just choose any set of such parameters. For example, a multi-compartment model parameterized in terms of (logarithms of) the rate constants associated with each exponential phase of disposition (e.g., λ_1, λ_2, etc., in (11.2)) would not be identifiable. This is because, without an ordering constraint on those rate constant parameters, each parameter would be free to represent any one of the various phases of disposition, and may thus represent different phases during different iterations of our MCMC sampler, which might lead to invalid inferences being drawn from the posterior samples. This type of unidentifiability is referred to as "flip-flop". The basic problem here is that there exist separate areas of parameter space that give rise to exactly the same model. The solution is to always choose parameterizations such that every single vector in $\mathbb{R}^p$ gives rise to a distinct PK profile.

When choosing a parameterization, it is worth bearing in mind that, ideally, we would like to relate various covariates (linearly) to our selected parameters. Thus, parameterizations with some physiologic interpretability, however tenuous, may be advantageous. (Note that the above issues also apply to the parameterization of the PD model.)

Because of the diversity of PD models and data types, there is little value here in discussing parameterizations for specific models. Since E-max models are quite widely used, however, we simply note that $\boldsymbol{\phi}'_{\cdot} = \{\ln E_{max}, \ln C_{50}, \ln \gamma\}$ is an appropriate parameterization for incorporating the Hill equation, $E = E_{max}C_e^{\gamma}/(C_{50}^{\gamma} + C_e^{\gamma})$, into the stochastic model described in (11.15)–(11.20) above.

Returning to pharmacokinetics, the following parameterization is usually appropriate for empirical compartmental systems:

$$\boldsymbol{\theta}'_i = \{\ell(\boldsymbol{\beta}_i), \ln \boldsymbol{\delta}_i, \ln \boldsymbol{\alpha}_i\} \tag{11.21}$$

where $\boldsymbol{\beta}_i$, $\boldsymbol{\delta}_i$ and $\boldsymbol{\alpha}_i$ are individual-specific row-vectors of relative bioavailabilities, disposition parameters, and absorption/input parameters, respectively. The $\boldsymbol{\beta}_i$ vector is empty unless more than one formulation of the drug is to be modelled, in which case a "reference" formulation must be chosen, the bioavailability of which (F_{ref}, say) cannot be estimated (because only its ratio with the initial volume of distribution can be identified). The elements of $\boldsymbol{\beta}_i$ then represent the bioavailabilities of the remaining formulations *relative to* the reference formulation. In cases where dosing histories involve IV doses, IV is normally chosen as the reference formulation and then an appropriate choice for $\ell(.)$ is the logistic function, i.e., $\ell(x) = \ln(x/(1-x))$, as any *relative* bioavailabilities must consequently lie in $(0, 1)$; otherwise $\ell(.) = \ln(.)$.

The $\boldsymbol{\delta}_i$ vector comprises the drug's clearance, any "distributional clearances" (e.g., $Q_{12} = Q_{21} = Q$ from Figure 11.2), and the volume of each compartment (except for when some compartments are ostensibly the same and ordering constraints on their volumes are required to make the model identifiable – we then parameterize in terms of volume differences). All of these disposition parameters are intrinsically scaled by the bioavailability of the reference formulation, e.g., CL/F_{ref}, Q/F_{ref}, since they all generally enter the system equations via flow-rate/volume ratios and

V_1 cannot be separated from F_{ref}. Some typical elements of $\boldsymbol{\alpha}_i$ are as follows: initial lag-times; absorption durations for zero-order models; and, for first-order models, the absorption rate constant k_a minus the rate constant associated with the first exponential phase of disposition, to avoid "flip-flop".

It is worth noting that the PK parameter vector should have the same meaning, and length, for all individuals, to avoid nonsense population assumptions in (11.16). It is therefore convenient if each individual's dosing history comprises the same set of absorption/input processes (and hence formulations). If this is not actually the case, however, because not all individuals received all formulations of the drug, then those individuals with incomplete data may be thought of as having received a number of "virtual" or "dummy" doses (with no associated data). The resulting samples for the corresponding "dummy" input parameters constitute predictive distributions for those individuals.

The parameterization of PBPK models depends very much on what information about the system/drug has already been measured and, also, what might realistically be learnt from the observed data. We first examine the situation where we simply wish to fit a single PBPK profile to whatever data are available. Normally we will have fairly accurate measurements regarding the values of each blood flow $Q_.$ and of each compartmental volume $V_.$; therefore, these may either be fixed (and assumed known) or assigned informative priors. Note, however, that all volumes should sum to the assumed body weight (assuming the body's density to be around 1), and all arterial blood flows should sum to the total cardiac output CO. One way of imposing such constraints is to parameterize in terms of fractions of the relevant total and then apply the type of sub-model normally used for constraining probability vectors; for example, [15]. In general, we may wish to be considerably less informative about other system parameters, e.g., $Kp_.$, V_{max}, k_m, k_a, and since these are typically defined on the positive real line, it seems appropriate, again, to parameterize in terms of their (natural) logarithms. Note that, with PBPK models, we have no control over "flip-flop" between any exponential absorption and disposition terms that might appear in the analytic solution since we do not actually know what that solution is. Aside from this, identifiability is rarely an issue when fitting single profiles as the level of information supplied about each $Q_.$ and $V_.$ identifies the associated compartment. In contrast, if we have population data and wish to allow inter-individual variability for each $Q_.$, $V_.$ and $Kp_.$ (which is unlikely) then it may be necessary to impose ordering constraints to distinguish between some compartments (e.g., "ADIPOSE" and "mu, bo, sk, te" in Figure 11.3).

11.3.4 Analysis

We typically analyze Bayesian population PK/PD models using a Gibbs-Metropolis hybrid sampler [7, 18, 10], as detailed below. At each iteration, random samples from the full conditional distributions of the following quantities are sought: $\boldsymbol{\zeta}$, σ^2, $\boldsymbol{\Omega}$, $\boldsymbol{\Sigma}$, $\boldsymbol{\mu}$, $\boldsymbol{\psi}$, each $\boldsymbol{\theta}_i$, each $\boldsymbol{\phi}_i$, and each censored y_{ij}. The full conditional distribution of $\boldsymbol{\zeta}$ cannot be derived until a model for the PD data and a corresponding prior for $\boldsymbol{\zeta}$ have been specified, but the remaining *population* parameters (σ^2, $\boldsymbol{\Omega}$, $\boldsymbol{\Sigma}$, $\boldsymbol{\mu}$ and $\boldsymbol{\psi}$) all have closed-form full conditionals from the same distributional families as their priors. Due to the non-linearity of the deterministic PK model, and the likely non-linearity of the PD model, closed form full conditionals for the random effects vectors $\boldsymbol{\theta}_i$ and $\boldsymbol{\phi}_i$ are not available. In order to draw samples for them during the analysis, we make use of a series of (univariate) adaptive "current-point" Metropolis-Hastings [18, 10] algorithms[4], which converge within the convergence of the encapsulating Gibbs sampler [22]. Let l index individual elements of $\boldsymbol{\theta}_i$ and $\boldsymbol{\phi}_i$. Candidate samples at iteration m for θ_{il} and ϕ_{il}, respectively, are drawn from the following proposal distributions:

$$\mathrm{N}(\theta_{il}^{(m-1)}, v_{il}); \quad \mathrm{N}(\phi_{il}^{(m-1)}, w_{il})$$

where $\theta_{il}^{(m-1)}$ and $\phi_{il}^{(m-1)}$ denote the $(m-1)$th samples for θ_{il} and ϕ_{il} respectively. The proposal variances v_{il} and w_{il} are initially set equal to very small values, e.g., 10^{-6}, to ensure rapid initial "drift" towards the target distribution's mode. They are then periodically adjusted based on each algorithm's recent acceptance rate with a view to eventually obtaining an acceptance rate of between 20 and 40 per cent for each variable (an intuitively reasonable compromise between frequency and size of movement). It is important to note that adaption must not be allowed to continue indefinitely, to ensure convergence of the underlying Markov chains.

The full conditional distribution of each censored y_{ij} is given by the right-hand side of (11.15), since that is the only distribution in the model involving the relevant quantity. Hence, at each iteration we are essentially imputing values for the missing data that directly inform about the values of individual-specific PK parameter vectors (and σ^2) through the fact that they always lie in the interval (l_{ij}, u_{ij}).

11.3.5 Prediction

The joint predictive distribution for new individuals' PK and PD parameters, $\boldsymbol{\theta}^*$ and $\boldsymbol{\phi}^*$ respectively, say, is given by

$$p(\boldsymbol{\theta}^*, \boldsymbol{\phi}^* | \mathbf{y}, \mathbf{e}) = \int \cdots \int p(\boldsymbol{\theta}^*, \boldsymbol{\phi}^* | \boldsymbol{\mu}, \boldsymbol{\Omega}, \boldsymbol{\psi}, \boldsymbol{\Sigma}) p(\boldsymbol{\mu}, \boldsymbol{\Omega}, \boldsymbol{\psi}, \boldsymbol{\Sigma} | \mathbf{y}, \mathbf{e}) d\boldsymbol{\mu} d\boldsymbol{\Omega} d\boldsymbol{\psi} d\boldsymbol{\Sigma} \tag{11.22}$$

where $\mathbf{y}$ and $\mathbf{e}$ denote all observed PK and PD data respectively. The right-hand side of (11.22) is the expectation under the posterior $p(\boldsymbol{\mu}, \boldsymbol{\Omega}, \boldsymbol{\psi}, \boldsymbol{\Sigma} | \mathbf{y}, \mathbf{e})$ of $p(\boldsymbol{\theta}^*, \boldsymbol{\phi}^* | \boldsymbol{\mu}, \boldsymbol{\Omega}, \boldsymbol{\psi}, \boldsymbol{\Sigma})$ and can thus be approximated by the mixture distribution

$$M^{-1} \sum_{m=1}^{M} p(\boldsymbol{\theta}^*, \boldsymbol{\phi}^* | \boldsymbol{\mu}^{(m)}, \boldsymbol{\Omega}^{(m)}, \boldsymbol{\psi}^{(m)}, \boldsymbol{\Sigma}^{(m)})$$

where $\boldsymbol{\mu}^{(m)}$, $\boldsymbol{\Omega}^{(m)}$, $\boldsymbol{\psi}^{(m)}$ and $\boldsymbol{\Sigma}^{(m)}$ denote the mth posterior samples for $\boldsymbol{\mu}$, $\boldsymbol{\Omega}$, $\boldsymbol{\psi}$ and $\boldsymbol{\Sigma}$, respectively, and M is the total number of such samples. According to the stochastic model defined in (11.15)–(11.20) above, we have that

$$\begin{aligned} p(\boldsymbol{\theta}^*, \boldsymbol{\phi}^* | \boldsymbol{\mu}^{(m)}, \boldsymbol{\Omega}^{(m)}, \boldsymbol{\psi}^{(m)}, \boldsymbol{\Sigma}^{(m)}) &= p(\boldsymbol{\theta}^* | \boldsymbol{\mu}^{(m)}, \boldsymbol{\Omega}^{(m)}) \times p(\boldsymbol{\phi}^* | \boldsymbol{\psi}^{(m)}, \boldsymbol{\Sigma}^{(m)}) \\ &= \mathrm{N}(\mathbf{Z}^* \boldsymbol{\mu}^{(m)}, \boldsymbol{\Omega}^{(m)}) \times \mathrm{N}(\mathbf{W}^* \boldsymbol{\psi}^{(m)}, \boldsymbol{\Sigma}^{(m)}) \end{aligned}$$

where $\mathbf{Z}^*$ and $\mathbf{W}^*$ are covariate design matrices that define the population of interest. Hence we can obtain samples from $p(\boldsymbol{\theta}^*, \boldsymbol{\phi}^* | \mathbf{y}, \mathbf{e})$ during the analysis via:

---

[4] Clearly other methods could be used instead. A multivariate Metropolis algorithm might improve mixing but is much harder to "tune" in practice.

$$\boldsymbol{\theta}^*_{(m)} \sim \mathrm{N}(\mathbf{Z}^*\boldsymbol{\mu}^{(m)}, \boldsymbol{\Omega}^{(m)}), \quad \boldsymbol{\phi}^*_{(m)} \sim \mathrm{N}(\mathbf{W}^*\boldsymbol{\psi}^{(m)}, \boldsymbol{\Sigma}^{(m)}), \quad m = 1, \ldots, M$$

Appropriate Bayesian utility/loss functions for enabling formal decision making will typically be specified in terms of "true" concentrations $C(.)$ or effects $E(.)$ [23]. Predictive distributions for these quantities can be derived simply by evaluating the relevant deterministic model component for each sample from $p(\boldsymbol{\theta}^*, \boldsymbol{\phi}^* | \mathbf{y}, \mathbf{e})$, i.e.,

$$C^*_{(m)} = C(\boldsymbol{\theta}^*_{(m)}), \quad E^*_{(m)} = E(\boldsymbol{\phi}^*_{(m)}; \boldsymbol{\theta}^*_{(m)}), \quad m = 1, \ldots, M$$

(where the dependence of $C(.)$ and $E(.)$ on both time and dosing history has been suppressed for notational convenience).

11.4 Implementation

As we have seen, the deterministic components of (Bayesian) population PK/PD models can be quite complex – indeed, in many cases, they cannot be expressed in closed form; in contrast, the stochastic components are fairly standard. Not only does each single dose require a potentially complex PK model but also each individual may receive many such doses, perhaps of different formulations of the drug, during the course of a clinical trial. All this complexity renders the model specification process, within any general purpose software package, both tedious and error-prone, to the point where, for many applications, a specialized interface for describing the problem at hand is considered a practical necessity.

We conclude this chapter with a brief discussion of two such interfaces, which both extend the WinBUGS framework [21, 14]. One other package that has been designed with (PB)PK/PD models in mind is MCSim [6].

11.4.1 PKBugs

The main purpose of the PKBugs interface [16, 13] is to simplify the specification of population PK/PD models by providing a means of translating what is a simple and intuitive shorthand format for describing complex dosing/event histories into a language that WinBUGS can understand. This format is the same as that conceived by the authors of NONMEM [4], that is, a rectangular data file with each row (or record) corresponding to an *event* (e.g., dose, observation) and each column, referred to as a *data item*, having a specific meaning (e.g., event time, amount of dose received). In order to describe how the software works, it is useful to first define a "standard" class of models. A "standard" model, in the context of PKBugs, is any model with the stochastic structure defined by (11.15)–(11.17), where the deterministic PK component $C(.)$ satisfies the following conditions. Only empirical models describing standard one-, two-, or three-compartment disposition kinetics (with input into and elimination from the central compartment) are permitted, but any number of doses with the following input characteristics may be combined: (i) intravenous; (ii) first-order; (iii) zero-order; (iv) first-order with initial lag; and (v) zero-order with initial lag. (The parameterization of $C(.)$ is that given by (11.21).) Standard models are specified in PKBugs via two simple steps: (i) data entry, where the entire event history for all individuals is loaded into the system so that it can be parsed; and (ii) basic user input through simple dialogue boxes and menu commands, during which the model structure, the hyperparameters, and suitable initial values for each stochastic variable are all defined. The model may then be analyzed directly using WinBUGS in the normal way. For more complex problems, the model should be specified as if it were standard and then the system can be instructed to generate equivalent WinBUGS code, which may be modified accordingly. An important design feature of such code is that it is virtually identical for all problems/data sets, because the vast majority of problem-specific detail is "hidden" within the block of data that is generated immediately beneath the model code. Thus, the code itself is concise and easy to follow.

In the context of this chapter, the most obvious use for this code generation facility is to enable linking of the specified population PK model to arbitrary PD models and data types. Indeed, the user now has the full generality of WinBUGS to hand and can exploit this in any way they choose. For example, it is straightforward to incorporate extra levels into the hierarchical model for modelling additional layers of variability [11, 12], or to replace normality assumptions with Student-t assumptions to provide robustness against outliers [24]. Alternatively, we may require a more sophisticated model for the residual error structure, or we might wish to acknowledge measurement error in some of our covariates [5], for instance.

11.4.2 WinBUGS Differential Interface

Here, we describe work in progress, which is towards implementing a differential equation solving interface within WinBUGS. Although the interface is being designed primarily for handling PBPK/PD models, there is clearly a much broader application area; therefore, this is a significant step forward for the software as a whole. Various integration routines and new BUGS-language constructs have already been implemented in a prototype version of the interface. For example, the system of ODEs required to describe the two-compartment model in Figure 11.2, with first-order input, say, is specified as follows:

```
D(C[1], t) <- (R - CL * C[1] - Q * C[1] + Q * C[2]) / V[1]
D(C[2], t) <- Q * (C[1] - C[2])/ V[2]
R <- F * Dose * ka * exp(-ka * t)
```

The numerical solution to the equations is accessed via syntax of the type:

```
model[1:n, 1:2] <- ode(C0[1:2], time[1:n], D(C[1:2], t),
                       origin, tol)
```

where `C0[.]` contains the initial conditions (`C0[1] <- 0; C0[2] <- 0` in this case), which pertain to the time given by `origin` (usually zero); `time[.]` is the grid of time points at which the numerical solution is required; `D(C[.], t)` specifies the system of ODEs to be solved (as above); and `tol` is the required level of accuracy. The next phase of development will entail the design of language constructs for representing arbitrarily complex input/absorption processes. A key design feature will be that the constructs facilitate automatic selection (by WinBUGS) of an appropriate method of integration for each specific problem.

References

[1] M. E. Andersen. A physiologically based toxicokinetic description of the metabolism of inhaled gases and vapors: analysis at steady state. *Toxicol. Appl. Pharmacol.*, 60:509–526, 1981.

[2] M. E. Andersen, H. J. Clewell, M. L. Gargas, F. A. Smith, and R. H. Reitz. Physiologically-based pharmacokinetics and the risk assessment for methylene chloride. *Toxicol. Appl. Pharmacol.*, 87:185–205, 1987.

[3] A. J. Bailer and D. A. Dankovic. An introduction to the use of physiologically based pharmacokinetic models in risk assessment. *Stat. Methods Med. Res.*, 6: 341–358, 1997.

[4] S. L. Beal and L. B. Sheiner. *NONMEM User's Guide, parts I-VII.* NONMEM Project Group, San Francisco, 1992.

[5] J. E. Bennett and J. C. Wakefield. Errors-in-variables in joint population pharmacokinetic/pharmacodynamic modelling. *Biometrics*, 57:803–812, 2001.

[6] F. Y. Bois and D. R. Maszle. MCSim: a Monte Carlo simulation program. *Journal of Statistical Software*, 2(9), 1997.

[7] S. Geman and D. Geman. Stochastic relaxation, Gibbs distributions and the Bayesian restoration of images. *IEEE Trans. Pattn. Anal. Mach. Intell.*, 6: 721–741, 1984.

[8] M. Gibaldi and D. Perrier. *Pharmacokinetics* (2nd Edition). Marcel Dekker, New York, 1982.

[9] W. R. Gilks and P. Wild. Adaptive rejection sampling for Gibbs sampling. *Appl. Statist.*, 41:337–348, 1992.

[10] W. K. Hastings. Monte Carlo sampling-based methods using Markov chains and their applications. *Biometrika*, 57:97–109, 1970.

[11] M. O. Karlsson and L. B. Sheiner. The importance of modelling inter-occasion variability in population pharmacokinetic analyses. *J. Pharmacokinet. Biopharm.*, 21:735–750, 1993.

[12] D. J. Lunn and L. J. Aarons. Markov chain Monte Carlo techniques for studying interoccasion and intersubject variability: application to pharmacokinetic data. *Appl. Statist.*, 46:73–91, 1997.

[13] D. J. Lunn, N. Best, A. Thomas, J. Wakefield, and D. Spiegelhalter. Bayesian analysis of population PK/PD models: general concepts and software. *J. Pharmacokinet. Pharmacodyn.*, 29:271–307, 2002.

[14] D. J. Lunn, A. Thomas, N. Best, and D. Spiegelhalter. WinBUGS – a Bayesian modelling framework: concepts, structure, and extensibility. *Stat. Comput.*, 10: 325–337, 2000.

[15] D. J. Lunn, J. Wakefield, and A. Racine-Poon. Cumulative logit models for ordinal data: a case study involving allergic rhinitis severity scores. *Stat. Med.*, 20:2261–2285, 2001.

[16] D. J. Lunn, J. Wakefield, A. Thomas, N. Best, and D. Spiegelhalter. *PKBugs User Guide Version 1.1.* Dept. Epidemiology and Public Health, Imperial College School of Medicine, London, 1999.

[17] M. Mayersohn and M. Gibaldi. Mathematical methods in pharmacokinetics. I. Use of the Laplace transform in solving differential rate equations. *Amer. J. Pharm. Ed.*, 34:608–614, 1970.

[18] N. Metropolis, A. W. Rosenbluth, M. N. Rosenbluth, A. H. Teller, and E. Teller. Equations of state calculations by fast computing machines. *J. Chem. Phys.*, 21:1087–1091, 1953.

[19] R. Natarajan and R. E. Kass. Reference Bayesian methods for Generalized Linear Mixed Models. *J. Am. Statist. Ass.*, 95:227–237, 2000.

[20] R. M. Neal. Markov chain Monte Carlo methods based on 'slicing' the density function. Technical Report 9722, Dept. of Statistics, University of Toronto, 1997.

[21] D. Spiegelhalter, A. Thomas, N. Best, and D. Lunn. *WinBUGS User Manual, Version 1.4*. Medical Research Council Biostatistics Unit, Cambridge, 2003.

[22] L. Tierney. Markov chains for exploring posterior distributions. *Ann. Statist.*, 22:1701–1762, 1994.

[23] J. C. Wakefield. An expected loss approach to the design of dosage regimens via sampling-based methods. *The Statistician*, 43:13–29, 1994.

[24] J. C. Wakefield, A. F. M. Smith, A. Racine-Poon, and A. E. Gelfand. Bayesian analysis of linear and non-linear population models by using the Gibbs sampler. *Appl. Statist.*, 43:201–221, 1994.

12

Assessing the Effectiveness of Bayesian Feature Selection

Ian T. Nabney[1], David J. Evans[1], Yann Brulé[1], and Caroline Gordon[2]

[1] Neural Computing Research Group, Aston University, Birmingham B4 7ET, UK.
i.t.nabney@aston.ac.uk

[2] Faculty of Medicine and Dentistry, University of Birmingham, Birmingham B15 2TT, UK.
p.c.gordon@bham.ac.uk

Summary. A practical Bayesian approach for inference in neural network models has been available for ten years, and yet it is not used frequently in medical applications. In this chapter we show how both regularization and feature selection can bring significant benefits in diagnostic tasks through two case studies: heart arrhythmia classification based on ECG data and the prognosis of lupus. In the first of these, the number of variables was reduced by two thirds without significantly affecting performance, while in the second, only the Bayesian models had an acceptable accuracy. In both tasks, neural networks outperformed other pattern recognition approaches.

12.1 Introduction

There are many strong theoretical reasons why the Bayesian framework for statistical inference is attractive. But for the hard-pressed practitioner, the question is whether Bayesian techniques outperform conventional maximum likelihood methods sufficiently to justify the extra effort they require for implementation and the additional training time required.

The purpose of this chapter is to examine this question through two medical case studies which use Automatic Relevance Determination (ARD), a Bayesian method for variable selection, to reduce the number of inputs to a non-linear model. Feature selection is an important tool in the medical domain, because causal links between symptoms or clinical measurements and disease are hard to establish, so it is often difficult to reason *a priori* about the relevance of particular inputs. Instead, it is common to take a large number of measurements to avoid missing out anything that might have a bearing on a diagnosis. Of course, a large number of inputs makes training a model more difficult, and can also affect the model's accuracy.

The second section of this chapter contains a description of the Bayesian techniques that we used. The third and fourth sections describe applications to arrhythmia classification based on ECG data and the diagnosis of lupus (an autoimmune disease) respectively. The final section summarises the main conclusions from these studies.

12.2 Bayesian Feature Selection

The Bayesian approach to statistical inference was introduced for neural networks in [14, 16, 15]. In this section we first give a brief overview of the Bayesian view of parameter estimation,[3] and then show how it can be used to select relevant input variables.

12.2.1 Bayesian Techniques for Neural Networks

Bayesian statistics is very simple in principle. Bayes' theorem tells us that the posterior density of a model's parameters $\boldsymbol{w}$, given a dataset $\mathcal{D}$, is given by

$$p(\boldsymbol{w}|\mathcal{D}) = \frac{p(\mathcal{D}|\boldsymbol{w})p(\boldsymbol{w})}{p(\mathcal{D})}, \tag{12.1}$$

where $p(\boldsymbol{w})$ is the prior, $p(\mathcal{D}|\boldsymbol{w})$ is the dataset likelihood (known as the *evidence* for $\boldsymbol{w}$), and $p(\mathcal{D})$ is a normalisation factor that ensures that the posterior density function integrates to 1. It is given by an integral over the parameter space:

$$p(\mathcal{D}) = \int p(\mathcal{D}|\boldsymbol{w}')p(\boldsymbol{w}')\, \mathrm{d}\boldsymbol{w}'. \tag{12.2}$$

Once the posterior has been calculated, every type of inference is made by integrating over this distribution. For example, to make a prediction at a new input $\boldsymbol{x}^*$, we calculate the prediction distribution $p(\boldsymbol{y}|\boldsymbol{x}^*, \mathcal{D})$ by the integral

$$p(\boldsymbol{y}|\boldsymbol{x}^*, \mathcal{D}) = \int p(\boldsymbol{y}|\boldsymbol{x}^*, \boldsymbol{w})p(\boldsymbol{w}|\mathcal{D})\, \mathrm{d}\boldsymbol{w}. \tag{12.3}$$

A point prediction uses the mean of this distribution, given by

$$E(\boldsymbol{y}|\boldsymbol{x}^*, \mathcal{D}) = \int \boldsymbol{y}\, p(\boldsymbol{y}|\boldsymbol{x}^*, \mathcal{D})\, \mathrm{d}\boldsymbol{y}, \tag{12.4}$$

while the variance of the prediction distribution (given by a similar integral) can be used to generate error bars. The problem is that evaluating integrals such as (12.2) and (12.4) is very difficult because they are only analytically tractable for a small class of prior and likelihood distributions. The dimensionality of the integrals is given by the number of model parameters, so simple numerical integration algorithms break down. This is why the use of approximations to the posterior (the evidence procedure [14]) and numerical methods for evaluating integrals (Monte Carlo methods combined with Markov Chain sampling [18]) play such a large role in the use of Bayesian methods with neural networks.

The prior probability distribution for the weights of a neural network[4] should embody our prior knowledge of the sort of network mappings that are "reasonable".

[3] See also Chapter 1

[4] A tutorial on multi-layer perceptrons in given in Chapter 3.

In general, we expect the underlying generator of our datasets to be smooth, and the network mapping should reflect this belief. A neural network with large weights will usually give rise to a mapping with large curvature, and so we favour small values for the network weights.

The requirement for small weights suggests a Gaussian prior distribution with zero mean of the form

$$p(\boldsymbol{w}) = \frac{1}{Z_W(\alpha)} \exp\left(-\frac{\alpha}{2}\|\boldsymbol{w}\|^2\right), \tag{12.5}$$

where α represents the *inverse* variance of the distribution and the normalisation constant is given by

$$Z_W(\alpha) = \left(\frac{2\pi}{\alpha}\right)^{W/2}. \tag{12.6}$$

Because α is a parameter for the distribution of other parameters (weights and biases), it is known as a *hyperparameter*. One of the strengths of the Bayesian formalism is that we can reason probabilistically with hyperparameters in a natural extension of inference for parameters.

The overall cost function for fitting a model is found by taking the negative log of (12.1). Ignoring the normalisation constant, which does not depend on the weights, the prior is equivalent to a weight error term (after taking the negative log) of the form

$$\alpha E_W = \frac{\alpha}{2}\|\boldsymbol{w}\|^2 = \frac{\alpha}{2}\sum_{i=1}^{W} w_i^2. \tag{12.7}$$

The log likelihood term is $-\log p(\mathcal{D}|\boldsymbol{w})$ and is given by the entropy or cross-entropy data error E_D for classification tasks, and by a scaled sum-of-squares error

$$\beta E_D = \frac{\beta}{2}\sum_{n=1}^{N}\{y(\boldsymbol{x}^n;\boldsymbol{w}) - t^n\}^2 \tag{12.8}$$

for regression tasks, where β represents the inverse variance of a Gaussian output noise model. Putting together (12.7) and (12.8), we derive the overall error (or misfit) function

$$E = S(\boldsymbol{w}) = \beta E_D + \alpha E_W. \tag{12.9}$$

In the case of a classification model, the coefficient β is omitted.

The *evidence* procedure is an iterative algorithm for determining optimal weights and hyperparameters. It is not a fully Bayesian approach because it searches for optimal hyperparameters instead of integrating them out; it is equivalent to the *type II maximum likelihood* method [1]. Nevertheless, it has given good results on many applications [21], and is considerably less computationally costly than fully Bayesian procedures such as Monte Carlo integration.

The aim of the evidence procedure is to find the most probable weights $\boldsymbol{w}_{MP}$, which involves optimising $S(\boldsymbol{w})$ for fixed α and β, and the most probable values of the hyperparameters α_{MP}, β_{MP}, which involves optimising the log evidence

$$\begin{aligned}\ln p(\mathcal{D}|\alpha,\beta) = &-\alpha E_W^{MP} - \beta E_D^{MP} - \frac{1}{2}\ln|\boldsymbol{A}| \\ &+ \frac{W}{2}\ln\alpha + \frac{N}{2}\ln\beta - \frac{N}{2}\ln(2\pi),\end{aligned} \tag{12.10}$$

as a function of α and β. This equation is derived by approximating the weight posterior distribution $p(\boldsymbol{w}|\alpha)$ by a Gaussian centered at $\boldsymbol{w}_{MP}$ with variance given by the inverse of $\boldsymbol{A}$, the Hessian of $S(\boldsymbol{w})$. The constants W and N represent the number of weights and data points respectively.

We can summarise the process as follows:

1. Choose initial values for the hyperparameters α and β. Initialise the weights in the network.
2. Train the network with a suitable optimisation algorithm to minimise the misfit function $S(\boldsymbol{w})$.
3. When the network training has reached a local minimum, the hyperparameters can be re-estimated with the following formulae:

$$\alpha^{\text{new}} = \frac{\gamma}{2E_W} \tag{12.11}$$

$$\beta^{\text{new}} = \frac{N-\gamma}{2E_D}, \tag{12.12}$$

where γ is defined as

$$\gamma = \sum_{i=1}^{W} \frac{\lambda_i}{\lambda_i + \alpha}. \tag{12.13}$$

In this equation, $\lambda_i + \alpha$ are the eigenvalues of $\boldsymbol{A}$. These re-estimation formulae can be iterated if desired. Note that although these formulae only apply when $S(\boldsymbol{w})$ is at a local minimum, it is possible to re-estimate the hyperparameters more frequently. However, the formulae use the eigenvalues of the Hessian matrix $\boldsymbol{A}$, so are computationally costly.
4. Repeat steps 2 and 3 until convergence of α and β.

The additional computational cost of the evidence procedure over standard maximum likelihood training can be significant. Standard error backpropagation to calculate network derivatives is $O(NW)$. The computation of the Hessian is $O(NW^2)$, and calculation of the eigenvalues (needed for the hyperparameter updates) is $O(W^3)$.

12.2.2 Automatic Relevance Determination

Selecting relevant input variables from a large set of possibilities is a common problem in applications of pattern analysis. Principal component analysis gives a reduced set of variables, but in an unsupervised way (i.e. it doesn't take account of the input-output mapping) while canonical variates is only applicable to linear classification and has an upper bound of $c-1$ for the number of variables created [6]. Selecting variables based on the magnitude of their correlation with the target variable is based only on linear relationships; frequently the importance of inputs is only revealed in a non-linear mapping. What is required is a way to determine the importance of each input to the outputs of a trained model.

The crudest method for doing this is to consider the magnitude of the weights fanning out from a particular input. However, this performs poorly in practice since if an input has no effect on the output, the weights leading from it can have arbitrary values. More well-founded are methods for measuring weight *saliency*, based on analysis of the Hessian matrix, that are used in weight pruning algorithms such as "optimal brain damage" [13] and "optimal brain surgery" [8]. However, these techniques can be difficult to interpret in a quantitative way.

In the Automatic Relevance Determination (ARD) framework, we associate a separate hyperparameter α_i with each input variable; this represents the inverse variance of the prior distribution of the weights fanning out from that input. During Bayesian learning it is possible to modify the hyperparameters; for example, using the evidence procedure, we find their optimal value, subject to some simplifying assumptions, using a modified form of the update rule (12.11). Because hyperparameters represent the inverse variance of the weights, a small hyperparameter value means that large weights are allowed, and we can conclude that the corresponding input is important. A large hyperparameter value means that the weights are constrained near zero, and hence the corresponding input is less important.

This still leaves open the question of deciding what a "large" hyperparameter value is (and this will depend on the measurement scale of the corresponding input; normalising inputs to zero mean and unit variance makes it easier to compare ARD hyperparameters), but it is certainly easy to decide on the relative importance of inputs.

12.3 ARD in Arrhythmia Classification

12.3.1 Clinical Context

The electrocardiogram (ECG) is an important non-invasive diagnostic tool for assessing the condition of the heart. Each beat is made up of a series of waves: P-wave, QRS complex, T-wave and occasionally a U-wave (see Figure 12.1). The signal morphology and timing are indicative of different clinical conditions: for example, changes in the ST segment suggest ischaemia (poor blood supply to heart muscle), while atrial fibrillation (multiple P-waves) indicates low cardiac output and often causes clots in the atria. In this study we analysed disturbances to the natural rhythm of the heart (arrhythmias), which may be caused by drugs or disease. Our interest is in separating normal sinus (or *supraventricular*) beats, which originate from the sino-atrial node or atria, from *ventricular* ectopic beats [4], which originate from the lower chambers, or ventricles.

Our goal was to evaluate the suitability of a range of pattern analysis algorithms for use in a device worn for 24 hours by the patient (such as the C.Net 2000 developed by Cardionetics Ltd. [7]). Such a device must be capable of analysing each heart beat (that is about 100,000 beats in a 24-hour test) for a large number of different patients without adaptation of the model parameters. In addition, since the device is worn during normal activities, it must be light and use small batteries [19]. This means that the computational demands of both feature extraction and classification must be scrutinised to minimise power consumption.

The ECG measures changes in the electric potential of different areas of the heart due to the *ionic flux* as charged chemicals move across cell walls. A muscle cell at rest is in a polarised state, so that the contents are negative relative to the cell membrane [4]. When the membrane receives enough negative charge, the cell depolarises and the muscle contracts about 0.02 to 0.04 seconds later. After depolarisation, the cell repolarises spontaneously over a rather longer time interval. The ECG records the passage of the depolarisation and repolarisation wave front

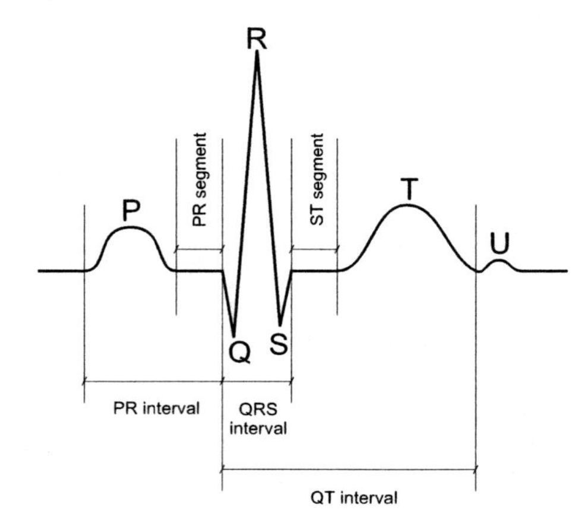

Fig. 12.1. Typical ECG with main features marked.

across the chambers of the heart. In our application, a single channel is measured using three electrodes (one for the earth) attached to the chest in the V4 position [4].

The ECG is conventionally divided into a sequence of waves:

P-wave: depolarisation of the atria (upper chambers), normally lasting at most 0.11 seconds.

QRS complex: depolarisation of the ventricles (lower chambers), normally lasting 0.05 to 0.1 seconds. The repolarisation of the atria happens at the same time, but this signal is swamped by that coming from the much larger ventricles. An initial negative wave is the Q-wave. The first positive deflection is the R-wave; this is usually the largest "spike" in the ECG and is used to determine the location of each beat. A following negative wave is the S-wave. If the signs of each part of the complex are reversed, this is called an inverted complex.

T-wave: repolarisation of the ventricles. This lasts less than 0.15 seconds.

U-wave: a much smaller wave may follow the T-wave; its function is not well understood and it is not relevant for this application.

This is the normal sequence of waves for a supraventricular beat. However, if the origin of a beat is in the ventricles, then there is usually no P-wave, and the QRS complex is much broader; these are the arrhythmia of interest for this application. There are two main morphologies of ventricular beat, which we have called *Vel* and *Ver*: examples of each are shown in Figure 12.2. The task is to separate supraventricular beats from ventricular ectopic beats using features extracted from their morphology.[5]

12.3.2 Benchmarking Classification Models

Single channel ECG was collected from 131 subjects using a digital data collection device at 100 Hz with the same frequency response characteristics as a C.Net 2000

[5] The differences between the two classes of ventricular beats have no clinical significance.

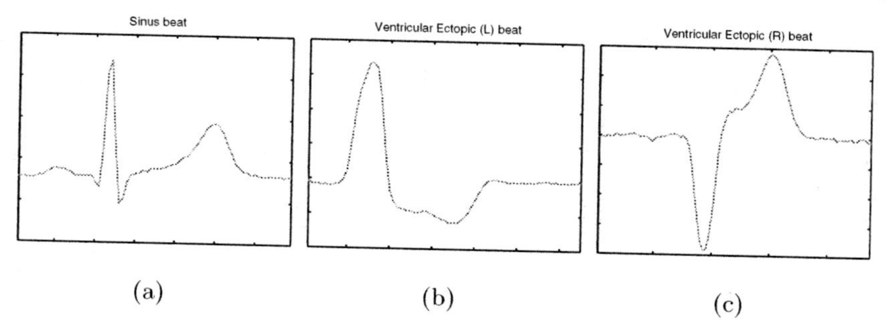

Fig. 12.2. Typical beats from (a) sinus, (b) *Vel* and (c) *Ver* classes.

ambulatory monitor. This was divided on a per-subject basis into training (35,403 beats), validation (11,800) and test (23,606) sets so that each dataset contains beats from separate subjects. The three classes of beat, supraventricular (including sinus) and two varieties of ventricular ectopic beats, had approximate prior probabilities 0.85, 0.05 and 0.10 respectively. Twenty-four time-domain features were extracted automatically from the data and normalised on a per-beat basis to reduce their subject specificity. These were chosen in consultation with experienced clinical cardiologists.

The problem was represented as a three-way classification since earlier experiments showed that this gives more accurate results than multiple two-way classification models. Early stopping was adequate to avoid overfitting, owing to the large quantity of training data. The classification models used were logistic regression (Generalised Linear Model, GLM), MLP and RBF neural networks [2]. The density models used were Gaussian Mixture Models (GMMs), Generative Topographic Mapping (GTM) [3], and Kohonen SOM [12], with one model per class. All model selection (e.g. number of hidden units) was performed using only the validation dataset. All the selected models were finally evaluated on the test set. Each model was trained five times with randomly initialised weights; in the case of the SOM and GTM this was a random perturbation of the weights following a PCA initialisation. The NETLAB toolbox[6] was used for all the experiments [17].

The classifiers were trained to model the Bayesian posterior distribution of the probability of a data point $\mathbf{x}$ belonging to class $\mathcal{C}_k$, formally written as $P(\mathcal{C}_k|\mathbf{x})$, the probability of $\mathcal{C}_k$ *given* an input vector, $\mathbf{x}$. The GLM, MLP and RBF models used a softmax output activation function to ensure that the outputs lay in the range $[0, 1]$ and summed to one.

For the density models we compute $P(\mathcal{C}_k|\mathbf{x})$ by modelling the class conditional density $P(\mathbf{x}|\mathcal{C}_k)$ (i.e. we train a model for each class) and then applying Bayes' theorem to compute the posterior distribution, $P(\mathcal{C}_k|\mathbf{x})$:

$$P(\mathcal{C}_k|\mathbf{x}) = \frac{P(\mathbf{x}|\mathcal{C}_k)P(\mathcal{C}_k)}{\sum_{i=1}^{K} P(\mathbf{x}|\mathcal{C}_i)P(\mathcal{C}_i)}. \tag{12.14}$$

Tables 12.1 and 12.2 contain the confusion matrices for the trained models. Confusion between the two ventricular classes is not important. Misclassifications of sinus beats as ventricular ectopics may lead to over-reporting of symptoms, but

[6] `http://www.ncrg.aston.ac.uk/netlab`

Table 12.1. Performance statistics for the classifiers. Confusion matrix entries are given as: median (min/max) over 5 seeds. Rows represent true classes sinus, *Vel*, *Ver*.

GLM: Mean err: 0.1593%; std err: 0.0110%		
19984 (19982/19985)	3 (2/5)	0 (0/0)
4 (3/4)	1159 (1159/1160)	25 (25/25)
0 (0/0)	5 (4/8)	2426 (2423/2427)

MLP: Mean err: 0.0153%; std err: 0.0038%		
19985 (19984/19985)	2 (2/3)	0 (0/0)
0 (0/0)	1187 (1187/1188)	1 (0/1)
0 (0/0)	0 (0/1)	2431 (2430/2431)

RBF Mean err: 0.1288%; std err: 0.0057%		
19981 (19981/19982)	5 (5/6)	0 (0/1)
1 (0/1)	1175 (1174/1176)	12 (12/13)
0 (0/0)	11 (11/13)	2420 (2418/2420)

misclassifications of ventricular beats as sinus (recorded in the first column below the first entry) are the most costly errors. These tables show that the most accurate model is the MLP, while the most accurate density model is the GTM.

Table 12.2. Performance statistics for the density models. Confusion matrix entries are given as: median (min/max) over 5 seeds. Rows represent true classes sinus, *Vel*, *Ver*.

SOM Mean err: 0.6219%; std err: 0.0746%		
19931 (19903/19945)	55 (40/84)	0 (0/2)
17 (4/48)	1132 (1096/1156)	28 (28/44)
0 (0/0)	42 (7/52)	2389 (2379/2424)

GTM Mean err: 0.1432%; std err: 0.0436%		
19971 (19970/19975)	15 (11/16)	1 (1/1)
4 (2/6)	1174 (1160/1184)	11 (0/22)
1 (1/1)	4 (2/7)	2426 (2423/2428)

GMM Mean err: 0.1805%; std err: 0.0311%		
19966 (19954/19971)	21 (16/33)	0 (0/1)
1 (0/4)	1179 (1164/1180)	8 (7/20)
1 (1/1)	4 (2/9)	2426 (2421/2428)

One of the two beats misclassified by the best MLP is shown in Figure 12.3; it can be seen that although it is a sinus beat (since there is a P-wave present and the timing is regular), the QRS complex is unusually broad and the T-wave (which is inverted) is relatively small; this morphology is probably that of a *fusion beat*, which is caused by concurrent sinus and ventricular excitation.

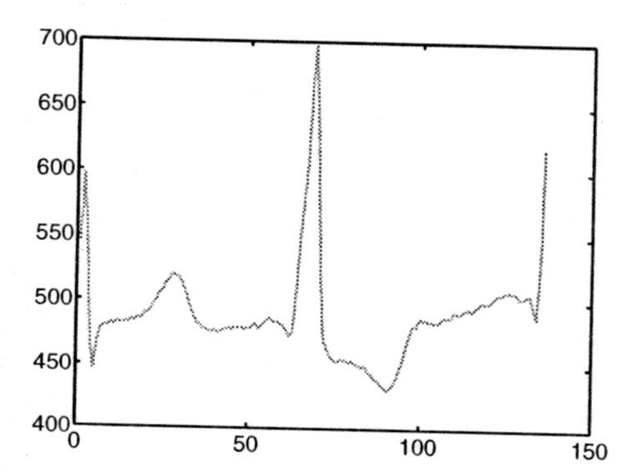

Fig. 12.3. Sinus beat misclassified by the MLP.

12.3.3 Variable Selection

Although the accuracy of the MLP classifier is excellent, it would be preferable if similar results could be achieved with fewer input variables. This is because ECG devices are powered by small batteries, and minimising power consumption is an important design goal.

We used two methods to select a smaller set of variables:

- feature extraction from raw input data;
- Automatic Relevance Determination.

The feature extraction process consisted of three steps. First, each beat was extracted from a raw ECG file by taking 75 samples around each R-wave peak. Then Principal Component Analysis (PCA) was applied to the beats from the training data. Finally, all the data was projected onto the first 5 principal components; this value was selected by visual inspection (see Figure 12.4(a)). Because we were using raw data, rather than preprocessed, the division into training, validation and test files was slightly different from the earlier experiments. However, it maintained the principle that all the data for each subject was contained in just one of the three subsets. We trained an MLP with 60 hidden units using the evidence procedure with separate priors for biases, first and second layer weights. Training runs were made with five different seeds for weight initialisation.

In the ARD experiments, we used an MLP with 40 hidden units[7] that was trained using the evidence procedure. Eighteen iterations were needed to achieve hyperparameter convergence; each consisted of 200 iterations of scaled conjugate gradient

[7] This number was constrained by memory limitations and the need to store the Hessian matrix of the network.

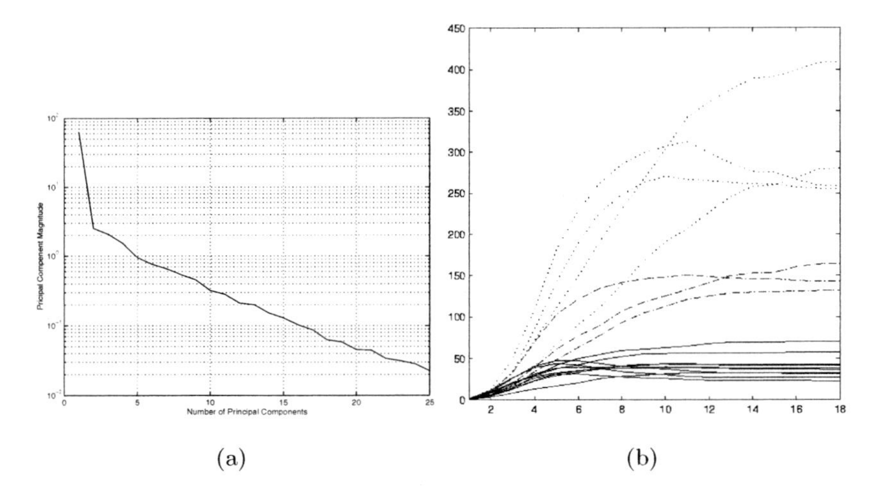

Fig. 12.4. (a) Principal values of ECG data. (b) Evolution of hyperparameter values during ARD training. $200 < \alpha < 400$ (*dotted line*), $100 < \alpha \leq 200$ (*dash-dotted line*), $\alpha \leq 100$ (*solid line*). All other hyperparameters diverged.

to optimise the network weights followed by ten iterations of the hyperparameter update equations [17].

Figure 12.4(b) shows the evolution of the hyperparameters during a typical training run. Five such runs were made with different seeds for weight initialisation. We then selected two subsets of input variables: those where the median hyperparameter value was less than 1000 (16 inputs) and those where the value was less than 100 (9 inputs). Two further sets of training runs (with five seeds in each case) were carried out for these networks. In the latter case, one hyperparameter diverged and there were effectively eight inputs.

The confusion matrices for both PCA and ARD networks are given in Table 12.3. Note that apart from misclassifications between the two ventricular ectopic classes, there are just one false positive and six false negatives for the ARD-MLP with nine inputs. All but one of the nine variables is a timing measure (i.e. measures the time between two events) with the exception being a peak height.

12.3.4 Conclusions

These results demonstrate that non-linear classification models offer significant advantages in ECG beat classification and that with a principled approach to feature selection, pre-processing, and model development, it is possible to get robust inter-subject generalisation even on ambulatory data. The MLP makes two false negative misclassifications. The dataset was sufficiently large that Bayesian regularisation was not needed to prevent over-fitting.

ARD has been applied successfully to reduce the number of inputs by two thirds without affecting significantly the model's accuracy; there were six false negatives and one false positive in a test set of 23,606 patterns. The experiment has also

Table 12.3. Performance statistics for MLP with reduced number of inputs. Confusion matrix entries are given as: median (min/max) over 5 seeds. Rows represent true classes sinus, *Vel*, *Ver*. PCA datasets are different from those used in other experiments.

ARD-MLP 16 inputs: Mean err: 0.0491%; std err: 0.0038%		
19983 (19983/19983)	4 (4/4)	0 (0/0)
0 (0/0)	1187 (1187/1187)	1 (1/1)
0 (0/0)	6 (6/8)	2425 (2423/2425)

ARD-MLP 9 inputs: Mean err: 0.0474%; std err: 0.0019%		
19981 (19981/19981)	6 (6/6)	0 (0/0)
1 (1/1)	1186 (1185/1186)	1 (1/2)
0 (0/0)	3 (3/3)	2428 (2428/2428)

PCA-MLP: 0.2119%; std err: 0.0215%		
13715 (13713/13718)	6 (6/7)	16 (12/17)
4 (4/11)	513 (506/513)	5 (5/5)
0 (0/0)	0 (0/0)	1033 (1033/1033)

highlighted that it may be necessary to apply ARD in an iterative way; a hyperparameter that had converged to a reasonable value in the experiment with 16 inputs diverged in the experiment with 9 inputs. The divergence was masked in the first experiment by the presence of other, even less important, inputs. Applying PCA to the original set of variables would not have been appropriate in this application, where the aim was to reduce the amount of computation required for the inputs. This is because applying the results of PCA requires *all* the original variables to be calculated followed by a linear transformation (which would therefore have needed more, rather than less, computation). The application of PCA to raw beat data gave less accurate results, showing that the cardiologist-selected features were effective.

12.4 ARD in Lupus Diagnosis

12.4.1 Clinical Context

Lupus is an autoimmune disease in which the patient's immune system creates antibodies which, instead of protecting the body from bacteria, viruses or other foreign matter, attack the person's own body tissues. This causes symptoms of fatigue, joint pain, muscle aches, anaemia, and possibly destruction of vital organs. Lupus is neither infectious nor contagious, and the cause is not known, though research has provided evidence implicating heredity, hormones, and infections. The disease lies dormant in the body until triggered by environmental factors.

Lupus mainly attacks women during their child-bearing years: in the UK, 1 in 750 women suffer from lupus, with the ratio of women to men being 9:1. There is no cure for lupus, but careful monitoring of the disease and a treatment program with medication adjusted to take account of symptoms enables the condition to be controlled, so most patients are able to live a normal life span.

The Birmingham lupus disease clinic was set up in 1989. Data is collected at every in-patient and out-patient visit according to a standard protocol, including clinical data, disease activity (the BILAG index [9]), and laboratory and medication data. This data is stored in a specially designed database called BLIPS: British Lupus Integrated Prospective System [10]. Assessments on 430 patients obtained during more than 7000 visits were available for analysis. This dataset shows that in Birmingham 1 in 2000 women suffer from the disease and the ratio of women to men is 14 to 1 [11]. The time between successive visits varies between three weeks and several years, with a mode of three months. The reason for this variation is that the doctor takes into account the severity of the disease in determining when the patient should be reassessed and how long the patient should continue with a certain treatment plan.

The key clinical variable is the doctor's evaluation of the level of disease activity in each body system. The British Isles Lupus Assessment Group (BILAG) have devised a scoring system based on patient history, examination and laboratory results [9, 10]. As well as general nonspecific features, seven systems are considered: mucocutaneous, neurological, musculoskeletal, cardiovascular and respiratory, vasculitis, renal, and haematological.

The BILAG index allocates a categorical score to each system: these are based on a sequence of structured questions to make the value more reproducible. This was later converted to a numerical system suitable for statistical analysis [20]. The scale is given in Table 12.4. The overall score for a patient is found by summing

Table 12.4. Scoring of the BILAG index

	Score	Interpretation
A	9	Requires disease-modifying treatment
B	3	Mild reversible problems requiring only symptomatic treatment
C	1	Stable mild disease
D or E	0	System previously affected but currently inactive or never involved

all the system scores. Of course, the validity of this is open to question, since the mapping from the ordinal scale of disease severity to the score numbers is arbitrary. The values were chosen to accord with clinical experience, some statistical analysis was carried out to validate the scheme, but this is unpublished.

The variables of most interest are the laboratory tests performed on each patient. Many of these tests are not measured routinely at every visit included in the study, so there was a significant fraction of missing data. Those that are reasonably prevalent include anti-double-stranded DNA antibody tests (F103E), C3 and C4 complement tests (F111, F112, F113), C-reactive protein (F119C), serum creatinine (F75), which is related to renal function, and ESR (F87). The most important treatment variable is F141, which represents the *change* in steroid dosage (coded as 1 for reduction, 2 for the same, 3 for increase, and 4 for starting). This is an important input for predictive models, since it is the main clinical intervention, and thus clearly has an impact on the subsequent progress of the disease. We also used two other therapeutic variables: F121 (the steroid dosage) and F133 (pulse cyclophosphamide).

The main clinical objective is to predict whether a particular patient will become ill with increased disease activity (known as a "flare"). Thus our goal was to develop a model that used laboratory tests to predict the disease activity at the following visit.

12.4.2 Linear Methods for Variable Selection

Our initial task was to determine objectively a good set of input variables for the task of predicting the BILAG score for a visit given the laboratory variables for the previous visit.

We first analysed the correlation matrix, and looked in particular at the correlation of the indicators Fxxx with the target variable. Other than two very specific renal indicators (F71 and F72), no variable had a correlation greater than 0.29 with the target variable. This strongly suggested that a linear model would not be very effective on this problem.

We then considered the possibility that there was a time lag between the indicators and target variable. To detect this, we considered the cross-correlation of each input with the target, using successive visits to construct a time series. Again, there were no correlations of significant magnitude.

In our final attempt to find informative input variables using linear methods, we applied Principal Component Analysis (PCA). In an experiment with all 31 input variables, the first 15 principal components were needed to explain just 80% of the variance. When restricted to just the 8 most important variables, as selected by clinical experts, the graph of variance explained against number of components is nearly a straight line. These results suggest that PCA is not extracting features that are significantly better than the original set of variables. Given that we are interested in explaining our results in terms of clinical indicators, there was no advantage in using these linear combinations.

12.4.3 Prognosis with Non-linear Models

The task was initially formulated as a regression problem: we set up the models to predict the value of the BILAG score (total or for a single system) at the next visit. As well as predicting the BILAG score y_{i+1} from the input variables $\boldsymbol{x}_i$, we also used a "difference" encoding to predict $y_{i+1} - y_i$ from $\boldsymbol{x}_i - \boldsymbol{x}_{i-1}$. The latter encoding was designed to test the hypothesis that *differences* in clinical measurements were related to *differences* in outcome.

We trained three different non-linear models: MLP (4, 8, 16, 32, and 64 hidden units), MLP with weight decay (same architecture as the MLP and weight decay $\alpha \in \{10^{-6}, 10^{-3}, 1, 10^3, 10^6\}$), and RBF with spherical Gaussian basis functions (4, 8, 16, 32, and 64 hidden units). We also trained a linear regression model as a benchmark. The dataset was divided into three subsets (training, validation and test) with all the visits for each patient confined to one subset. All data with a gap of six months between the tests and the next visit was removed, as it was felt that a predictive model would not be appropriate in such cases.

The results for all these models were very poor. Figure 12.5 shows typical results on test data, which show that there is virtually no correlation between the predictions and the target values. The fact that this performance was also repeated on the training and validation datasets shows that it is not a matter of a flaw in the training process, but that there is no underlying mapping from the input to output variables.

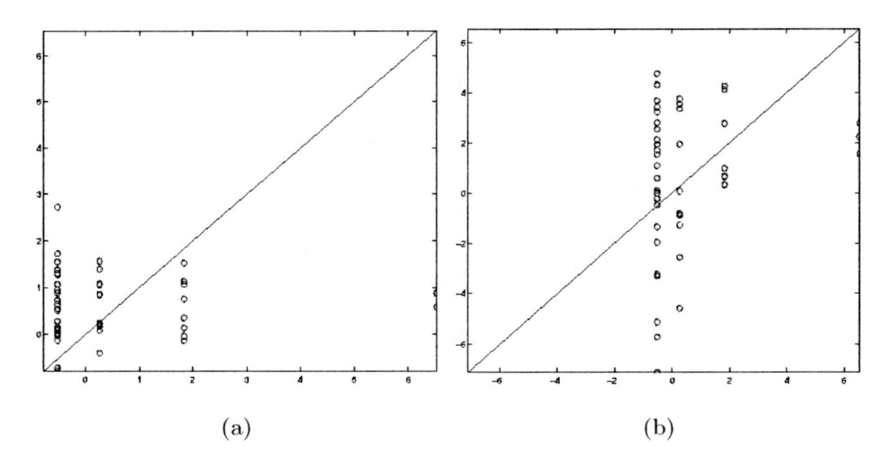

(a) (b)

Fig. 12.5. Predicting the renal BILAG score: predicted value (y-axis) against true value (x-axis). The ideal model would give points along the line $y = x$. (a) Linear regression. (b) RBF with 16 hidden units.

One plausible explanation for these poor results is that the numeric BILAG scores are not reliable enough to use as targets. Therefore, we decided to recast the problem as a classification task. Although there are four different BILAG scores we decided to reduce the problem to just two categories: a significant flare-up of the disease (scores 3 and 9), and all other outcomes (scores 0, 1). For the total BILAG score we first used a score of 10 or above as a threshold to discriminate between the classes. However, again this can be problematic due to the influence of low system scores on the total, so instead we required at least three systems to have a score of three or greater.

This representation gave rise to difficulties because of the relatively small number of visits with a flare of the disease. The fraction of visits with a flare varied from 0.02 (neurological) to 0.19 (musculo-skeletal). A model trained on a dataset with such a small fraction of examples from one class is unlikely to generate reliable estimates of the conditional class probabilities $P(C_k|\boldsymbol{x})$. To circumvent this, we trained on a *balanced* dataset (i.e. one with approximately equal numbers of examples from both classes) and then rescaled the model outputs using the following formula, derived from Bayes' theorem (see [2] Section 6.5):

$$P(C_k|\boldsymbol{x}) \propto \frac{P(C_k^b|\boldsymbol{x})P(C_k)}{P(C_k^b)}, \tag{12.15}$$

where $P(C_k^b|\boldsymbol{x})$ is the output of the model trained on the balanced dataset, $P(C_k)$ is the true prior probability of class C_k (estimated by the true fraction of examples belonging to C_k) and $P(C_k^b)$ is the prior probability of class C_k in the balanced training set. After the values $P(C_k|\boldsymbol{x})$ have been computed for each class C_k, they are normalised to sum to 1.

We trained a similar set of models as in the regression problem, except we replaced linear regression by logistic regression and the MLP output units used a logistic function rather than equality. The error function was changed from sum-of-squares to cross-entropy, so that it still represented the negative log likelihood of the data.

If a prognostic model were used clinically, it would be used in an advisory way. For this reason, it is possible to leave doubtful cases to be classified by a medical expert. Such cases arise where the posterior class probability $P(C_k|\boldsymbol{x})$ is close to 0.5. Therefore we used a *rejection threshold*:

$$\text{if } \max_k P(C_k|\boldsymbol{x}) \begin{cases} \geq \theta & \text{classify } \boldsymbol{x} \\ < \theta & \text{reject } \boldsymbol{x} \end{cases} \tag{12.16}$$

where $0.5 < \theta < 1$. The larger the value of θ, the smaller the number of patterns that are classified.

When assessing the performance of the models on the validation data, the threshold was moved from 0.5 to 1.0 in steps of 0.1. For each model we selected the threshold that represented the best compromise between obtaining the lowest false positive rate and reject fraction, and the highest true positive rate.

Table 12.5 shows the results on the test data for the best model (selected using the validation data) for each body system. The cardiorespiratory and neurological systems had too few examples of flares to be valid. Clearly these results are still a long way from providing us with a model that would be useable in a clinical situation.

Table 12.5. Results of the best classification model. TP is the true positive rate just on the classified (i.e. unrejected) examples, TPt, is the true positive rate over all the examples, FP is the false positive rate.

	TP	TPt	FP	Rejected
General	0.86	0.60	0.33	0.28
Renal	0.73	0.73	0.39	0.00
Haema	0.82	0.73	0.37	0.20
Muco	0.44	0.28	0.43	0.46
Muscu	0.62	0.35	0.54	0.36
Vasc	0.54	0.43	0.45	0.16

12.4.4 Bayesian Variable Selection

At this point in the project we decided that to improve the performance of our prognostic models we would have to revisit the variable selection question. As linear methods had failed to provide any useful information, we decided to apply ARD to ensure that the variables selected were relevant both to the task and the model. We used an MLP trained with the evidence procedure to perform variable selection for the total BILAG score. The variables that were included in the study were the eight selected by our domain expert, and an additional two variables (F133 and F75) which we thought were of limited relevance. These were included to give us a benchmark for the threshold hyperparameter value and also to assess whether the results of ARD are sensible.

We ran the ARD process for both regression and classification models: the results are contained in Table 12.6. The results on the regression problem are disappointing;

Table 12.6. Hyperparameter values after ARD. Regression (row 1), classification (row 2) and classification on reduced set (row 3). See Section 12.4.1 for a description of variables. F121, F141 and F133 are related to drug therapy, and all the others are laboratory tests.

F103E	F111	F112	F113	F119C	F87	F121	F141	F133	F75
0.00	0.00	0.00	0.00	0.00	0.00	0.00	0.00	0.00	0.00
1800	133	35	55	39	99	18	6	26	222
–	–	5.58	3.12	10.08	–	27.84	4.65	99.79	–

the hyperparameters for all the variables are small, and so it is impossible to select a useful subset of variables.

However, the results on the classification problem (row 2) are more interesting. A subset of six variables (F112, F113, F119C, F121, F141, and F133) have significantly smaller hyperparameter values than the rest. We therefore carried out a second ARD experiment with the inputs restricted to just this set (row 3). This enabled us to distinguish an even smaller subset of four variables (F112, F113, F119C, and F141) that were the most relevant for this task. We note that none of the additional variables are included in this set, which is reassuring. It is also interesting that F141 (representing the change in steroid dosage) is more useful than F121 (representing the level of steroid dosage).

To assess the value of this result, we trained all four model types with just these four variables as inputs. The graphical results can be seen in Figure 12.6. The rejection rate was between 0.1 and 0.15 for the RBF, and around 0.02 for the other models. The graphs show that the MLP is the model which performs best, achieving a true positive rate of 0.98 and a false positive rate of 0.075. This is similar to the MLP with weight decay, but superior to logistic regression (true positive 0.82, false positive 0.08) and much better than the RBF. More details on these results can be found in [5].

12.4.5 Conclusions

This application has shown that ARD can be a vital tool in the data analyst's toolbox, as simpler methods of variable selection gave no useful information, and it was only after the smaller set of most relevant variables had been found that we

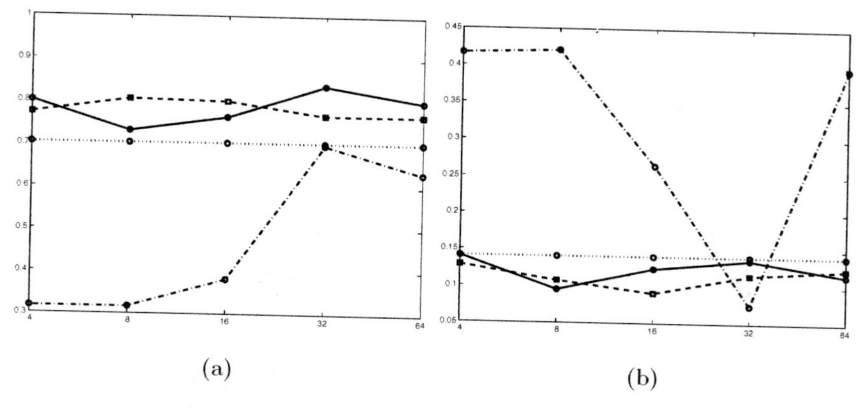

Fig. 12.6. Results of classifiers trained on reduced set of input variables. x-axis represents numbers of hidden units. Logistic regression (*dotted line*), MLP (*solid line*), MLP with weight decay (*dashed line*), RBF (*dash-dotted line*). (a) True positive rate. (b) False positive rate.

were able to develop models with some potential for real application. The variables that were selected can be justified from clinical knowledge, but the real strength of the technique is that it enabled us to reject variables that might be disease-related, but that were poor predictors of the clinical outcome. If the approach were extended to each system, then it would probably be possible to reduce the number of clinical tests (thus reducing costs) while also providing the clinicians with a useful support tool for guiding their diagnosis. The therapeutic inputs were included to see if they were confounding variables, and to assess the reliability and effectiveness of the laboratory tests under realistic conditions. The fact that one of these variables was selected by ARD is strong evidence that it is an important factor in reliable predictions.

The poor performance of the regression models (both with the full set of inputs, and when applying ARD) suggests that the numerical BILAG scores (which are based on clinical judgements) are not very reliable, and that a two-class discrimination may be all that can be reproducibly measured across a large number of clinics.

12.5 Conclusions

The two case studies have demonstrated that Bayesian methods for feature selection are a practical proposition and can give genuinely useful results that could not be obtained by other means. In the ECG study, very high accuracy levels were maintained while the number of input variables was reduced by two thirds. In the lupus study, it was only by using ARD that we were able to train a model which had an acceptable level of accuracy.

In both studies, a multi-stage application of ARD gave the best results. This seems to be because the presence of very large hyperparameters masks the differences between smaller ones. A second run of ARD, excluding the inputs corresponding to large hyperparameters, identifies the irrelevant variables from the smaller subset.

The computational effort for the ARD training runs was about 40 times as large as standard maximum likelihood training (in the ECG study, an MLP training run of 4 hours became about 7 days using ARD[8]); the ratio of training times depends on the number of iterations needed for the hyperparameters to converge, the number of weights, and linearly on the number of training set patterns. This is a significant drawback, but the procedure is feasible on modern PCs.

Acknowledgments

ITN and DJE would like to thank Cardionetics Ltd. for supporting the Cardionetics Institute of Bioinformatics, under whose auspices the ECG study was carried out.

ITN, YB and CG would like to thank Lupus UK for supporting the Birmingham lupus cohort and Deva Situnayeke for contributing patients and advice.

References

[1] J. O. Berger. *Statistical Decision Theory and Bayesian Analysis.* Springer-Verlag, New York, 2nd edition, 1985.

[2] C. M. Bishop. *Neural Networks for Pattern Recognition.* Oxford University Press, 1995.

[3] C. M. Bishop, M. Svensén, and C. K. I. Williams. GTM: The Generative Topographic Mapping. *Neural Computation*, 10(1):215–235, 1996.

[4] J. Boutkan. *A Guide to Electrocardiography.* Macmillan, 1972.

[5] Y. Brulé. Lupus prognosis: a clinical study. Master's thesis, Aston University, Birmingham, UK, 2000.

[6] C. Chatfield and A. J. Collins. *Introduction to Multivariate Analysis.* Chapman and Hall, 1980.

[7] L. Gamlyn, P. Needham, S. M. Sopher, and T. J. Harris. The development of a neural network-based ambulatory ECG monitor. *Neural Computing and Applications*, 8:273–278, 1999.

[8] B. Hassibi and D. G. Stork. Second order derivatives for network pruning: optimal brain surgeon. In S. J. Hanson, J. D. Cowan, and C. L. Giles, editors, *Advances in Neural Information Processing Systems*, volume 5, pages 164–171, San Mateo, CA, 1993. Morgan Kaufmann.

[9] E. M. Hay, P. A. Bacon, C. Gordon, D. A. Isenberg, P. Maddison, M. L. Snaith, D. P. M. Symmons, N. Viner, and A. Zoma. The BILAG index: a reliable and valid instrument for measuring clinical disease activity in systemic lupus erythematosus. *Quart. J. Medicine*, 86:447–458, 1993.

[10] D. A. Isenberg and C. Gordon. From BILAG to BLIPS. Disease activity assessment in lupus: past, present and future. *Lupus*, 9:651–654, 2000.

[11] A. E. Johnson, C. Gordon, R. G. Palmer, and P. A. Bacon. The prevalence and incidence of systemic lupus erythematosus in Birmingham, UK, related to ethnicity and country of birth. *Arthritis Rheum.*, 38:551–558, 1995.

[8] Experiments were carried out on an 865 MHz Pentium PC running Linux.

[12] T. Kohonen. *Self-Organizing Maps*. Springer-Verlag, Berlin, 1995.
[13] Y. Le Cun, J. S. Denker, and S. A. Solla. Optimal brain damage. In D. S. Touretzky, editor, *Advances in Neural Information Processing Systems*, volume 2, pages 598–605, San Mateo, CA, 1990. Morgan Kaufmann.
[14] D. J. C. MacKay. Bayesian interpolation. *Neural Computation*, 4(3):415–447, 1992.
[15] D. J. C. MacKay. The evidence framework applied to classification networks. *Neural Computation*, 4(5):720–736, 1992.
[16] D. J. C. MacKay. A practical Bayesian framework for back-propagation networks. *Neural Computation*, 4(3):448–472, 1992.
[17] I. T. Nabney. *Netlab: Algorithms for Pattern Recognition*. Springer-Verlag, London, 2002.
[18] R. M. Neal. *Bayesian Learning for Neural Networks*. Lecture Notes in Statistics: Number 118. Springer-Verlag, New York, 1996.
[19] P. Standing, M. Dent, A. Craig, and B. Glenville. Changes in referral patterns to cardiac out-patient clinics with ambulatory ECG monitoring in general practice. *Brit. J. Cardiol.*, 6:394–398, 2001.
[20] T. Stoll, C. Gordon, B. Seifert, K. Richardson, J. Malik, P. A. Bacon, and D. A. Isenberg. Consistency and validity of patient administered assessment of quality of life by the mos sf-36; its association with disease activity and damage in patients with systemic lupus erythematosus. *J. Rheum*, 24:1608–1614, 1997.
[21] H. H. Thodberg. Ace of Bayes: application of neural networks with pruning. Technical Report 1132E, The Danish Meat Research Institute, Maglegaardsvej 2, DK-4000 Roskilde, Denmark, 1993.

13

Bayes Consistent Classification of EEG Data by Approximate Marginalization

Peter Sykacek, Iead Rezek, and Stephen Roberts

University of Oxford, Dept. of Engineering Science, Oxford, UK
{psyk,irezek,sjrob}@robots.ox.ac.uk

Summary. This chapter proposes a generative model and a Bayesian learning scheme for a classifier that takes uncertainty at all levels of inference into account. Classifier inputs will be uncertain if they are estimated, for example using a preprocessing method. Classical approaches would neglect the uncertainties associated with these variables. However, the decisions thus found are not consistent with Bayesian theory. In order to conform with the axioms underlying the Bayesian framework, we must incorporate all uncertainties into the decisions. The model we use for classification treats input variables resulting from preprocessing as latent variables. The proposed algorithms for learning and prediction fuse information from different sensors spatially and across time according to its certainty. In order to get a computationally tractable method, both feature and model uncertainty of the preprocessing stage are obtained in closed form. Classification requires integration over this latent feature space, which in this chapter is done approximately by a Markov chain Monte Carlo (MCMC) method. Our approach is applied to classifying cognitive states from EEG segments and to classification of sleep spindles.

13.1 Introduction

Once we opt for decision analysis within a Bayesian framework, we must do this throughout the entire process. The approach studied in this chapter assumes that we are given some segments of time series, each labelled as being in one of K possible states. Such a setting is typically found in biomedical diagnosis, where successive segments of biosignals have to be classified. Usually, the number of samples within the segments is large. However, the information contained in a segment is often represented by a much smaller number of features. Such problems are typically solved by splitting the whole problem into two parts: a preprocessing method that extracts some features and a classifier.

Using Bayesian inference for each part is common practice. For preprocessing it has been considered among many others by [1] and [2]. A review of recent developments is provided by [3]. The situation in post-processing is similar: see e.g. [4], [5] or [6] for a summary. We could follow these lines and apply Bayesian techniques to both stages of the decision process separately. However this would mean establishing a non-probabilistic link between preprocessing and classification. Such a link does not allow feature or model uncertainty, as found by Bayesian preprocessing, to have an influence on the beliefs reported by the classifier. In a Bayesian sense this is equivalent to approximating the *a-posteriori* probability density over feature variables by a delta peak and ignoring the uncertainty in the stochastic model used for preprocessing.

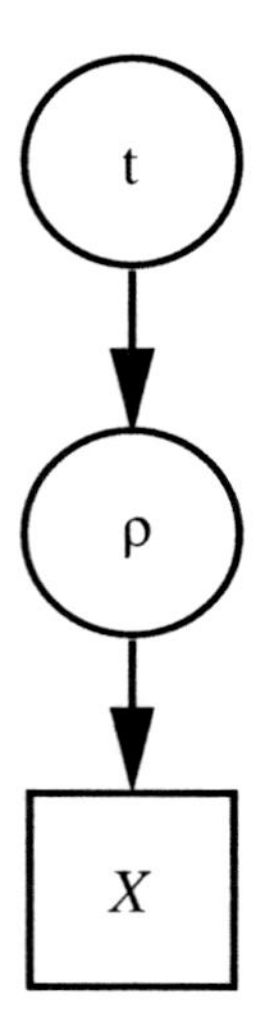

Fig. 13.1. A directed acyclic graph for the hierarchical model. We used t to denote the unknown state variable of interest, ρ is a latent (unobserved) variable representing features from preprocessing and $\mathcal{X}$ denotes a segment of a time series. Circles indicate latent variables, whereas the square indicates that $\mathcal{X}$ is an observed quantity.

A model that allows for a probabilistic link between preprocessing and post-processing has to have a structure similar to the directed acyclic graph (DAG) shown in Figure 13.1. The key idea is to treat the features obtained by preprocessing as latent variables. The link between ρ and $\mathcal{X}$ represents preprocessing, which has to be carried out in a Bayesian setting. The model used in this chapter for preprocessing is a lattice filter representation of an auto regressive (AR) model. The coefficients of this model are the well-known reflection coefficients as commonly used in speech processing [7]. We give a short summary of our derivation of "Bayesian reflection coefficients" in section 13.2. So far approaches using a probabilistic structure, similar to the DAG in Figure 13.1, have focused on marginalising out input uncertainties. The main emphasis in [8] and [9] is to derive a predictive distribution for regression models where input uncertainty is taken into account. In a Bayesian sense this approach is the only way of consistent reasoning if perfect knowledge of inputs is not available. We provide a similar analysis for classification problems. However our approach goes further:

- We allow for different uncertainties at different inputs. This leads to predictions that are dominated by inputs that are more certain. Using generative models to link t and ρ, the model provides information about the *true* input values of less certain sensors. Using several sensors will lead to "Bayesian sensor fusion". The use of a generative model gives us the additional benefit that we can use unlabelled data for parameter inference as well.
- Another extension of the work reported in [8] and [9] is that we take the model uncertainty, inherent to all preprocessing methods, into account. Model uncertainty is represented by the *a-posteriori* probability of the model conditional on the corresponding data segment, $\mathcal{X}$.

In the following sections of the chapter, we derive a Bayesian solution for lattice filter AR-models that captures both feature and model uncertainty. We show that marginalising out latent variables in a static DAG indeed performs sensor fusion such that predictions depend more on certain information. Equipped with this theoretical insight, we propose a DAG and inference scheme that is well suited for time series classification. We assume a first order Markov dependency among class labels of interest and derive MCMC updates that sample from the joint probability distribution over latent variables and model coefficients. The experimental section of this chapter provides a synthetic experiment to illustrate the idea and provides then a quantitative evaluation using the proposed method for sleep spindle classification and as a classifier in a brain–computer interface experiment.

13.2 Bayesian Lattice Filter

The lattice filter is a representation of an auto regressive (AR) model [7]. Its parameters are the so-called refection coefficients, below denoted as r_m. Equation (13.1) shows an AR model, where $x[t]$ is the sample of a time series at time t, a_μ is the μ-th AR coefficient of the m-th order AR model and $e[t]$ the forward prediction error, which we assume to be independently identically distributed (i.i.d.) Gaussian with zero mean and precision (inverse variance) β.

$$x[t] = -\sum_{\mu=1}^{m} x[t-\mu]a_\mu + e[t] \tag{13.1}$$

The autocovariance function, which is the sufficient statistic of a stationary Gaussian noise AR model, is invariant to the direction of time [7]. The corresponding backward prediction model thus shares the same parameters.

$$x[t-m] = -\sum_{\mu=1}^{m} x[t+1-\mu]a_\mu + b[t] \tag{13.2}$$

To derive Bayesian reflection coefficients, we assume that N data points, $\mathcal{X} = \{x[1], \ldots, x[N]\}$, are available to estimate the model. We denote the m-th order AR coefficients as $\boldsymbol{\varphi}_m$, summarise the forward prediction errors $e[t]$ as $\boldsymbol{\epsilon}_m$ and all backward prediction errors $b[t]$ as $\boldsymbol{b}_m$. Applying the backward time shift operator q^{-1} on $\boldsymbol{b}_m$, linear regression onto the forward prediction errors, $\boldsymbol{\epsilon}_m$, defines the likelihood of the m-th order AR coefficients and the $m+1$-th reflection coefficient r_{m+1}.

$$\begin{aligned} p(\mathcal{X}|r_{m+1}, \beta, \boldsymbol{\varphi}_m) &= (2\pi)^{-0.5N}\beta^{0.5N} \\ &\times \exp\left(-0.5\left(\boldsymbol{\epsilon}_m + r_{m+1}q^{-1}\boldsymbol{b}_m\right)^{\mathsf{T}}\left(\boldsymbol{\epsilon}_m + r_{m+1}q^{-1}\boldsymbol{b}_m\right)\right) \end{aligned} \tag{13.3}$$

Since we use this model to represent segments of biological time series, we know with certainty that the underlying AR-process must be stable. As the reflection coefficients of a stable model have to be within the interval $[-1, 1]$, we may use a flat prior within this range. Thus the uninformative proper prior over reflection coefficients is $p(r_{m+1}) = 0.5$. Another parameter which appears in the likelihood expression of the lattice filter model is the noise level β. The noise level is a scale parameter and following [10] we use the Jeffreys' prior, $p(\beta) = 1/\beta$.

In order to obtain the posterior distribution over the $m+1$-th reflection coefficient r_{m+1}, the Bayesian paradigm requires us to treat both the m-th order AR coefficients, $\boldsymbol{\varphi}_m$, and the noise level, β, as nuisance parameters and integrate them out. We may simplify calculations considerably by assuming a sharply peaked posterior over $\boldsymbol{\varphi}_m$. This results in an order recursive estimation, where we condition on the forward and backward prediction errors that result from the most probable coefficients.

$$p(r_{m+1}|\mathcal{X}) = \frac{1}{\sqrt{2\pi}s}\exp\left(-\frac{1}{2s^2}(r_{m+1} - \hat{r}_{m+1})^2\right) \tag{13.4}$$

as the posterior distribution of the $m+1$-th order reflection coefficient, in which

$$\hat{r}_{m+1} = -\frac{\boldsymbol{\epsilon}_m^{\mathsf{T}} q^{-1}\boldsymbol{b}_m}{\boldsymbol{b}_m^{\mathsf{T}}\boldsymbol{b}_m} \tag{13.5}$$

represents the most probable value of the reflection coefficient and,

$$s^2 = \frac{1-(\hat{r}_{m+1})^2}{(N-1)}, \tag{13.6}$$

the corresponding variance. We finally need to update the forward and backward prediction errors, to account for the $m+1$-th reflection coefficient.

$$\begin{aligned} \boldsymbol{\epsilon}_{m+1} &= \boldsymbol{\epsilon}_m + \hat{r}_{m+1}q^{-1}\boldsymbol{r}_m \\ \boldsymbol{r}_{m+1} &= q^{-1}\boldsymbol{r}_m + \hat{r}_{m+1}\boldsymbol{\epsilon}_m \end{aligned} \tag{13.7}$$

Our analysis will also consider the uncertainty about the lattice filter model, by allowing for two explanations of the data $\mathcal{X}$. We assume that the data is either modelled by an M-th order lattice filter or that it is white noise. This uncertainty is captured by the posterior probability $P(I_M|\mathcal{X})$, where $I_M \equiv 1$ denotes the lattice filter explanation and $I_M \equiv 0$ denotes the white noise case. The Bayesian model evidence (marginal likelihood) of the M-th order lattice filter model, $I_M \equiv 1$, is then

$$\begin{aligned} p(\mathcal{X}|I_M \equiv 1) = 0.5\pi^{-\frac{N}{2}}\Gamma(\frac{N}{2})\sqrt{2\pi s} \\ \times \left((\boldsymbol{\epsilon}_{M-1} + \hat{r}_M \boldsymbol{b}_{M-1})^{\mathsf{T}}(\boldsymbol{\epsilon}_{M-1} + \hat{r}_M \boldsymbol{b}_{M-1})\right)^{-\frac{N}{2}} . \end{aligned} \quad (13.8)$$

Comparing the M-stage lattice filter model with the Bayesian evidence of explaining the data as white noise gives a measure of model uncertainty if we allow for these two explanations only. We obtain the evidence of a white noise explanation by integrating out the noise level β. We indicate the corresponding model by I_0 and get

$$p(\mathcal{X}|I_M \equiv 0) = \pi^{-\frac{N}{2}}\Gamma(\frac{N}{2})\left(\boldsymbol{\epsilon}_0^{\mathsf{T}}\boldsymbol{\epsilon}_0\right)^{-\frac{N}{2}} , \quad (13.9)$$

where $\boldsymbol{\epsilon}_0$ refers to the 0-order model residuals (the original time series). Using equal priors for both models, the *a-posteriori* probability of the m-th reflection coefficient compared with a white noise explanation is

$$P(I_M \equiv 1|\mathcal{X}) = \frac{p(\mathcal{X}|I_M \equiv 1)}{p(\mathcal{X}|I_M \equiv 1) + p(\mathcal{X}|I_M \equiv 0)}. \quad (13.10)$$

We use $P(I_M|\mathcal{X})$ to measure the uncertainty of modelling the data by an M-th order lattice filter, when we allow for a white noise explanation as the other possibility. Our motivation for this two-model hypothesis is our intent to model electroencephalography (EEG) data. EEG is often contaminated by muscle artefacts, which result in measurements that are very similar to white noise.

Equations (13.4), (13.5) and (13.6) imply that the underlying processes are dynamically stable systems since they do not allow reflection coefficients to be outside the interval $[-1, 1]$. Since we intend to model the distributions in the latent feature space by a mixture of Gaussian distributions, we have to resolve a mismatch between the domain of the posterior over M-th order lattice filter coefficients, $\boldsymbol{r} \in [-1, 1]^M$ and the domain of the Gaussian mixture model, which requires $\boldsymbol{\rho} \in \mathbb{R}^M$. To resolve the problem, we follow [11] and map using Fisher's z-transform

$$\boldsymbol{\rho} = \operatorname{arctanh}(\boldsymbol{r}), \quad (13.11)$$

which we use henceforth as representation of the feature space. Using error analysis [12], we can approximate the posterior distribution over the transformed reflection coefficients ρ_m by

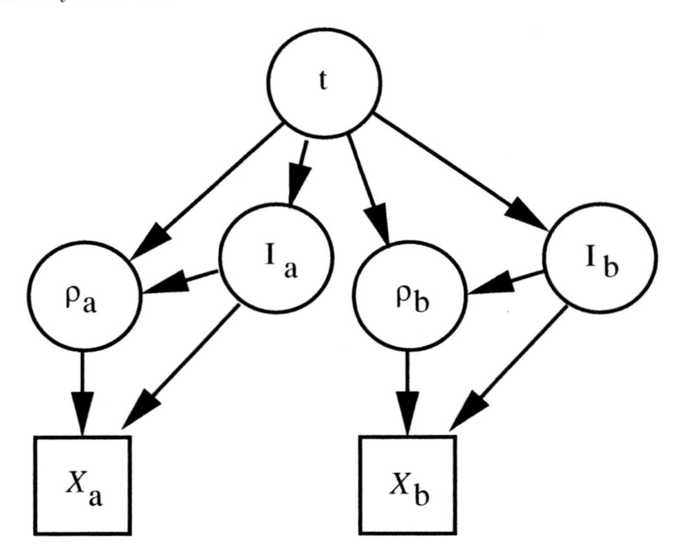

Fig. 13.2. A directed acyclic graph that captures both parameter uncertainty as well as model uncertainty in preprocessing. We used t to denote the unknown state variable of interest, ρ_a and ρ_b are two latent variables representing the true values of features estimated by preprocessing. Both $\mathcal{X}_a$ and $\mathcal{X}_b$ are the corresponding segments of a time series. The latent binary indicator variables I_a and I_b control the dependency of the data segments on the latent variables.

$$p(\rho_m|\mathcal{X}) = \frac{1}{\sqrt{2\pi}}\sqrt{\lambda}\exp\left(-\frac{1}{2}\lambda(\rho_m - \hat{\rho}_m)^2\right) \tag{13.12}$$

where $\hat{\rho}_m = \text{arctanh}(\hat{r}_m)$ and $\lambda = (N-1)(1-\hat{r}_m^2)$.

13.3 Spatial Fusion

In our case the input uncertainty is a result of the limited accuracy of feature estimates as obtained by preprocessing. If we know that the model used in preprocessing is the *true* model that generated the time series $\mathcal{X}$, the approach taken by [8] and [9] would be sufficient. However, as argued in Section 13.2, we do not know whether the model used during preprocessing is the *true* one and we have to consider feature as well as model uncertainty. Thus inference has to be carried out with a DAG that allows for both feature *and* model uncertainty. Sensor fusion will only take place if different sensors are conditionally dependent on the state of interest. In order to take this into account, we have to extend the DAG structure as shown in Figure 13.2. We introduce binary indicator variables I_a and I_b that control the conditional dependency of the observed data segments $\mathcal{X}_a$ and $\mathcal{X}_b$ on the latent variables ρ_a and ρ_b respectively.

The DAG in Figure 13.2 illustrates the dependency between a state variable t, latent variables ρ_a and ρ_b and the corresponding segments of a time series $\mathcal{X}_a$ and $\mathcal{X}_b$. The dependency is controlled by two model indicator variables, I_a and I_b, one for each sensor. Both models, I_a and I_b, representing particular stages of a lattice filter, are *probable* explanations of the corresponding time series $\mathcal{X}_a$ and $\mathcal{X}_b$.

During preprocessing we allow for two possible explanations of each segment of the time series. With probability $P(I_a|\mathcal{X}_a)$, the latent variable ρ_a is conditional on both the time series $\mathcal{X}_a$ *and* the state variable t. However, with probability $1 - P(I_a|\mathcal{X}_a)$, $\mathcal{X}_a$ is pure white noise and does not require ρ_a. In this case, we have to condition on t only. Loosely speaking, we deal with a problem of "probably missing values". However this interpretation of Figure 13.2 tells us that we need to use the following definition of the conditional probability density of $\mathcal{X}_a$

$$p(\mathcal{X}_a|\rho_a, I_a) = \begin{cases} p(\mathcal{X}_a|\rho_a, I_a \equiv 1) \\ p(\mathcal{X}_a|I_a \equiv 0). \end{cases} \tag{13.13}$$

Depending on the value of I_a, we introduce a conditional independence between the data, $\mathcal{X}_a$ and the true feature value ρ_a which is not seen in the DAG in Figure 13.2. When changing indices, we get the same statements for the *latent* variable ρ_b.

As previously mentioned, we want to predict the belief of state t conditional on *all* available information. This is the observed time series $\mathcal{X}_a$ and $\mathcal{X}_b$ as well as all training data $\mathcal{D}$ observed so far. Although we will not state this explicitly, *all* beliefs are also conditional on training data $\mathcal{D}$. This is a requirement that humans apply intuitively: whenever a clinical expert wants to monitor a new recording of some biological time series they have prior expectations about the range they should use.

In order to provide deeper insight into the model illustrated in Figure 13.2, we will infer both the *a-posteriori* probability $P(t|\mathcal{X}_a, \mathcal{X}_b)$ and the *a-posteriori* probability density $p(\rho_a|\mathcal{X}_a, \mathcal{X}_b)$. Using Bayes' theorem, we express $P(t)p(\rho_a|t)$ as $p(\rho_a)P(t|\rho_a)$ and $P(t)p(\rho_b|t)$ as $p(\rho_b)P(t|\rho_b)$. Conditioning on $\mathcal{X}_a$ and $\mathcal{X}_b$, the DAG in Figure 13.2 implies that

$$\begin{aligned} &p(t, \rho_a, I_a, \rho_b, I_b|\mathcal{X}_a, \mathcal{X}_b) = \\ &\frac{P(t|\rho_a, I_a)P(t|\rho_b, I_b)p(\rho_a|I_a, \mathcal{X}_a)p(I_a|\mathcal{X}_a)p(\rho_b|I_b, \mathcal{X}_b)p(I_b|\mathcal{X}_b)p(\mathcal{X}_a)p(\mathcal{X}_b)}{P(t)p(\mathcal{X}_a, \mathcal{X}_b)}. \end{aligned} \tag{13.14}$$

As none of the variables on the left side of the conditioning bar in (13.14) are observed, we use marginal inference. We obtain $P(t|\mathcal{X}_a, \mathcal{X}_b)$ by plugging (13.13) into (13.14) and integrating out ρ_a, I_a, ρ_b and I_b:

$$P(t|\mathcal{X}_a, \mathcal{X}_b) = \frac{p(\mathcal{X}_a)p(\mathcal{X}_b)}{p(\mathcal{X}_a, \mathcal{X}_b)P(t)} \times \sum_{I_a} \int_{\rho_a} P(t|\rho_a, I_a)p(\rho_a|I_a, \mathcal{X}_a)P(I_a|\mathcal{X}_a)d\rho_a \times \sum_{I_b} \int_{\rho_b} P(t|\rho_b, I_b)p(\rho_b|I_b, \mathcal{X}_b)P(I_b|\mathcal{X}_b)d\rho_b. \quad (13.15)$$

The naïve Bayes structure of the DAG in Figure 13.2 allows us to expand $P(t|\rho_a, I_a) = \frac{P(t|\rho_a)P(t|I_a)}{P(t)}$, which equivalently holds for sensor b. The influence of feature uncertainty on the probability of the state t is most easily seen if we assume perfect knowledge of the preprocessing model:

$$P(t|\mathcal{X}_a, \mathcal{X}_b) \propto \frac{1}{P(t)} \int_{\rho_a} P(t|\rho_a)p(\rho_a|\mathcal{X}_a)d\rho_a \int_{\rho_b} P(t|\rho_b)p(\rho_b|\mathcal{X}_b)d\rho_b.$$

This expression shows that the probability $P(t|\mathcal{X}_a, \mathcal{X}_b)$ is dominated by $\mathcal{X}_a$, if ρ_a is, under its posterior, more informative about class t.[1] At a first glance we might expect that higher accuracy should dominate and this seems counter-intuitive. However, perfect knowledge does not help if the extracted feature is equally likely for different classes. Thus although known with less precision, a variable might dominate if it allows on average for better discrimination. The other extreme is that we know that $\mathcal{X}_a$ and $\mathcal{X}_b$ are white noise. In this case we get $P(I_a \equiv 0|\mathcal{X}_a) = 1$ and $P(I_b \equiv 0|\mathcal{X}_b) = 1$ and thus

$$P(t|\mathcal{X}_a, \mathcal{X}_b) \propto \frac{P(t|I_a)P(t|I_b)}{P(t)}.$$

This is a very intuitive result, as without parameters ρ_a and ρ_b the model indicators I_a and I_b are the only information about class t.

If we are interested in the *a-posteriori* distribution over one of the latent spaces, say (I_a, ρ_a), we have to apply similar manipulations. Assuming that the continuous parameter ρ_a is a point in $\mathbb{R}^M$, (I_a, ρ_a) lies in $I_a \equiv 1 \times \rho_a \in \mathbb{R}^M \bigcup I_a \equiv 0 \times \rho_a \in \mathbb{R}^0$, where the dimension of ρ_a in the second case is zero. The posterior is then

$$p(\rho_a, I_a|\mathcal{X}_a, \mathcal{X}_b) = \frac{p(\mathcal{X}_a)p(\mathcal{X}_b)}{p(\mathcal{X}_a, \mathcal{X}_b)} \times \sum_t \left[\frac{P(t|\rho_a, I_a)p(\rho_a|I_a, \mathcal{X}_a)P(I_a|\mathcal{X}_a)}{P(t)} \times \sum_{I_b} \int_{\rho_a} P(t|\rho_b, I_b)p(\rho_b|I_b, \mathcal{X}_b)P(I_b|\mathcal{X}_b)d\rho_b \right]. \quad (13.16)$$

[1] The same argument holds for the other sensor $\mathcal{X}_b$.

By exchanging marginalisation over (I_b, ρ_b) with marginalisation over (I_a, ρ_a), we obtain the corresponding *a-posteriori* density over the feature space (I_b, ρ_b) .

We should now point out that we did not follow an exact Bayesian scheme, since this requires us to use all available information. The derivations presented so far deviate slightly, since the probabilistic dependency between t and the latent variables ρ_a and ρ_b allows, via the conditional distributions $p(\rho_a|t)$ and $p(\rho_b|t)$, for information flow between the two sensors. Hence irrespective of whether we know t or not, we will have information about ρ_a and ρ_b that goes beyond the "stability prior" adopted in the last section. However, the problem is that using this information, we can not derive any expressions analytically as was done there. Instead we have to resort to MCMC techniques for the entire analysis including preprocessing [11]. Even with modern computers, this is still a very time consuming procedure. A qualitative argument shows that this approximation will in practical situations not effect the results dramatically. The usual settings in preprocessing will lead to *a-posteriori* densities over coefficients that, compared with the priors, are sharply peaked around the most probable value.[2] In this case using either a uniform prior in the range $[-1, 1]$, or the more informative prior provided via t does not make a big difference.

As a last step it remains to provide an abstract formulation of an inference procedure of model coefficients for the DAG shown in Figure 13.2. In order to make life easier, we assume for now that we are given only labelled samples. A generalisation to include also unlabelled samples is provided in the next section. Assuming to know the *true* values of features and states, conventional model inference would condition on training data, $\mathcal{A} = \{\rho_{a,i} \forall i\}$, $\mathcal{B} = \{\rho_{b,i} \forall i\}$ and $\mathcal{T} = \{t_i \forall i\}$. Denoting all model coefficients jointly by $\boldsymbol{w}$, inference would lead to $p(\boldsymbol{w}|\mathcal{A}, \mathcal{B}, \mathcal{T})$. In our setting the $I_{a,i}$, $I_{b,i}$, $\rho_{a,i}$ and $\rho_{b,i}$ are latent variables and we can not condition on them. Instead we would like to condition on the corresponding $\mathcal{X}_{a,i}$ and $\mathcal{X}_{b,i}$. Such conditioning can not be done directly. Assuming independence of observations, the DAG in Figure 13.2 implies the likelihood to be

$$\begin{aligned} p(\mathcal{T}, \mathcal{A}, I_A, \mathcal{X}_A, \mathcal{B}, I_B, \mathcal{X}_B|\boldsymbol{w}) &= \\ &= \prod_i p(t_i, \rho_{a,i}, I_{a,i}, \mathcal{X}_{a,i}, \rho_{b,i}, I_{b,i}\mathcal{X}_{b,i}|\boldsymbol{w}) \\ &= \prod_i \left[\frac{P(t_i|\rho_{a,i}, I_{a,i}, \boldsymbol{w})P(t_i|\rho_{b,i}, I_{b,i}, \boldsymbol{w})}{P(t_i|\boldsymbol{w})} \right. \\ &\quad \left. \times p(\rho_{a,i}|I_{a,i}, \mathcal{X}_{a,i})p(I_{a,i}|\mathcal{X}_{a,i})p(\rho_{b,i}|I_{b,i}, \mathcal{X}_{b,i})p(I_{b,i}|\mathcal{X}_{b,i}) \right], \end{aligned} \tag{13.17}$$

[2] As can be seen from Equation (13.6), this is just a matter of the number of samples used to estimate the feature values.

where we use $I_A = \{I_{a,i} \forall i\}$, $\mathcal{X}_A = \{\mathcal{X}_{a,i} \forall i\}$, $I_B = \{I_{b,i} \forall i\}$ and $\mathcal{X}_B = \{\mathcal{X}_{b,i} \forall i\}$ and make the dependency on model parameters $\boldsymbol{w}$ explicit. We finally get the posterior over model coefficients $\boldsymbol{w}$ by multiplication with a prior $p(\boldsymbol{w})$ and marginalising out all $\rho_{a,i}$, $I_{a,i}$, $\rho_{b,i}$ and $I_{b,i}$.

$$
\begin{aligned}
p(\boldsymbol{w}|\mathcal{T}, \mathcal{X}_A, \mathcal{X}_B) \propto p(\boldsymbol{w}) \prod_i \Bigg[& \frac{1}{P(t_i)} \\
& \times \sum_{I_{a,i}} \int_{\rho_{a,i}} P(t_i|\rho_{a,i}, I_{a,i}, \boldsymbol{w}) P(I_{a,i}|\mathcal{X}_{a,i}) p(\rho_{a,i}|I_{a,i}, \mathcal{X}_{a,i}) d\rho_{a,i} \\
& \times \sum_{I_{b,i}} \int_{\rho_{b,i}} P(t_i|\rho_{b,i}, I_{b,i}, \boldsymbol{w}) P(I_{b,i}|\mathcal{X}_{b,i}) p(\rho_{b,i}|I_{b,i}, \mathcal{X}_{b,i}) d\rho_{b,i} \Bigg]
\end{aligned}
\quad (13.18)
$$

Expression (13.18) is just proportional to the posterior since we still need to normalize. In general neither the integrals nor the normalisation constants in (13.15), (13.16) or (13.18) will be analytically tractable. In all practical problems we will have to apply MCMC methods.

The model in this section illustrates that marginalising out variables and model uncertainty leads to predictions that are dominated by information that allows for reliable discrimination. However the DAG is not optimally suited for classification of biomedical time series. As our interest is classification of adjacent segments of a time series, we can improve on the DAG in Figure 13.2 by allowing for additional temporal dependencies. In the following section we propose a model which allows for a first order Markov dependency among additional discrete latent variables, d_i, and thus for information flow across time. We propose Bayesian inference by sampling from the joint probability density over latent variables and model coefficients.

13.4 Spatio-temporal Fusion

A DAG structure that allows spatio-temporal sensor fusion is obtained by imposing a conditional dependency among adjacent state variables and to spatially different sensors. Sensor fusion is then achieved very naturally by treating this DAG within the Bayesian framework. Bayesian preprocessing will assess both model and coefficient uncertainties. Marginalising out these uncertainties will lead to beliefs about states that are less affected by less reliable information. Such an approach can go even further: it allows one to infer the expected feature values which for unreliable segments will differ from the values obtained from preprocessing alone. This requires that the architecture contains a generative model. Thus, as a by-product, we will be able to use labelled as well as unlabelled data during model inference.

13.4.1 A Simple DAG Structure

This subsection proposes a DAG structure that allows spatio-temporal sensor fusion. Measured in terms of model complexity (number of free parameters), we aim at a simple solution. Assuming that we want to solve a classification task, we regard the class labels as the state of interest. In order to exploit temporal correlations among successive classifications we propose a model that has the latent indicator variables d_i and the class labels t_i connected to form a first order Markov chain. The idea behind linking the class labels t_i is that in cases where one of the state values of d_i corresponds to a high uncertainty state (i.e. with similar probabilities $P(t_i|d_i)$ for all t_i) this gives us additional information about the class label. Furthermore, we assume conditional independence between all latent variables depending on each state variable. Figure 13.3 shows a DAG structure imposed by these assumptions. Training data consists of labelled as well as unlabelled segments of a time series. Unobserved states are represented by circles and the observed states by squares. We have already decided about the latent variables $\rho_{i,j}$ and indicator

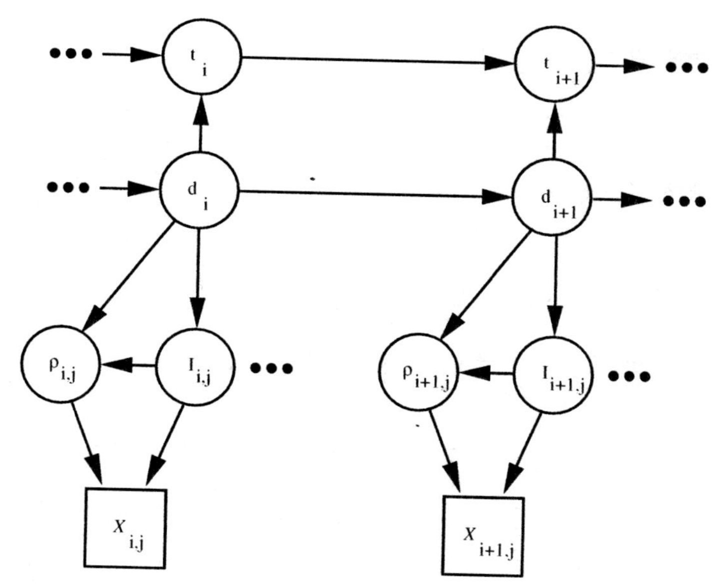

Fig. 13.3. A directed acyclic graph for spatio-temporal sensor fusion: the DAG assumes a first order Markov dependency among states d_i and conditional on these, independence of the latent variables $\rho_{i,j}$. We used t_i to denote the unknown state variables of interest (i.e. the class labels of the segments under consideration), which are linked with a second Markov chain. The idea behind this second chain is that it allows us to resolve ambiguity which might be caused by a high uncertainty state. Both $\rho_{i,j}$ and $I_{i,j}$ are latent variables, representing feature and model uncertainty from preprocessing. Finally $\mathcal{X}_{i,j}$ denote the corresponding segments of a time series.

variables $I_{i,j}$: they are stages in an AR-lattice filter and $\mathcal{X}_{i,j}$ are the corresponding segments of a time series. It remains to decide about the generative model between the state variables d_i and the latent variables $\rho_{i,j}$ and $I_{i,j}$. In our case the $\rho_{i,j}$ are continuous variables and the generative model will be implemented as diagonal Gaussian distributions,

$$p(\rho_{i,j}|d_i) = \mathcal{N}(\rho_{i,j}|\boldsymbol{\mu}_{j,d}, \boldsymbol{\lambda}_{j,d}), \tag{13.19}$$

with mean $\boldsymbol{\mu}_{j,d}$ and precision $\boldsymbol{\lambda}_{j,d}$. The model indicator $I_{i,j}$ is given a multinomial-1 distribution

$$p(I_{i,j}|d_i) = \mathcal{M}n(I_{i,j}|\boldsymbol{\Pi}_{j,d}), \tag{13.20}$$

where $\boldsymbol{\Pi}_{j,d}$ are the binary probabilities observing either one of the two preprocessing models given state d_i. Model inference will be based on a Markov chain Monte Carlo (MCMC) method. We thus need to consider the likelihood function, design a DAG that shows the relations during inference, specify convenient priors and, as a final step, formulate the MCMC updates.

13.4.2 A Likelihood Function for Sequence Models

As already mentioned, we are interested in a fully Bayesian treatment of the model. This can be done as soon as we are able to formulate a normalized likelihood function and priors. We are dealing with a sequence model, where the likelihood is usually (see [13], pp. 150) formulated via paths that are possible sequences of latent states:

$$\begin{aligned} P(\mathcal{D}, \Pi_d, \Pi_t|\boldsymbol{w}) = {} & P(d_1) \prod_j p(\rho_{1,j}, I_{1,j}|d_1) P(t_1|d_1) \\ & \times \prod_{i=2}^{N} \left(P(d_i|d_{i-1}) P(t_i|d_i, t_{i-1}) \prod_j p(\rho_{i,j}, I_{i,j}|t_i) \right). \end{aligned} \tag{13.21}$$

In (13.21) we used $\mathcal{D}$ to denote a realisation of all latent variables $\rho_{i,j}$ and model indicators $I_{i,j}$. A sequence of latent variables d_i is denoted as Π_d and a sequence of labels is denoted by Π_t. Note that for the second sequence not all paths are possible since we have to visit all given labels. We thus obtain the likelihood

$$P(\mathcal{D}, \mathcal{T}|\boldsymbol{w}) = \sum_{\Pi_d, \Pi_t} P(\mathcal{D}, \Pi_d, \Pi_t|\boldsymbol{w}), \tag{13.22}$$

where $\mathcal{T}$ denotes the observed class labels. If several independent sequences are used to infer model coefficients, the overall likelihood is the product of several expressions like (13.22). In order to obtain a final expression of the likelihood of model coefficients we have to plug Equations (13.19) and (13.20) into Equation (13.22). It is evident that the resulting likelihood is highly nonlinear and parameter inference had to be done by carrying out Metropolis–Hastings updates. The conventional way to maximize such likelihood functions is to apply the expectation maximisation (EM) algorithm [14] which was introduced for HMMs in [15]. The sampling algorithm proposed in the next subsection uses similar ideas. We use both Gibbs updates and Metropolis–Hastings updates to draw samples from the *a-posteriori* distribution over model coefficients and latent variables.

13.4.3 An Augmented DAG for MCMC Sampling

The likelihood function associated with the probabilistic model in Figure 13.3 is highly non-linear in the model coefficients and we have to use MCMC methods to infer them. As already indicated, we want to use Gibbs updates wherever possible. Only such variables that do not allow Gibbs moves will be updated with Metropolis–Hastings steps. Following the ideas of the EM procedure, we introduce latent indicator variables, d_i, which indicate the kernel number of the Gaussian prior over the latent variables $\rho_{i,j}$.

Figure 13.4 shows a DAG that results from the DAG in Figure 13.3 when augmented with all coefficients of the probabilistic model and the hyper-parameters of the corresponding priors. In order to keep the graph simple, Figure 13.4 displays only those variables that we need to derive the MCMC updates for inference. In particular we illustrate only one observation model. Other sensors are indicated by dots.

The state variable d_i is conditionally dependent on its predecessor and on the transition probability $\boldsymbol{T}$. Class labels, t_i, depend on the state variable and on the preceding label t_{i-1}. The state conditional transition probabilities are summarized by $\boldsymbol{W}$. For both the transition probabilities, $\boldsymbol{T} = P(d_i|d_{i-1})\ \forall\ d_i, d_{i-1}$, and prior allocation probabilities, $\boldsymbol{W} = P(t_i|d_i, t_{i-1})$ $\forall\ d_i, t_i, t_{i-1}$, we use a Dirichlet prior. Conditional on the latent state d_i, we have the observation model for the latent variables $\rho_{i,j}$ and the corresponding model indicator $I_{i,j}$. The observation model for $I_{i,j}$ is a multinomial-one distribution with observation probabilities $\boldsymbol{\Pi}_j = P(I_{i,j}|d_i)\ \forall\ I_{i,j}, d_i$. These probabilities are given a Dirichlet prior using δ_{Π} as prior counts. Except that we do not infer the number of kernels, the model for $\rho_{i,j}$ is largely identical to the model used by [16] for their one-dimensional mixture of Gaussians analysis with varying number of kernels. The means μ_j are given a normal prior with mean ξ_j and precision κ_j. Each component has its own precision (inverse variance) λ_j. In order to avoid problems with singular solutions the variances are coupled with hyper-parameters α and β_j. The latter, β_j, has itself a Gamma prior. This hierarchical prior specification allows for informative priors without introducing large dependencies on the values of the hyper-parameters. The difference between our observation model and the one used in [16] is that $\rho_{i,j}$ are latent variables, with the time series $\mathcal{X}_{i,j}$ being conditionally dependent on $\rho_{i,j}$ and $I_{i,j}$.

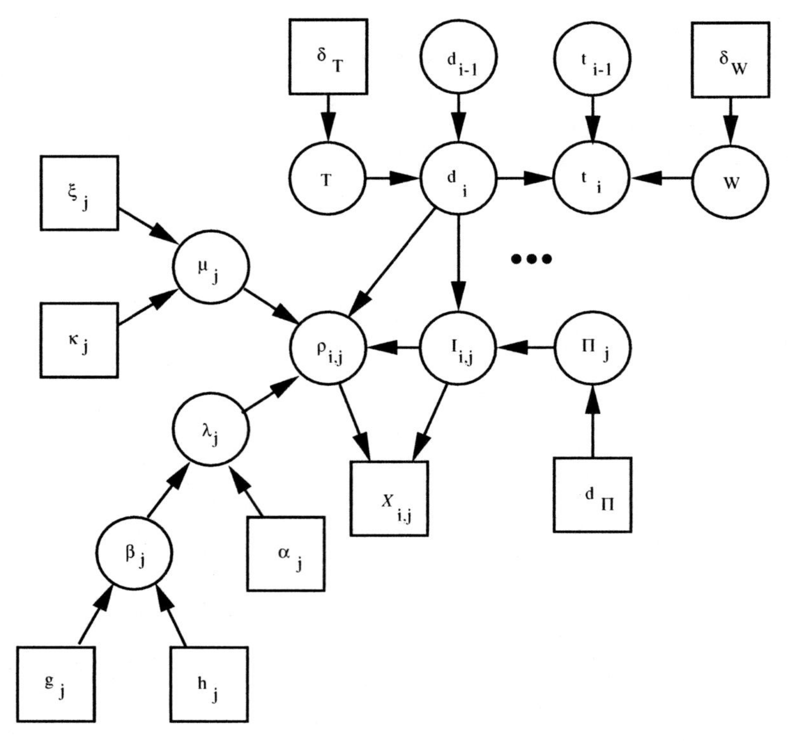

Fig. 13.4. A DAG for parameter inference. In order to keep it simple, the DAG shows only one of the observation models for $\rho_{i,j}$, $I_{i,j}$ one pair of latent variables d_{i-1}, d_i, and one pair of class labels, t_{i-1}, t_i. We use three dots to indicate that there could be more sensors. The DAG shows transition probabilities for the states, $\boldsymbol{T} = P(d_i|d_{i-1}) \; \forall \; d_i, d_{i-1}$ and for the class labels $\boldsymbol{W} = P(t_i|d_i, t_{i-1}) \; \forall \; d_i, t_i, t_{i-1}$. The multinomial observation model for the model indicator is specified by $\boldsymbol{\Pi}_j = P(I_{i,j}|d_i) \; \forall \; I_{i,j}, d_i$. Finally we have a hierarchical model for specifying the observation model for the lattice filter coefficients specified by $\boldsymbol{\mu}_j$ and $\boldsymbol{\lambda}_j$. As before, square nodes denote observed quantities and circles are latent variables. However there is an exception since during model inference some of the t_i are observed.

13.4.4 Specifying Priors

In order to be able to derive an MCMC scheme to sample from the *a-posteriori* distributions of model coefficients and latent variables, we need to specify the functional form as well as the parameters of all priors from the DAG in Figure 13.4. Gibbs sampling requires full conditional distributions from which we can draw efficiently. The full conditional distributions are the distributions of model coefficients when conditioning on all other model coefficients, latent variables and data. Apart from the EM-like idea to introduce latent variables, tractable distributions will be obtained by using so-called conjugate priors, as discussed in [17].

In order to allow Gibbs updates for most of the parameters, we use the following prior specification:

- Each component mean, $\mu_{j,d}$, is given a Gaussian prior: $\mu_{j,d} \sim \mathcal{N}_1(\xi_j, \kappa_j^{-1})$.
- The precision is given a Gamma prior: $\lambda_{j,d} \sim \Gamma(\alpha, \beta_j)$.
- The hyper-parameter, β_j, gets a Gamma hyper-prior: $\beta_j \sim \Gamma(g, h)$.
- The transition probabilities for the latent kernel indicators, $\boldsymbol{T}_d$, get a Dirichlet prior: $\boldsymbol{T}_d \sim \mathcal{D}(\delta_T^1, \ldots, \delta_T^D)$, with D denoting the number of kernels.
- The transition probabilities for the class labels, $\boldsymbol{W}_{k,d}$, get a Dirichlet prior: $\boldsymbol{W}_{k,d} \sim \mathcal{D}(\delta_W^1, \ldots, \delta_W^K)$, with K denoting the number of class labels.
- The observation probabilities of the model indicators, $\boldsymbol{\Pi}_d$ get a Dirichlet prior: $\boldsymbol{\Pi}_d \sim \mathcal{D}(\delta_\Pi^1, \ldots, \delta_\Pi^D)$, with D denoting the number of kernels.

The quantitative settings are similar to those used in [16]: values for α are between 1 and 2, g is usually between 0.2 and 1 and h is typically between $1/R_{max}^2$ and $10/R_{max}^2$, with R_{max} denoting the largest input range. The mean, μ_j, gets a Gaussian prior centred at the midpoint, ξ_j, with inverse variance $\kappa_j = 1/R_j^2$, where R_j is the range of the j-th input. The multinomial priors of the prior allocation counts and the prior transition counts are set up with equal probabilities for all counters. We set all prior counts, i.e. for δ_T, δ_W and δ_Π to 1, which gives the most uninformative proper prior.

13.4.5 MCMC Updates of Coefficients and Latent Variables

The prior specification proposed in the last subsection enables us to use mainly Gibbs updates. The latent variables $\rho_{i,j}$ however need to be sampled via more general Metropolis–Hastings updates. The main difficulty is that we regard "input" variables as being latent. In other words: conventional approaches condition on the $\rho_{i,j}$, whereas our approach regards them as random variables which have to be updated as well.

We will first summarise the Gibbs updates for the model coefficients. The expressions condition on hyperparameters, other model coefficients, hidden states, class labels and the latent representation of preprocessing (i.e. $\rho_{i,j}$ and $I_{i,j}$). During model inference we need to update all unobserved variables of the DAG, whereas for predictions we update only the variables shown in the DAG in Figure 13.3. The updates for the model coefficients are done using full conditional distributions, which have the same functional forms as the corresponding priors. These full conditionals follow previous publications [11], with some modifications required by the additional Markov dependency between successive class labels.

Update of the transition probabilities, $\boldsymbol{T}$

The full conditional of the transition probabilities $\boldsymbol{T}_{d_i}[d_{i+1}] = P(d_{i+1}|d_i)$ is a Dirichlet distribution. The expression depends on the prior counts, δ_T, and on all hidden states, d_i.

$$\boldsymbol{T}_d \sim \mathcal{D}(\delta_T + n^d_{d,1}, \ldots, \delta_T + n^d_{d,D}), \quad (13.23)$$

with $n^d_{d,1}, \ldots, n^d_{d,D}$ denoting the number of transitions from state $d_i = d$ to $d_{i+1} = \{1, \ldots, D\}$. The prior probability of the hidden states $\boldsymbol{P}_T$ is the normalised eigenvector of $\boldsymbol{T}$ that corresponds to the eigenvalue 1.

Update of the transition probabilities for class labels, $\boldsymbol{W}$

The full conditional of the transition probabilities, $\boldsymbol{W}_{d_i,t_{i-1}}[t_i] = P(t_i|d_i, t_{i-1})$ is a Dirichlet distribution. These transition probabilities are conditional on both the previous class label and the current state. We thus obtain the posterior counts, $n^\tau_{d,t}$, by counting transitions from class label τ to class label t, given the current latent state is d. The transition probability is a Dirichlet distribution.

$$\boldsymbol{W}^\tau_d \sim \mathcal{D}(\delta_W + n^\tau_{d,1}, \ldots, \delta_T + n^\tau_{d,K}). \quad (13.24)$$

Conditional on d, the prior probability of the class labels $\boldsymbol{P}_{W,d}$ is the normalised eigenvector of $\boldsymbol{W}_d$ that corresponds to the eigenvalue 1.

Update of the observation probability of model orders, $\boldsymbol{\Pi}_j$

The full conditional of the observation probabilities of model order $\Pi_j[d_i, I_{i,j}] = P(I_{i,j}|d_i, j)$ is a Dirichlet distribution. The expression depends on the prior counts, δ_Π, on the model indicators $I_{i,j}$ and on the state d_i. Each sensor j has its own set of probabilities $\boldsymbol{P}_j$.

$$\boldsymbol{\Pi}_{j,d} \sim \mathcal{D}(\delta_P + n^{I_j}_{d,0}, \ldots, \delta_P + n^{I_j}_{d,I_{\max}}), \quad (13.25)$$

where $n^{I_j}_{d,I}$ denotes the number of cases in which $I_{i,j} \equiv I$ and $d_i \equiv d$.

Updating the Gaussian observation model

We use a separate Gaussian observation model for the latent features $\boldsymbol{\rho}_{i,j}$ of each sensor j. Each observation model needs three updates.

The full conditional of the kernel mean, $\boldsymbol{\mu}_j$, is a Normal distribution. The expression depends on the hyperparameters κ_j and ξ_j, on the hidden states d_i, on the model indicators $I_{i,j}$, on the covariance matrix $\boldsymbol{\lambda}_j$ and on the latent coefficients $\boldsymbol{\rho}_{i,j}$.

$$\boldsymbol{\mu}_{j,d}[k] \sim \mathcal{N}(\hat{\mu}_{j,d}[k], \sigma^\mu_{j,d}[k]) \quad (13.26)$$

with

$$\hat{\mu}_{j,d}[k] = (n^\mu_{j,d}[k]\boldsymbol{\lambda}_{j,d}[k,k] + \boldsymbol{\beta}_j[k])^{-1}(n^\mu_{j,d}[k]\boldsymbol{\lambda}_{j,d}[k,k]\bar{\boldsymbol{\rho}}_{d,j}[k] + \kappa_j[k]\xi_j[k])$$
$$\sigma^\mu_{j,d}[k] = (n^\mu_{j,d}[k]\boldsymbol{\lambda}_{j,d}[k,k] + \boldsymbol{\beta}_j[k])^{-1},$$

where we use index k to denote the k-th dimension of the latent vector $\boldsymbol{\rho}_{i,j}$. The dependency of Equation (??) on $I_{i,j}$ is implicit in

$$n^{\mu}_{j,d}[k] = \sum_{i|I_{i,j}\equiv 1} \delta(d_i \equiv d)$$

and in

$$\bar{\boldsymbol{\rho}}_{d,j}[k] = \frac{1}{n^{\mu}_{j,d}[k]} \sum_{i|I_{i,j}\equiv 1} \delta(d_i \equiv d)\boldsymbol{\rho}_{i,j}[k].$$

The full conditional of the kernel covariance, $\boldsymbol{\lambda}_{j,d}[k]$, is a Gamma distribution. The expression depends on the hyperparameter α_j and $\boldsymbol{\beta}_j$, on the hidden states, d_i, on the corresponding kernel mean $\boldsymbol{\mu}_{j,d}[k]$ and on the model indicators $I_{i,j}$.

$$\boldsymbol{\lambda}_{j,d}[k] \sim \Gamma(\hat{\alpha}, \hat{\beta}) \tag{13.27}$$

with

$$\hat{\alpha} = \alpha_j + \frac{n^{\mu}_{j,d}[k]}{2}$$
$$\hat{\beta} = \boldsymbol{\beta}_j[k] + \frac{1}{2} \sum_{i|I_{i,j}\equiv 1} \delta(d_i \equiv d)(\boldsymbol{\rho}_{i,j}[k] - \boldsymbol{\mu}_{j,d}[k])^2$$

The full conditional of the hyperparameter $\boldsymbol{\beta}_j$ depends on the hyper-hyper-parameters g_j and $\boldsymbol{h}_j$, on α_j and on $\boldsymbol{\lambda}_{j,d}$.

$$w\boldsymbol{\beta}_j[k] \sim \Gamma(g_j + D\alpha_j, \boldsymbol{h}_j[k] + \sum_d \boldsymbol{\lambda}_{j,d}[k]) \tag{13.28}$$

13.4.6 Gibbs Updates for Hidden States and Class Labels

Updating d_i

The full conditionals for d_i are multinomial-one distributions. The first state has no preceding state d_0. We thus use the unconditional prior probability of the state, $P_T(d_1)$ instead of $T_{d_0}[d_1]$.

$$d_i \sim \mathcal{M}n(1, \{P(d_i|\ldots)\ \forall\ d_i = 1\ldots D\}) \tag{13.29}$$

with

$$P(d_1|\ldots) = \frac{P_T[d_1]T_{d_1}[d_2]P_{W,d_1}[t_1]\prod_j p(\boldsymbol{\rho}_{1,j}, I_{1,j}|d_1)}{\sum_{d_1} P_T[d_1]T_{d_1}[d_2]P_{W,d_1}[t_1]\prod_j p(\boldsymbol{\rho}_{1,j}, I_{1,j}|d_1)}$$
$$P(d_{i\neq 1}|\ldots) = \frac{T_{d_{i-1}}[d_i]T_{d_i}[d_{i+1}]W_{d_i,t_{i-1}}[t_i]\prod_j p(\boldsymbol{\rho}_{i,j}, I_{i,j}|d_i)}{\sum_{d_i} T_{d_{i-1}}[d_i]T_{d_i}[d_{i+1}]W_{d_i,t_{i-1}}[t_i]\prod_j p(\boldsymbol{\rho}_{i,j}, I_{i,j}|d_i)}$$

For the last state of the Markov chain, the successor d_{i+1} does not exist and the expression of the probability, $P(d_{i\neq 1}|\ldots)$, does not include the term $T_{d_i}[d_{i+1}]$.

Updating t_i

Unknown class labels, t_i, are updated by multinomial-one distributions.

$$T_i \sim \mathcal{M}n(1, \{P(t_i|\ldots) \; \forall \; t_i = 1..K\}) \tag{13.30}$$

with

$$\begin{aligned} P(t_1|\ldots) &= \frac{P_{W,d_1}[t_1]W_{d_2,t_1}[t_2]}{\sum_{t_1} P_{W,d_1}[t_1]W_{d_2,t_1}[t_2]} \\ P(t_i \neq 1|\ldots) &= \frac{W_{d_i,t_{i-1}}[t_i]W_{d_{i+1},t_i}[t_{i+1}]}{\sum_{t_i} W_{d_i,t_{i-1}}[t_i]W_{d_{i+1},t_i}[t_{i+1}]} \end{aligned}$$

Since class label t_{i+1} does not exist for the last segment, we have to remove the term $W_{d_{i+1},t_i}[t_{i+1}]$ when expressing the corresponding probability $P(t_i|\ldots)$.

13.4.7 Approximate Updates of the Latent Feature Space

We finally have to formulate updates for the latent feature space, i.e. for the variables $\boldsymbol{\rho}_{i,j}$ and $I_{i,j}$. These updates involve the posteriors formulated in Equations (13.10) and (13.12) and are drawn from the "joint conditional" distribution $p(I_{i,j}, \boldsymbol{\rho}_{i,j}|\ldots) \propto p(I_{i,j}, \boldsymbol{\rho}_{i,j}|\mathcal{X}_{i,j})p(d_i|I_{i,j}, \boldsymbol{\rho}_{i,j})$. We draw from $p(I_{i,j}, \boldsymbol{\rho}_{i,j}|\ldots)$ by first proposing from $(I'_{i,j}, \boldsymbol{\rho}'_{i,j}) \sim p(I_{i,j}, \boldsymbol{\rho}_{i,j}|\mathcal{X}_{i,j})$ and then accepting $(I'_{i,j}, \boldsymbol{\rho}'_{i,j})$ by a Metropolis–Hastings acceptance probability. We draw model indicator $I'_{i,j}$ from $p(I_{i,j}|\mathcal{X}_{i,j})$ which is a multinomial-one distribution.

$$I'_{i,j} \sim \mathcal{M}n(1, \{P(I_{i,j}|\mathcal{X}_{i,j})), \tag{13.31}$$

with $P(I_{i,j}|\mathcal{X}_{i,j})$ defined in Equation (13.10). Using the indicator variable we then propose $\boldsymbol{\rho}'_{i,j}$.

$$\boldsymbol{\rho}'_{i,j} \sim \begin{cases} \forall I'_{i,j} \equiv 1 : \boldsymbol{\rho}'_{i,j} \sim p(\boldsymbol{\rho}_{i,j}|\mathcal{X}_{i,j}) \\ \forall I'_{i,j} \equiv 0 : \boldsymbol{\rho}'_{i,j} = [\,], \end{cases} \tag{13.32}$$

where $p(\boldsymbol{\rho}_{i,j}|\mathcal{X}_{i,j})$ is a product of the distributions in Equation (13.12) and the second case denotes the white noise case, in which the latent parameter $\boldsymbol{\rho}'_{i,j}$ has dimension zero. In order to get a sample from the full conditional distribution, we have to calculate the acceptance probability

$$P_a = \min\left(1, \frac{P(d_i|\boldsymbol{\rho}'_{i,j}, I'_{i,j})}{P(d_i|\boldsymbol{\rho}_{i,j}, I_{i,j})}\right) notag \tag{13.33}$$

where

$$P(d_i|\boldsymbol{\rho}'_{i,j}, I'_{i,j}) = \begin{cases} \forall I'_{i,j} \equiv 1 : \frac{p(\boldsymbol{\rho}'_{i,j}|\boldsymbol{\mu}_{j,d_i}, \boldsymbol{\lambda}_{j,d_i})\Pi_{d_i,j}[I'_{i,j}]}{\sum_{d_i} p(\boldsymbol{\rho}'_{i,j}|\boldsymbol{\mu}_{j,d_i}, \boldsymbol{\lambda}_{j,d_i})\Pi_{d_i,j}[I'_{i,j}]} \\ \forall I'_{i,j} \equiv 0 : \frac{\Pi_{d_i,j}[I'_{i,j}]}{\sum_{d_i} \Pi_{d_i,j}[I'_{i,j}]} \end{cases}$$

and accept the new values of the latent features $(I'_{i,j}, \boldsymbol{\rho}'_{i,j})$ according to this probability. We would like to point out that this scheme is an approximation to the exact updates of the latent space since the proposal distributions in Equations (13.10) and (13.12) do not consider the correct prior which would be the mixture distribution $P(d_i)p(\boldsymbol{\rho}_{i,j}|d_i)p(I_{i,j}|d_i)$. Instead we use the priors specified in Section 13.2. However, we argue that the difference is not large if the number of samples is sufficient since in this case the likelihood by far outweighs the prior.

13.4.8 Algorithms

Model inference

Algorithm 1 *Pseudo-code for sweeps during model inference.*

$\forall\, d$	initialise$(\boldsymbol{W}_d, \boldsymbol{T}_d)$	
$\forall\, j$	initialise$(\boldsymbol{\beta}_j)$	
$\forall\, j, d$	initialise$(\boldsymbol{\mu}_{j,d}, \boldsymbol{\lambda}_{j,d}, \boldsymbol{\Pi}_{j,d})$	
$\forall\, i$	initialise(d_i, t_i)	% only missing t_i are initialised
$\forall\, i, j$	initialise$(I_{i,j}, \boldsymbol{\rho}_{i,j})$	

sweepcounter=0

REPEAT

$\forall\, d$	update$(\boldsymbol{T}_d)$	% according to Equation (13.23)
$\forall\, d$	update$(\boldsymbol{W}_d)$	% according to Equation (13.24)
$\forall\, j, d$	update$(\boldsymbol{\Pi}_{j,d})$	% according to Equation (13.25)
$\forall\, j, d$	update$(\boldsymbol{\mu}_{j,d})$	% according to Equation (??)
$\forall\, j, d$	update$(\boldsymbol{\lambda}_{j,d})$	% according to Equation (13.27)
$\forall\, j$	update$(\boldsymbol{\beta}_j)$	% according to Equation (13.28)
$\forall\, i, j$	$(\boldsymbol{\rho}'_{i,j}, I'_{i,j}) \sim p(I_{i,j}, \boldsymbol{\rho}_{i,j}\vert\mathcal{X}_{i,j})$	% according to Eqns. (13.10) and (13.12)
	accept$(\boldsymbol{\rho}'_{i,j}, I'_{i,j})$ with P_a	% according to Equation (13.33)
$\forall\, i$	update(d_i)	% according to Equation (13.29)
$\forall\, i$	if t_i missing	
	update(t_i)	% according to Equation (13.30)

inc(sweepcounter)

sample[sweepcounter]=$\{\boldsymbol{T}_d, \boldsymbol{W}_d, \boldsymbol{\Pi}_{j,d}, \boldsymbol{\mu}_{j,d}, \boldsymbol{\lambda}_{j,d}\ \forall j, d\}$

UNTIL (sweepcounter > maxcount)

For model inference we start the MCMC scheme by drawing initial model parameters from their priors. We initialize all $(I_{i,j}, \boldsymbol{\rho}_{i,j}) \sim p(I_{i,j}, \boldsymbol{\rho}_{i,j}|\mathcal{X}_{i,j})$ with samples drawn from the posteriors in Equations (13.10) and (13.12) and all unobserved states d_i are drawn from the prior probabilities $P(d_i)$. The class labels of unlabelled segments are drawn from their prior $P(t_i|d_i)$ as well. After this initialisation we update according to the full conditionals and in the case of feature updates according to the single component Metropolis–Hastings step. Pseudo-code of these updates is shown in Algorithm 1.

Predictions

Algorithm 2 *Pseudo-code for sweeps during predictions.*

$\forall\ i$ initialise(d_i, t_i)
$\forall\ i, j$ initialise$(I_{i,j}, \boldsymbol{\varphi}_{i,j})$
sweepcounter=0
expcounter=0
REPEAT
  inc(sweepcounter)
  $\{\boldsymbol{T}_d, \boldsymbol{W}_d, \boldsymbol{\Pi}_{j,d}, \boldsymbol{\mu}_{j,d}, \boldsymbol{\lambda}_{j,d}\ \forall j, d\}$ = sample[sweepcounter]
  $\forall\ i, j$ $(\boldsymbol{\rho}'_{i,j}, I'_{i,j}) \sim p(I_{i,j}, \boldsymbol{\rho}_{i,j}|\mathcal{X}_{i,j})$ % according to Eqns. (13.10) and (13.12)
    accept$(\boldsymbol{\rho}'_{i,j}, I'_{i,j})$ with P_a % according to Equation (13.33)
  $\forall\ i$ update(d_i) % according to Equation (13.29)
  $\forall\ i$ update(t_i) % according to Equation (13.30)
  if sweepcounter > burnincounter
    $P(t_i) = P(t_i) + 1$
    expcounter = expcounter + 1
UNTIL (sweepcounter > maxcount)
$\forall\ t_i$ $P(t_i) = P(t_i)/$expcounter

In order to get consistent estimates of the beliefs of the states, predictions have to be marginalized over $\rho_{i,j}$ and $I_{i,j}$. The integrals need to be solved numerically. We use all samples drawn from the posterior in order to allow the $\rho_{i,j}$ of the test data to converge. All sample expectations are then taken after allowing for a burn-in period. Apart from beliefs about states, we can also obtain expectations from all latent variables - most interestingly from the $I_{i,j}$ and $\rho_{i,j}$.

Predictions are based on an approximation of the *a-posteriori* distribution of class labels, t_i, latent allocations, d_i and latent variables, $\rho_{i,j}$. We initialize the latent variables d_i and the class labels t_i by drawing according to the respective prior probabilities. The initial $(I'_{i,j}, \boldsymbol{\rho}'_{i,j}) \sim p(I_{i,j}, \boldsymbol{\rho}_{i,j}|\mathcal{X}_{i,j})$ are drawn from the posteriors in Equations (13.10) and (13.12). The coefficients are then updated using full conditional distributions for t_i and d_i and the single component Metropolis–Hastings step for $(I_{i,j}, \rho_{i,j})$. During each round of Algorithm 2, we use the next sample from the Markov chain obtained during parameter inference. We are interested in obtaining the probabilities of class labels t_i and expected values of the latent variables $(I_{i,j}, \rho_{i,j})$. We estimate these quantities by averaging after having allowed for a burn-in period.

Assessing convergence

Although in theory MCMC algorithms can approximate arbitrary distributions, the difficulty is that there is a random error inherent to the approach. This means that we need to estimate how many samples from the posterior we need in order to be able to approximate the desired value with sufficient accuracy. Different approaches to obtain such estimates are discussed at length in the MCMC literature (e.g. [18] and [19]). Although all suggested approaches can diagnose non-convergence, there is no way that allows to assess convergence with certainty. We thus need to treat quoted numbers with caution. Despite this difficulty, it is important to have at least a rough idea about how many samples to draw. The suggested methods follow two different strategies.

- Along the lines of [20], we can compare the samples obtained from multiple runs.
- As is suggested in [21], we can use one run and apply Markov chain theory to assess how many samples we need to discard at the beginning to get estimates that are independent of the starting value and how many samples we need to converge to a sufficiently accurate result.

Although there are cases where the second case might fail to diagnose slow convergence, [19] points out that the multiple chain approach is less efficient since we have to wait more than once until the Markov chain visits a high probability region. The model proposed in this work has definitely a very complicated structure, such that initial convergence might be slow. We thus apply the method suggested in [21] to the likelihood of the class labels we calculate from the Markov chain. We should point out that we cannot use the model coefficients directly since the mixture model is not identified and label switching might give a wrong sense of the actual mixing. Calculations suggest that we should draw around $15,000$ samples which is confirmed by observing virtually no difference in probabilities obtained from repeated runs.

13.5 Experiments

This section evaluates the proposed method on two biomedical classification problems. The first experiment classifies in segments of sleep EEG, whether sleep spindles are present or not. We use this data because it reflects a problem of very unbalanced class labels. For the second experiment we apply the proposed method to classification of cognitive states of segments of EEG recordings. In this case the cognitive experiments have been designed to obtain data with balanced class labels.

13.5.1 Data

Classification of sleep spindles

Sleep spindles are an important phenomenon in sleep EEG. This experiment uses data recorded from the standard 10–20 electrodes F4, C4 and P4 [22, 23] that were recorded against averaged ear potential. The sampling frequency used here was 102.4 Hz. This data is segmented into segments of 0.625 seconds duration such that we get 16 segments for a 10 second recording. A segment is labelled as containing a spindle if more than half of the segment shows spindle activity. This setup results in a prior probability for "spindle" to be roughly $P_{\text{spindle}} = 0.15$. We use data from two different subjects, each containing 7 minutes of sleep EEG that was marked for sleep spindles by a human expert. Figure 13.5 shows the second reflection coefficient and a 1 standard deviation error bar for 30 seconds of data calculated according to Equation (13.12). The classification experiment uses two datasets from different subjects. For every electrode we extract three reflection coefficients, including the standard deviation and the probability of the model compared against a white noise explanation. We report within subject results, evaluated on 672 data points using 6-fold cross-validation.

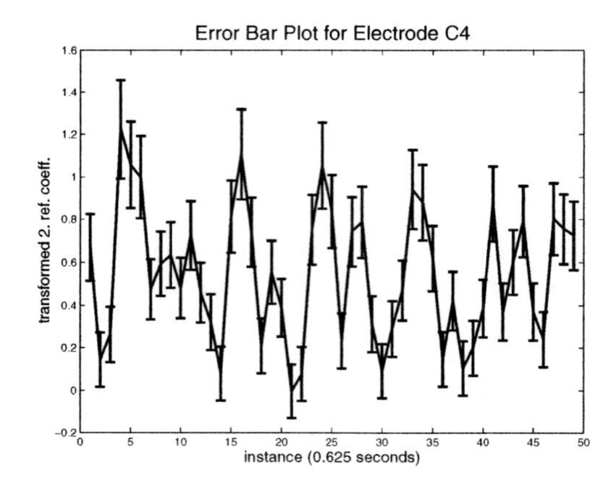

Fig. 13.5. The transformed reflection coefficient and corresponding 1 standard deviation error bar for 30 seconds of sleep EEG recorded from electrode C4. Positive peaks in the plot correspond to spindle activity.

Classification of cognitive tasks

The data used in these experiments is EEG recorded from 10 young, healthy and untrained subjects while they perform different cognitive tasks. We classify two task pairings: auditory–navigation and left motor–right motor imagination. The recordings were taken from 3 electrode sites: T4, P4 (right

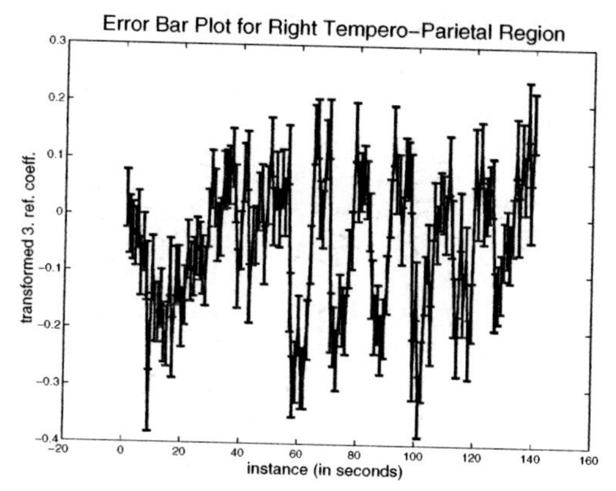

Fig. 13.6. Transformed reflection coefficient plus minus one standard deviation for 140 seconds of cognitive EEG recorded in the right tempero-parietal region from electrodes T4 and P4. The rhythmicity in the second half of the experiment corresponds to alternating cognitive states.

tempero-parietal for spatial and auditory tasks), C3' , C3" (left motor area for right motor imagination) and C4' , C4" (right motor area for left motor imagination). Note that these electrodes are 3 cm anterior and posterior to the electrode positions C3 and C4, as defined in the classical 10–20 electrode setup [22, 23]. The ground electrode was placed just lateral to the left mastoid process. The data were recorded using amplification gain of 10^4 and fourth order band pass filter with pass band between 0.1 Hz and 100 Hz. These signals were sampled with 384 Hz and 12-bit resolution. Each cognitive experiment was performed 10 times for 7 seconds. Figure 13.6 shows the second reflection coefficient and a 1 standard deviation error bar for 140 seconds of data from the right tempero-parietal region calculated according to Equation (13.12). We extract for both electrodes three reflection coefficients, the standard deviation and the probability of the model compared against a white noise explanation. We report within subject results, evaluated on 140 data points using 5-fold cross-validation.

13.5.2 Classification Results

The classification results reported in this section have been obtained by drawing $15,000$ samples from the posterior distribution of the class labels t_i in the test data. This allows us to estimate the posterior probability over class labels and hence predict the Bayes optimal class label. Figure 13.7 shows the posterior probabilities for spindle events for the data used above to illustrate preprocessing results. Figure 13.8 shows the probability for cognitive state "auditory" for the data used above to illustrate the preprocessing result. To quantify the results, we obtain independent predictions for all data and cal-

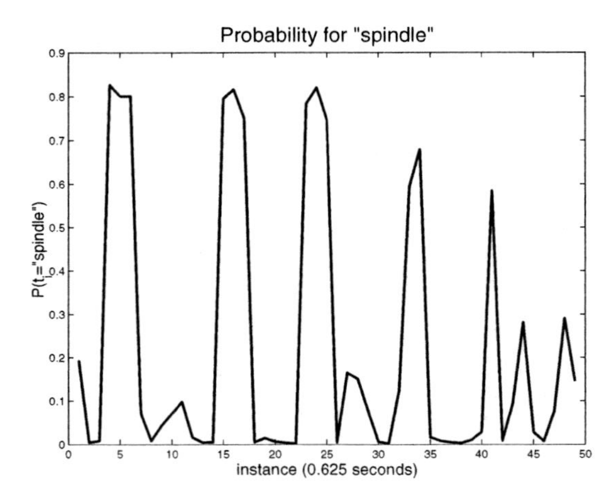

Fig. 13.7. Probabilities of "spindle" for the parameters shown in Figure 13.5.

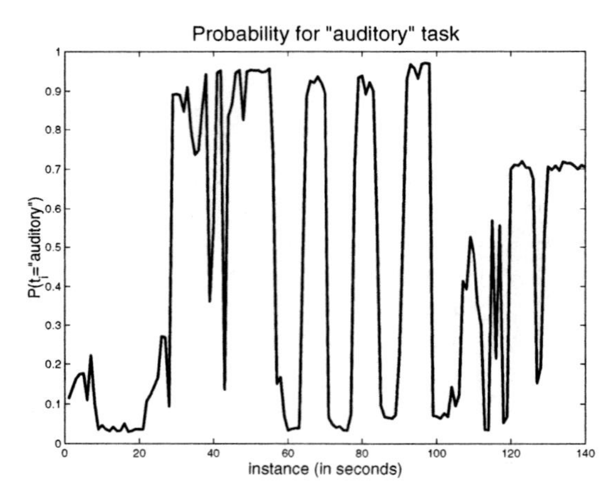

Fig. 13.8. Probability for cognitive state "auditory" for the parameters shown in Figure 13.6.

culate the expected generalisation accuracies. For the cognitive experiments this is an average across 10 subjects. The predictions are done on a one second basis to get a situation similar to reality in brain–computer interface experiments, where predictions have to be done in real time. The results on spindle classification are averaged over two subjects. The overall generalisation accuracies are shown in Table 13.1. We can also obtain a more general picture by looking at the receiver operator characteristics (ROC) curves shown in Figure 13.9.

Table 13.1. Generalisation accuracies for sleep spindle data and two cognitive experiments.

Data	Accuracy
Spindle	93%
left/right	66%
aud./navig.	80%

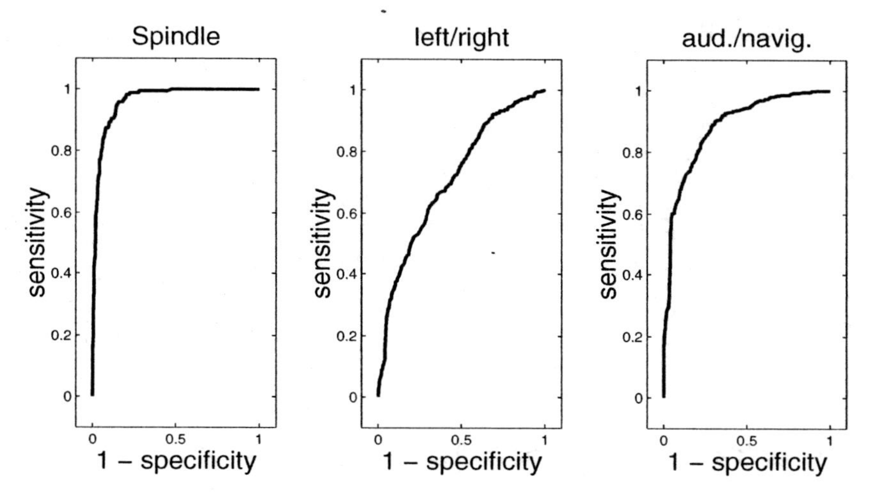

Fig. 13.9. Receiver operator characteristics (ROC) curve for the three different problems used in this chapter. Plot "spindle" shows the ROC curve for classification of sleep spindles. Plot "left/right" shows the ROC curve for classifying left/right movement imagination. The last plot, "aud./navig." shows the ROC curve when classifying the auditory versus navigation task.

13.6 Conclusion

Applications of machine learning to biomedical problems often separate feature extraction from modelling the quantity of interest. In a probabilistic sense this must be regarded as an approximation to the exact approach, which should model the quantities of interest as *one* joint distribution similar to the DAG in Figure 13.1. To further illustrate this idea, we consider the problem of time series classification which is often found in medical monitoring and diagnosis applications. By time-series classification, we mean the problem of classifying subsequent segments of time-series data. Examples of that kind are: sleep staging which is usually based on recordings of brain activity (EEG), muscle activity (EMG) and eye movements (EOG); scoring of vigilance, which is again based on EEG; or classifying heart diseases from ECG. The examples used in this chapter to illustrate the proposed approach are classifying of sleep spindles and classifying cognitive activity. The latter is used as part of a brain–computer interface. The spatio-temporal nature of these problems is very likely to introduce both spatial and temporal correlations. We thus propose a probabilistic model with dependencies across space and time. For model inference and to obtain probabilities of class labels, we have to solve marginalisation integrals. In this chapter this is done by Markov chain Monte Carlo methods. Algorithms 1 and 2 are approximations of [11], where we use exact inference and allow for different model orders of the latent feature space. The advantage of the approximation proposed here is a significantly reduced computational cost without losing much accuracy.

Acknowledgments

P. Sykacek is currently funded by the BUPA foundation (Grant No. F46/399). We want to thank our colleagues Prof. Stokes and Dr. Curran, for providing the cognitive data and Prof. Rappelsberger and Dr. Trenker for providing the sleep spindles.

References

[1] G. E. P. Box and G. M. Jenkins. *Time Series Analysis, Forecasting and Control.* Holden-Day, Oakland, CA, 1976.
[2] G. L. Bretthorst. Bayesian analysis I: Parameter estimation using quadratur NMR models. *Journal of Magnetic Resonance*, 88:533–551, 1990.
[3] J. J. K. Ó Ruanaidh and W. J. Fitzgerald. *Numerical Bayesian Methods Applied to Signal Processing.* Springer-Verlag, New York, 1995.
[4] D. J. C. MacKay. Bayesian interpolation. *Neural Computation*, 4:415–447, 1992.
[5] D. J. C. MacKay. The evidence framework applied to classification networks. *Neural Computation*, 4:720–736, 1992.
[6] R. M. Neal. *Bayesian Learning for Neural Networks.* Springer, New York, 1996.
[7] L. Ljung. *System Identification, Theory for the User.* Prentice-Hall, Englewood Cliffs, NJ, 1999.
[8] W. A. Wright. Bayesian approach to neural-network modelling with input uncertainty. *IEEE Trans. Neural Networks*, 10:1261–1270, 1999.
[9] P. Dellaportas and S. A. Stephens. Bayesian analysis of errors-in-variables regression models. *Biometrics*, 51:1085–1095, 1995.
[10] H. Jeffreys. *Theory of Probability.* Clarendon Press, Oxford, 3rd edition, 1961.
[11] P. Sykacek and S. Roberts. Bayesian time series classification. In T. G. Dietterich, S. Becker, and Z. Gharamani, editors, *Advances in Neural Processing Systems 14*, pages 937–944. MIT Press, 2002.

[12] M. Abramowitz and I. A. Stegun. *Handbook of Mathematical Functions with Formulas, Graphs and Mathematical Tables.* Dover, New York, 1965.

[13] S. Brunak and P. Baldi. *Bioinformatics.* MIT Press, Cambridge, MA, 1998.

[14] A. P. Dempster, N. M. Laird, and D. B. Rubin. Maximum likelihood from incomplete data via the EM algorithm (with discussion). *Journal of the Royal Statistical Society series B*, 39:1–38, 1977.

[15] L. E. Baum, T. Petrie, G. Soules, and N. Weiss. A maximization technique occurring in the statistical analysis of probabilistic functions of Markov chains. *Annals of Mathematical Statistics*, 41:164–171, 1970.

[16] S. Richardson and P. J. Green. On Bayesian analysis of mixtures with an unknown number of components. *Journal Royal Stat. Soc. B*, 59:731–792, 1997.

[17] J. M. Bernardo and A. F. M. Smith. *Bayesian Theory.* Wiley, Chichester, 1994.

[18] W. R. Gilks, S. Richardson, and D. J. Spiegelhalter (ed.). *Markov Chain Monte Carlo in Practice.* Chapman & Hall, London, 1996.

[19] C. P. Robert and G. Casella. *Monte Carlo statistical methods.* Springer, New York, 1999.

[20] A. Gelman and D. B. Rubin. Inference from iterative simulations using multiple sequences (with discussion). *Statist. Sci.*, 7:457–511, 1992.

[21] A. E. Raftery and S. M. Lewis. Implementing MCMC. In W. R. Gilks, S. Richardson, and D. J. Spiegelhalter, editors, *Markov Chain Monte Carlo in Practice*, pages 115–130. Chapman & Hall, London, 1996.

[22] H. H. Jasper. Report of the committee on methods of clinical examination in electroencephalography. *Clinical Neurophysiology*, 10:370–1, 1958.

[23] H. H. Jasper. Appendix to report of the committee on methods of clinical examination in EEG: the ten-twenty electrode system of the International Federation of Electroencephalography. *Clinical Neurophysiology*, 10:371–375, 1958.

14

Ensemble Hidden Markov Models with Extended Observation Densities for Biosignal Analysis

Iead Rezek and Stephen Roberts

University of Oxford, Dept. of Engineering Science, Oxford, UK
{irezek,sjrob}@robots.ox.ac.uk

Summary. Hidden Markov Models (HMM) have proven to be very useful in a variety of biomedical applications. The most established method for estimating HMM parameters is the maximum likelihood method which has shortcomings, such as repeated estimation and penalisation of the likelihood score, that are well known. This paper describes a variational learning approach to try and improve on the maximum-likelihood estimators. Emphasis lies on the fact that for HMMs with observation models that are from the exponential family of distributions, all HMM parameters and hidden state variables can be derived from a single loss function, namely the Kullback-Leibler divergence. Practical issues, such as model initialisation and choice of model order, are described. The paper concludes with application of three types of observation model HMMs to a variety of biomedical data, such as EEG and ECG, from different physiological experiments and conditions.

14.1 Introduction

Hidden Markov models (HMMs), introduced in Section 2.3.4 and Section 10.11.4, are well-established tools with widespread use in biomedical applications. They have been applied to sleep staging [3], non-stationary biomedical signal segmentation [16], brain–computer interfacing [13], and of course speech [24]. Their strength lies in the fact that they are capable of modelling sudden changes in the dynamics of the data, a situation frequently observed in physiological data. Another crucial factor is their ability to segment the data into informative states in a completely unsupervised fashion. When very little about the underlying physiological state is known *a priori*, unsupervised methods are a useful way forward.

The most established method of training the parameters of a HMM uses the maximum-likelihood framework [17, 24]. The methods leads to simple parameter update equations. There are, however, some problems with the maximum-likelihood approach. Leaving the Bayesian argument aside, maximum-likelihood estimators are comparatively slow in their convergence.

From our experience, maximum *a posteriori* estimators are considerably faster, presumably because the priors somewhat smooth the likelihood surface and thus optimisation homes in quicker on a local maximum. Also, in maximum-likelihood estimation, special care must be taken not to over-fit the data. To avoid this, models of different complexity must be repeatedly estimated and the residuals computed and penalised for complexity of the model until an optimal model is found. While some heuristics may well be available to overcome such a computationally expensive approach they nonetheless remain expensive [23] and the finiteness of training data means that larger models cannot be computed without running into computational problems, such as near-singular covariance matrices.

These drawbacks of maximum-likelihood base estimation of HMM parameters have lead us to investigate Bayesian approaches to learning model parameters and structures. Unlike maximum likelihood estimators, which estimate a single value for the parameters, a Bayesian estimator results in a distribution for the HMM parameters and thus confidence measure for the model. In computing this distribution, which is known as the posterior, the Bayesian estimator requires the likelihood of the data under the model and the prior distributions of the model parameters. The priors in Bayesian approaches play a role similar to information gathered from previously collected data [7] and thus allow us to overcome the problems of singularities in the presence of limited actual training data. In addition, if new data does not support the hypothesized model complexity, posterior densities of the model parameters will be no different from their prior densities, which in effect results in an automatic pruning process. The main difficulty of Bayesian methods tends to be of a mathematical nature. Complex models can quickly become mathematically intractable, i.e. integrating out nuisance parameters becomes impossible. This is often resolved by the use of sampling approaches to estimate the posterior densities [20]. Analytic approximations also exist. They might lead to slightly inferior solutions when compared with sampling, as they often seek only *local* maxima. Being analytic, however, we expect them to converge must faster than sampling estimators.

In this chapter we describe the use of an analytical approximation to the exact Bayesian posterior densities by means of the variational framework. This framework provides a unified view of estimating all unknown HMM variables - parameters and hidden states [12]. We will describe how update equations can be obtained for a wide range of HMMs with various observation densities. We finally apply the HMMs to biomedical data, such as electrocardiogram derived R-wave interval series, respiration recordings and electroencephalographic signals (EEG).

14.2 Principles of Variational Learning

Chapters on variational calculus can be found in many mathematics textbooks, yet their use in statistics, briefly mentioned in Section 2.3.6, is relatively recent (see [8] and [10] for excellent tutorials). In essence, the aim is to minimise a cost function which, in this case, is the Kullback-Leibler (KL) divergence [2]. The KL divergence measures a distance between two distributions, say Q and P, by the integral[1]

$$\mathcal{F} = D(Q(H)||P(H,V)) = \int Q(H) \log \frac{Q(H)}{P(H|V)} \,\mathrm{d}S + \log P(V) \,. \quad (14.1)$$

Here, the distributions $Q(H)$ and $P(H|V)$ are defined over the set of all hidden variables H, such as parameters or hidden states, conditioned on the observed data V.

The choice of cost function, like that of the squared error, is primarily influenced by its practicability, i.e. it often results in simple solutions. One way of achieving this, in the case of the KL divergence, is to stay within the group of the exponential family and to approximate the full but intractable posterior probability density $P(H|V)$, which parameterises the true model, by a simpler but tractable distribution, $Q(H)$. Minimising or differentiating the KL divergence with respect to the approximate posterior distribution, $Q(H)$, results in simple equations, which are often coupled and thus need to be re-estimated in an iterative fashion.

By approximating the full posterior, one can enjoy some of the benefits of Bayesian analysis, such as full Bayesian model estimation and automatic penalties for over-complex models to avoid over-fitting. Note, the first term on the right-hand side in equation (14.1) is always non-negative, and thus the divergence is a bound to the true log-probability of the data $P(V)$. This means that optimal model selection takes place within the class of approximated and thus suboptimal models.

The simplest of all approximations to the true posterior distribution, $P(H|V)$, can be obtained by assuming that, if one is given a set of hidden variables $H = \{H_1, \ldots, H_N\}$, the Q-distribution factorises

$$Q(H) = \prod_{i=1}^{T} Q(H_i) \,, \quad (14.2)$$

with the additional obvious constraint that the distributions integrate to unity, that is $\int Q(H_i)\, dH_i = 1$. This assumption is known as the as the "mean-field" assumption. Under the mean-field assumption, the distributions $Q(H_i)$ which maximise the KL divergence (14.1) can be shown [6] to have the general form

[1] Physicists have noted that the same function occurs in statistical mechanics and therefore often refer to it as minimising the so-called variational free energy [9].

$$Q(H_i) = \frac{1}{Z} \exp \int Q(\bar{H}_i) \log P(H_i|\bar{H}_i) \mathrm{d}\bar{H}_i \; , \tag{14.3}$$

where $\bar{H}_i = H \setminus H_i$ is the set of all hidden variables H excluding H_i and Z is just a normalisation constant. For completeness, we repeat the derivation of the model-free form (14.3) of [6] in Appendix A.

There is, in principle no reason to restrict oneself to the independence assumption of the H_i. One can easily define H_i to be actually a subset of variables forming a partition of H. In this chapter for instance, we form such a partition by grouping all HMM variables into the set of hidden state variables and the set of HMM model parameters (governing the probability of observing the datum at a particular time instance and the probability of transit to the next time step). The actual set of model parameters we denote by $\theta = \{\theta_1, \ldots, \theta_M\}$ and the set of hidden state variables by $S = \{S_0, \ldots, S_T\}$. The hidden state variables, S form one partition within the overall set of variables and are updated jointly. In contrast the members of the set of HMM model parameters, θ, are assumed to be independent from one another. With these assumptions, the approximating distribution $Q(H)$ may be expressed as

$$Q(H) \triangleq Q(S)Q(\theta) = Q(S_0) \prod_{t=1}^{T} Q(S_t|S_{t-1}) \prod_{j=1}^{M} Q(\theta_j). \tag{14.4}$$

This is useful because the distribution $Q(S)$ has the structure of a simple chain. This makes it tractable and an exact updating scheme can be found jointly for all $Q(S_t)$.

Finally, we make one further assumption. Models of different structures or sizes, e.g. state space dimensions or observation model order, are taken to be independent from one another. The set of all model sizes is denoted by A and a particular model size is indexed with a. We can then write the posterior probability of all model sizes A and unknown variables in the following form

$$P(S, \theta, A) = \prod_{a=1}^{A} P(S|a)P(\theta|a)P(a) \; , \tag{14.5}$$

where each factor, $P(S|a)P(\theta|a)P(a)$, corresponds to a different model size. Assuming that all model structures in A are equally likely, the posterior model probability can be computed as

$$Q(a) \propto \exp\{-\mathcal{F}_a\} \; , \tag{14.6}$$

where $\mathcal{F}_a$ is the KL divergence of the entire model for a fixed model size, i.e.

$$\mathcal{F}_a = \iint Q(S|a)Q(\theta|a) \log \frac{Q(S|a)Q(\theta|a)}{P(S, V, \theta, a)} \mathrm{d}S\mathrm{d}\theta \; . \tag{14.7}$$

The assumption is primarily chosen to make it easier to select a particular model, which will be the model with the smallest KL divergence between the true and approximate model distribution. In general, such an assumption should be used with caution as models are very likely to overlap significantly. However, this assumption is used widely though in a different form. It is identical to the assumption of uniform priors over model structures.

14.3 Variational Learning of Hidden Markov Models

Consider a set of T random variables, $S = \{S_1, \ldots, S_t, \ldots, S_T\}$. Each random variable can take on one of, say M, discrete values, $S_t = \{s_1, \ldots, s_M\}$. If we impose, for $t > 0$ a probability on observing the variable S_t that is conditioned on the value of the variable S_{t-1} and denote this probability by $P(S_t|S_{t-1})$, one obtains a Markov Chain since $P(S_t|S_{t-1})$ is known as the Markov property. A Hidden Markov process supposes further that what is actually observed are not the individual S_t, but a corrupted version of them. The variables S_t are thus hidden from the observer and the observations, say X_t are dependent on the variable S_t. This probability distribution over the entire sequence of observations $X = \{X_1, \ldots, X_t, \ldots, X_T\}$ and states $S = \{S_1, \ldots, S_t, \ldots, S_T\}$ then takes the mathematical form of

$$P(S, X) = P(S_0) \prod_{t=1}^{T} P(S_t|S_{t-1}) P(X_t|S_t) \, . \tag{14.8}$$

The state transition probability, $P(S_t|S_{t-1})$ is a multinomial (i.e. discrete) distribution, encoded in an $M \times M$ matrix since there are M possible values S_t can take for every value S_{t-1} has taken. These probabilities are denoted by $\pi_{t_{t-1}}$ and are assumed to be independent of the time t, i.e. we assume the Markov chain is homogeneous. The initial state probability S_0 is parameterised by π_0 and is also a multinomial with M probability values. The value M is called the state space dimension. The probability $P(X_t|S_t)$ is called the observation probability and is parameterised by θ_{Obs}. Its form depends on the assumed observation model, which in the case of a Gaussian corrupted Markov chain is simply a set of M Gaussian densities, one for each value of S_t.

The speech community represents a HMM graphically, shown in Figure 14.1(a) for a HMM with $M = 2$, by representing each state a variable S_t can take by a vertex. The transitions from one state into the next are depicted by arcs and labelled with the probability of making the transition. Unlike the state space representation of the HMM, the graphical model representation, shown in Figure 14.1(b), depicts the HMM using vertices for the state variables S and observations X. This has its origin in interpreting the HMM as a Bayesian network in which all random variables are assigned a vertex. Observed (a.k.a. instantiated) random variables have shaded vertices. Arrows between vertices represent statistical relationships between the random variables. The functional form of the relationship is often left out and results in ambiguities. A factor graph makes the functional form of variable dependencies clearer. Such a graph is shown in Figure 14.1(c).

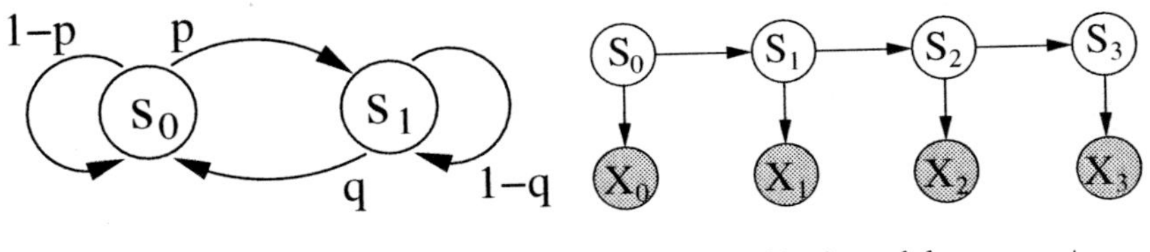

(a) State space representation of a HMM

(b) Graphical model representation of a HMM

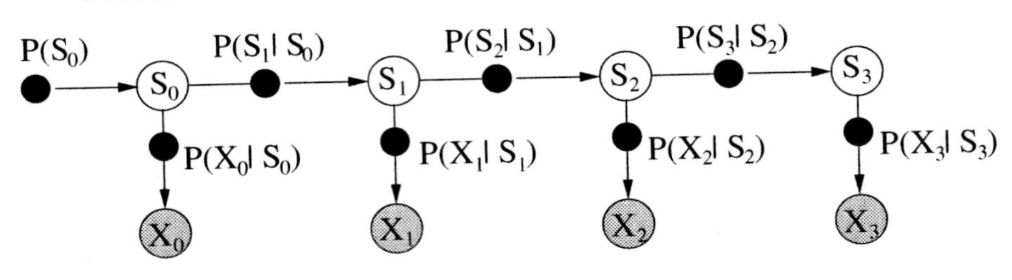

(c) Factor graph representation of a HMM

Fig. 14.1. A HMM represented graphically. Subfigures (b) and (c) represent the HMM with four unrolled time slices. Shaded nodes denote observed random variables.

The concepts of variational learning described in the previous section can be readily applied to a first order hidden Markov model. We assume a HMM of length T, state space dimension M, hidden state variables, $S = \{S_1, \ldots, S_T\}$, and observations $X = \{X_1, \ldots, X_T\}$, transition model and the observation model. The HMM parameters θ, consist of $\pi_{t_{t-1}}$ which determine the state transition probability $P(S_t|S_{t-1})$, π_0 which parameterise the initial state probability $P(S_0)$ and θ_{Obs} which describe the observation probabilities $P(X_t|S_t)$. The full true posterior probability of the model is then given by

$$\begin{aligned} P(S, X, \theta) &= P(S, X|\theta)P(\theta) && (14.9) \\ &\triangleq P(S, X|\pi_{t_{t-1}}, \pi_0, \theta_{\text{Obs}})P(\pi_{t_{t-1}}, \pi_0, \theta_{\text{Obs}}) && (14.10) \\ &= P(S_0|\pi_0) \prod_{t=1}^{T} P(S_t|S_{t-1}, \pi_{t_{t-1}})P(X_t|S_t, \theta_{\text{Obs}}) \\ &\qquad P(\pi_{t_{t-1}})P(\pi_0)P(\theta_{\text{Obs}}) \,. && (14.11) \end{aligned}$$

What remains to apply the cost function (14.1) is the distribution which approximates the full posterior probability $P(S, X, \theta)$. First, we assume that all the HMM model parameters, θ (i.e. all variables but the state space variables) are independent (mean field assumption). Second, all the hidden state variables are grouped together and are governed by one distribution $Q(S)$. With these assumptions, the resulting KL divergence (14.1) then becomes

$$\mathcal{F} = \int \cdots \int Q(S) \ \ Q(\pi_{t_{t-1}})Q(\pi_0)Q(\theta_{\text{Obs}}) \\ \log \frac{Q(S)Q(\pi_{t_{t-1}})Q(\pi_0)Q(\theta_{\text{Obs}})}{P(S, X, \pi_{t_{t-1}}, \pi_0, \theta_{\text{Obs}})} \ \mathrm{d}S\mathrm{d}\theta \ . \quad (14.12)$$

This KL divergence can now be minimised individually with respect to the distributions, $Q(S), Q(\pi_{t_{t-1}}), Q(\pi_0)$ and $Q(\theta_{\text{Obs}})$. In the two following sections we first update divergence (14.12) with respect to the distribution of the hidden states, $Q(S)$, to show that it leads to the well-known Baum-Welch or forward-backward recursions. Then the cost function (14.12) is minimised with respect to $Q(\theta_{\text{Obs}})$. The minimisation depends on the functional form of the observation model, $Q(\theta_{\text{Obs}})$, and is shown for different types of observation models, such as Gaussian and linear observation models.

14.3.1 Learning the HMM Hidden State Sequence

We begin by optimising the KL divergence (14.12) with respect to the distribution over all hidden states, $Q(S)$. Using the mean-field update equation (14.3), the optimal posterior distribution over all hidden states, $Q(S)$, can be computed by replacing all HMM parameters θ for $\bar{H}_i$ in equation (14.3), to give

$$Q(S) \propto \exp \int Q(\theta) \log P(S, X, \theta)\mathrm{d}\theta \quad (14.13)$$

Of interest, however, is not so much the global distribution, $Q(S)$, but the marginal distributions, $Q(S_t)$, and the joint hidden state probabilities, $Q(S_t, S_{t+1})$. They can be calculated using the well-known Baum-Welch or forward-backward recursions.

The justification for using the forward-backward recursions comes from the fact that they are the result of minimising equation (14.12) with respect to the individual hidden state probabilities, $Q(S_t)$, and the joint hidden state probabilities, $Q(S_t, S_{t+1})$. To see this, assume all other Q-distributions are held constant and parameterised by $\tilde{\theta}$ which are the values calculated during previous iterations. Then, the KL divergence (14.12) simplifies to

$$\mathcal{F} = \int Q(S) \log \frac{Q(S)}{\tilde{P}(S, X)} \ \mathrm{d}S + const \ , \quad (14.14)$$

where

$$\tilde{P}(S, X) = \int Q(\theta) \log P(S, X, \theta) \ \mathrm{d}\theta \ , \quad (14.15)$$

and the constant includes all terms not involving S. To further minimise the divergence (14.14), additional consistency and normalisation constraints are needed. One set of constraints simply ensures that all Q-distributions normalise to 1. In addition, consistency (or holonomic) constraints are required which ensure that marginalising $Q(S_t, S_{t-1})$ with respect to $Q(S_t)$ gives the same result as marginalising $Q(S_t, S_{t+1})$. These additional constraints are added to the KL divergence (14.14) with the usual Lagrangian multipliers. The simple structure of the hidden state chain permits an analytic solution to equation (14.14) in form of iterative computations of the Lagrangian multipliers. The detailed steps starting from optimising the KL divergence (14.14) leading up to the Baum-Welch recursions are given in Appendix B.

For simplicity, in the following we assume the Baum-Welch recursions have been applied and yield the marginal and joint distributions $Q(S_t)$ and $Q(S_t, S_{t-1})$, respectively. We make use of the notation introduced in [17], specifically we denote the probability of the state variable S_t taking one of the M values $m = 1, 2, \ldots, M$, by

$$\gamma_t(m) = Q(S_t = m|X) \ . \tag{14.16}$$

Further, we denote the joint probability of variable S_t taking value n and S_{t-1} taking value m, by

$$\xi_t(m, n) = Q(S_t = n, S_{t-1} = m|X) \ . \tag{14.17}$$

14.3.2 Learning HMM Parameters

The updated probabilities of the hidden state variables result in values of $\gamma_t(m)$ and $\xi_t(m, n)$ (see previous section) for each time instance t. In order to obtain an analytic solution for the HMM parameters after substituting into equation (14.3), we need to choose appropriate prior distributions, $P(\theta)$, for the HMM parameters, θ. To obtain analytic solutions, the prior distributions, $P(\theta)$, are required to be conjugate distributions. The approximate posterior distributions $Q(\theta)$ will then be functionally identical to the prior distributions (i.e. a Gaussian prior density is mapped to a Gaussian posterior density). Apart from the parameters of the observation model, which will be discussed later, for the HMM these conjugate prior distributions are as given in [1]. For the initial state probability π_0, we use an M-dimensional Dirichlet density

$$Dir(\pi_0) = \frac{\Gamma(\sum_l \kappa_l)}{\prod_l \Gamma(\kappa_l)} \prod_{m=1}^{M} \pi_{0_m}^{\kappa_m - 1} \ , \tag{14.18}$$

and, for the transition probabilities, π_m, $M \times M$-dimensional Dirichlet densities

$$Dir(\pi_{t_{t-1}}) = \prod_{m=1}^{M} \frac{\Gamma(\sum_l \lambda_{m_l})}{\prod_l \Gamma(\lambda_{m_l})} \prod_{n=1}^{M} \pi_{m_n}^{\lambda_{m_n} - 1} \ . \tag{14.19}$$

Based on these assumptions, minimisation of the KL divergence with respect to the posterior distributions $Q(\pi_{t_{t-1}})$ and $Q(\pi_0)$ leads to posterior initial state and transition probabilities that are again Dirichlet distributed and have parameters, respectively,

$$\tilde{\kappa}_m = \gamma_{t=0} = m + \kappa_m; \tag{14.20}$$

$$\tilde{\lambda}_{m_n} = \sum_t \xi_t(m,n) + \lambda_{m_n} \,. \tag{14.21}$$

The hyperparameters κ and λ are fixed and typically set to integer values just greater than 1, reflecting the fact that little is known *a priori* about the initial state and state transition probabilities.

14.3.3 HMM Observation Models

What remains to specify is the probability of the observation given the state at time t, $P(X_t|S_t)$. Determining it will also force our hands in determining the prior distributions of the parameters governing the observation model, $P(X_t|S_t)$. The choice of $P(X_t|S_t)$ is also very much dependent on the application. The two classic and simplest of all cases assume the Markov chain is corrupted by additive Gaussian noise or that the observations are discrete. In the latter case, the observation model is simply a multinomial while in the former the observation model is (multivariate) Gaussian. Many others have, of course, been suggested in the HMM's long history. Among them are Poisson densities for count processes [11], and linear models (spectral or autoregressive) for use in, say EEG modelling [16], along with more complex models such as "independent component" models [15].

The Gaussian observation model

For observations which, conditional on the state, are Gaussian distributed,

$$P(X_t|S_t = m) = P(X_t|\mu_m, C_m) \tag{14.22}$$

where $\mu = \{\mu_1, \ldots, \mu_M\}$ and $C = \{C_1, \ldots, C_M\}$ are the normal distribution mean vectors and precision matrices, respectively. The conjugate densities [1] for the means μ_m, are K-dimensional Normal densities ($m = 1, \ldots, M$)

$$P(\mu_m) \propto e^{-\frac{1}{2}(\mu-\mu_{m_0})^{\mathsf{T}} C_{m_0} (\mu-\mu_{m_0})}, \tag{14.23}$$

and for the precisions C_m, K-dimensional Wishart densities ($m = 1, \ldots, M$)

$$P(C_m) \propto |C_m|^{\alpha_m - \frac{K+1}{2}} e^{-\mathrm{tr}(B_m C_m)} \tag{14.24}$$

Inserting these densities into (14.12) and subsequent minimisation leads to update equations for the parameters of the posterior densities of the means and precisions. The posterior means follow normal densities $q(\mu_m) \sim \mathcal{N}(\tilde{\mu}_{m0}, \tilde{C}_{m0})$, with parameters

$$\tilde{\mu}_{m0} = (\bar{\gamma}_m \tilde{\alpha}_m \tilde{B}_m^{-1} + C_{m0})^{-1} (\tilde{\alpha}_m \tilde{B}_m^{-1} \bar{x}_m + C_{m0}\mu_{m0}); \quad (14.25)$$

$$\tilde{C}_{m0} = (\tilde{\gamma}_m \tilde{\alpha}_m \tilde{B}_m^{-1} + C_{m0}) \quad (14.26)$$

where $\bar{x}_m = \sum_{t=1}^{T} \gamma_t(m) x_t$ and $\bar{\gamma}_m = \sum_{t=1}^{T} \gamma_t(m)$.

Similarly, the posterior precisions follow a Wishart density, $q(C_m|\tilde{\alpha}_m, \tilde{B}_m) \sim \mathcal{W}(\tilde{\alpha}_m, \tilde{B}_m)$, with parameters

$$\tilde{\alpha}_m = \frac{1}{2}\bar{\gamma}_m + \alpha_m; \quad (14.27)$$

$$\tilde{B}_m = \frac{1}{2}\sum_t^T \gamma_t(m)(x_t - \tilde{\mu}_{m0})(x_t - \tilde{\mu}_{m0})^\top + \frac{1}{2}\bar{\gamma}_m \tilde{C}_{m0}^{-1} + B_m \quad (14.28)$$

The Poisson observation model

The choice of Gaussian observation model depends on the data and, hence, might not be appropriate. Particularly, when dealing with count data, such as the RR interval series obtained from the ECG signal, Gaussian observation models are only applicable after some preprocessing of the data, such as interpolation [21]. To avoid this we demonstrate the variational estimation of a Poisson observation model for HMMs. In this case, the observation density is

$$P(X_t|S_t = m, \mu) = e^{-x_t \mu_m} (x_n \mu_m)^{y_t} \frac{1}{y_t!} \quad (14.29)$$

where, each of the M states has a Poisson distribution with parameter μ_m. The data points $y_1, \ldots, y_T$ are counts while the values x_t are called the exposure of the t-th unit, i.e. a fraction of the unknown parameter of interest μ_m [4]. The prior for the parameter of the Poisson distribution is chosen to be conjugate, which is a Gamma density ($m = 1, \ldots, M$)

$$P(\mu_m) \propto \mu_m^{\alpha_0 - 1} \exp\{\beta_0 \mu_m\}. \quad (14.30)$$

The optimised Q-distribution for the Poisson rate of state m are also Gamma, with parameters

$$Q(\mu_m) \sim \mathcal{G}(\tilde{\alpha}_0, \tilde{\beta}_0)$$

$$\tilde{\alpha}_0 = \sum_t \gamma_{tm} y_t + \alpha_0 \quad (14.31)$$

$$\tilde{\beta}_0 = \sum_t \gamma_{tm} x_t + \beta_0 \quad (14.32)$$

The multivariate linear observation model

The final model described here is the multivariate linear observation model. It is particularly useful when, for instance, auto-regressive features are to be extracted from EEG signals and later segmented using a HMM with Gaussian observation models. It is clear that if the process of feature extraction and segmentation can be combined the results are much improved [22]. Further, if the linear model has sinusoids as basis functions, one can use the HMM to segment the signal based on its spectral content. Without any major mathematical complications, we can also assume that a short data segment can be described with the same linear model. The model then becomes a matrix variate linear model, in which a segment of multivariate data forms an observation matrix that is modelled by a linear model. The model is best described as a graphical model shown in Figure 14.2.

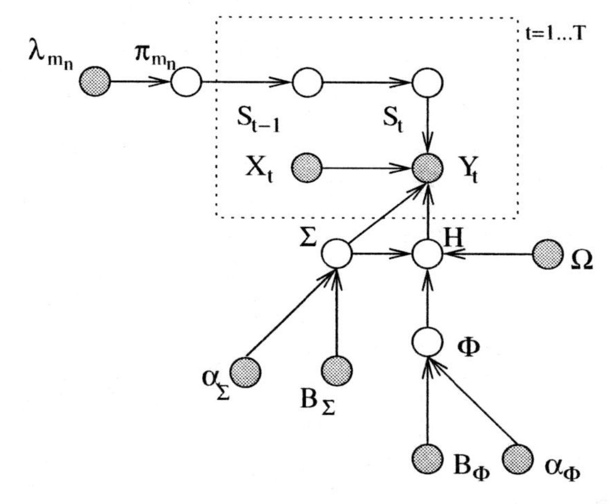

Fig. 14.2. Directed graph of a HMM with a matrix-variate linear observation model for observations Y and basis functions X.

For observation Y_t and basis functions X_t, the linear observation model is given as

$$P(Y_t - H_m X_t | S_t = m) = \mathcal{N}_{d,u}(0, \Sigma_m, I_u) \tag{14.33}$$

where $\mathcal{N}_{d,u}$ is a $d \times u$-matrix variate normal density function [5], $H = \{H_m\} \quad \forall m = \{1, \ldots, M\}$ and I_u is a $u \times u$ identity matrix. For example, assume a multivariate autoregressive (AR) model of order p which models a d-variate observation $\mathbf{y}_t$. The past samples can be concatenated in a matrix, $x_t \stackrel{\text{def}}{=} [\mathbf{y}_{t-1}^{\mathsf{T}}, \ldots, \mathbf{y}_{t-p}^{\mathsf{T}}]^{\mathsf{T}}$. Thus $\mathbf{y}_t \in \mathbb{R}^d$ is a d-variate response vector at time t, $\mathbf{x}_t \in \mathbb{R}^{dp}$ is a dp-variate basis vector at time t. $\bar{H}_p \in \mathbb{R}^{d \times d}$ is the matrix of model coefficients, $H \in \mathbb{R}^{d \times dp}$ is a partitioned matrix composed of the coefficient matrices at lag p. If, furthermore, the samples are grouped into segments, indexed by n, each of which contains u samples of $\mathbf{y}_t$, one can construct a matrix with u response- and u basis-vectors, i.e.

$$Y_n = \left[\mathbf{y}_{(n-1)u}, \ldots, \mathbf{y}_{nu}\right] \tag{14.34}$$

$$X_n = \left[\mathbf{x}_{(n-1)u}, \ldots, \mathbf{x}_{nu}\right] . \tag{14.35}$$

The final form of the linear model takes the form $Y_n = HX_n$ the residuals of which are Gaussian distributed, thus giving equation (14.33), with index t replaced by n.

The prior densities for the coefficient matrices H_m are assumed to be a $d \times dp$-matrix variate normal densities, $\mathcal{N}_{d,dp}(\Omega, \Sigma_m, \Phi_m)$, with mean Ω and precisions Σ_m and Φ_m. The prior for residual precisions Σ_m and the coefficient precisions Φ_m are Wishart densities [1], $\mathcal{W}_d(\alpha_\Sigma, B_\Sigma)$ and $\mathcal{W}_{dp}(\alpha_\Phi, B_\Phi)$, with shape/scale parameters α_Σ/B_Σ and α_Φ/B_Φ, respectively.

The posterior density of the model coefficients, H_m, is a $d \times dp$ matrix variate Normal density with mean $\tilde{\Omega}$ and precision matrices $\tilde{\Sigma}_m, \tilde{\Phi}_m$ computed by

$$\tilde{\Omega}_m^\top = \tilde{\Phi}_m^{-1}\left(\sum_n \gamma_{nm} X_n Y_n^\top + \tilde{\alpha}_{\Phi m} \tilde{B}_{\Phi m}^{-1} \Omega^\top\right) \tag{14.36}$$

$$\tilde{\Sigma}_m = \tilde{\alpha}_{\Sigma m} \tilde{B}_{\Sigma m}^{-1} \tag{14.37}$$

$$\tilde{\Phi}_m = \sum_n \gamma_{nm} X_n X_n^\top + \tilde{\alpha}_{\Phi m} \tilde{B}_{\Phi m}^{-1} \tag{14.38}$$

The posterior of the residual variances, Σ_m, is a Wishart density with shape and scale parameters computed by

$$\begin{aligned}
\tilde{\alpha}_{\Sigma m} &= \frac{1}{2}\left(\sum_n u\gamma_{nm} + dp + 2\alpha_\Sigma\right) \\
\tilde{B}_{\Sigma m} &= \frac{1}{2}\sum_n \gamma_{nm}\left[(Y_n - \tilde{\Omega}_m X_n)(Y_n - \tilde{\Omega}_m X_n)^\top + \mathrm{tr}\left(X_n X_n^\top \tilde{\Phi}_m^{-1}\right)\tilde{\Sigma}_m^{-1}\right] \\
&\quad + \frac{1}{2}\left(\tilde{\Omega}_m - \Omega_m\right)\tilde{\alpha}_{\Phi m}\tilde{B}_{\Phi m}^{-1}\left(\tilde{\Omega}_m - \Omega_m\right)^\top + \frac{1}{2}\mathrm{tr}\left(\tilde{\alpha}_{\Phi m}\tilde{B}_{\Phi m}^{-\top}\tilde{\Phi}_m^{-1}\right)\tilde{\Sigma}_m^{-1} + B_\Sigma
\end{aligned} \tag{14.39}$$

The posterior model coefficient variances, Φ_m, also follow a Wishart density with parameters

$$\begin{aligned}
\tilde{\alpha}_{\Phi m} &= \frac{d}{2} + \alpha_\Phi \\
\tilde{B}_{\Phi m} &= \frac{1}{2}(\tilde{\Omega}_m - \Omega)^\top \tilde{\alpha}_{\Sigma m}\tilde{B}_{\Sigma m}^{-1}(\tilde{\Omega}_m - \Omega) + \frac{1}{2}\mathrm{tr}(\tilde{\alpha}_{\Sigma m}\tilde{B}_{\Sigma m}^{-1}\tilde{\Sigma}_m^{-1})\tilde{\Phi}_m^{-1} + B_\Phi
\end{aligned} \tag{14.40}$$

14.3.4 Estimation

Having obtained the update equations for the observation models and the state transition probabilities, estimation then follows the familiar fashion of iteratively computing the HMM hidden state sequence (equivalent to the E-step in the Maximum Likelihood EM framework) and the HMM parameter posterior distributions (equivalent to M-step). This is repeated until convergence is reached. Convergence is measured by the actual value of the KL divergence (14.12) and the estimation is terminated when (14.12) no longer changes significantly. The mathematical form of the KL divergence (14.12) will obviously depend on the type of model, which here means the type of observation model. The complete formulae, for each of the three observation model HMMs, are listed in Appendix C.

Choice of model size

The iterations are run for a fixed HMM state space dimension and observation model order (number of basis function coefficients in the linear observation model). Estimation is then repeated for different settings and the value of the KL divergence (14.12) recorded. The smallest achievable value of (14.12), according to equation (14.6), results in the highest probability for the particular choice of model.

As an example, data was generated from two bi-variate AR processes, with AR-coefficient matrices of the first model set to $A_{lag=1} = [0.4, 1.2; 0.3, 0.7]$ and $A_{lag=2} = [0.35, -0.3; -0.4, -0.5]$. The second model coefficient matrices were set to $A_{lag=1} = [0.4, 0; 0, 0.7]$ and $A_{lag=2} = [0.35, -0.3; -0.4, -0.5]$. The intercept vector was set to a zero vector and the noise variance matrix to $C = [1.00, 0.50; 0.50, 1.50]$. Figure 14.3(a) shows the KL divergence values for different settings of linear model order and hidden state space dimension. The most probable model size is shown in Figure 14.3(b) and peaks at the expected model size.

Under certain conditions, the state space dimension need not be estimated as above. If the observation model is correct, for example the dimensions of the Gaussian observation model match those of the clusters in the data or the linear model order is the true order, one can exploit the fact that the state transition probabilities factorise, i.e. $P(S_t|S_{t-1}) = \prod_{m=1}^{M} P(S_t|S_{t-1} = m)$. The state space dimension, M, can now be set to an arbitrarily large value and the HMM is estimated just once. States that are not visited by the model will automatically collapse to be equal to their prior distributions. One can thus read out most likely hidden state dimensions from the number of distinct state values in the hidden state sequence.

This effect is shown in Figure 14.4. The HMM was started with $M = 6$ and the number of distinct states monitored at each step of the iteration.

Observation model parameter distributions can also be automatically set to their prior distributions, provided the mathematical formulation of model

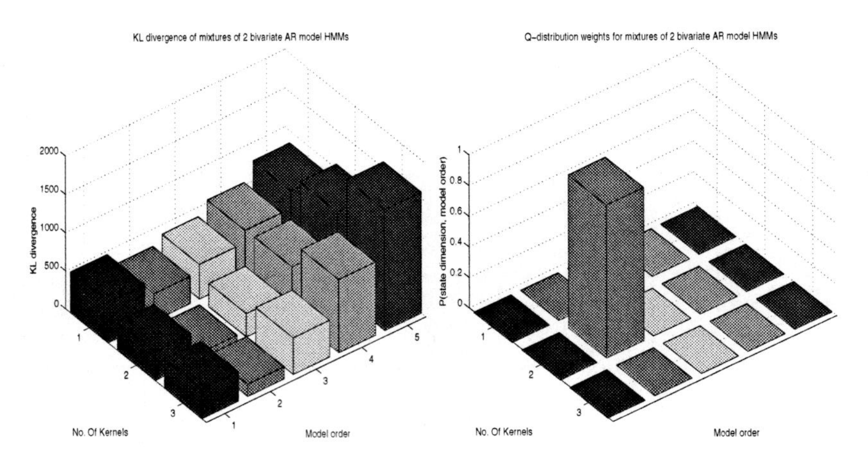

(a) KL divergence for bivariate AR model

(b) Posterior of model for bivariate AR model

Fig. 14.3. KL divergences for mixtures of AR models.

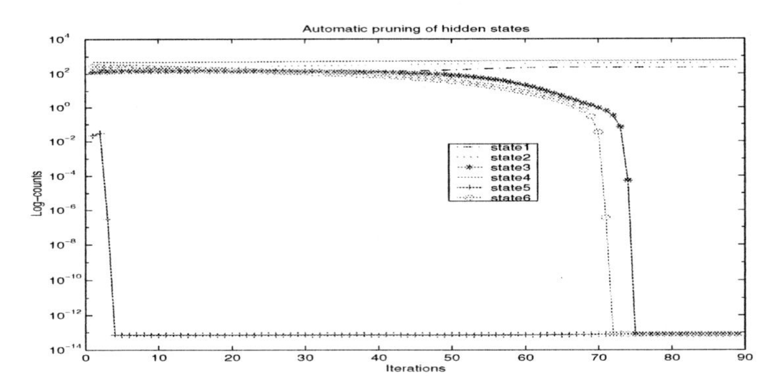

Fig. 14.4. The collapse of the state space dimension during the estimation.

is in a factorised form. For instance, if the linear model description was in terms of reflection rather than autoregressive coefficients, the mean field assumptions leads to an estimator which automatically prunes out all states and model coefficients (and thus model orders) not supported by the data. This is not always possible; however,some engineering short-cuts can be used to quickly home in on the true observation model size. For example, in the linear observation model's current form one can investigate the eigen-spectrum of the linear model parameters' scale matrix $\tilde{B}_{\Phi_m}$. The number of non-zero eigenvalues are an indication of the model order. Also, looking at the distance between the model coefficient matrices of each state, $\|H_i - H_j\|$ for different

$i \neq j$ and $i, j = 1, \ldots, M$, might give some indication as to the preferred number of hidden states. An example of the use of the eigen-spectrum is shown in Figure 14.5. As the model order is increased, the eigenvalues clearly shallow off at the correct model order. The coefficients themselves are relatively close to zero - below 10% of the largest coefficient. Ignoring numerical stability, the Bayesian treatment avoids again the singularities of maximum likelihood methods.

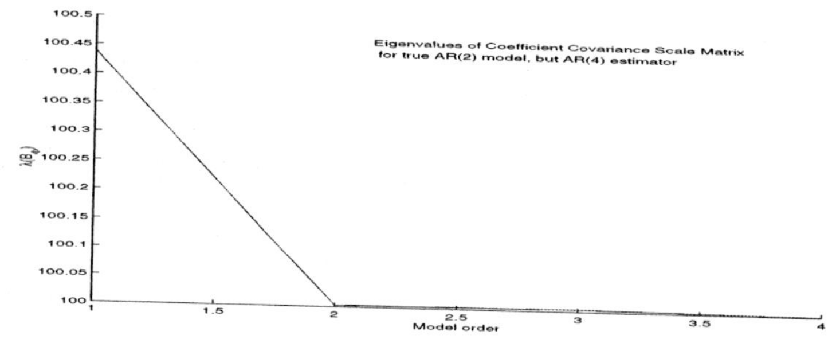

Fig. 14.5. Eigen-spectrum of the coefficient precision posterior density scale parameter B_{Φ} for a univariate AR model.

Model initialisation

Evidently, there are various ways of initialising the HMM and all depend on the observation model. The simplest initialisation is the random initialisation of the hidden state probabilities. The estimation then begins by estimating the HMM model parameters, thus avoiding to a large extent manual setting of HMM parameters. In practice, however, there is often the desire to keep the number of iterations, till convergence is reached, to a minimum. To achieve that, more educated "guesses" have to be made as far as the model parameters are concerned. This can be done in some cases by making use of the data to set the parameters and begin with the estimation of the hidden state probabilities. We illustrate this below for the Gaussian and linear autoregressive observation models.

The Gaussian observation model can be initialised by running a few iterations of the (much faster) K-means algorithm or Gaussian mixture EM on the training data. The obtained cluster centres can be assigned to the posterior means, $\tilde{\mu}_m$, of the HMM observation model means. The means' posterior precision matrices, $\tilde{C}_{m_0}$, are set all equal to the covariance of the total training data. The parameters of the posterior Wishart density for the observation model precision matrices consist of the shape parameter $\tilde{\alpha}_m$ and the scale parameter $\tilde{B}_m$. The value of $\tilde{\alpha}_m$ is set to the half the dimensionality of the training data, while $\tilde{B}_m$ is set to the total training data covariance matrix scaled up by $\tilde{\alpha}_m$. Practice has shown this to be the most robust initialisation procedure; robust, that is, in the sense that it is least sensitive to cluster shapes and data range.

The observation model priors are generally set to be as flat as possible. The observation model means have an associated Gaussian prior with mean and covariance parameters set to the median and squared range of the training data, respectively.

The Poisson observation model is initialised at random. Conditioned on each state, we randomly select a sample from the data. The sample size itself is also drawn randomly. The shape, $\tilde{\alpha}_0$, and scale parameters, $\tilde{\beta}_0$, of the posterior Gamma distribution are then set to the sum of the sample counts and exposure, respectively.

For the experiment described below, the observation model prior shape and scale parameters are set to a minimum of 1 count per interval, i.e. $\alpha_0 = 1$, and and an average rate of 60 beats per minute, respectively.

The linear autoregressive observation model is initialised in three steps. First, an initial data segment is used to calculate the values of the AR-coefficient variances and the residual noise variance. Second, with the use of the variances obtained in the first step, a multivariate Kalman filter is applied to the entire training data.[2] Finally, the so obtained AR-coefficients are segmented using a few iterations of K-means, say.

The posterior density of the model coefficients, H_m, is a matrix variate Gaussian. Its mean, $\tilde{\Omega}_m$ is set the the K-means cluster centres. The covariance matrices, $\tilde{\Sigma}_m$ and $\tilde{\Phi}_m$ are set, respectively, to the estimates of the residual noise variance and AR-coefficient variances of step one above. The posterior of the residual noise variances, Σ_m, is a Wishart density. Its scale parameter is set to $\frac{1}{2}d+1$, i.e. half the residual noise dimensionality incremented by 1. The shape parameter is set to the residual noise variance multiplied by the Wishart density's scale parameter. Similarly, the posterior of the model coefficients, Φ_m, also follow a Wishart density. Its scale parameter is set to $\frac{1}{2}dp + 1$, that is half the product of the linear model order and training data dimension and incremented by 1. The shape parameter is set to the AR coefficient variances of step one above, multiplied by the Wishart density's scale parameter.

The priors for the linear observation model assumes a standardised training data set, i.e. the data is detrended and its variance normalised to unity. The prior for the linear model coefficients, H_m, is thus set to have a mean of zero. The scale coefficient, B_Σ, of the prior for the noise precision Σ_m, is set to unity and the shape coefficient α_Σ to the dimension of the noise precision. The prior of the linear model coefficient precisions is assumed to be more accurate than the noise precision. The scale, B_Φ, is set to one order of magnitude larger than

[2] If the training data is very large, experience has shown that a simple segmentation of the data and estimation of the AR coefficient matrices is faster than the Kalman filter approach, yet equally useful.

B_{Σ}, while the shape is set to the dimension of the coefficient space (model order $\times$ data dimensionality).

14.4 Experiments

14.4.1 Sleep EEG with Arousal

The first application to medical time series analysis demonstrates the use of the variational HMM to features extracted from a section of electroencephalogram data. The recordings were taken from a subject during a sleep experiment. The study looked at changes of cortical activity during sleep in response to external stimuli (e.g. from a vibrating pillow under the subject's head). The fractional spectral radius (FSR) measure and spectral entropy [19] were computed for consecutive non-overlapping windows of one second length. In Figure 14.6, the model clearly shows a preference for a 3-dimensional state space. Figure 14.7 shows a 10-minute section of data with the corresponding Viterbi state sequence. The data is segmented into the following regimes: wake (state 2, first 90 s of the recording), deeper sleep (state 1) and light sleep (state 3) which is clearly visible at sleep onset ($t \approx 90$ s) and at the arousal ($t \approx 200$ s).

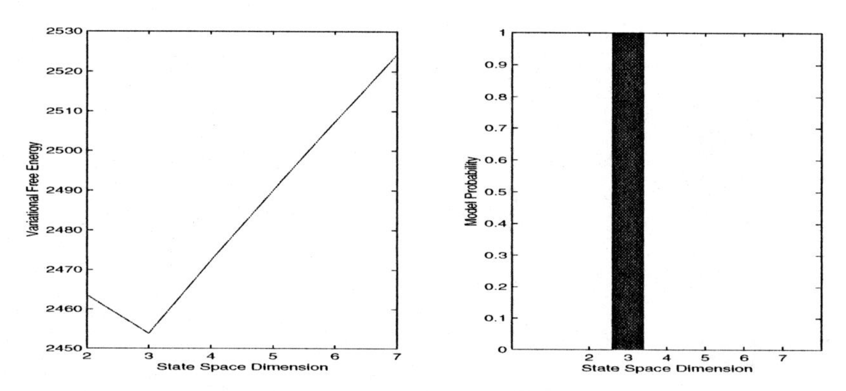

Fig. 14.6. State space dimension selection

14.4.2 Whole-Night Sleep EEG

In the following example we study the use of the HMM in segmenting EEG recordings for sleep staging. The data was recorded from one female subject exhibiting poor sleep quality during an 8-hour session in a sleep laboratory. The data was manually scored by three different sleep experts based on the standard Rechtschaffen and Kales (R&K) system [18]. The majority vote was

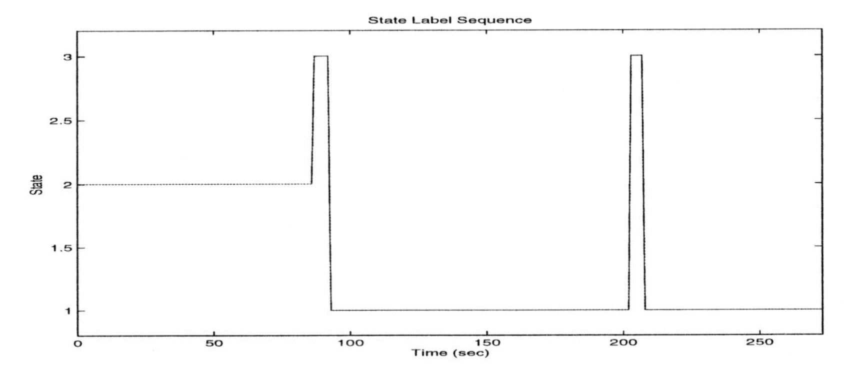

Fig. 14.7. HMM sleep EEG segmentation

then taken, to overcome disagreements between manual labels, resulting in a consensus score.

The data used here was recorded at the electrode sites $C4$ [14] using a 200 Hz sampling rate. The state space dimension was set to 7, corresponding to the number of states according to R&K. The confusion matrix (Table 14.1) based on the consensus score shows, however, that only 4 states are used by the HMM. One such state corresponds clearly to deep sleep, i.e. sleep stage 4. Corresponding somewhat less strongly, are state 2 of the HMM with the lighter sleep stages 2 and 3. Class 3 of the HMM is predominantly visited when the subject resides in REM sleep, according to the experts. It is interesting to note that the HMM exhibits the same difficulty humans face when trying to distinguish REM sleep from light sleep (stages 1 and 2). Finally, the weakest association between the HMM and human labels is observed in HMM class 4. Seemingly mostly connected with the Wake state, much overlap also exists between it and sleep stage 2, hence the significance of this last class is uncertain.

The table is best summarised by the estimated HMM state sequence. Figure 14.8 shows the hypnogram with a filtered Viterbi state sequence (using an 11-th order median filter). The filtering is justified by noting that human labels are over a 30 s long data segment and are based on the occurrence of a particular distinctive feature within that time period. The algorithm, on the other hand, calculates the label based on the most frequent class for that segment, on a one-second resolution.

14.4.3 Periodic Respiration

We also applied the HMM to features extracted from a section of Cheyne Stokes (CS) Data, [3] consisting of one EEG recording and a simultaneous

[3] A breathing disorder in which bursts of fast respiration are interspersed with breathing absence.

Table 14.1. HMM Gaussian observation confusion matrix

HMM Class	Manual sleep score S4	S3	S2	S1	REM	Movement	Wake
Class 1	0.9086	0.0600	0.0092	0	0	0.0222	0
Class 2	0.1014	0.1978	0.6889	0.0060	0	0.0060	0
Class 3	0	0	0.2191	0.1561	0.6027	0.0118	0.0103
Class 4	0	0.1250	0.2159	0.1477	0	0	0.5114

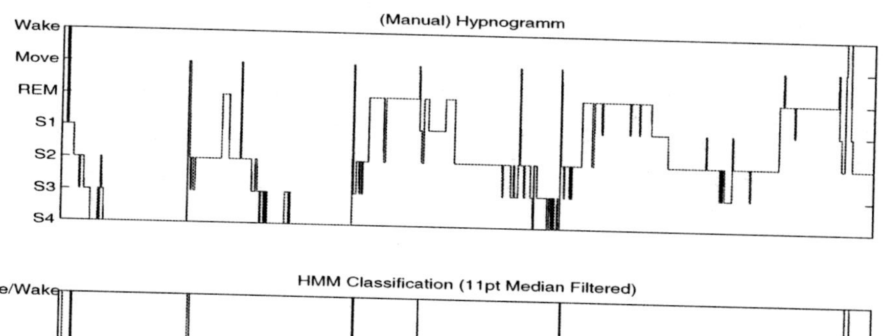

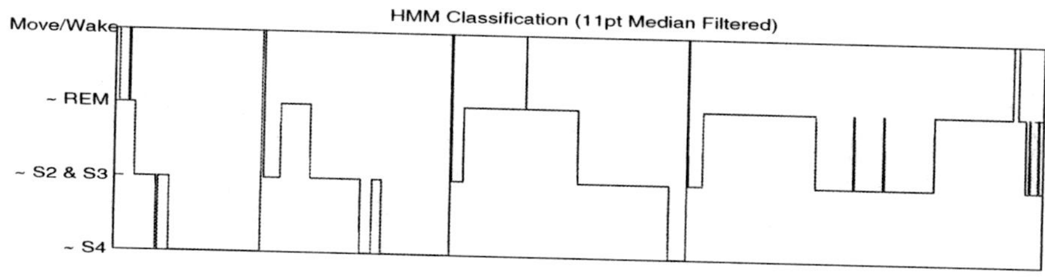

Fig. 14.8. Manual and estimated sleep segmentation of 1 night sleep EEG.

respiration recording, both sampled at 128 Hz. The fractional spectral radius (FSR) [19], was computed from consecutive non-overlapping windows of two seconds length for the EEG and respiration signals separately. The features thus extracted jointly formed a 2-dimensional feature space to which the HMM was then applied. As seen in Figure 14.9, the model clearly shows a preference for a 4-dimensional state space. Figure 14.10 shows a data section with the corresponding Viterbi state sequence. The data is segmented predominantly into the following regimes: segments of arousal from sleep, wake state with rapid respiration, and two sleep states different only in the EEG micro-structure.

14.4.4 Heartbeat Intervals

In order the apply the Poisson model of the HMM, we took a sequence of RR-intervals, obtained from the RR-Data base at UPC, Barcelona. A subject (Identifier RPP1, Male, Age: 25 years, Height: 178cm, Weight: 70kg) underwent a controlled respiration experiment. While sitting, the subject took six

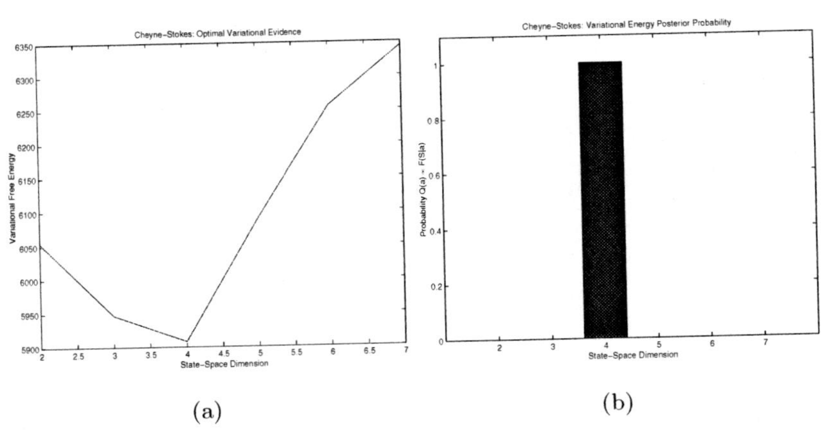

Fig. 14.9. Model order for CS-data: variational free energy and model probability.

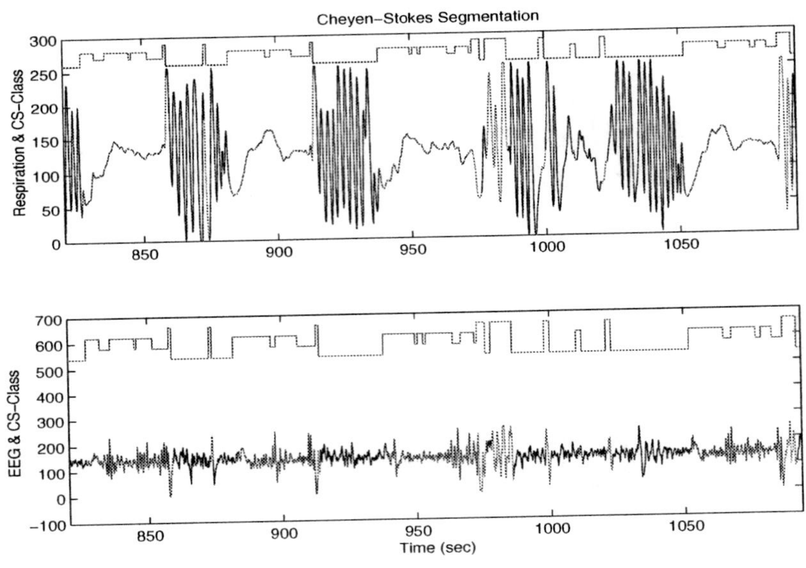

Fig. 14.10. CS-data: respiration and EEG signals with their respective segmentation.

deep breaths between 30 and 90 seconds after recording onset (ECG signal sampling rate is 1 kHz). The optimal segmentation was found to be three states and is shown in Figure 14.11. The top plot depicts the original RR-interval time series and the middle plot the state labels resulting from the Viterbi path. The segmentation based on the Viterbi path is shown in the bottom plot. A change in state dynamics is clearly visible in the state sequence between 30 and 90 seconds, i.e. the period during with the subject took deep breaths. The state dynamics parallel those observed in the heart-rate signal, obtained from the RR-intervals by interpolation. The difference, however, is that the state sequence is essentially a smoothed version of the heart-rate signal as several heart-rate levels will fall into one state. In addition, no interpolation as such is done, i.e. the HMM derives the heart rate statistically, which is in deep contrast to traditional heart-rate analysis.

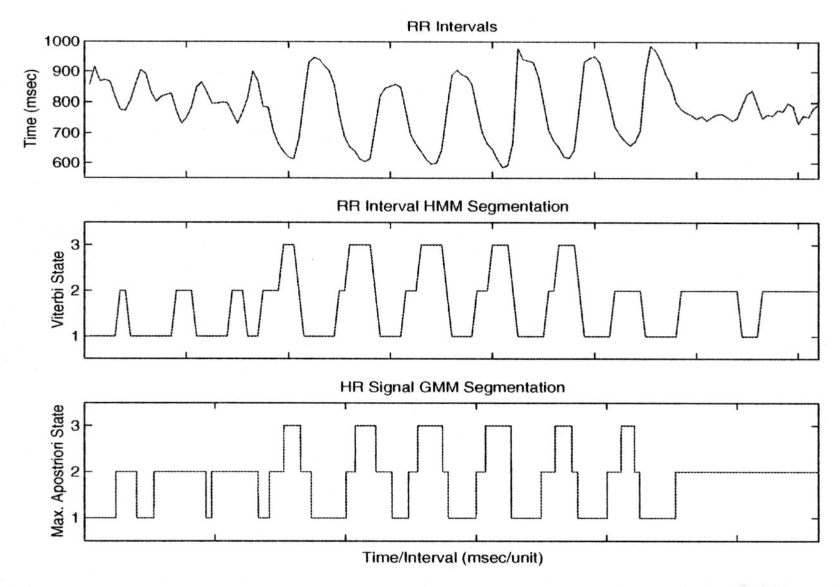

Fig. 14.11. HMM 3-stage Viterbi segmentation for subject RPP1 during controlled respiration experiments.

14.4.5 Segmentation of Cognitive Tasks

The idea of the brain–computer interface (BCI) experiment is that we infer the unknown cognitive state of a subject from his brain signals which we record via surface EEG. The data in this study were obtained with an ISO-DAM system using a gain of 10^4 and a fourth order band pass filter with pass band between 0.1 Hz and 100 Hz and sampled at 384 Hz with 12-bit resolution.

The BCI experiments were done by several young, healthy and untrained subjects who performed auditory imagination and imagined spatial navigation tasks. Each task was done for 7 seconds with an experiment consisting of 10 repetitions of alternating these tasks. The recordings were taken from two electrode sites: T4, P4. The ground electrode was placed just lateral to the left mastoid process.

We train the HMM with a linear observation model on the EEG of one subject. We used the first five repetitions for the auditory imagination and imagined spatial navigation task and computed the Viterbi path for two further repetitions of each task. Thus 70 s of data constituted the training data, while the test data was 28 s long. The Viterbi path for the (optimal) three-state model is shown in Figure 14.12. The experiment shows that there is a clear change in state dynamics between the different cognitive tasks. We obtain one model almost entirely allocated to the auditory task and two models that are almost exclusively used in the navigation task.

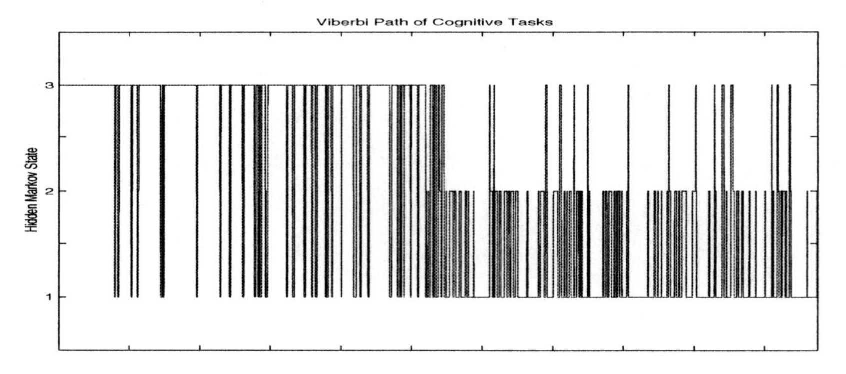

Fig. 14.12. HMM 3-stage Viterbi segmentation for two cognitive tasks, corresponding to the first and second half of the recoding, respectively (total duration 28 s).

14.5 Conclusion

The goal of the variational approach applied to learning HMMs was, first, to improve in some aspect of the traditional maximum likelihood method and, second, to find a unifying view of for deriving all variables, hidden states and parameters. In most cases, the existence of priors densities over the parameters resulted in an improved stability of the model. In some cases the automatic pruning effects of the estimators, which being completely consistent with the theory, is a nice added feature. By deriving all update equations from one single cost function, it has also become clear that the maximum likelihood method is a point estimate in the model parameters, while actually Bayesian in the hidden state space. The variational approach, on the other hand, is consistent from a theoretical point of view and it casts light on the mathematical origin of the Baum-Welch recursions.

While the variational estimators have so far proved to be much more robust than the maximum likelihood based estimators, they also come with a price, i.e. the number of parameters increased considerably. It is no longer enough to estimate single parameter values, but also their distributions. In practice this means that estimator initialisation is considerably more involved.

The examples presented in this chapter do not permit any conclusions as to the quality of the estimator, for example with regards to stability of the solutions found or sensitivity to initial conditions and priors. Much is left to understand the estimators better, however, the initial results seem quite promising.

Acknowledgments

The authors would like to thank R. Conradt for her invaluable contributions to this research and L. Pickup for her help in typesetting. I.R. is supported by the UK EPSRC to whom we are most grateful. We also like to thank Dr. M.A.García González from the Electronic Engineering Department at the Polytechnique University of Catalonia in Barcelona for providing the RR-interval recording (available at `http://petrus.upc.es/~wwwdib/people/GARCIA_MA/database/main.htm`).

A Model Free Update Equations

Following [6] we re-derive the model free variational learning functionals for continuous distributions.

In general we aim to estimate the following KL divergence

$$\begin{aligned} D(q\|p) \triangleq \mathcal{F} &= \int Q(S) \log \frac{Q(S)}{P(S|X)} \,\mathrm{d}S \\ &= \int Q(S) \log \frac{Q(S)}{P(S,X)} \,\mathrm{d}S - \log P(X), \end{aligned}$$

where $\log P(X)$ is the data log-likelihood. The second form makes clear that $D(q\|p)$ is bounded from below by $\log P(X)$ and attains $\log P(X)$ only if

$$D(Q(S)\|P(S|X)) = 0 \ ,$$

i.e. $Q(S) = P(S|X)$). Given a set of variables $S = \{S_1, \ldots, S_T\}$, in the mean field scenario we assume that

$$Q(S) = \prod_i^T Q(S_i).$$

The set S incorporates all possible variables, hidden variables and "hidden" parameters alike. Without loss, we split the set S in the form $S = \{S_i, \bar{S}_i\}$, where $\bar{S}_i = \{S_1, \ldots, S_{i-1}, S_{i+1}, \ldots, S_T\}$, so that $Q(S) = Q(S_i)Q(\bar{S}_i)$ and $P(S,X) = P(S_i, X|\bar{S}_i)P(\bar{S}_i)$. In all cases we have the additional constraint that $\int Q(S_i) \,\mathrm{d}S_i = 1$. Thus, we are seeking to minimise

$$\mathcal{F}(S) = \int Q(S) \log \frac{Q(S)}{P(S,X)} \,\mathrm{d}S + \sum_{i=1}^T \lambda_i \left(\int Q(S_i) \,\mathrm{d}S_i - 1 \right).$$

Under the mean field assumption this can be expanded and simplified to

$$\begin{aligned} \mathcal{F}(S) \triangleq & \int Q(\bar{S}_i) \log Q(\bar{S}_i) \,\mathrm{d}\bar{S}_i - \int Q(\bar{S}_i) \log P(\bar{S}_i) \,\mathrm{d}\bar{S}_i + \\ & \int Q(S_i) \log Q(S_i) \,\mathrm{d}S_i - \int Q(\bar{S}_i) \log P(S_i, X|\bar{S}_i) \,\mathrm{d}\bar{S}_i + \\ & \sum_{i=1}^T \lambda_i \left(\int Q(S_i) \,\mathrm{d}S_i - 1 \right). \end{aligned}$$

Thus,

$$\frac{d\mathcal{F}(S)}{dQ(S_i)} = \log(Q(S_i)) + 1 - \int Q(\bar{S}_i) \log P(\bar{S}_i, X|\bar{S}_i) \,\mathrm{d}\bar{S}_i + \lambda_i = 0.$$

Integrating the above expression within symmetric integration bounds we obtain a solution for λ_i,

$$\exp(-1-\lambda_i)^{-1} = \int \exp\left(\int Q(\bar{S}_i)\log P(S_i, X|\bar{S}_i)\,\mathrm{d}\bar{S}_i\right)\mathrm{d}S_i,$$

which can be inserted into the partial the solution for the functional $Q(S_i)$ to obtain

$$Q(S_i) = \frac{1}{\int \exp\left(\int Q(\bar{S}_i)\log P(S_i, X|\bar{S}_i)\,\mathrm{d}\bar{S}_i\right)\,\mathrm{d}S_i} \exp\left(\int Q(\bar{S}_i)\log P(S_i, X|\bar{S}_i)\,\mathrm{d}\bar{S}_i\right)$$

or, in short,

$$Q(S_i) \propto \exp \int Q(\bar{S}_i)\log P(S_i, X|\bar{S}_i)\,\mathrm{d}\bar{S}_i.$$

In deriving these equations we found the derivative of $F(S)$ using the total differential and thus partial derivatives. Therefore, in optimising one distribution $Q(S_i)$, all others are held constant.

B Derivation of the Baum-Welch Recursions

We start with the KL divergence (14.41), again denoting the entire set of hidden state variables by $S = \{S_1, \ldots, S_T\}$ and all the observations by $X = \{X_1, \ldots, X_T\}$:

$$\mathcal{F} = \int Q(S)\log\frac{Q(S)}{P(S)}\mathrm{d}S \tag{14.41}$$

$$= \int Q(S)\log Q(S)\mathrm{d}S - \int Q(S)\log P(S)\mathrm{d}S \tag{14.42}$$

where the first integral in equation (14.42) is just the entropy, denoted by $H(S)$. For a HMM,

$$P(S, X) = P(S_0)\prod_{t=1}^{T} P(S_t|S_{t-1})P(X_t|S_t) = \prod_{t=1}^{T}\frac{P(X_t, S_t, S_{t-1})}{P(S_{t-1})}$$

For ease of notation, it is sufficient for the moment to assume that each node S_t has an associated datum X_t, and we omit the extra variable X_t in the notation of the joint distribution. Thus

$$P(S) = P(S_0)\prod_{t=1}^{T}\frac{P(S_t, S_{t-1})}{P(S_{t-1})},$$

and identically for the Q joint distribution:

$$Q(S) = Q(S_0) \prod_{t=1}^{T} \frac{Q(S_t, S_{t-1})}{Q(S_{t-1})}.$$

Substituting into equation (14.42), and abbreviating $l(S) = \log P(S)$, we have

$$\mathcal{F} = H(S) - \sum_{t=1}^{T} \int Q(S_t, S_{t-1}) l(S_t, S_{t-1}) \mathrm{d}S_{t-1}^{t} + \sum_{t=1}^{T-1} \int Q(S_t) l(S_t) \mathrm{d}S_t$$

where the entropy term is

$$H(S) = \sum_{t=1}^{T} \int Q(S_t, S_{t-1}) \log Q(S_t, S_{t-1}) \mathrm{d}S_{t-1}^{t} - \sum_{t=1}^{T-1} \int Q(S_t) \log Q(S_t) \mathrm{d}S_t.$$

Before minimising $\mathcal{F}$ there are some additional constraints required to obtain a consistent solution. These relate to the fact that it must be possible to integrate out over one of the variables in the all of the joint distributions and be left with an identical marginal distribution:

$$\int Q(S_t, S_{t-1}) \mathrm{d}S_{t-1} = Q(S_t) = \int Q(S_t, S_{t+1}) \mathrm{d}S_{t+1}$$

Introducing Lagrange multipliers for each of these constraints, the full expression for $\mathcal{F}$ becomes

$$\begin{aligned} \mathcal{F} = & \sum_{t=1}^{T} \int Q(S_t, S_{t-1}) \log Q(S_t, S_{t-1}) \mathrm{d}S_{t-1}^{t} - \sum_{t=1}^{T-1} \int Q(S_t) \log Q(S_t) \mathrm{d}S_t - \\ & \sum_{t=1}^{T} \int Q(S_t, S_{t-1}) l(S_t, S_{t-1}) \mathrm{d}S_{t-1}^{t} + \sum_{t=1}^{T-1} \int Q(S_t) l(S_t) \mathrm{d}S_t + \\ & \lambda_{t,t-1}(S_t) \Big(Q(S_t) - \sum_{S_{t-1}} Q(S_t, S_{t-1}) \Big) + \\ & \mu_{t,t-1}(S_{t-1}) \Big(Q(S_{t-1}) - \sum_{S_t} Q(S_t, S_{t-1}) \Big). \end{aligned}$$

Differentiating with respect to $Q(S_t, S_{t-1})$

$$Q(S_t, S_{t-1}) = \frac{1}{z_{t,t-1}} e^{l(S_t, S_{t-1})} e^{\lambda_{t,t-1}(S_t)} e^{\mu_{t,t-1}(S_{t-1})} \tag{14.43}$$

where the constants of integration have been re-written in the form of a scaling factor $\frac{1}{z}$. Likewise, differentiating with respect to the marginals, $Q(S_t)$,

$$Q(S_t) = \frac{1}{z_t} e^{l(S_t)} e^{\lambda_{t,t-1}(S_t)} e^{\mu_{t+1,t}(S_t)} \tag{14.44}$$

There are two joint distributions defined over $Q(St)$, namely $Q(S_t, S_{t-1})$ and $Q(S_t, S_{t+1})$. By marginalising out S_{t-1} and S_{t+1} in (14.43),

$$Q(S_t) = \sum_{S_{t-1}} \frac{1}{z_{t,t-1}} e^{l(S_t,S_{t-1})} e^{\lambda_{t,t-1}(S_t)} e^{\mu_{t,t-1}(S_{t-1})} \quad (14.45)$$

and

$$Q(S_t) = \sum_{S_{t+1}} \frac{1}{z_{t+1,t}} e^{l(S_{t+1},S_t)} e^{\lambda_{t+1,t}(S_{t+1})} e^{\mu_{t+1,t}(S_t)} \quad (14.46)$$

Equating the expressions for $Q(S_t)$ from (14.44) and (14.46) one can solve for the first Lagrange multiplier,

$$e^{\lambda_{t,t-1}(S_t)} = z_t e^{-l(S_t)} \sum_{S_{t+1}} \frac{1}{z_{t+1,t}} e^{l(S_{t+1},S_t)} e^{\lambda_{t+1,t}(S_{t+1})} \quad (14.47)$$

and, similarly, equating the expressions for $Q(S_t)$ from (14.44) and (14.45):

$$e^{\mu_{t+1,t}(S_t)} = z_t e^{-l(S_t)} \sum_{S_{t-1}} \frac{1}{z_{t,t-1}} e^{l(S_t,S_{t-1})} e^{\mu_{t,t-1}(S_{t-1})} \quad (14.48)$$

Substituting $\beta(t)$ for $e^{\lambda_{t,t-1}(S_t)}$ in (14.47) gives

$$\beta(t) = \frac{1}{z_t} \sum_{S_{t+1}} P(S_{t+1}|S_t)\beta(t+1),$$

and substitution of $\alpha(t) = e^{\mu_{t+1,t}(S_t)} P(S_t)$ in (14.48) gives

$$\alpha(t) = z_t \sum_{S_{t-1}} P(S_t|S_{t-1})\alpha(t-1)$$

Finally, restating (14.43) using $\alpha(t)$ and $\beta(t)$ leads to the well-known equation of the joint distributions

$$\begin{aligned} Q(S_t, S_{t-1}) &= \frac{1}{z_{t,t-1}} e^{l(S_t,S_{t-1})} e^{\lambda_{t,t-1}(S_t)} e^{\mu_{t,t-1}(S_{t-1})} \\ &= \frac{1}{z_{t,t-1}} P(S_t, S_{t-1})\beta(t) \left(\frac{\alpha(t-1)}{P(S_{t-1})} \right) \\ &= \frac{1}{z_{t,t-1}} P(S_t|S_{t-1})\beta(t)\alpha(t-1) \end{aligned}$$

C Complete KL Divergences

To monitor the convergence of the variational algorithm and to test for the best model order/size, requires the calculation of the complete KL divergence (14.12), given the data. The general overall KL divergence (14.12) can be split into the following three terms,

$$\mathcal{F} = \underbrace{-\int q(S)q(\theta) \log P(X, S|\theta) \, \mathrm{d}S \, \mathrm{d}\theta}_{\text{average log-likelihood}} + \underbrace{\int q(S) \log q(S) \, \mathrm{d}S}_{\text{negative entropy}} + \underbrace{\int q(\theta) \log \frac{q(\theta)}{P(\theta)} \, \mathrm{d}\theta}_{\text{KL divergence}} \tag{14.49}$$

All terms vary depending on the observation model, with the exception of the negative entropy term, which only changes if the HMM topology changes. The KL divergence measures the divergence between the prior and approximate posterior distributions. Since all the models here are within the exponential family, the mathematical form of many KL divergence terms occurs repeatedly. Hence we list these forms separately and refer back to them when needed.

C.1 Negative Entropy

The neg-entropy term for HMMs is

$$H_{_{HMM}} = H(S_{t=0}) + \sum_{t=1}^{T} H(S_t|S_{t-1}) \tag{14.50}$$

$$= \sum_{t=1}^{T} H(S_t, S_{t-1}) - H(S_t) \tag{14.51}$$

C.2 KL Divergences

The KL divergence in equation (14.49) measures the divergence between the prior and approximate posterior distributions. Many of them occur repeatedly. Given two densities, Q and P, which have parameters indexed by q and p, and using the notation of [1] and [5], the KL divergences between two Dirichlet, Wishart and multi-variate Normal densities are given as follows:

- Between two Dirichlet densities

$$D_{\mathcal{D}ir}(q\|p) = \log \left(\frac{\Gamma(\sum_{l=1}^{k} \alpha_{ql})}{\Gamma(\sum_{l=1}^{k} \alpha_{pl})} \right) + \sum_{l=1}^{k} \log \frac{\Gamma(\alpha_{pl})}{\Gamma(\alpha_{ql})} + \sum_{l=1}^{k} (\alpha_{ql} - \alpha_{pl}) \left(\Psi(\alpha_{ql}) - \Psi\left(\sum_{l=1}^{k} \alpha_{ql} \right) \right) \tag{14.52}$$

- Between two Gamma densities

$$D_{\mathcal{G}}(q\|p) = \log \frac{\Gamma(\alpha_p)}{\Gamma(\alpha_q)} + (\alpha_q - \alpha_p)\Psi(\alpha_q) + \alpha_q \log \frac{\beta_q}{\beta_p} + \alpha_q \left(\beta_p \beta_q^{-1} - 1 \right) \tag{14.53}$$

- Between two Wishart densities

$$D_{\mathcal{W}}(q\|p) = \sum_{l=1}^{k} \log \frac{\Gamma(\frac{1}{2}(2\alpha_p + 1 - l))}{\Gamma(\frac{1}{2}(2\alpha_q + 1 - l))} + (\alpha_q - \alpha_p) \sum_{l=1}^{k} \Psi\left(\frac{2\alpha_q + 1 - l}{2}\right)$$
$$+\alpha_q \log \frac{|B_q|}{|B_p|} + \alpha_q \left(\mathrm{tr}\left(B_p B_q^{-1}\right) - k\right) \tag{14.54}$$

- Between two multivariate Normal densities

$$D_{\mathcal{M}v\mathcal{N}}(q\|p) = \frac{1}{2}\left(\log \frac{\lambda_q}{\lambda_p} - 1 + \lambda_p \lambda_q^{-1} + (\mu_q - \mu_p)^{\mathsf{T}} \lambda_p (\mu_q - \mu_p)\right) \tag{14.55}$$

- Between two $m \times n$ matrix variate Normal densities

$$D_{\mathcal{M}a\mathcal{V}\mathcal{N}}(q\|p) = \frac{1}{2}\left\{n \log \frac{|\Sigma_q|}{|\Sigma_p|} + m \log \frac{|\Phi_q|}{|\Phi_p|} + \mathrm{tr}\left(\Phi_p \Phi_q^{-1}\right) \mathrm{tr}\left(\Sigma_p \Sigma_q^{-1}\right)\right.$$
$$\left. + \mathrm{tr}\left(\Sigma_p \left(M_q - M_p\right) \Phi_p \left(M_q - M_p\right)^{\mathsf{T}}\right) - nm\right\} \tag{14.56}$$

C.3 Gaussian Observation HMM

The average log-likelihood term in (14.49) for Gaussian observation models is given as

$$\begin{aligned}
\mathcal{L}_{avg} = & \sum_m \gamma_{t_0} \Psi(\tilde{\lambda}_{0_m}) - \bar{\gamma}_0 \Psi(\sum_l \tilde{\lambda}_{0_l}) + \\
& \sum_{m,n} \bar{\xi}(m,n) \Psi(\tilde{\lambda}_{m_n}) - \sum_n \bar{\bar{\xi}}(n) \Psi(\sum_l \tilde{\lambda}_{l_n}) + \\
& T \log(2\pi)^{\frac{K}{2}} + \frac{1}{2} \bar{\gamma}_m \bar{\Psi}_{\tilde{\alpha}_m} - \frac{1}{2} \bar{\gamma}_m \log |\tilde{B}_m| - \\
& \frac{1}{2} \sum_t \gamma_{t_m} (x_t - \tilde{\mu}_{m_0})^{\mathsf{T}} \tilde{\alpha}_m \tilde{B}_m (x_t - \tilde{\mu}_{m_0}) - \frac{1}{2} \bar{\gamma}_m \mathrm{tr}\left(\tilde{\alpha}_m \tilde{B}_m \tilde{C}_{m_0}\right)
\end{aligned} \tag{14.57}$$

where

$$\begin{aligned}
\bar{\gamma}_0 &= \sum_m \gamma_{0_m} , \\
\bar{\gamma}_m &= \sum_t \gamma_{t_m} , \\
\bar{\xi}(m,n) &= \sum_t \xi_t(m,n) , \\
\bar{\bar{\xi}}(n) &= \sum_t \sum_m \xi_t(m,n) ,
\end{aligned} \tag{14.58}$$

and

$$\bar{\Psi}_{\tilde{\alpha}_m} = \sum_k \Psi\left(\frac{1}{2}(2\tilde{\alpha}_m + 1 - k)\right) . \tag{14.59}$$

C.4 Poisson Observation HMM

The average log-likelihood term for a Poisson observation HMM can be shown to be

$$\mathcal{L}_{avg} = \sum_{m,n} \gamma_{nm} \left[-x_n \tilde{\alpha}_m \tilde{\beta}_m + y_n \log(x_n) + y_i \left(\Psi(\tilde{\alpha}_m) - \log(\tilde{\beta}_m)\right) - \log(y_n!)\right] \tag{14.60}$$

The KL divergence between the approximate posterior density $Q(\mu_m)$, with parameters $\tilde{\alpha}_0, \tilde{\beta}_0$, and the prior $P(\mu_m)$, with parameters α_0, β_0, is a standard Gamma density divergence $D_{\mathcal{G}}(Q(\mu_m)\|P(\mu_m))$, given by equation (14.53).

C.5 Linear Observation Model HMM

The average log-likelihood term for the HMMs with linear observation models is given as

$$\begin{aligned}
\mathcal{L}_{avg} = & -N\frac{du}{2}\log(2\pi) - \frac{u}{2}\sum_m \bar{\gamma}_m \log|\tilde{B}_{\Sigma m}| \\
& + \sum_m \bar{\gamma}_m \left(\Psi(\tilde{\rho}_m) - \Psi(\sum_{m=1}^{M} \tilde{\rho}_m) + \frac{u}{2}\sum_{l=1}^{d} \Psi\left(\frac{1}{2}(2\tilde{\alpha}_{\Sigma m} + 1 - l)\right)\right) \\
& - \sum_{n,m} \left\{\gamma_{nm} \ \frac{1}{2}\mathrm{tr}\left(\tilde{\alpha}_{\Sigma m}\tilde{B}_{\Sigma m}^{-1}(Y_n - \tilde{\Omega}_m X_n)(Y_n - \tilde{\Omega}_m X_n)^{\mathsf{T}}\right)\right\} \\
& - \frac{1}{2}\sum_m \tilde{\alpha}_{\Sigma m} \ \mathrm{tr}\left(\tilde{B}_{\Sigma m}^{-1}\tilde{\Sigma}_m^{-1}\right)\sum_n \gamma_{nm} \ \mathrm{tr}\left(X_n X_n^{\mathsf{T}} \tilde{\Phi}_m^{-1}\right)
\end{aligned} \tag{14.61}$$

The KL divergences are given as

$$\begin{aligned}
D(Q(\theta)\|P(\theta)) = & \sum_m \left\langle D_{\mathcal{M}a\mathcal{V}\mathcal{N}}(Q(H_m)\|P(H_m|\Sigma_m, \Phi_m))\right\rangle_{Q(\Sigma_m,\Phi_m)} && (14.62) \\
& + \sum_m D_{\mathcal{W}}(Q(\Sigma_m)\|P(\Sigma_m)) && (14.63) \\
& + \sum_m D_{\mathcal{W}}(Q(\Phi_m)\|P(\Phi_m)) && (14.64) \\
& + D_{\mathcal{D}ir}(Q(\boldsymbol{\kappa})\|P(\boldsymbol{\kappa})) && (14.65)
\end{aligned}$$

where divergences (14.63), (14.64) and (14.65) are given by (14.54), (14.54) and (14.52), respectively, and divergence (14.62) is given by

$$\begin{aligned}
&\Big\langle D_{\mathcal{M}a\mathcal{VN}}(Q(H_m)\|P(H_m|\Sigma_m,\Phi_m))\Big\rangle_{Q(\Sigma_m,\Phi_m)} \\
&\quad=\frac{1}{2}\Big\{(dp)\log|\tilde{\Sigma}_m| + d\log|\tilde{\Phi}_m| - d^2p \\
&\quad - (dp)\left(\sum_{l=1}^{d}\Psi\left(\frac{2\tilde{\alpha}_{\Sigma m}+1-l}{2}\right) - \log|\tilde{B}_{\Sigma m}|\right) \\
&\quad - d\left(\sum_{l=1}^{dp}\Psi\left(\frac{2\tilde{\alpha}_{\Phi m}+1-l}{2}\right) - \log|\tilde{B}_{\Phi m}|\right) \\
&\quad + \operatorname{tr}\left(\tilde{\alpha}_{\Phi m}\tilde{B}_{\Phi m}^{-1}\tilde{\Phi}_m^{-1}\right)\operatorname{tr}\left(\tilde{\alpha}_{\Sigma m}\tilde{B}_{\Sigma m}^{-1}\tilde{\Sigma}_m^{-1}\right) \\
&\quad + \operatorname{tr}\left(\tilde{\alpha}_{\Sigma m}\tilde{B}_{\Sigma m}^{-1}(\tilde{\Omega}_m-\Omega)\tilde{\alpha}_{\Phi m}\tilde{B}_{\Phi m}^{-1}(\tilde{\Omega}_m-\Omega)^{\mathsf{T}}\right)\Big\}
\end{aligned} \tag{14.66}$$

References

[1] J.M. Bernardo and A.F.M. Smith. *Bayesian Theory.* John Wiley and Sons, 1994.

[2] T.M. Cover and J.A. Thomas. *Elements of Information Theory.* John Wiley & Sons, New York, 1991.

[3] A. Flexer, G. Dorffner, P. Sykacek, and I. Rezek. An automatic, continuous and probabilistic sleep stager based on a hidden Markov model. *Applied Artificial Intelligence*, 16(3):199–207, 2002.

[4] A. Gelman, J.B. Carlin, H.S. Stern, and D.B. Rubin. *Bayesian Data Analysis.* Chapman & Hall/CRC, 2000.

[5] A.K. Gupta and D.K. Nagar. *Matrix Variate Distributions.* Monographs and Surveys in Pure and Applied Mathematics. Number 104. Chapman & Hall/CRC, 2000.

[6] M. Haft, R. Hofmann, and V. Tresp. Model-independent mean field theory as a local method for approximate propagation of information. *Computation in Neural Systems*, 10:93–105, 1999.

[7] D. Heckerman. A tutorial on learning with Bayesian networks. Technical Report MSR-TR-95-06, Microsoft Research, 1995.

[8] T.S. Jaakkola. Tutorial on variational approximation methods. In M. Opper and D. Saad, editors, *Advanced Mean Field Methods: Theory and Practice.* MIT Press, 2000.

[9] T.S. Jaakkola and M.I. Jordan. Improving the mean field approximation via the use of mixture distributions. In M.I. Jordan, editor, *Learning in Graphical Models.* Kluwer Academic Press, 1997.

[10] M.I. Jordan, Z. Ghahramani, T.S. Jaakkola, and L.K. Saul. An introduction to variational methods for graphical models. In M.I. Jordan, editor, *Learning in Graphical Models.* Kluwer Academic Press, 1997.

[11] B. Kemp. *Model-based monitoring of human sleep stages.* PhD thesis, Twente University of Technology, The Netherlands, 1987.

[12] D.J.C. MacKay. Ensemble learning for hidden Markov models. Technical Report, Cavendish Laboratory, 1998.

[13] B. Obermeier, C. Guger, C. Neuper, and G. Pfurtscheller. Hidden Markov models for online classification of single trial EEG. *Pattern Recognition Letters*, 22:1299–1309, 2001.

[14] C. Pastelak-Price. Das internationale 10-20-System zur Elektrodenplazierung: Begründung, praktische Anleitung zu den Meßschritten und Hinweise zum Setzen der Elektroden. *EEG-Labor*, 5:49–72, 1983.

[15] W.D. Penny, R. Everson, and S.J. Roberts. Hidden Markov independent component analysis. In M. Girolami, editor, *Advances in Independent Component Analysis*. Springer Verlag, 2000.

[16] W.D. Penny and S.J. Roberts. Dynamic models for nonstationary signal segmentation. *Computers and Biomedical Research*, 32(6):483–502, 1999.

[17] L. R. Rabiner. A tutorial on hidden Markov models and selected applications in speech recognition. *Proceeding of the IEEE*, 77(2):257–284, 1989.

[18] A. Rechtschaffen and A. Kales (eds). *A manual of standardized terminology, techniques and schoring system for sleep stages in human subjects.* US Public Health Service, US Government Printing Office, Washington DC, 1968.

[19] I. Rezek and S.J. Roberts. Stochastic complexity measures for physiological signal analysis. *IEEE Transactions on Biomedical Engineering*, 44 (9):1186–1191, 1998.

[20] C.P. Robert, T. Rydén, and D.M. Titterington. Bayesian inference in hidden Markov models through the reversible jump Markov chain Monte Carlo method. *Journal of the Royal Statistical Society, Series B*, 62(1): 57–75, 2000.

[21] O. Rompelman, J.B. Snijders, and C. van Spronsen. The measurement of heart rate variability spectra with the help of a personal computer. *IEEE Transactions on Biomedical Engineering*, 29:503–510, 1982.

[22] P. Sykacek and S.J. Roberts. Bayesian time series classification. In T.G. Dietterich, S. Becker, and Z. Ghahramani, editors, *Advances in Neural Information Processing Systems*, volume 14, 2001.

[23] N. Ueda, R. Nakano, Z. Ghahramani, and G.E. Hinton. SMEM algorithm for mixture models. *Neural Computation*, 12(9):2109–2128, 2000.

[24] S. Young, G. Evermann, D. Kershaw, G. Moore, J. Odell, D. Ollason, V. Valtchev, and P. Woodland. *The HTK Book*. Entropic, 1995.

15

A Probabilistic Network for Fusion of Data and Knowledge in Clinical Microbiology

Steen Andreassen[1], Leonard Leibovici[2], Mical Paul[2], Anders D. Nielsen[1], Alina Zalounina[1], Leif E. Kristensen[3], Karsten Falborg[3], Brian Kristensen[4], Uwe Frank[5], and Henrik C. Schønheyder[6]

[1] Center for Model-Based Medical Decision Support, Aalborg University, Fredrik Bajers Vej 7 C1, DK-9220 Aalborg East, Denmark
{sa,nielsen}@miba.auc.dk, az@mi.auc.dk

[2] Department of Medicine, Beilinson Campus, Rabin Medical Center, 49100 Petah-Tiqva, Israel
leibovic@post.tau.ac.il, mica@inter.net.il

[3] Judex Datasystemer, Lyngvej 8, DK-9000 Aalborg
{lek,kf}@judex.dk

[4] Department of Clinical Microbiology, Aarhus University Hospital, Nørrebrogade 44, DK-8000 Århus C, Denmark
bkr@miba.auc.dk

[5] Freiburg Universiy Hospital, Institut für Umweltmedizin und Krankenhaushygiene, Hugstetter Straße 55, D-79106 Freiburg, Germany
ufrank@iuk3.ukl.uni-freiburg.de

[6] Department of Clinical Microbiology, Aalborg Hospital, P.O. Box 365, DK - 9100 Aalborg, Denmark
u19212@aas.nja.dk

Summary. A problem in clinical microbiology is that of inappropriate antibiotic therapy. Various decision-support systems have been proposed to aid physicians in this domain, and we discuss the *a priori* advantages of using a probabilistic network over other approaches. The Treat project uses a probabilistic network to combine clinical signs, symptoms and laboratory results, and we discuss the problem of obtaining probabilities for the network. Finally, we consider how such a system can be tested in clinical practice and outline the results of our tests.

15.1 Introduction

Decision-support systems that provide advice on selection of antibiotics for bacterial infections have a long history going back to the Mycin system [17]. This long-standing interest in antibiotic therapy is not without reason: infections are a frequent cause of death, but the risk of death can be substantially reduced by appropriate antibiotic therapy [13]. In current clinical practice, about a third of patients with moderate to severe infections receive inappropriate antibiotic therapy resulting in increased morbidity, extended hospital stay, and increased mortality [11]. Of more importance for the role of decision-support systems, it can be noted that testing of decision-support systems indicates that antibiotic therapy can be improved beyond current clinical practice. Based on this assumption, partners in four countries – Denmark, Germany, Italy, and Israel – have embarked on the Treat project, with the aim of producing and testing a system that can improve antibiotic therapy beyond current clinical practice.

In this chapter we will first outline the considerations surrounding the institution of antibiotic therapy in clinical practice. We will then describe how we have translated these considerations into a decision-support system, called Treat, for selection of antibiotic therapy. The decision-support system is implemented using *causal probabilistic networks* (CPNs)[7] to calculate the probabilities of a range of events relevant to the selection of antibiotic therapy. Decision theory is then used to perform a cost-benefit analysis based on these probabilities, which results in advice on antibiotic therapy. The steps in the decision process will be illustrated through an example; namely, a patient with a urinary tract infection. As the example unfolds, it will provide an informal opportunity to describe the fusion of data of different types; for example, results of the physical examination of the patient, results of laboratory tests, and the results from cultures of the pathogens found in the blood stream. In this context, we have reserved the word "data" for information about a specific patient. The example will also provide an opportunity to discuss the fusion of knowledge. In this context, the word "knowledge" is reserved for information that can be applied across a population of patients. The knowledge used in CPNs is causal: it may be structural (e.g., that pathogens cause infection or that antibiotics may cure an infection), or it may be quantitative, typically represented in the form of a conditional probability. It will become apparent that the causal representation of knowledge allows a clear separation between the many types of knowledge required to build the system. This separation between different types of knowledge also makes it possible to divide the knowledge into two different types: knowledge that is assumed to be universally applicable, and knowledge that is specific for a given hospital and that may even change over time.

Some consideration on the testing of medical decision-support systems will be given and the results obtained so far from testing of the decision-support system will be described. The results are promising, and this provides some room for speculations on the reasons for this apparent success.

The structured approach that is possible with CPNs provides a high degree of modularity to the system. This makes it easier to construct the system and, perhaps more importantly, it makes the system robust to changes in the

[7] "Causal probabilistic network" is one of the synonyms for "Bayesian network" (see Section 10.9).

medical environment and increases maintainability. Changes in the prevalence of pathogens, the resistance to certain antibiotics, or the cost and availability of certain antibiotics are readily accommodated.

15.2 Institution of Antibiotic Therapy

The purpose of Treat is to assist in the selection of antibiotic therapy for moderate to severe infections, with either bacteria or fungi as the pathogen. This section will outline the process that in clinical practice leads to the decision on antibiotic therapy.

The relevant groups of patients are either patients with community-acquired infections, which are admitted to hospital with symptoms compatible with an infection, or patients with hospital-acquired infections, which are already hospitalized but, in the course of their hospitalization, develop symptoms of infection. In the following, we shall say that these patients with systemic symptoms of infection have varying degrees of sepsis. Some of them only have mild infections and, accordingly, only have some of the symptoms of sepsis (e.g., fever), some have all the symptoms associated with generally accepted definitions of sepsis [5], and the most severely affected patients are in a state of septic shock.

The attending clinician will usually draw a blood sample for culture from these patients in the hope that the pathogen(s) can be isolated from the blood sample. Per year, the number of blood samples drawn from "septic" patients is about 1800 per 100,000 inhabitants. This can be compared with the yearly incidence in the USA of 375 per 100,000 inhabitants that fulfil the clinical definition of sepsis [3]. In 10%–20% of the blood samples, which corresponds to about 200 cases per 100,000 inhabitants, bacteria are isolated. In these bacteraemic patients, the identity and the resistance of the pathogens to antibiotics can be determined, typically 2–3 days after the blood sample is drawn. Meanwhile, the clinician will institute the so-called empirical antibiotic treatment based on the data available at the time the blood sample was drawn.

The Treat system is designed to help in the later stages of treatment as the microbiological information becomes available. We shall limit our attention to the empirical treatment and the so-called semi-empirical treatment, which typically is instituted within two days of the onset of the infectious episode when microbiological results become available.

The components of the process leading to the decision on empirical treatment are [14]:

1. Assessment of sepsis
2. Determining the most likely site of infection
3. Identifying the most probable pathogen(s)
4. Choosing the antibiotic therapy with the best balance between cost (including purchase, side effects and ecological impact on future resistance) and gain (including increase in life expectancy and reduction of bed-days).

15.3 Calculation of Probabilities for Severity of Sepsis, Site of Infection, and Pathogens

This section will use a typical case of urinary tract infection to illustrate how the CPN can be used to calculate the probabilities for severity of sepsis, site of infection, and pathogens. This requires the fusion of many different types of data about the patient, some derived from the anamnesis, some from the physical examination, and some from the results of laboratory tests. The case example will also make it clear that many types of knowledge about infectious diseases are required to construct the CPN. The knowledge may be derived from textbooks or from a general understanding of the causal relations between the variables in the CPN, or it may be derived from case databases.

15.3.1 Patient Example (Part 1)

A 28-year-old female with fever and chills was referred to the Rabin Medical Center in Israel by her general practitioner. At the time of arrival at the hospital, no further details were available. In the outpatient clinic, she was questioned about her underlying conditions, the presence of implanted devices, and the presence of other current conditions. The answers are given in Figure 15.1 in the field labelled "Background conditions". Blood pressure and heart rate were measured, and a blood sample was taken. Apart from the fever and chills, all findings were normal with the exception of elevated values for leucocytes, neutrophils and creatinine, as shown in Figure 15.1 in the field labelled "Sepsis presentation".[8]

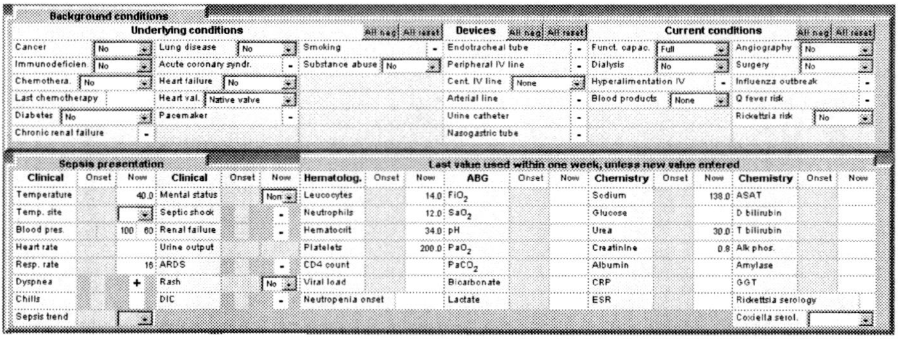

Fig. 15.1. Background conditions and sepsis presentation for the patient at the time of admission to the hospital.

[8] Coloured versions of the figures in this chapter are available from `http://robots.ox.ac.uk/~parg/pmbmi.html`

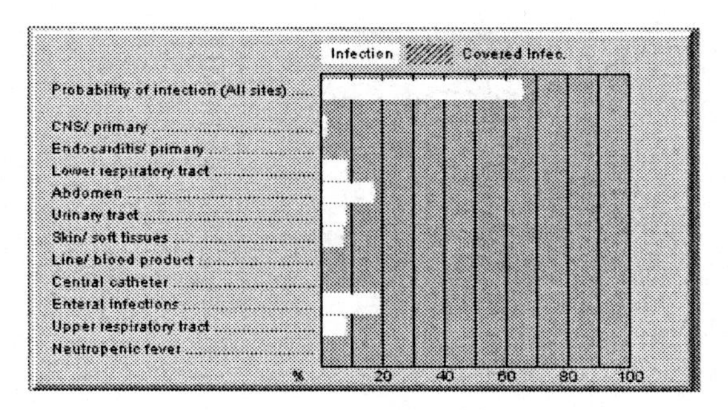

Fig. 15.2. The probability of infection and its distribution on the 11 possible sites of infection, given background conditions and sepsis presentation for the patient at the time of admission.

With this information entered, Treat can provide a preliminary opinion on the probability of an infection and the probability of the infection originating from each of the 11 sites of infection being considered by Treat. It can be seen from Figure 15.2 that the evidence in favour of an infection has not completely convinced Treat about the presence of an infection. The probability of infection is 64%, and this probability mass is distributed over seven out of the 11 potential sites of infection. The distribution on sites of infection mainly reflects the *a priori* probability of the different sites, except that the blood-sample results show that the patient is not neutropenic, and the absence of peripheral or central intravenous lines eliminates these as possible sites of infection. The absence of a visible bar for endocarditis does not reflect that this probability is zero: it merely reflects the low *a priori* probability of that condition.

The highest likelihood seen is for gastroenteritis and abdominal infections; therefore, an anamnesis and a physical examination were performed focusing on these sites. The findings were all negative, as indicated in Figure 15.3. With these findings entered, Treat almost excludes abdominal infection and gastroenteritis, as given in Figure 15.4.

The remaining part of the physical examination is now complete. All findings were negative, except for the urinary tract where the patient had dysuria and increased frequency of micturition and complained about flank tenderness (Figure 15.5(a)). With these findings, Treat ascribed close to 100% probability of a urinary tract infection and probabilities close to 0% for the other sites of infection (Figure 15.5(b)). The probabilities over the sites may add up to more than 100% because of the possibility of two simultaneous infections. In the present case there is, however, only evidence for a single site; namely, the urinary tract.

At this time, a blood sample was taken and sent to the microbiology laboratory for culture. A urine sample was also taken and analysed, and it showed microscopic hematuria and the presence of leucocytes in the urine (Figure

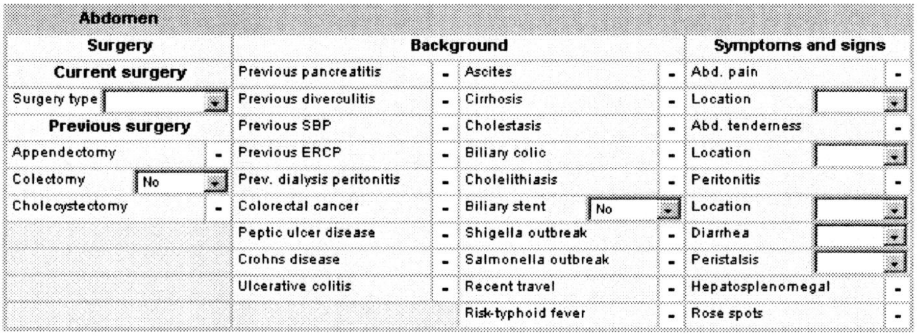

Abdomen
Surgery
Background
Symptoms and signs
Current surgery
Surgery type
Previous surgery
Appendectomy
Colectomy
No
Cholecystectomy
Previous pancreatitis
Previous diverculitis
Previous SBP
Previous ERCP
Prev. dialysis peritonitis
Colorectal cancer
Peptic ulcer disease
Crohns disease
Ulcerative colitis
Ascites
Cirrhosis
Cholestasis
Biliary colic
Cholelithiasis
Biliary stent
No
Shigella outbreak
Salmonella outbreak
Recent travel
Risk-typhoid fever
Abd. pain
Location
Abd. tenderness
Location
Peritonitis
Location
Diarrhea
Peristalsis
Hepatosplenomegal
Rose spots

Fig. 15.3. Anamnesis and results of the physical examination for abdominal infection and gastroenteritis.

Infection
Covered Infec.
Probability of infection (All sites)
CNS/ primary
Endocarditis/ primary
Lower respiratory tract
Abdomen
Urinary tract
Skin/ soft tissues
Line/ blood product
Central catheter
Enteral infections
Upper respiratory tract
Neutropenic fever
%
20
40
60
80
100

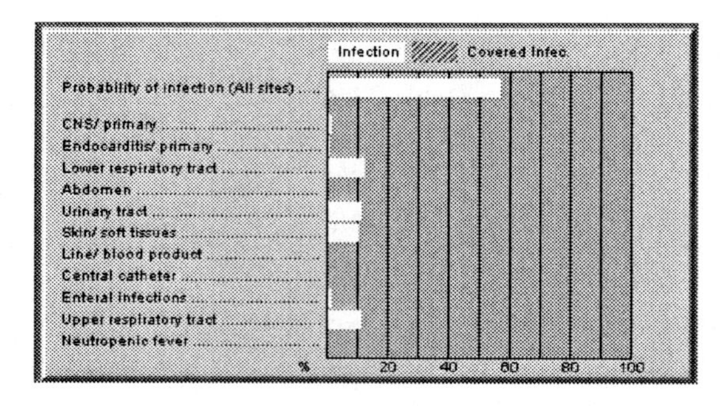

Fig. 15.4. The distribution of probability of infection over the sites when it is known that all findings related to the abdomen are negative.

15.6(a)). This reinforced the belief of a urinary tract infection, but since this already had a probability very close to 100% it made no difference. The absence of nitrites in the urine was puzzling because the pathogens listed in Figure 15.6(b) produce nitrite, except for "Enterococcus sp." and "Staphylococcus saprophyticus"; however, the sensitivity of the nitrite test was quite low (corresponding to a high rate of false negative findings) and the absence of nitrites was, therefore, only quite weak evidence against the majority of the pathogens. It was, however, enough to reduce the probability of most of the pathogens slightly and to allow the probability of the non-nitrite-producing pathogens, *Enterococcus sp.* and *Staphylococcus saprophyticus*, to increase, as shown in Figure 15.6(b).

15.3.2 Fusion of Data and Knowledge for Calculation of Probabilities for Sepsis and Pathogens

The calculation of all the probabilities mentioned above is performed by a CPN. In its present form, the CPN contains about 8500 nodes, each node

Symptoms and signs							
Dysuria	+	Frequency	+	Incontinence	-	Urogenital procedure	-
Suprapubic pain	-	Flank pain tenderness	+	Gross hematuria	-		

(a)

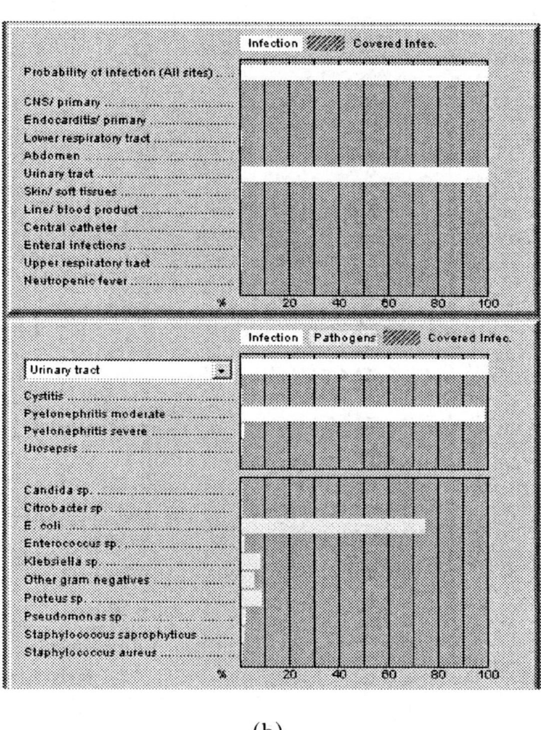

(b)

Fig. 15.5. (a) Findings related to the urinary tract excluding the urinalysis. (b) Upper panel: The distribution of probability of infection over the sites when the physical examination has been completed. Middle panel: The distribution of probability over four diagnoses related to urinary tract infection, cystitis, moderate and severe pyelonephritis, and urosepsis. Lower panel: The distribution of probabilities over the nine groups of pathogens considered for the urinary tract.

representing a discrete stochastic variable. The nodes are connected by directed links. The topology of the graph consisting of the nodes and links reflects the constructors' opinion about the causal relations within the CPN. A node that receives a link from another node is called a *child*, and a node from which the link originates is called a *parent*. Each node has an associated table of conditional probabilities: the probability of the states in the node given its parents. These tables form the quantitative substance of the CPN. The topology of the CPN encodes a set of independence properties, the

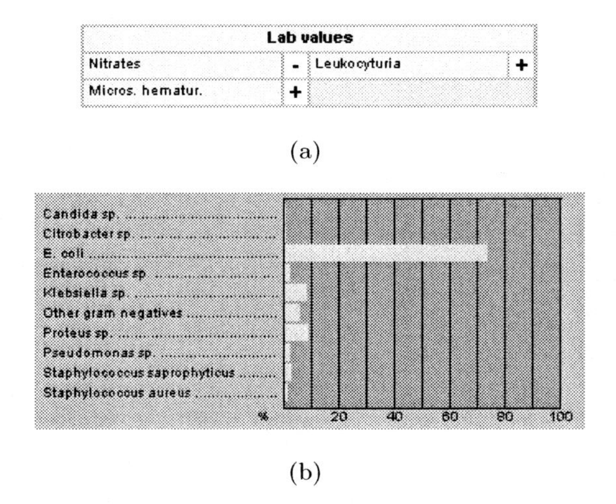

(a)

(b)

Fig. 15.6. (a) Findings from the urinalysis. (b) The distribution of probabilities over the nine groups of pathogens considered for the urinary tract.

so-called d-separation properties [16] and, in combination with the tables of conditional probabilities and the axioms of probability theory, it is possible to calculate the marginal probabilities of all nodes in the CPN when the states of some of the nodes in the CPN are known [10] (see Chapter 2 for more details). In Treat, the commercially-available inference machine Hugin [4][9] is used to construct the CPN and calculate the marginal probabilities of the individual nodes (see Section 16.5.1). In general, Hugin handles CPNs with discrete stochastic variables, although continuous variables can be handled in some special cases. We have chosen only to use discrete stochastic variables, and the variables that are naturally continuous (e.g., body temperature) must, therefore, be converted to discrete variables. This is done by dividing the domains of the variables into intervals; for example, in the case of temperature, into five intervals (Figure 15.7).

In principle, this solves all problem of data fusion, or rather, it becomes equivalent to finding an appropriate topology and conditional probability tables for the CPN. Thereafter, axioms of probability theory, embodied in the inference machine provided by Hugin, provide the data fusion. This observation changes the focus from fusion of data to fusion of knowledge, where we use knowledge to designate the combination of topology and conditional probability tables. We shall now illustrate the fusion of data and knowledge through a small example. The example chosen is the calculation of the distribution of probability over the states of sepsis.

The structure of the CPN in Figure 15.8 contains several postulates about the causes of the 11 signs and symptoms at the bottom of the figure. It con-

[9] `http://www.hugin.com/`

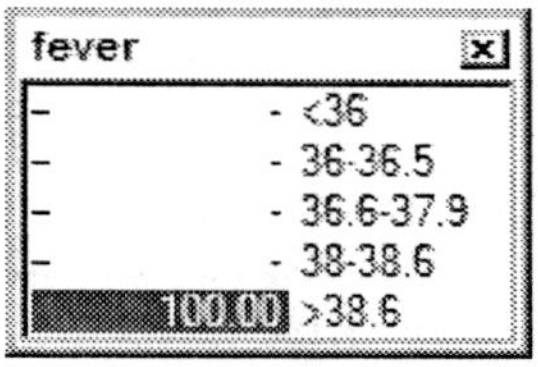

Fig. 15.7. The continuous stochastic variable "fever" is converted into a discrete variable by dividing its domain into five intervals. The bars indicate the current distribution of probabilities over the states of the node. The state ">36.8" has been observed, giving it a 100% probability. The state is said to be instantiated to the value ">36.8".

tains the postulate that there is an unobservable stochastic variable *sepsis*, and that the sepsis may be caused by infection in a number of different sites in the body; for example, gastrointestinal infections, urinary tract infections, or lung infections. In turn, sepsis may cause the signs and symptoms, such as fever and chills, but this is mediated through four factors labelled "Fact_fever", "Fact_alb_ESR", "Fact_leuco_creat" and "Shock". The word "Sepsis" refers to the fact that, in this condition, sites in the body that are normally sterile may contain pathogens. In the CPN, the concept of sepsis is used to designate a collection of signs and symptoms that represent a state of increased activity of the immune system. This use of the concept was not invented by the constructors of the CPN but is a clinically well-established concept. The four factors mediating the immune response to the 11 signs and symptoms were, however, invented by the constructors. The 11 signs and symptoms could have been direct children of sepsis, but this would have been equivalent to a "naive Bayes" assumption. A naive Bayes assumption contains the proposition that the children are conditionally independent, given the parent (see Figure 10.2). Since there will usually be some dependence between the children, it is well known that this assumption leads to overconfidence in the conclusions that are drawn [6], essentially because the effect of correlated variables is exaggerated. This can be avoided by introducing an intermediate layer of variables. The four intermediate factors were found by factor analysis, and, together, they explain more than 80% of the variance in the dependent variables [11]. The data required for this exercise were obtained from the Rabin bacteraemia database and normal values from the literature. It is also very interesting that although the four intermediate factors are statistical constructs, they probably have a high degree of physical reality. For example, the fever factor "Fact_fever" can essentially be mapped onto the plasma level of interleukin-6 [11], one of the factors that are known to mediate the immune system's inflammatory systemic response.

The probabilities shown in Figure 15.8 correspond to the situation in the CPN when the data on background conditions and sepsis presentation are instantiated in the CPN. It can be seen from the probabilities that the fever

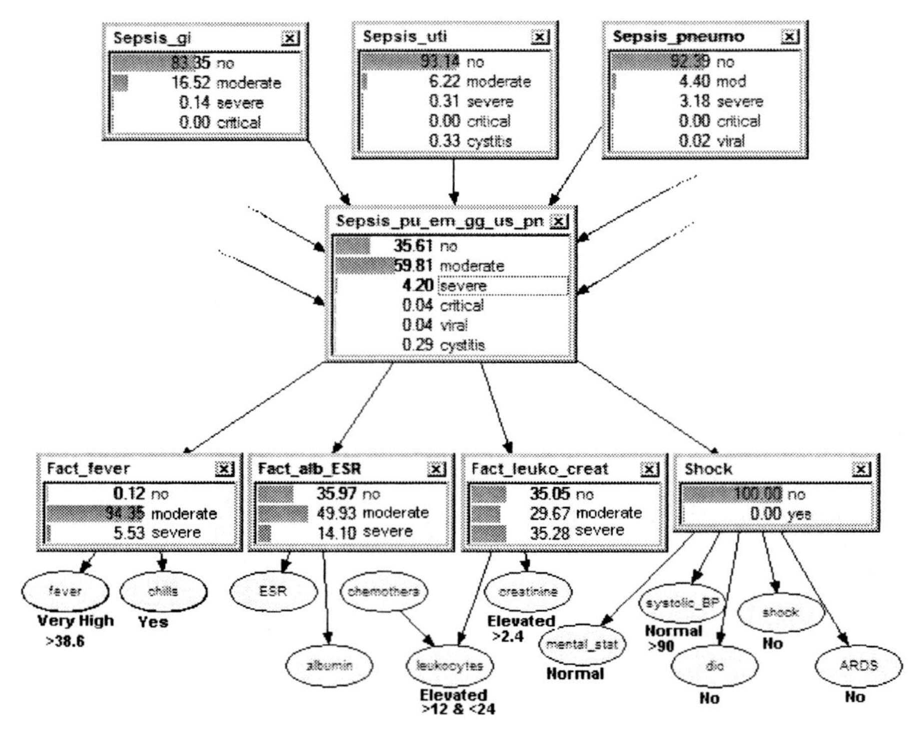

Fig. 15.8. The calculation of the distribution of probabilities over the states of sepsis. The eight nodes at the top are shown with the monitors open, i.e. such that the state probabilities can be seen. For the 12 nodes at the bottom only their name and the state to which they are instantiated are shown.

factor is allowed to reach a quite high probability of "moderate" or "severe" without this being reflected in a similarly high probability of the states different from "no" in the sepsis node. This is an example of the intermediate factors serving to eliminate the errors that would have been produced by the naive Bayes assumption.

In conclusion, this example has shown how data from several sources (e.g., background condition and sepsis presentation) can be integrated. Missing data is not a problem in the CPN methodology, and this eliminates the need for schemes for filling in missing data items. The example deals with data that are bound to concepts of physiology. We will assume that the clinical expression of an infection is independent of geography, and the structure and conditional probabilities will thus be applied by all partners in the Treat project.

15.4 Calculation of Coverage and Treatment Advice

15.4.1 Patient Example (Part 2)

The information about the patient that can reasonably be collected within a few hours has now been collected and it is time to initiate treatment. At this time there is no microbiological information about the patient's infection, and the uncertainty about which pathogen(s) caused the infection is correspondingly large. For this reason, the treatment initiated at this time is usually referred to as the empirical treatment. Figure 15.9 ranks a number of treatments, with chloramphenicol as the top-ranking treatment. The numbers given in the left-most column are the coverages. The *coverage* provided by a treatment is defined as the probability that the treatment can eliminate the activity of the pathogen(s) causing the infection. It can be seen that the treatment preferred by Treat is not the treatment giving the highest probability of coverage. The coverage provided by chloramphenicol is 62%, while, for example, the treatment ranked second by Treat, a combination of ofloxacin and chloramphenicol, provides a coverage of 89%.

To choose a treatment, it is necessary to consider both the *cost* of the treatment and the *benefit* of the treatment. In Treat, the balance between cost and benefit of a treatment is done by a decision-theoretic approach. It can be seen from Figure 15.9 that the costs of chloramphenicol are much smaller than the costs of the combination therapy of ofloxacin plus chloramphenicol.

Table 15.1 gives the three components of cost. The first component is *price*, which is the cost of purchasing the drug, with an addition of the cost of disposables and the labour costs. The second component is the *cost of side-effects* causing acute and chronic morbidity. Among the adverse effects included were nephrotoxicity and *Clostridium difficile*-related diarrhoea. This cost is based on a meta-analysis of the costs of toxic side-effects elicited by gentamycin and imipenem [20], supplemented by numbers from a similar meta-analysis for ampicillin, cefuroxime, cefotaxime, and ceftazidime (Leibovici, personal communication). For the remaining antibiotics, the cost of side-effects was extrapolated from these numbers.

The third component of cost is *ecological cost*, which was calculated from a simple model that contains a number of assumptions; primarily, that the rate of rise of resistance to a drug is proportional to the consumption of the drug, to the present level of resistance, and to a proportionality constant that is characteristic for the drug. This proportionality constant was derived from resistance data from the Rabin database combined with data on drug consumption at Rabin. Combined with an assumption of unchanged antibiotic policy over the next two years, this can be translated into an increased risk of non-covering treatment of future patients, which, in turn, can be translated into an associated increase in mortality. This calculation provides an estimate of the risk for the population as a whole, but to this risk must be added the increased risk for the patient currently being treated in case of a recurring infection in that patient. This risk was estimated using a similarly simple model. The risks for the population and for the individual patient were added, and the result of the calculation is represented in Table 15.1 as the ecological risk.

Table 15.1. The components of cost and treatment benefit, calculated for an empirical treatment with an average duration of two days. The treatments are (N) "no treatment", (C) "chloramphenicol", and (O+C) "ofloxacin plus chloramphenicol". The abbreviated column names have the following meanings: "Eff", side-effect cost; "Eco", ecological cost; "Cvg", percentage coverage; "Mort", percentage mortality; "BD", *BedDayBenefit*; "Surv", *SurvivalBenefit*.

Treatment	Costs				Benefits					*Cost-Benefit*
	Price	Eff	Eco	Total	Cvg	Mort	BD	Surv	Total	
N	0	0	0	0	0	1.21	0	0	0	0
C	29	44	43	116	62.3	1.01	654	501	1155	1039
O+C	42	62	585	689	88.7	0.93	931	712	1643	954

The benefits of the treatment are divided into the bed-day benefit and the survival benefit.

The *bed-day benefit* is calculated from the equation

$$BedDayBenefit =$$
$$(Infection_{NoTreat} - Infection_{Treat}) \times SavedBedDays \times BedDayCost.$$

In this equation, *SavedBedDays* is an estimate of the number of bed-days saved by covering antibiotic treatment of a patient with moderate to severe infection, and *BedDayCost* is the average cost per bed-day of a patient residing outside the intensive care unit. *SavedBedDays* was estimated as 3 days from the Rabin bacteraemia database (Leibovici, personal communication), and *BedDayCost* was estimated as 350 Euro for a patient at Rabin Medical Center. $Infection_{NoTreat}$ represents the probability of infection, which corresponds to the total length of the bar labelled "Probability of infection (All sites)" in Figure 15.9(c), including the hatched area. $Infection_{Treat}$ represents the probability that a given treatment will not cover the infection, corresponding to the blue part of the bar labelled "Probability of infection (All sites)". In Figure 15.9(a), the black square next to the treatment "Chloramphenicol" indicates that the coverage given in Figure 15.9(c) relates to the treatment "Chloramphenicol". Note that the coverages given in the left-most column in Figure 15.9(a) are calculated for each treatment as the ratio

$$Coverage_{Treat} = Infection_{Treat}/Infection_{NoTreat}.$$

We can now calculate *BedDayBenefit* for chloramphenicol,

$$BedDayBenefit = (100\% - 37.7\%) \times 3 \times 350 \text{ Euro} = 654 \text{ Euro},$$

as given in Table 1.

The *survival benefit* is calculated from the equation:

$$SurvivalBenefit = (Mortality_{NoTreat} - Mortality_{Treat}) \times ALE \times CLY.$$

ALE is the average life-year expectancy for this group of patients and is assumed to be 5 years [13]. CLY is the value used to express the intrinsic value of a life-year, and it is assumed to be 50,000 Euro per life-year, approximately the cost of maintaining a patient for one year on haemodialysis [15]. $Mortality_{NoTreat}$ is the probability of the patient dying within 30 days provided he is given no treatment or non-covering treatment. $Mortality_{Treat}$ is the probability of the patient dying, provided he is given a certain treatment. For each treatment, including no treatment, the CPN calculates the probability of dying. If desired, the probabilities can be displayed by selecting "Mortality" instead of "Coverage", as illustrated in Figure 15.9(b). We can now calculate the survival benefit from the equation given above; for example, for chloramphenicol, we have

$$SurvivalBenefit = (1.21\% - 1.01\%) \times 5 \times 50000 \text{ Euro} = 501 \text{ Euro}.$$

The total benefit, calculated as the sum of the $BedDayBenefit$ and the $SurvivalBenefit$, is 1155 Euro for chloramphenicol. To finish the cost-benefit analysis, we subtract the total costs from the total benefit:

$$CostBenefit = 1155 \text{ Euro} - 116 \text{ Euro} = 1039 \text{ Euro}.$$

For the combination of ofloxacin plus chloramphenicol, the treatment ranked second by Treat, the $CostBenefit$ is 954 Euro. Because this is less than that for chloramphenicol, Treat prefers chloramphenicol. The ofloxacin-plus-chloramphenicol treatment has a substantially higher benefit (1643 Euro), but this is more than compensated for by its higher cost (689 Euro).

The treatment recommended by Treat is not necessarily the treatment that will be given to the patient. The attending clinician may consult Treat, but this, of course, does not oblige him to follow the advice given by Treat. In this particular case study, the clinician preferred to give the patient ofloxacin plus chloramphenicol, presumably aiming at the higher coverage provided by this treatment.

Thirty-six hours later, a notification for positive blood cultures was received, with growth of streptococci in four blood culture bottles. Streptococci fall in the group of pathogens labelled "Enterococci sp." in Figure 15.10, and this, therefore, provides strong support for an enterococcal infection. This gives a major change in the pathogen probabilities, and the advice provided by Treat for the so-called semi-empirical treatment instantiated at this time is, therefore, also different from the advice for the empirical treatment. Ampicillin is the recommended treatment, and it provides a coverage of 85% at a fairly low cost. This completes the patient example.

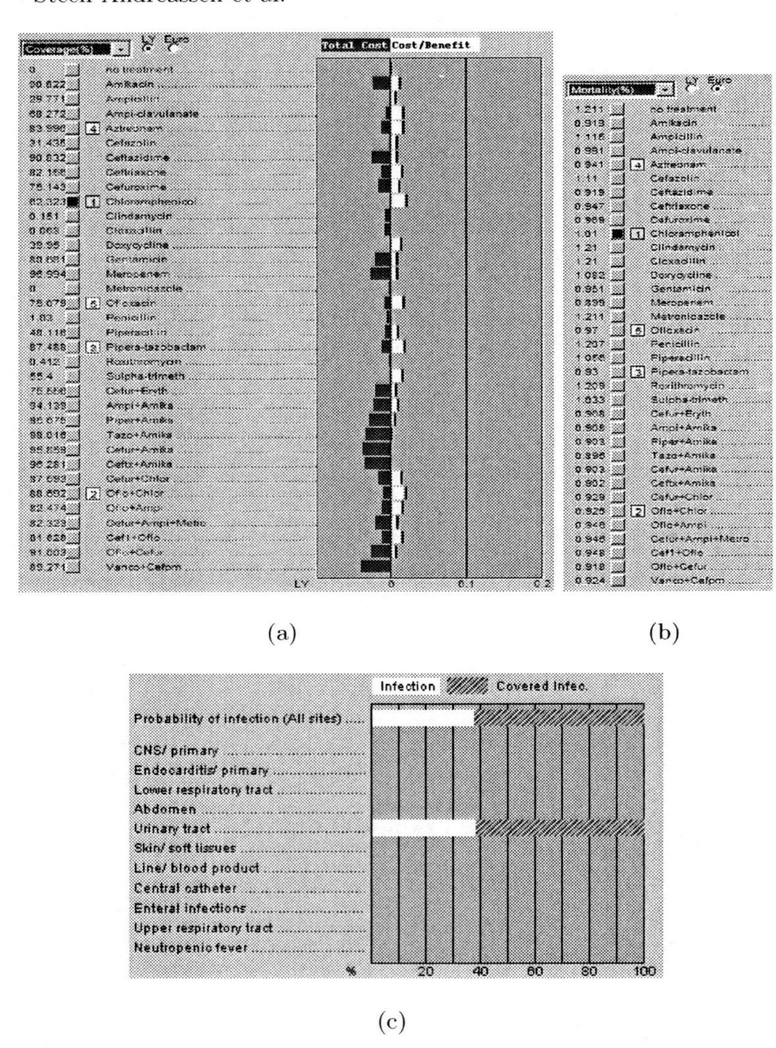

(a) (b)

(c)

Fig. 15.9. (a) Advice on empirical treatment provided by Treat. From left to right, the columns contain the probability of coverage provided by each treatment, the ranking given by Treat (numbers in small boxes), and an abbreviated name for the treatment. The orange bars give the total cost of each treatment, the distance from the bottom of the orange bar to the fat line gives the benefit provided by the treatment, and the green bar thus gives the cost minus benefit, if this is positive. Costs and benefits are given in life-years (LY). (b) Thirty-day mortalities calculated for each treatment. (c) Probability of infection, distributed over sites. The total length of the bars (blue + hatched) gives the probability of infection prior to the treatment, the blue part of the bar indicating the probability of leaving the infection uncovered, and the hatched part indicating the probability of covering the infection. The coverages are given for the treatment chloramphenicol.

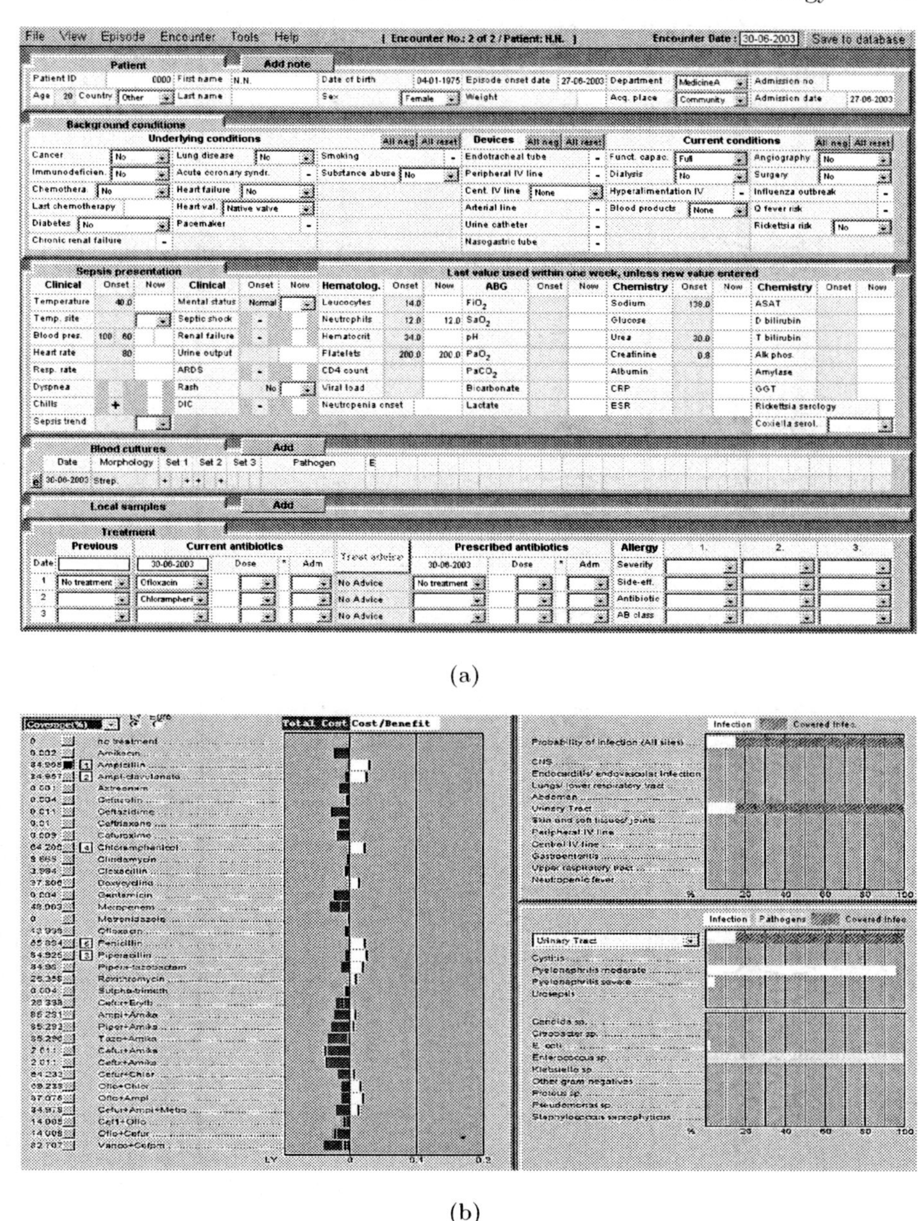

Fig. 15.10. (a) A complete view of the main data-entry screen in the Treat system at the time where the semi-empirical treatment is instantiated. (b) The analysis provided by Treat.

15.4.2 Fusion of Data and Knowledge for Calculation of Coverage and Treatment Advice

A number of assumptions have been embedded in the topology of the CPN. These assumptions include the assumption that infections are caused by pathogens (bacteria, fungi, or viruses), and that infections may cause symptoms, both local to the site of infection and systemic responses, as already discussed. It is also assumed that antibiotics exert their effects on infections by reducing the activity of the pathogens, and that this, in turn, makes the infection and its symptoms subside. These assumptions are hardly controversial, but they dictate the basic topology of the CPN. How this translation from the assumption to the topology is performed has been described in previous publications [1, 2, 11].

The starting point for the calculation of coverage is the distribution of probabilities over the different pathogens that may cause the infection at each site. Here, we shall briefly consider an example of knowledge required to calculate the coverage for a given treatment. In turn, the coverage forms the basis for the decision-theoretic calculation of advice by Treat, as illustrated in the patient example discussed above.

The knowledge required takes the form of a matrix that contains the susceptibilities for each of the 40 groups of pathogens considered in Treat. The *susceptibility* of a pathogen to an antibiotic is the probability that the activity of a pathogen can be eliminated by the given antibiotic. This susceptibility also depends on the place of acquisition of the infection. Hospital-acquired infections tend to be less susceptible to antibiotics than infections acquired in the community; therefore, the place of acquisition is also an entry in the matrix of susceptibilities.

The susceptibilities differ between countries and even between hospitals in the same country. It is believed that it is the consumption of antibiotics that drives the reduction in susceptibilities that can be observed in many places, and it is this assumption that provided the model for the calculation of the ecological cost; however, at a given hospital, at a given point in time, we need to provide estimates of susceptibilities to allow the CPN to calculate the probability that a given treatment will cover. This is in striking contrast to the conditional probabilities that must be provided to calculate the probability of sepsis. These conditional probabilities were assumed to be universally applicable, independent of time and place.

The hospitals included in the clinical trial of the Treat system have compiled databases with susceptibilities of most of the relevant pathogens for a number of antibiotics. Even though these databases may contain several thousand cases, complications still arise. Some of the groups of pathogens are not frequently occurring, and some pathogens may only be tested for their susceptibility to a small number of antibiotics. As a consequence, a matrix of susceptibilities can contain a minority of entries with high counts; for example, several hundred cases where the pathogen *Escherichia coli* had its susceptibility tested to the antibiotic ampicillin. Most of the entries are in a poor state, and the susceptibility must be decided on the basis of a few, or even zero, observed cases. We have chosen a Bayesian approach, where a prior distribution is specified for the susceptibility. It is practical to use beta distributions as the priors and to update the posterior distributions using Dirichlet learning [18] (Chapter 1). These prior distributions may be based on observations from the literature, on databases from other clinical sites, or on the knowledge that, for example, some antibiotics will always be ineffective against certain pathogens. As more local data become available, the probability distributions are updated using Bayes' theorem, and the impact of the prior distributions decreases.

15.5 Calibration Databases

The discussion of the conditional probability tables has revealed that they can be divided into two groups. The first group, which is by far the largest, consists of conditional probabilities that we assume to be independent of time and place. Typically, these conditional probabilities are hard-wired into the CPN. A single example has been discussed: the conditional probabilities required for the assessment of the state of sepsis.

Conditional probabilities in the other group are assumed to be specific for each participating hospital, and they may change over time. These conditional probabilities are placed in calibration databases that can be compiled into the CPN. The most important of the calibration databases is the calibration database for susceptibilities, which has already been discussed. Other calibration databases are those that describe the prevalence of pathogens, the mortalities associated with the infections, the treatments available at the hospital, and their cost components. The constants in the cost-benefit analysis (e.g., the cost of a bed-day) must also be specified by each hospital.

In addition to these calibration databases that influence the basic reasoning of the system, there are also a number of more trivial calibration databases. These contain information about the names of the hospital departments, the antibiotics available at the hospital pharmacy, the antibiotics used for testing of susceptibilities, and text strings and other information that at least partially allow the texts available in the system to be made specific for the hospital or adapted to the local language and that allow measurements to be converted between different unit systems. In the clinical example of a patient with a urinary tract infection, the calibration databases were calibrated to Rabin Medical Center. This implies that if the Treat system is applied with a different set of calibration databases, then the advice will be different. In particular, differences across Europe in susceptibilities will lead to substantially different advice.

15.6 Clinical Testing of Decision-support Systems

A decision-support system must be tested under realistic clinical conditions. At this point in time, three different evaluations of the Treat system have been planned. The first type of evaluation involves the retrospective testing of the system on case databases. The second type of evaluation is a non-interventional test, where the data are collected prospectively, but where the advice from the Treat system is not made available to the attending clinician. The third type of evaluation is a randomized clinical trial, where the advice from Treat is made available to the attending clinician before he decides on the antibiotic therapy. These three types of evaluation will provide answers to a range of different questions.

The retrospective testing allows the quality of the advice provided by Treat to be evaluated against current clinical practice and against the recommendations of the local guidelines for antibiotic use. The results can, if positive, provide some assurance that the system can provide sound advice.

The non-interventional evaluation can be used to test aspects of the clinical acceptability of Treat. The provision of sound advice is an important consideration, and the non-interventional testing provides an opportunity to assess the soundness of the advice when the system is used under conditions that approximate routine clinical conditions; however, the system may also fail if the user interface is inappropriate, if computing time is too long, or if the required data collection does not fit into the work flow of the departments involved.

The randomized clinical trial can be initiated provided the results from the preceding two types of evaluation are positive. The design of a trial of a decision-support system is not straightforward and is fraught with a number of methodological pitfalls [7]. Some of the methodological problems stem from the fact that, for the testing of a decision-support system like Treat, it is not practical to perform a blinded study. Other problems are derived from problems with the randomization. The behaviour of the participating clinicians is likely to be modified through the use of Treat, and, therefore, a randomization of patients is not possible. Instead, we have chosen to randomize the participating departments. This requires that a reasonable number of departments are participating, and currently the trial is planned with 12 departments in Israel, Germany and Italy.

15.7 Test Results

In the Treat project, a non-interventional trial of Treat has been completed. Preliminary results show promising results with significant improvements in coverage and substantial reductions of costs [19]. A randomised controlled clinical trial will be concluded in late 2004. The retrospective testing has been done using a unique access to databases compiled by the partners. A database of bacteraemia for the years 1992–1996 was available for the County of Northern Jutland. Data from 1992–1994 were used to calibrate the decision-support system to local patterns of susceptibility of the pathogens to antibiotics and to local prevalences of the pathogens. Data from 1995–1996 (1597 cases) were used to test the system.

Results of the retrospective testing [8, 9] were as follows. The treatment given in clinical practice provided coverage in 60.8% of the cases. Had the clinicians followed the guidelines in the *List of Pharmaceuticals* provided by the Danish Medical Association, an average coverage of 92.7% would have been achieved, and had the advice of Treat been followed, the coverage would have been even higher: 94.6%.

The costs that would have been incurred by following the guidelines were 45% higher than the cost of the current clinical practice. According to the cost-benefit analysis, this increase in cost would have been more than paid for since the benefit would have increased by 47%, and the cost-benefit by 48%.

The costs that would have been incurred by following the Treat advice were 35% higher than the costs of the current clinical practice, but actually lower than the cost of following the guidelines. The benefit was 52% of clinical practice and the cost-benefit was 54% of clinical practice, both somewhat better than the guidelines.

The main observation is thus that a 48% improvement can be obtained simply by following the guidelines, which were actually only adhered to in 17% of the cases. A further modest but statistically significant 6% increase in cost-benefit can be obtained by following the advice of Treat. We have found these results promising enough to proceed with the planning of the next two phases, the non-interventional testing and the controlled clinical trial.

15.8 Discussion

The aim of the Treat project is to develop a medical decision-support system based on a probabilistic model of infectious diseases. As part of the project, the system will be tested in four European countries. It is too early to speculate on the ultimate success of the system. A retrospective trial in Denmark has indicated that the advice from the system may be a useful improvement over current clinical practice [9]. This result cannot necessarily be extrapolated to other countries, since the problems in antibiotic therapy are quite different in the participating countries. In Denmark, the level of susceptibility to antibiotics is higher than in most other countries. Should it turn out that the Treat system is capable of providing useful advice in all the participating countries, this must be seen as an indication of the flexibility of the method chosen to construct the system. Some encouragement can be derived from the fact that a system developed by one of the partners for use in Israel prior to the Treat project was capable of providing advice that also represented a substantial improvement over clinical practice [12].

The previously developed system only performed well in the hospital where it was designed. This provided part of the motivation for the Treat project, including the separation of knowledge into universal knowledge and knowledge that changes with time and place. The development of the concept of calibration databases for the Treat system represents an attempt to isolate the knowledge that needs to be calibrated to each hospital.

Should the system prove to be successful, we believe the success can be ascribed to several factors:

1. It is difficult for a clinician to know about all the factors that may influence the prevalence of pathogens; for example, in a urinary tract infection, does the presence of a catheter increase or decrease the probability of an *E. coli* infection?
2. Even if the clinician can keep track of these factors, and thus produce realistic estimates of pathogen probabilities, the calculation of coverage of a treatment not only requires an updated knowledge of susceptibilities, but it also requires that the fairly complicated multiplication of pathogen probabilities with susceptibilities is performed correctly. This is certainly done much better by a computer.
3. Finally, the choice of antibiotic therapy depends on a balancing of costs against benefits. The clinician may disagree with the weighting performed by the system, but it will give him information that he can use in forming his own decision.

The comparison of clinical practice with the recommendations by the Danish guidelines and with the Treat advice revealed that Treat was quite close to the guidelines. Perhaps the Treat system can also, in the future, be seen as a system that can assist verification of antibiotic policies and guidelines.

Acknowledgments

This work was supported by a grant from the European Commission for the TREAT-project under the IST programme (IST-1999-11459), a grant from the Danish Technical Research Council (2051-01-0011), a grant from the PhD programme at Aalborg Hospital, Denmark and a grant from the Scandinavian Society for Antimicrobial Therapy. The Bacteraemia Register at the Department of Clinical Microbiology was supported by grants from the County of Northern Jutland and Det Obelske Familiefond.

References

[1] S. Andreassen, L. Leibovici, H.C. Schønheyder, B. Kristensen, C. Riekehr, A.G. Kjær, and K.G. Olesen. A decision theoretic approach to empirical treatment of bacteraemia originating from the urinary tract. In W. Horn,

editor, *Lecture Notes in Artificial Intelligence, Vol. 1620*, pages 197–206. Springer-Verlag, Berlin, 1999.

[2] S. Andreassen, C. Riekehr, B. Kristensen, H.C. Schønheyder, and L. Leibovici. Using probabilistic and decision-theoretic methods in treatment and prognosis modeling. *Artificial Intelligence in Medicine*, 15:121–134, 1999.

[3] D.C. Angus, W.T. Linde-Zwirble, J. Lidicker, G. Clermont, J. Carcillo, and M.R. Pinsky. Epidemiology of severe sepsis in the United States: analysis of incidence, outcome, and associated costs of care. *Critical Care Medicine*, 29:1303–1310, 2001.

[4] Hugin Expert (anonymous). *Hugin System Introduction, version 5.1.* Hugin Expert A/S, Aalborg, 1997.

[5] R.C. Bone. Toward a theory regarding the pathogenesis of the systemic inflammatory response syndrome: What we do and do not know about cytokine regulation. *Critical Care Medicine*, 24:163–172, 1996.

[6] R.O. Duda and P.E. Hart. *Pattern Classification and Scene Analysis.* Wiley, New York, 1973.

[7] C.P. Friedman and J.C. Wyatt. *Evaluation Methods in Medical Informatics. Computers and Medicine.* Springer-Verlag, New York, 1998.

[8] B. Kristensen, S. Larsen, H.C. Schønheyder, L. Leibovici, M. Paul, U. Frank, and S. Andreassen. A decision support system (DSS) for antibiotic treatment improves empirical treatment and reduces costs. In *Proceedings of 41st Interscience Conference on Antimicrobial Agents and Chemotherapy (ICAAC)*, page 476, Illinois, 2001. American Society for Microbiology.

[9] B. Kristensen, C.H. Riekehr, H.C. Schønheyder, S. Larsen, J. Klitgaard, A. Zalounina, L. Leibovici, U. Frank, and S. Andreassen. Empirical antibiotic treatment of bacteraemia: Evaluation of a Bayesian decision model against clinical practice and guidelines. (Submitted), 2004.

[10] S.L. Lauritzen and D.J. Spiegelhalter. Local computation with probabilities on graphical structures and their application to expert systems (with discussion). *Journal of the Royal Statistical Society, Series B*, 50 (2):157–224, 1988.

[11] L. Leibovici, M. Fishman, H.C. Schønheyder, C. Riekehr, B. Kristensen, I. Shraga, and S. Andreassen. A causal probabilistic network for optimal treatment of bacterial infections. *IEEE Transactions on Knowledge and Data Engineering*, 12(4):517–528, 2000.

[12] L. Leibovici, V. Gitelman, Y. Yehezkelly, O. Poznanski, G. Milo, M. Paul, and P. Ein-Dor. Improving empirical antibiotic treatment: Prospective, non-intervention testing of a decision support system. *Journal of Internal Medicine*, 242:395–400, 1997.

[13] L. Leibovici, Z. Samra, H. Konigsberger, M. Drucker, S. Ashkenazi, and S.D. Pitlik. Long-term survival following bacteraemia or fungemia. *Journal of the American Medical Association*, 274:807–812, 1995.

[14] L. Leibovici, I. Shraga, and S. Andreassen. How do you choose antibiotic treatment? *British Medical Journal*, 318:1614–1616, 1999.

[15] T.R. Maschoreck, M.C. Sørensen, M. Andresen, I.M. Høgsberg, P. Rasmussen, and J. Søgård. Omkostningsanalyse af dialysebehandlingen på Odense Universitetshospital og Sønderborg Sygehus. *Ugeskr Læger*, 160: 7418–7424, 1998.

[16] J. Pearl. *Probabilistic Reasoning in Intelligent Systems: Networks of Plausible Reasoning.* Morgan Kaufmann, San Mateo, CA, 1988.

[17] E. Shortliffe. *Computer-Based Medical Consultations: MYCIN.* North Holland, New York, 1976.

[18] D.J. Spiegelhalter and S.L. Lauritzen. Sequential updating of conditional probabilities on directed graphical structures. *Networks*, 20:579–605, 1990.

[19] E. Tacconelli, M. Paul, M.A. Cataldo, N. Almanasreh, A. Zalounina, A. Nielsen, S. Andreassen, U. Frank, R. Cauda, and L. Leibovici. A computerized decision support system (TREAT) to reduce inappropriate antibiotic therapy of bacterial infection. *Proceedings at 14th European Congress of Clinical Microbiology and Infectious Diseases*, 10(3):4 (abstract), 2004.

[20] A.P. Wilson, A.J Bint, A.M. Glenny, L. Leibovici, and T.E. Peto. Meta-analysis and systematic review of antibiotic trials. *Journal of Hospital Infections*, 43:S211–S214, 1999.

16

Software for Probability Models in Medical Informatics

Richard Dybowski

InferSpace, 143 Village Way, Pinner HA5 5AA, UK.
richard@inferspace.com

Summary. The purpose of this chapter is to make the reader aware of some of the software packages available that can implement probability models connected with medical informatics. The modelling techniques considered are logistic regression, neural networks, Bayesian networks, class-probability trees, and hidden Markov models.

16.1 Introduction

Several developments over the past 10 years have impacted significantly on software for probabilistic models. Three of these are the substantial advances made in computing technology, the explosive growth of the Internet, and the rise of open-source software.

The 45-fold increase in CPU speed witnessed during the 1990s[1] has enabled a number of computationally-intensive techniques to be readily available to the data analyst. These techniques include optimizations (such as parameter estimation and evolutionary computation [19, 16]), Monte Carlo simulations (particularly bootstrap methods [18, 15] and MCMC sampling [23]), and advanced computer graphics for data visualization [34, 9].

The Internet has enabled those with common interests to communicate with each other via discussion groups. The existence of these virtual forums for software packages allows the users of those packages to readily provide technical support and offer new developments. Furthermore, through the existence of the World Wide Web, a number of free, peer-reviewed, online journals have appeared, such as *Journal of Statistical Software* and *Journal of Machine Learning Research*. Furthermore, several conferences, such as *Uncertainty in Artificial Intelligence* and *Neural Information Processing Systems*, have made their proceedings available online at no charge.

The Internet has also been crucial to the creation and evolution of the open-source movement, which we now describe.

---

[1] Moore's Law states that the computer industry doubles the power of microprocessors every 18 months.

16.2 Open-source Software

The usual economics of software development is that a business organization produces an item of computer software and sells it to those wishing to have it, with the buyers of the product having no control over its development. However, during the 1990s, an alternative economic model for software development emerged called Open Source [37, 2].

The basic principle of *open-source software development* is that the human-readable computer program underlying the software (the *source code*) is available to everyone. This is in stark contrast to the situation with proprietary software, in which only the company producing the software can modify it. Because of the availability of the source code, a large syndicate of interested users can make the improvements they wish to see in the software. The proposed improvements are vetted by a hierarchically coordinated group of volunteer programmers and incorporated in the next release of the software [36, 20]. Thus, a subset of users sort out known problems and eventually get the functionality they require. The most famous example of this approach to software development is the success of the Linux operating system [52].

An important device in maintaining the open-source status of software is the use of open-source licences [42], such as the *GNU General Public License* (GPL) [47]. This legally-binding document ensures that any item of software covered by it remains open source. The license allows people to modify the source code of GPL software, but any modified software they distribute is also covered by the GPL. A person may distribute GPL software for free or sell it for profit, but they cannot sell it under a restrictive license, for that would inhibit development of the software within the open-source framework. Other open-source licences include the *Artistic Licence*, the *Apache License*, and the *Python License*.

We will bring to the reader's attention open-source software relevant to the theme of this chapter.

Cautionary Note:

Most public-domain software (open-sourced, freeware, and shareware) has not been rigorously tested; therefore, it is more likely to contain programming bugs than commercially-developed software.

16.3 Logistic Regression Models

[Logistic regression was featured in Sections 3.3 and 10.4.]

There are many statistics packages competing with each other, ranging from the more advanced packages, such as S-Plus, designed for professional statisticians, to the more user-friendly packages, such as Data Desk, for non-specialists. All the major commercial statistics packages – such as Genstat, GLIM, SAS, S-Plus, SPSS, and Statistica – provide some means of fitting logistic models to data, although there is some package-to-package variation in the functionality and diagnostics available.[2] [3] This is not surprising given that some packages were designed, at least initially, for specific types of users. For example, SPSS was designed for social scientists, whereas GLIM was designed for those requiring generalized linear models.

Collett [12, Chap. 9] compared the logistic regression capabilities of six packages; however, given that his review was written in 1991, some of his comments may no longer apply.

16.3.1 S-Plus and R

S-Plus is one of the most sophisticated statistics packages available [10, 49, 50].[4] It is based on the S language [3], and is supported by an active discussion group. Harrell [25] has contributed substantially to the S-Plus code pertaining to regression. This includes routines for contemporary statistical techniques such as bootstrapping for model validation. The GLIB S-Plus package by Raftery and Volinsky [40] aids the use of model-averaged logistic regression (Section 10.5).

Example 1. The logistic regression model

$$\text{logit}(p(Kyphosis = 1|Age, Number, Start)) = \beta_0 + \beta_1 Age + \beta_2 Number + \beta_3 Start$$

can be fitted to the `kyphosis` data set [10] using the S-Plus code

```
kyph.glm <- glm(Kyphosis ~ Age + Number + Start,
                family = binomial, data = kyphosis)
```

where `glm` is the generalized linear modelling function. The regression coefficients and associated standard errors can be viewed using the command `summary(kyph.glm)`

```
Coefficients:
                   Value Std. Error   t value
(Intercept) -2.03693225 1.44918287 -1.405573
        Age  0.01093048 0.00644419  1.696175
     Number  0.41060098 0.22478659  1.826626
      Start -0.20651000 0.06768504 -3.051043
```

Given a new vector of values `xnew` for Age, $Number$ and $Start$, the command

```
predict(kyph.glm, newdata = xnew, type = "response")
```

provides the estimated probability $p(Kyphosis = 1|\texttt{xnew})$ from the regression model. $\triangleleft$

---

[2] Updated links to software and discussion groups featured in this chapter are available from the website `http://robots.ox.ac.uk/~parg/pmbmi.html`.

[3] Comparisons between a number of mathematical and statistical packages – such as Gauss, Mathematica, Matlab, and S-Plus – are available at the *Scientific Web* website: `http://www.scientificweb.com/ncrunch/`

[4] `http://www.insightful.com/`

In our opinion, the best open-source statistics package is *R* [28], a language and environment for statistical computing and graphics.[5] It is very similar to S-Plus, but not identical to it; however, a lot of code written for S-Plus can be run unchanged within the R environment; for example, the `glm` and `predict` commands of Example 1 are available in R. One of the advantages of R over S-Plus is that the graphics capability of R is generally superior to that available from S-Plus.

The evolution of R (the *R Project*) is managed by a group of coordinated teams. There are a number of discussion groups associated with these teams, including a highly effective support forum. There is also a very good online journal called *R-News* for the R community.

16.3.2 BUGS

[MCMC methods were featured in Chapters 2 and 10.]

BUGS (Bayesian inference Using Gibbs Sampling) [45] generates the necessary code to perform MCMC sampling from a model specification supplied by a user.[6] The syntax is an extension of the S langauge.

The original format (*Classic BUGS*) has a command-line interface that provides univariate Gibbs sampling and a simple Metropolis-within-Gibbs routine. A more recent version (*WinBUGS*) provides a GUI for use with Windows, and it has a more sophisticated univariate Metropolis sampler. Although there is, as yet, no version of WinBUGS for the Linux or Unix platforms, WinBugs can be run within these platforms by using an emulator such as Wine.

A wide range of S-Plus and R routines (*CODA*) supplement BUGS by providing diagnostics and plots for MCMC analysis and convergence checks.

Example 2. In this example, adapted from Spiegelhalter et al. [44], WinBUGS is used to estimate the regression coefficients of a random-effects logistic regression model that allows for over-dispersion. The data consist of N plates for which, in the ith plate, there were r_i positive outcomes out of n_i units. The hierarchical structure of the model is

$$\begin{aligned} r_i &\sim Binomial(p_i, n_i) \\ \text{logit}(p_i) &= \beta_0 + \beta_1 x_{1,i} + \beta_2 x_{2,i} + \beta_{12} x_{1,i} x_{2,i} + b_i \\ \beta_0, \beta_1, \beta_2, \beta_{12} &\sim Normal(0, 10^6) \\ b_i &\sim Normal(0, \tau^{-1}) \\ \tau &\sim Gamma(10^{-3}, 10^{-3}) \end{aligned}$$

for which the corresponding BUGS code can be written as

```
model{
   for(i in 1:N){
      r[i] ~ dbin(p[i],n[i])
      logit(p[i]) <- beta0 + beta1*x1[i] + beta2*x2[i] +
                          beta12*x1[i]*x2[i] + b[i]
```

[5] http://www.r-project.org/

[6] http://www.mrc-bsu.cam.ac.uk/bugs/

```
        b[i] ~ dnorm(0.0,tau)
    }
    beta0 ~ dnorm(0.0,1.0E-6)
    beta1 ~ dnorm(0.0,1.0E-6)
    beta2 ~ dnorm(0.0,1.0E-6)
    beta12 ~ dnorm(0.0,1.0E-6)
    tau ~ dgamma(0.001,0.001)
}
```

Following a "burn in" using 1000 samples, 9000 samples from the posterior distribution of the parameters provided the following estimates:

	β	SE
(intercept)	−0.5496	0.1927
x_1	0.0772	0.307
x_2	1.356	0.2773
x_1x_2	−0.823	0.4205

◁

Several specialized versions of BUGS have been developed for specific domains. One of these is *PKBugs*, which was designed to provide hierarchical pharmacokinetic and pharmacodynamic models. Further details of PKBugs, along with an example, are given in Chapter 11.

Another MCMC package is *Hydra* [51], a suite of Java libraries. Although it does provide a range of MCMC samplers, its use requires some familiarity with the Java language.

16.4 Neural Networks

[Neural networks were featured in Chapters 3 and 12, and Section 10.6.]

There are at least 35 commercial packages and 47 freeware/shareware packages for neural computation. James [29] provides a review of some of the commercial packages, and a tabular comparison of 12 packages is given in Table 16.1. Some of the major mathematical packages, such as Mathematica, and Matlab, have neural-network toolboxes designed specifically for them. This also true of some of the statistical packages, including S-Plus and Statistica; however, in our opinion, the toolbox with the most functionality is an open-sourced package called Netlab.

16.4.1 Netlab

Netlab was developed to accompany the seminal book *Neural Networks for Pattern Recognition* by Chris Bishop [4], and, in our experience, it has the best functionality of any neural-network package.[7]

Matlab [27] is a powerful commercial software package for performing technical computations,[8] and Netlab is a collection of open-source routines designed to be

[7] `http://www.ncrg.aston.ac.uk/netlab/`

[8] `http://www.mathworks.com/`

executed within the Matlab environment. In addition to being open-sourced, Netlab contains a powerful collection of routines for neural computation, including routines for Bayesian computations, latent-variable models (such as Generative Topographic Mapping [48]), and Gaussian processes [22]. Nabney [33] has written an excellent textbook and manual for Netlab, which provides many worked examples based on Bishop's book.

Example 3. The topology of a classification multilayer perceptron (MLP) with a single hidden layer is defined by the number of input nodes `nin` for the feature vectors $\mathbf{x}$, the number of hidden nodes `nhidden`, and the number of output nodes `nout` for the conditional class probabilities $p(y = k|\mathbf{x})$. With these structural values, an MLP can be created in Matlab by using the Netlab `mlp` routine; for example,

```
nin = 4; nhidden = 6; nout = 1;
alpha = 0.1;  % weight-decay coefficient
net = mlp(nin, nhidden, nout, 'logistic', alpha);
```

The string `'logistic'` specifies that the logistic function is to be used for the output-node activation function.

The `mlp` routine initializes the network weights to random values; however, the command `net = mlpinit(net, prior)` can be used to randomly select the weights from a zero-mean Gaussian distribution with covariance `1/prior`.

If a data set consists of input-target pairs $(\mathbf{x}_i, y_i)$, the MLP can now be trained for, say, 1000 cycles using the quasi-Newton optimization algorithm:

```
options = foptions; options(14) = 1000; % algorithm options
[nnet, options] = netopt(net, options, xdata, ydata, 'quasinew');
```

where `xdata` is the matrix of $\mathbf{x}_i$ values, and `ydata` is the vector of the y_i values associated with `xdata`. Forward propagation of a new feature vector `xnew` along the trained network is performed with

```
cpd = mlpfwd(nnet, xnew);
```

which estimates the conditional probability distribution $p(y|\texttt{xnew})$. ◁

16.4.2 The Stuttgart Neural Network Simulator

A limitation of Netlab is that it does not provide networks specifically for the construction of temporal neural networks. In contrast, the Stuttgart Neural Network Simulator (SNNS), supports time-delay networks (TDNN), Jordan networks, Elman networks, and extended hierarchical Elman networks.[9]

16.5 Bayesian Networks

[Bayesian networks were featured in Chapters 2 and 4 and Section 10.9.]

As a result of the large interest in Bayesian networks (BNs), many software packages have been designed to support BN development. We are aware of at least eight

[9] `http://www-ra.informatik.uni-tuebingen.de/SNNS/`

commercial and 30 academic BN packages, with at least 20 of the latter providing source code. Kevin Murphy has compiled an extensive table that summarizes the features of 37 BN packages. A modified version of this table is shown in Table 16.2. Korb and Nicholson [30] have made a detailed comparison of 12 packages, including Bayes Net Toolbox, Hugin, Bayesware Discoverer, and Tetrad.

Table 16.1. Summary of some academic and commercial software for neural-network development. The "Code" column states whether the source code is available (N ≡ no). If it is, the language used is given. The "GUI" column states whether a GUI is available (Y ≡ yes). The "RBF" column states whether radial basis function networks can be developed. The "*t*" column states whether temporal (dynamic) networks can be developed beyond the use of delay vectors. The "B" column states whether Bayesian neural techniques can be used. The "Free" column states whether the software is free (R ≡ only a restricted version is free).

Package	Developer	Code	GUI	RBF	*t*	B	Free
BrainMaker	California Scientific Software	N	Y	N	N	N	N
Mathematica Neural Networks	Wolfram Research	Mathematica	N	Y	Y	N	N
Matlab Neural Network Toolbox [24]	The MathWorks	Matlab	Y	Y	Y	Y [a]	N
Netlab [33]	I.T. Nabney et al.	Matlab	N	Y	N	Y [b]	Y
NeuralWorks	NeuralWare	N	Y	Y	Y	N	R
NeuroSolutions [38]	NeuroDimension	N	Y	Y	Y	N	R
NuRho	soNit.biz	N	Y	N	N	N	R
PDP++ [35]	R.C. O'Reilly et al.	C++	Y	N	Y	N	Y
SNNS	University of Stuttgart	C	Y	Y	Y	N	Y
Statistica Neural Networks	StatSoft	N	Y	Y	N	N	R
ThinksPro	Logical Designs Consulting	N	Y	Y	Y	N	R
Tiberius	P. Brierley	VB/Excel [c]	Y	N	N	N	R

[a] Bayesian regularization.
[b] Includes the evidence framework and MCMC-based approximation.
[c] Backpropagation code also available in Fortran 90 and Java.

Table 16.2. Summary of some academic and commercial software for BN development (adapted from Murphy [32], reprinted with permission). The "Code" column states whether the source code is available (N ≡ no). If it is, the language used is given. The "CVN" column states whether continuous-valued nodes can be accommodated (N ≡ restricted to discrete-valued nodes; Y ≡ yes and without discretization; D ≡ yes but requires discretization). The "GUI" column states whether a GUI is available. The "$\boldsymbol{\theta}$" column states whether parameter learning is possible. The "$\mathcal{G}$" column states whether structure learning is possible. The "Free" column states whether the software is free (R ≡ only a restricted version is free).

Package	Developer	Code	CVN	GUI	$\boldsymbol{\theta}$	$\mathcal{G}$	Free
BayesBuilder	SNN Nijmegen	N	N	Y	N	N	R
BayesiaLab	Bayesia	N	D	Y	Y	Y	R
Bayesware Discoverer	Bayesware	N	D	Y	Y [a]	Y [a]	R
BN PowerConstructor	J. Cheng	N	N	Y	Y	Y [b]	Y
BNT [32]	K. Murphy	Matlab/C	Y	N	Y	Y	Y
BNJ	W.H. Hsu et al.	Java	N	Y	N	Y	Y
BUGS [45]	MRC/Imperial College	N	Y	Y	Y	N	Y
CoCo [1] [c]	J.H. Badsberg	C/Lisp	N	Y	Y	Y	Y
Deal [6]	S.G. Bøttcher et al.	R	Y [d]	Y	Y	Y	Y
GDAGsim [53]	D. Wilkinson	C	Y [e]	N	N	N	Y
GRAPPA	P.J. Green	R	N	N	N	N	Y
Hugin	Hugin Expert	N	Y	Y	Y	Y	R
Hydra [51]	G. Warnes	Java	Y	Y	Y	N	Y
JavaBayes [14]	F.G. Cozman	Java	N	Y	N	N	Y
MIM [17] [f]	Hypergraph Software	Y	Y	Y	Y	Y	R
MSBNx [26]	Microsoft	N	N	Y	N	N	R
Netica	Norsys Software	N	Y	Y	Y	N	R
Tetrad [43]	P. Spirtes et al.	N	Y	N	Y	Y	Y
WebWeaver	Y. Xiang	Java	N	Y	N	N	Y

[a] Uses the "bound and collapse" algorithm [41] to learn from incomplete data.
[b] Uses Cheng's three-phase construction algorithm [11].
[c] Analyzes associations between discrete variables of large, complete, contingency tables.
[d] Restricted to conditional Gaussian BNs.
[e] Restricted to Gaussian BNs.
[f] Provides graphical modelling for undirected graphs and chain graphs as well as DAGs.

16.5.1 Hugin and Netica

The best-known commercial packages for BN development are Hugin and Netica.[10]

Hugin (Hugin Expert) has an easy-to-use graphical user interface (GUI) for BN construction and inference (Figure 16.1).[11] It supports the learning of both BN parameters and BN structures from (possibly incomplete) data sets of sample cases. The structure-learning is done via the PC algorithm [46]. APIs (application programmers interfaces) are available for C, C++ and Java, and an Active-X server is provided. These enable the inference engine to be used within other programs. Hugin is compatible with the Windows, Solaris and Linux platforms.

Like Hugin, *Netica* (Norsys Software) supports BN construction and inference through an advanced GUI.[12] It has broad platform support (Windows, Linux, Sun Sparc, Macintosh, Silicon Graphics, and DOS), and APIs are available for C, C++, Java, and Visual Basic. Netica enables parameters (but not structures) to be estimated from (possibly incomplete) data; however, although the functionality of Netica is less than that of Hugin, it is considerably less expensive.

16.5.2 The Bayes Net Toolbox

In 1997, Kevin Murphy started to develop the *Bayes Net Toolbox* (BNT) [32] in response to weaknesses of the BN systems available at the time.

BNT is an open-sourced collection of Matlab routines for BN (and influence diagram) construction and inference, including *dynamic probability networks.*[13] It allows a wide variety of probability distributions to be used at the nodes (e.g., multinomial, Gaussian, and MLP), and both exact and approximate inference methods are available (e.g., junction tree, variable elimination, and MCMC sampling).

Both parameter and structure estimation from (possibly incomplete) data are supported. Structures can be learnt from data by means of the K2 [13] and IC/PC [46] algorithms. When data are incomplete, the structural EM algorithm can be used.[14]

Example 4. In BNT, a directed acyclic graph (DAG) is specified by a binary-valued matrix $\{e_{i,j}\}$, where $e_{i,j} = 1$ if a directed edge goes from node i to node j. For the DAG shown in Figure 16.1(a), this adjacency matrix is obtained by

```
N = 4; % Number of nodes
dag = zeros(N,N); % Initially no edges
C = 1; S = 2; R = 3; W = 4; % IDs for the four nodes
dag(C,[R S]) = 1; dag(R,W) = 1; dag(S,W)=1; % Edges defined
```

Next, the type of nodes to be used for the BN are defined:

```
discrete_nodes = 1:N; % All nodes are discrete-valued
nodesizes = 2*ones(1,N); % All nodes are binary
bnet = mk_bnet(dag,node_sizes,'discrete', discrete_nodes);
```

---

[10] Hugin and Netica also support the development of influence diagrams.

[11] http://www.hugin.com/

[12] http://www.norsys.com/

[13] http://www.ai.mit.edu/~murphyk/Software/BNT/bnt.html

[14] See Section 2.3.6 and Section 4.4.5.

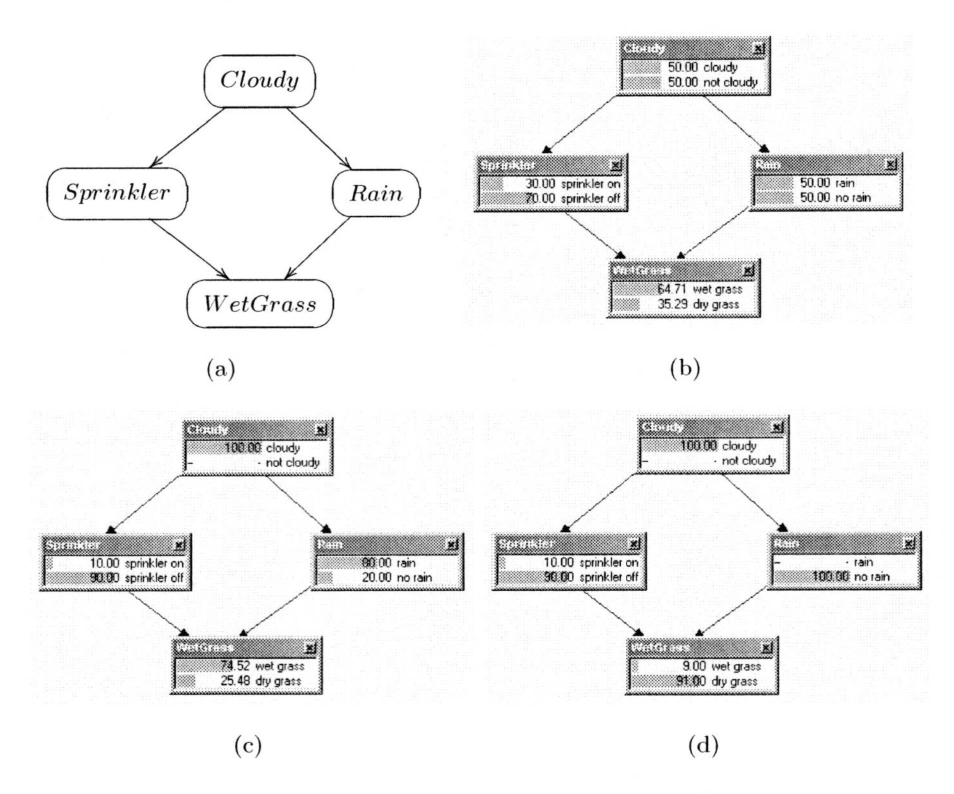

Fig. 16.1. (a) A DAG for the classic "wet grass" scenario. (b) A Hugin rendering of this DAG. The histograms show the probability distributions at each node X, which, initially, are the prior probabilities $p(X)$. (c) $Cloudy = true$; consequently, the probabilities are updated to the posterior distributions $p(X|Cloudy = true)$. (d) $Cloudy = true$ and $Rain = false$; therefore, the probability distributions are updated to $p(X|Cloudy = true, Rain = false)$.

(In BNT, $false = 1$ and $true = 2$.) The BN definition is completed by defining the conditional probability distribution at each node. For this example, binomial distributions are used, and the values are entered manually. If $V_1, \ldots, V_n$ are the parents of node X, with sizes $|V_1|, \ldots, |V_n|$, the conditional probability distribution $p(X|V_1, \ldots, V_n)$ for node X can be defined as follows:

```
CPT = zeros(|V1|, ..., |Vn|, |X|);
CPT(v1, ..., vn, x) = p(X = x|V1 = v1, ..., Vn = vn);
··· repeated for each p(x|v1, ..., vn)
bnet.CPD{X} = tabular_CPD(bnet, X, 'CPT', CPT);
```

We can perform inferences with this BN. To enter the evidence that $Cloudy = true$ and find the updated probability $p(WetGrass = true|Cloudy = true)$ via the junction-tree algorithm, we can use

```
evidence = cell(1,N); evidence{C} = 2; % Cloudy = true
engine = jtree_inf_engine(bnet); % Use junction-tree algorithm
[engine, loglikelihood] = enter_evidence(engine, evidence);
marg = marginal_nodes(engine, W); % p(W|Cloudy = true)
prob = marg.T(2); % p(W = 2|Cloudy = true)
```

An alternative to the above manual approach is to let BNT learn the probabilities from available data. To obtain the maximum-likelihood estimates of the probabilities from a complete data set `data`, we can first initialize the probabilities to random values,

```
seed = 0; rand('state', seed);
bnet.CPD{C} = tabular_CPD(bnet, C, 'CPT', 'rnd');
bnet.CPD{R} = tabular_CPD(bnet, R, 'CPT', 'rnd');
bnet.CPD{S} = tabular_CPD(bnet, S, 'CPT', 'rnd');
bnet.CPD{W} = tabular_CPD(bnet, W, 'CPT', 'rnd');
```

and then apply

```
bnet = learn_params(bnet, data);
```

◁

There are some limitations to BNT. Firstly, it does not have a GUI. Secondly, BNT requires Matlab to run it. It would be better if a version of BNT was developed that is independent of any commercial software. Furthermore, Matlab is a suboptimal language in that it is slow compared with C, and its object structure is less advanced than that of Java or C++. The desire to overcome these drawbacks was the motivation behind the OpenBayes initiative.

16.5.3 The OpenBayes Initiative

Although there are a number of software packages available for constructing and computing graphical models, no single package contains all the features that one would like to see, and most of the commercial packages are expensive. Therefore, in order to have a package that contains the features desired by the BN community, InferSpace launched the *OpenBayes* initiative in January 2001, the aim of which was to prompt the building of an open-sourced software environment for graphical-model development.

There have been other BN-oriented open-source initiatives, such as Fabio Cozman's *JavaBayes* system.

16.5.4 The Probabilistic Networks Library

In late 2001, Intel began to develop an open-sourced C++ library called the *Probabilistic Networks Library* (PNL), which initially closely modelled the BNT package.[15] PNL has been available to the public since December 2003.

[15] `http://www.ai.mit.edu/~murphyk/Software/PNL/pnl.html`

16.5.5 The gR Project

In September 2002, the *gR* project was conceived, the purpose of which is to develop facilities in R for graphical modelling [31].[16] The project is being managed by Aalborg University.

The software associated with the gR project includes (i) *Deal* [6], for learning conditionally Gaussian networks in R, (ii) *mimR*, an interface from R to MIM (which provides graphical modelling for undirected graphs, DAGs, and chain graphs [17]), and (iii) an R port for *CoCo* [1], which analyzes associations within contingency tables. The ability of R (and S-Plus) to interface with programs written in C++ means that Intel's PNL could become a powerful part of the gR project.

16.5.6 The VIBES Project

The use of variational methods for approximate reasoning in place of MCMC sampling is gaining interest (Chapter 14). In a joint project between Cambridge University and Microsoft Research, a system called *VIBES* (Variational Inference for Bayesian Networks) [5] is being developed that will allow variational inference to be performed automatically on a BN specified through a GUI.

16.6 Class-probability trees

[Class-probability trees were featured in Section 10.10.]

Two of the original tree-induction packages are *C4.5* [39] and *CART* [7]. C4.5 has been superseded by *C5.0*, which, like its Windows counterpart *See5*, is a commercial product developed by RuleQuest Research.[17]

CART introduced the concept of surrogate splits to enable trees to handle missing data (Section 10.10). It is available as a commercial package from Salford Systems.[18]

Class-probability trees can also be created by several statistical packages. These facilities include the S-Plus `tree` function and the R `rpart` function. An advantage of the `rpart` function is that it can use surrogate variables in a manner closely resembling that proposed by Breiman et al. [7].

Example 5. The R function `rpart` can grow a tree from the kyphosis data used in Example 1:

```
kyph.tree <- rpart(Kyphosis ~ Age + Number + Start,
                   data=kyphosis, parms=list(split='gini'))
```

In this example, the Gini index of class heterogeneity has been used. The information-theoretic entropy measure is also available. Figure 16.2 shows a visualization of the tree obtained with

```
plot(kyph.tree); text(kyph.tree, use.n=TRUE)
```

[16] `http://www.r-project.org/gR/gR.html`
[17] `http://www.rulequest.com/`
[18] `http://www.salford-systems.com/`

A new feature vector of values **xnew** can be dropped down the tree in order to estimate $p(Kyphosis = 1|\texttt{xnew})$ from a leaf node. This is done using

```
predict(kyph.tree, newdata = xnew)
```

◁

In Section 10.10.2, we described Buntine's approach to Bayesian trees [8]. His ideas are implemented in the *IND* package, which can now be obtained (along with the source code) from the NASA Ames Research Center under a NASA software usage agreement.[19]

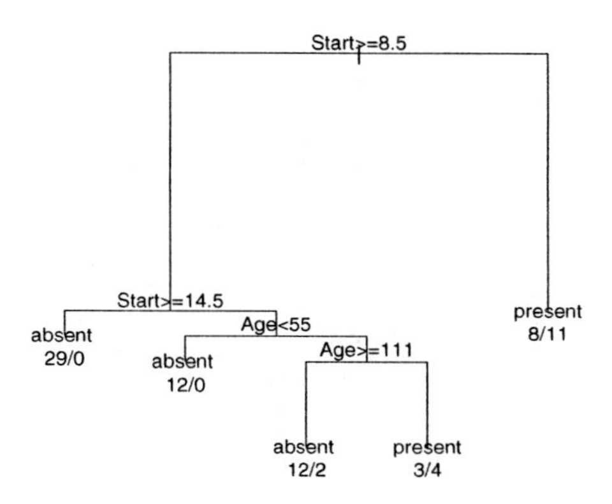

Fig. 16.2. Plot obtained when the R function **rpart** was used to grow a tree (Example 5). At each split, the left branch corresponds to the case when the split criterion is true for a given feature vector, and the right branch to when the criterion is false. Each leaf node is labelled with the associated classification followed by the frequency of the classes "absent" and "present" at the node (delimited by "/").

16.7 Hidden Markov Models

[Hidden Markov models were featured in Chapter 14 and Sections 10.11.4, 2.2.2, 4.4.7 and 5.10.]

A Hidden Markov model (HMM) consists of a discrete-valued hidden node S linked to a discrete- or continuous-valued observed node X. Figure 16.3 shows the model "unrolled" over three time steps: $\tau = 1, 2, 3$.

Although the majority of statistical software packages enable classical time-series models, such as ARIMA, to be built, tools for modelling with HMMs are not a standard feature. This is also true of mathematical packages such as Matlab and Mathematica.

[19] **http://ic.arc.nasa.gov/projects/bayes-group/ind/IND-program.html**

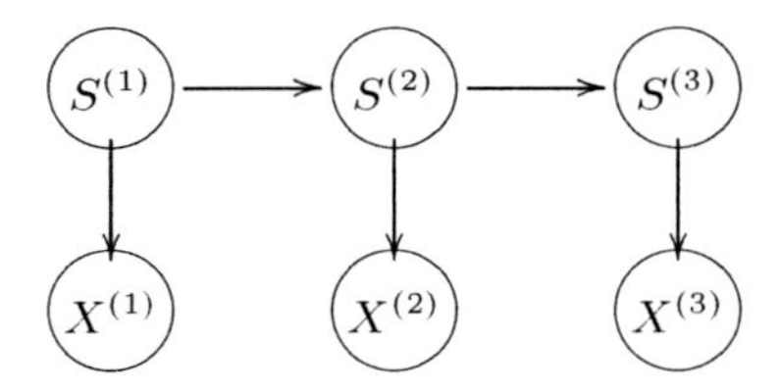

Fig. 16.3. A graphical representation of an HMM. The model is defined by the probability distributions $p(S^{(1)})$, $p(S^{(\tau+1)}|S^{(\tau)})$, and $p(X^{(\tau)}|S^{(\tau)})$. The last two distributions are assumed to be the same for all time slices $\tau \geq 1$.

16.7.1 Hidden Markov Model Toolbox for Matlab

Kevin Murphy has written a toolbox for developing hidden HMMs with Matlab.[20] Tools for this purpose are also available within his BNT package (Section 16.5.2). We illustrate the HMM toolbox with the following example.

Example 6. Suppose we wish to classify a biomedical time series $\mathbf{x} = \{x^{(1)}, x^{(2)}, \ldots, x^{(T)}\}$ by assigning it to one of K classes (for example, K physiological states). We assume that a time series is generated by an HMM associated with a class, there being a unique set of HMM parameters $\boldsymbol{\theta}_k$ for each class k. The required classification can be done probabilistically by assigning a new time series $\mathbf{x}_{\text{new}}$ to the class k for which $p(\boldsymbol{\theta}_k|\mathbf{x}_{\text{new}})$ is maximum.

For each of the K classes of interest, we can train an HMM using a sample (`data_k`) of time series associated with class k. The standard method is to use the EM algorithm to compute the MLE $\hat{\boldsymbol{\theta}}_k$ of $\boldsymbol{\theta}_k$ with respect to `data_k`:

```
[LL, prior_k, transmat_k, obsmat_k] =
 dhmm_em(data_k, prior0, transmat0, obsmat0, 'max_iterations',10);
```

where `prior0`, `transmat0`, `obsmat0` are initial random values respectively corresponding to the prior probability distribution $p(S^{(1)})$, the transition probability matrix $p(S^{(\tau+1)}|S^{(\tau)})$, and the observation probability matrix $p(X^{(\tau)}|S^{(\tau)})$. The resulting MLEs for these probabilities are given by `prior_k`, `transmat_k`, and `obsmat_k`, which collectively provide $\hat{\boldsymbol{\theta}}_k$.

From $\hat{\boldsymbol{\theta}}_k$, the log-likelihood $\log p(\texttt{x\_new}|\hat{\boldsymbol{\theta}}_k)$ for a new time series `x_new` can be obtained using

```
loglik = dhmm_logprob(x_new, prior_k, transmat_k, obsmat_k)
```

which can be related to $p(\hat{\boldsymbol{\theta}}_k|\texttt{x\_new})$ by Bayes' theorem. $\triangleleft$

Acknowledgments

We would like to thank Paulo Lisboa and Peter Weller for their careful reading and constructive comments on an earlier draft of this chapter.

We are grateful to Kevin Murphy for allowing us to use data from his website *Software Packages for Graphical Models/Bayesian Networks*[21] for Table 16.2.

[20] `http://www.ai.mit.edu/~murphyk/Software/HMM/hmm.html`

[21] `http://www.ai.mit.edu/~murphyk/Software/BNT/bnsoft.html`

References

[1] J.H. Badsberg. *An Environment for Graphical Models.* PhD dissertation, Department of Mathematical Sciences, Aalborg University, 1995.

[2] J.M.G. Barahona, P.D.H. Quiros, and T. Bollinger. A brief history of free software and open source. *IEEE Software*, 16(1):32–33, 1999.

[3] R.A. Becker, J.M. Chambers, and A.R. Wilks. *The New S Language.* Wadworth & Brooks/Cole, Pacific Grove, CA, 1988.

[4] C.M. Bishop. *Neural Networks for Pattern Recognition.* Clarendon Press, Oxford, 1995.

[5] C.M. Bishop, D. Spiegelhalter, and J. Winn. VIBES: A variational inference engine for Bayesian networks. In *Advances in Neural Information Processing Systems 9*, MIT Press, Cambridge, MA, 2003.

[6] S.G. Bottcher and C. Dethlefsen. Deal: A package for learning Bayesian networks. Technical report, Department of Mathematical Sciences, Aalborg University, 2003.

[7] L. Breiman, J.H. Friedman, R.A. Olshen, and C.J. Stone. *Classification and Regression Trees.* Chapman & Hall, New York, 1984.

[8] W. Buntine. *A Theory of Learning Classification Rules.* PhD dissertation, School of Computing Science, University of Technology, Sydney, February 1990.

[9] S.K. Card, J.D. Mackinlay, and B. Shneiderman. *Readings in Information Visualization: Using Vision to Think.* Morgan Kaufmann, San Fransisco, CA, 1999.

[10] J.M. Chambers and T.J. Hastie. *Statistical Models in S.* Wadsworth & Brooks/Cole Advanced Books & Software, Pacific Grove, CA, 1992.

[11] J. Cheng and R. Greiner. Learning Bayesian belief network classifiers: Algorithms and systems. In E. Stroulia and S. Matwin, editors, *Proceedings of the 14th Canadian Conference on Artificial Intelligence*, Lecture Notes in Computer Science, pages 141–151, Springer-Verlag,New York, 2001.

[12] D. Collett. *Modelling Binary Data.* Chapman & Hall, London, 1991.

[13] G.F Cooper and E. Herskovits. A Bayesian method for the induction of probabilistic networks from data. *Machine Learning*, 9:309–347, 1992.

[14] F.G. Cozman. The JavaBayes system. *The ISBA Bulletin*, 7(4):16–21, 2001.

[15] A.C. Davidson and D.V. Hinkley. *Bootstrap Methods and Their Applications.* Cambridge University Press, Cambridge, 1997.

[16] K.A. De Jong. *Evolutionary Computation: A Unified Approach.* MIT Press, Cambridge, MA, 2003.

[17] D. Edwards. *Introduction to Graphical Modelling.* Springer-Verlag, New York, 2nd edition, 2000.

[18] B. Efron and R.J. Tibshirani. *An Introduction to the Bootstrap.* Chapman & Hall, New York, 1993.

[19] D.B. Fogel. *Evolutionary Computation: Toward a New Philosophy of Machine Intelligence.* IEEE Press, New York, 1995.

[20] K. Fogel. *Open Source Development with CVS.* Coriolis, Scottsdale, AZ, 1999.

[21] N. Friedman. The Bayesian structural EM algorithm. In G.F. Cooper and S. Moral, editors, *Proceedings of the 14th Conference on Uncertainty in Artificial Intelligence*, pages 129–138, Morgan Kaufmann, San Francisco, CA, 1998.

[22] M.N. Gibbs. *Bayesian Gaussian Processes for Regression and Classification.* PhD dissertation, Department fo Computing Science, University of Cambridge, 1997.

[23] W.R. Gilks, S. Richardson, and D.J. Spiegelhalter, editors. *Markov Chain Monte Carlo in Practice.* Chapman & Hall, London, 1996.

[24] M.T. Hagan, H.B. Demuth, and M. Beale. *Neural Network Design.* PWS Publishing, Boston, 1996.

[25] F.E. Harrell. *Regression Modeling Strategies.* Springer, New York, 2001.

[26] E. Horvitz, D. Hovel, and C. Kadie. MSBNx: A component-centric toolkit for modeling and inference with Bayesian networks. Technical Report MSR-TR-2001-67, Microsoft Research, Redmond, WA, July 2001.

[27] B.R. Hunt, R.L. Lipsman, and J.M. Rosenberg. *A Guide to MATLAB: For Beginners and Experienced Users.* Cambridge University Press, Cambridge, 2001.

[28] R. Ihaka and R. Gentleman. R: a language for data analysis and graphics. *Journal of Computational and Graphical Statistics*, 5:299–314, 1996.

[29] H. James. Editorial. *Neural Computing and Applications*, 5:129–130, 1997.

[30] K.B. Korb and A.E. Nicholson. *Bayesian Artificial Intelligence.* CRC Press, London, 2003.

[31] S.L. Lauritzen. gRaphical models in R. *R News*, 3(2):39, 2002.

[32] K.P. Murphy. The Bayes Net Toolbox for Matlab. *Computing Science and Statistics*, 33:331–350, 2001, The Interface Foundation of North America.

[33] I.T. Nabney. *NETLAB: Algorithms for Pattern Recognition.* Springer, London, 2002.

[34] G.M. Nielson, H. Hagan, and H. Müller. *Scientific Visualization: Overviews, Methodologies, and Techniques.* IEEE Computer Society, Los Alamitos, CA, 1997.

[35] R.C. O'Reilly and Y. Munakata. *Computational Explorations in Cognitive Neuroscience.* MIT Press, Cambridge, MA, 2000.

[36] R.C. Pavlicek. *Embracing Insanity: Open Source Software Development.* SAMS, Indianapolis, IN, 2000.

[37] B. Perens. The Open Source definition. In C. DiBona and S. Ockman, editors, *Open Sources: Voices From the Open Source Revolution*, pages 171–188. O'Reilly & Associates, Sebastopol, CA, 1999.

[38] J.C. Principe, N.R. Euliano, and W.C. Lefebvre. *Neural and Adaptive Systems.* John Wiley, New York, 2000.

[39] J.R. Quinlan. *C4.5: Programs for Machine Learning.* Morgan Kaufman, San Mateo, CA, 1993.

[40] A.E. Raftery and C. Volinsky, 1999. *Bayesian Model Averaging Home Page* [WWW]. Available from: http://www.research.att.com/ volinsky/bma.html [accessed 9 July 1999].

[41] M. Ramoni and P. Sebastiani. Learning Bayesian networks from incomplete databases. Technical Report KMI-TR-43, Knowledge Media Institute, Open University, February 1997.

[42] D.K. Rosenberg. *Open Source: The Unauthorized White Papers.* M & T Books, Foster City, CA, 2000.

[43] R. Scheines, P. Spirtes, C. Glymour, and C. Meek. *TETRAD II: Tools for Discovery.* Lawrence Erlbaum Associates, Hillsdale, NJ, 1994.

[44] D. Spiegelhalter, A.Thomas, N. Best, and W. Gilks. *BUGS: Bayesian inference Using Gibbs Sampling.* MRC Biostatistics Unit, Cambridge, 1996.

[45] D.J. Spiegelhalter, A. Thomas, and N.G. Best. *WinBUGS Version 1.2 User Manual.* MRC Biostatistics Unit, Cambridge, 1999.

[46] P. Spirtes, C. Glymour, and R. Scheines. *Causation, Prediction, and Search.* MIT Press, Cambridge, MA, 2nd edition, 2001.

[47] R. Stallman. The GNU Operating System and the Free Software Movement. In C. DiBona and S. Ockman, editors, *Open Sources: Voices From the Open Source Revolution*, pages 53–70. O'Reilly & Associates, Sebastopol, CA, 1999.

[48] M. Svensén. *GTM: The Generative Topographic Mapping.* PhD dissertation, Neural Computing Research Group, Aston University, April 1998.

[49] W.N. Venables and B.D. Ripley. *Modern Applied Statistics with S-Plus.* Springer, New York, 3rd edition, 1999.

[50] W.N. Venables and B.D. Ripley. *S Programming.* Springer, New York, 2000.

[51] G.R. Warnes. HYDRA: a Java library for Markov chain Monte Carlo. *Journal of Statistical Software*, 7: issue 4, 2002.

[52] M. Welsh, M.K. Dalheimer, and L. Kaufman. *Running Linux.* O'Reilly & Associates, Sebastopol, CA, 3rd edition, 1999.

[53] D.J. Wilkinson and S.K.H. Yeung. A sparse matrix approach to Bayesian computation in large linear models. *Computational Statistics and Data Analysis*, 44:423–516, 2004.

A

Appendix: Conventions and Notation

Table A.1: Conventions.

X	(i.e., upper case) refers to a random variable
x	(i.e., lower case) refers to a value. x also refers to a random variable in Chapters 1, 2, 4, 5, 6, 8, and 9
$\mathbf{X}$	(i.e., bold upper case) refers to a matrix of random variables or values. $\mathbf{X}$ also refers to a vector of random variables in Chapter 10
$\mathbf{x}$	(i.e., bold lower case) refers to a vector of random variables or values

Table A.2: Abbreviations used frequently.

ANN	artificial neural network
ARD	Automatic Relevance Determination
BN	Bayesian (belief) network
DAG	directed acyclic graph
ECG	electrocardiogram
EEG	electroencephalogram
EM	expectation-maximization
HMM	hidden Markov model
MAP	maximum a posteriori
MCMC	Markov chain Monte Carlo
MLE	maximum likelihood estimate

continued on next page

continued from previous table	
MLP	multilayer perceptron
PCA	principal component analysis
PD	pharmacodynamics
PK	pharmacokinetics
RBFNN	radial basis function neural network

Table A.3: Non-Greek notation used frequently.

$\mathcal{B}(a, b)$	beta distribution with parameters a and b
$Bernoulli(p)$	Bernoulli distribution with success probability p
$\mathcal{D}$	data
$Dir(\alpha_1, \ldots, \alpha_n)$	Dirichlet distribution with parameters $\alpha_1, \ldots, \alpha_n$
$E(\boldsymbol{\theta})$	error function with respect to parameters $\boldsymbol{\theta}$
$\mathcal{E}$	expectation operator
$Gamma(\alpha, \beta)$; $\mathcal{G}(\alpha, \beta)$	gamma distribution with coefficients α and β
$KL(A, B)$; $D(A\|\|B)$	Kullback–Leibler divergence between A and B
ℓ	logistic function
L	set of leaf nodes of a tree in Chapter 4
$\mathcal{M}$	model or structure
$Normal(\mu, \nu)$; $N(\mu, \nu)$; $\mathcal{N}(\mu, \nu)$	Normal distribution with mean μ and variance ν
$\mathrm{MVN}_p(\boldsymbol{\mu}, \boldsymbol{\Sigma})$; $\mathcal{M}_p(\boldsymbol{\mu}, \boldsymbol{\Sigma})$	p-dimensional multivariate Normal distribution with mean $\boldsymbol{\mu}$ and variance $\boldsymbol{\Sigma}$
$p(A)$; $P(A)$	probability of A [1]
$p(A\|B)$; $P(A\|B)$	probability of A given knowledge of B
$\mathbf{q}$	parameter vector (alternative notation to $\boldsymbol{\theta}$)
$\mathbb{R}$	the set of real numbers

continued on next page

[1] p (and P) denotes different functions for different arguments; e.g., $p(X)$ and $p(Y)$ are different functions.

continued from previous table

S	hidden state; i.e., the random variable associated with a hidden node in a Bayesian network. S denotes a tree topology in Chapters 4 and 5 [2]
$\mathcal{S}$	a set, sequence, or vector of hidden states
$\mathrm{tr}(\mathbf{A})$	trace of matrix $\mathbf{A}$
$\mathsf{Var}(X)$; $Var(X)$	variance of X
$\mathcal{W}(\alpha, \mathbf{\Sigma})$	Wishart distribution with parameters α and $\mathbf{\Sigma}$
$\mathbf{w}$	vector of neural-network weights in Chapter 3. $\mathbf{w}$ denotes branch lengths in a phylogenetic tree in Chapters 4, 5, and 6

Table A.4: Greek notation used frequently.

β	regression coefficient
$\boldsymbol{\beta}$	vector of regression coefficients
$\delta(x)$	delta function [3]
$\delta_{i,k}$	Kronecker delta
$\Gamma(x)$	gamma function [4]
$\Gamma(\alpha, \beta)$	gamma distribution with coefficients α and β
$\boldsymbol{\theta}$	parameter vector (alternative notation to $\mathbf{q}$)
μ	mean of a univariate normal distribution
$\boldsymbol{\mu}$	mean of a multivariate normal distribution
σ	standard deviation
$\mathbf{\Sigma}$	covariance matrix
$\Omega[\xi]$	sample space for ξ

[2] Chapter 5 combines both notations in that the tree topology corresponds to the hidden state of an HMM, hence S is both a hidden state and a tree topology.

[3] $\delta(0) = \infty$, $\delta(x) = 0$ if $x \neq 0$, and $\int_{-\infty}^{\infty} \delta(x)dx = 1$

[4] $\int_0^\infty \exp(-t)t^{x-1}dt$. For integer n, $\Gamma(n+1) = n!$

Table A.5: Other mathematical conventions and symbols used frequently.

$\tilde{X}$	approximate value of X
$\binom{N}{k}$	combination of k from N [5]
$\|\mathbf{A}\|$; $\det(\mathbf{A})$	determinant of matrix $\mathbf{A}$
$n!!$	double factorial of n [6]
$x \in A$	x is an element of set A
$\triangleleft$	end of example
$\square$	end of proof
$\hat{X}$	estimated value of X (usually an MLE)
$\langle X \rangle$	expectation of X
$\forall x$	for all values of x
$\nabla f(\mathbf{x})$	gradient at $f(\mathbf{x})$
$A \perp B$	A is independent of B
$A \perp B \mid C$	A is independent of B given C
$A \cap B$	intersection of sets A and B
$A \setminus B$	set A minus set B
$\|A\|$	number of elements in set or vector A
$A \subseteq B$	A is a subset of B
$\mathbf{A}^{\mathsf{T}}$; $\mathbf{A}^{\dagger}$	transposition of vector or matrix $\mathbf{A}$
$A \cup B$	union of sets A and B

[5] $\binom{N}{k} = \frac{N!}{k!(N-k)!}$ for integer N, k, but $\binom{N}{k} = \frac{\Gamma(N+1)}{(k+1)\Gamma(N-k+1)}$ for continuous N, k

[6] $n!! = n \times (n-2) \times (n-4) \times \ldots \times 3 \times 1$ for n odd, and $n!! = n \times (n-2) \times (n-4) \times \ldots \times 4 \times 2$ for n even.

Index

A-optimality, 226
AIDS, 84, 86, 88, 147
ALARM system, 320
ANOVA, 226
apoptosis, 289
approximating a posterior distribution, 420, 421
Archea, 192
Automatic Relevance Determination, 316, 375

backpropagation, 14
batch learning, 72
Baum-Welch, 425
Bayes Net Toolbox, 480, 481
Bayes' theorem, 4, 10, 299, 372, 397, 398, 400
BayesBuilder, 480
BayesiaLab, 480
Bayesian information criterion, 41, 53
Bayesian model selection, 421
Bayesian networks, 239, 241, 317, 452, 478
  conditional Gaussian networks, 320
  construction, 321, 322
  dynamic, 251, 252, 317
  example, 18
  Gaussian networks, 320
  greedy search, 322
  hidden states, 46
  inference, 318
  introduction to, 17
  junction-tree algorithm, 52, 319
  loopy belief propagation, 320
  missing data, *see* missing data, Bayesian networks
  parameters, 25, 26
  Pearl's message passing algorithm, 52, 116
  quickscore algorithm, 319
  structure, 17, 26
  synonyms, 317
Bayesian statistics, 10, 63, 130, 298, 352, 356, 360, 363, 365, 367, 372, 391, 393–398, 400, 403, 405, 407, 408, 411, 412, 416
  axioms, 391
  Bayes factor, 304
  computations, 300
  conjugate priors, 403
  decision, 391
  evidence, 395
  full conditional distributions, 405, 407, 408
  Gibbs sampling, 403
  hierarchical models, 306
  inference, 391, 400, 403, 405, 407, 408, 416
  Jeffreys' prior, 394
  logistic regression, 302
  marginal likelihood, 395
  marginalisation, 392, 397, 398, 400, 416
  model averaging, 299
  model uncertainty, 395–398, 400
  modelling, 396
  neural networks, 311

parameter averaging, 299
parameter inference, 400
parameter uncertainty, 394, 396–398, 400, 411, 412
posterior probability, 393, 394, 397, 398, 400, 405, 407, 408
prediction, 397, 416
preprocessing, 392–395, 416
prior probability, 363, 365, 394, 403
Dirichlet, 321
uninformative, 299
theory, 391
tree induction, 325
uncertainty, 391, 392, 396–398, 400
updating, 299
Bayesware Discoverer, 480
BCI, 393
beta distribution, 11, 12
BIC, *see* Bayesian information criterion
BILAG index, 382
binary dummy variables, 69
bioavailability, 354, 364
birth weight, 302, 324
BLAST, 258
BN PowerConstructor, 480
BNJ, 480
bootstrapping, 281
in phylogenetics, 127–129
comparison with Bayesian posterior probabilities, 208
comparison with MCMC, 134
example, 9
illustration of, 8
introduction, 8
parametric, 158
shortcomings of, 129
brain computer interface, *see* BCI
BrainMaker, 479
BUGS, 476, 480

C4.5, 484
C5.0, 484
CART, 484
causal Markov assumption, 38, 246
Chapman-Kolmogorov equation, 107, 114, 115, 140
Cheyne Stokes respiration, 436
class-probability trees, 484
classical statistics, *see* statistics
classification, 60, 66, 234, 391, 396, 400, 413, 416
probabilistic classification, 66
static, 396
time series, 400
clinical trial, 468
clustering, 234, 241
neighbour joining, 96, 98, 126, 159
shortcomings of, 98
UPGMA, 93–95, 129
CoCo, 480, 484
codon position, 136, 140
coefficient of variation, 219
cognitive tasks, 439
combining information, *see* sensor fusion
compensatory substitutions, *see* RNA
conjugate distributions, 426
conjugate prior, *see* prior probability
consensus tree, *see* phylogenetic tree
cost-benefit analysis, 463
covariation, *see* RNA
cross-validation, 75
curse of dimensionality, 77
cytokines, 289

d-separation, *see* DAG
DAG, 18, 392, 396, 397, 400, 402, 403, 405
arcs, *see* edges
child, 17
clique, 52
d-separation, 22–24, 246
edges, 17
equivalence classes, 35, 38, 39, 251
explaining away, 22
Markov blanket, 19, 179, 246
Markov neighbours, 245
neighbourhood, 35
nodes, 17
order relations, 246
parent, 17
separator relations, 246
v-structure, 35, 38
vertices, *see* nodes
data conditioning, 327
Deal, 480, 484
decision boundary, 61
decision regions, 61

decision-support systems, 451
delta method, 219
deoxyribonucleic acid, *see* DNA
desiderata for models, 297
detailed balance, *see* Markov chain
diagnosis, 391
directed acyclic graph, *see* DAG
discrete gamma distribution, *see* gamma distribution
diseases
  acute abdominal pain, 317
  arrhythmia, 375
  brain tumours, 333
  breast cancer, 305, 320
  cervical cancer, 308
  cyanosis, 320
  epilepsy, 332
  hepatitis, 326
  lupus, 382
  multiple sclerosis, 314
  Parkinson's disease, 314
  sepsis, 453
  urinary tract infection, 309, 455
distance between sequences, *see* genetic distances
DNA, 87
  base pairs, 212
  coding versus non-coding, 136
  deletions, 45
  double helix, 212
  gaps, 45, 135
  hybridization, 212
  indels, 45
  insertions, 45
  multiple sequence alignment, 45, 88, 89, 147
  mutations, 86
  pairwise sequence alignment, 45, 46
  replication, 86
  sequencing, 84, 87
DNAML, *see* likelihood method in phylogenetics
double helix, *see* DNA
dynamic programming, 48, 50

E-score, *see* BLAST
E-step, *see* EM algorithm
E. *coli*, 194
EEG, *see* electroencephalogram
electrocardiogram, 375
electroencephalogram, 328, 330, 332, 336, 391, 395, 411–413
  artefacts, 395
  cognitive tasks, 391, 412, 413
  electrode positions, 10-20 system, 411, 412
  sleep, 391, 411
  sleep spindles, 391, 411, 413
EM algorithm, 52, 274
  applied to HMMs, 49
  E-step, 44, 274
  for detecting recombination, 175
  illustration of, 44
  introduction to, 43
  M-step, 44, 275
  structural EM algorithm, 53, 125, 322
empirical models, 352, 353, 367
entropy, 194
epidemiology, 83
epoch, 72
equivalence classes, *see* DAG
eukaryotes, 192
evidence procedure, 41, 304, 373
evolution, 83
evolutionary distances, *see* genetic distances
exogenous variables, 272, 273
expectation maximization algorithm, *see* EM algorithm
extreme value theory, 338

false discovery rate (FDR), 233
family wise error rate (FWER), 232
feature extraction, *see* preprocessing
feature space, 61
feature vector, 60
filters
  autoregressive, 327
  Kalman–Bucy, 328
  linear, 327
Fisher information matrix, 41
Fisher's z-transform, 395
Fitch-Margoliash algorithm, 159
fixation, 196
forensic science, 83
free energy, 194, 195
frequentist statistics, *see* statistics

G+C-content, 140, 141
gamma distribution
  discrete, 136
GDAGsim, 480
gene, 212
  expression, 212
  expression data, 211, 269, 288
gene conversion, 184, 185
general time-reversible model, *see* nucleotide substitutions
generalisation accuracy, 411–414, 416
  cross validation, 411, 412
generative model, 393, 396, 400
genetic distances, 91, 99, 159
  additivity, 97
  corrected, 93
  saturation of, 93
genetic networks, 239, 269
Gibbs sampling, 177, 178, 304, 316
Gibbs-Metropolis hybrid sampler, 365
GLIB, 304, 475
gR, 484
gradient ascent, 120, 121
GRAPPA, 480
greedy optimization, 120, 121

H*aemophilus influenzae*, 87
Hastings ratio, *see* Markov chain Monte Carlo
Heart Beat Intervals, 437
hepatitis-B virus, 45
Hidden Markov Model Toolbox for Matlab, 486
hidden Markov models, 335–338, 400, 402, 423, 486
  Bayesian HMMs, 176
  coupled, 337
  derivation of Baum-Welch recursions, 443
  emission probabilities, 47–49
  estimation of observation model size, 431
  estimation of state space dimension, 431
  factor graph representation, 424
  factorial HMM, 180
  for detecting recombination, 171, 173, 174, 183, 186
  for modelling rate variation in phylogenetics, 138
  forward-backward algorithm, 50, 425
  Gaussian observation model, 427, 447
  graphical model representation, 423
  illustration of, 47
  initial state probability, 423, 426
  introduction to, 44
  KL divergences, 445
  linear observation model, 448
  negative entropy, 446
  observation model, 423
  Poisson observation model, 448
  state space representation, 423
  state transition probability, 423, 426
  transition probabilities, 47–49
  Viterbi algorithm, 48, 175
HIV, 84, 86, 150
HKY85 model, *see* nucleotide substitutions
HMMs, *see* hidden Markov models
homologous nucleotides, 88
Hugin, 458, 480, 481
human immunodeficiency virus, *see* HIV
hybridization, *see* DNA
Hydra, 477, 480
hyperparameters, 12, 174
hyperthermophiles, 140
hypothesis testing, 283, 285
  null hypothesis, 282
hysteretic oscillator, 258

image analysis
  median filter, 215
  morphological opening, 215
  top-hat filter, 215
IND, 485
independence
  conditional, 20, 23
  marginal, 21, 23
independent component anaylsis, 329
  blind source separation, 329
inference, 3, 4
inflammation response, 289
intensive care, 301
interleukin, 289
Internet, 473
intervention versus observation, 39

JavaBayes, 480
junction-tree algorithm, *see* Bayesian networks

Kalman filter, 276
Kalman gain matrix, *see* Kalman filter
Kalman smoother, 275
kernel function, 309
Kimura model, *see* nucleotide substitutions
Kullback-Leibler (KL) divergence, 43, 51, 164, 330
  Dirichlet density, 446
  Gamma density, 446
  matrix variate Normal density, 447
  multivariate Normal density, 447
  Wishart density, 447

Laplace approximation, 42
latent space, 398, 400, 416
latent variable, 391, 392, 396
ligand, 258
likelihood, 5, 11, 402
  marginal, 27
  of a phylogenetic tree, 111
likelihood method in phylogenetics, 104
  Bayesian inference, 130
  comparison with parsimony, 118
  DNAML, 122, 126
  maximum likelihood, 120
  peeling algorithm, 116, 174
  quartet puzzling, 123, 124, 126
linear dynamical systems, *see* state-space models
linlog-function, 222
localization assays, 262
loess normalization, 227
log-transformation, 219
logistic regression, 65, 301, 474
long branch attraction, *see* phylogenetics, parsimony method
loop design, 226

M-step, *see* EM algorithm
magnetic resonance imaging, 329
maize actin genes, 185
MammoNet, 320
MAP estimate, *see* maximum a posteriori estimate

Markov blanket, *see* DAG
Markov chain
  aperiodic, 29
  detailed balance, 30
  ergodic, 29
  homogeneous, 106, 110
  illustration of, 29
  irreducible, 29
  non-homogeneous, 139
  non-stationary, 139
  stationary, 110
  stationary distribution, 29
Markov chain Monte Carlo, 28, 300, 315, 391, 398, 400, 402, 403, 405, 407–411, 416
  algorithms, 409, 410
  applied to HMMs, 177
  comparison with bootstrapping, 134
  convergence, 33, 179, 411
  convergence test, 36, 255
  for detecting recombination, 163
  full conditional distributions, 405, 407, 408
  Gibbs sampling, 403, 405, 407, 408
  Hastings ratio, 33, 35, 248
  hybrid, 315
  illustration of, 32
  in phylogenetics, 131, 200
  Metropolis algorithm, 33, 315
  Metropolis-Hastings algorithm, 31, 33, 403, 408
  proposal moves in tree space, 133
  reversible jump MCMC, 54, 332
  sweeps, model inference, 409
  sweeps, model prediction, 410
Markov Chain sampling, 372
Markov neighbours, *see* DAG
Markov relations, *see* DAG, Markov neighbours
Mathematica Neural Networks, 479
Matlab, 477
Matlab Neural Network Toolbox, 479
maximum a posteriori, 299, 420
maximum a posteriori estimate, 13
maximum chi-squared method, 152
  illustration of, 152, 153
  shortcoming of, 155
maximum likelihood, 65, 298, 419
maximum likelihood estimate, 5, 13, 43

maximum parsimony, *see* phylogenetics, parsimony method
MCMC, *see* Markov chain Monte Carlo
mean field approximation, 53, 421
median filter, *see* image analysis
metabolism, 358, 359
metric, 96
  of a tree, 97
Metropolis algorithm, *see* Markov chain Monte Carlo
Metropolis-Hastings algorithm, *see* Markov chain Monte Carlo
microarrays, 211, 269
  cDNA-array, 213
  background, 216
  channel, 213
  differential expression, 228
  dye swap, 226
  eigenarray, 234
  eigengene, 234
  flagging, 224
  gridding, 216
  housekeeping genes, 225
  landing lights, 216
  MA-plot, 223
  mismatch, 213
  normalization, 222
  oligonucleotide arrays, 213
  perfect match, 213
  probe, 212
  quantile normalization, 228
  rank invariant set of genes, 228
  SAM, 233
  simulated gene expression data, 258, 259
  spiking, 225
  spot, 216
  target, 212
  technical replicates, 224, 282
  transformation, 218
MIM, 480, 484
minimum description length, 42
missing data, 298
  Bayesian networks, 322
  cold-deck imputation, 310
  data augmentation, 310
  distinction of parameters, 310
  EM algorithm, 310
  hot-deck imputation, 310
  ignorability, 310
  imputation, 310
  missing at random, 310
  multiple imputation, 310
  neural networks, 310
  tree-based models, 324
mixed model, 226
mixture models, 229
mixture of Gaussians model, 332
mixtures of variational distributions, 422
ML estimate, *see* maximum likelihood estimate
model selection, 281, 305
molecular clock, 95, 96
molecular phylogenetics, *see* phylogenetics
morphological opening, *see* image analysis
MSBNx, 480
multi-layer perceptron, 307
multinomial distribution, 243

naïve Bayes, 316, 396–398, 400, 459
neighbour joining, *see* clustering
Netica, 480, 481
Netlab, 477, 479
neural networks, 59–78, 307, 477
  1-in-c coding, 69
  activation functions, 61
  back-propagation algorithm, 63
  balanced data set, 78
  bias–variance trade-off, 74
  committee of networks, 77, 313
  conjugate-gradients algorithm, 73
  early stopping, 75
  error function, 69, 307
    cross-entropy, 69
  error surface, 70
  evidence framework, 75, 312
  generalization, 74
  global minimum, 70
  gradient descent, 70, 73
  hyperparameters, 312
  learning rate, 70
  local minima, 75
  McCulloch-Pitts neuron, 59
  missing data, *see* missing data, neural networks

moderated output, 311
momentum, 73
multi-layer perceptron, 62–63, 67–78
back-propagation algorithm, 70–72
forward propagation, 72
hidden nodes, 62, 77
training, 69–73
number of exemplars, 78
over-fitting, 74
preprocessing, 77
probabilistic neural networks, 309
quasi-Newton algorithm, 68, 73
radial basis functions, 309
random restarts, 77
regularization, 74, 307
single-layer perceptron, 61
softmax, 69
weight decay, 68, 75
NeuralWorks, 479
NeuroSolutions, 479
novelty detection, 78, 338
nucleotide substitutions, 92
general time-reversible model, 199
HKY85 model, 110, 112, 173, 199
Kimura model, 107, 108, 112, 173, 199
mathematical model, 104–106, 139
for RNA, 197
rate heterogeneity, 136
rate matrix, 107, 110
reversibility condition, 112, 199
Tamura model, 140
transitions, 105, 198
transversions, 105, 198
nucleotides, 87
NuRho, 479
Neisseria, 147, 184

Occam factor, 27
open-source software, 474
GNU General Public License, 474
Linux, 474
OpenBayes, 483
order relation, *see* DAG
outgroup, *see* phylogenetic tree
over-fitting, 14, 28

p-value, 155, 231
adjusted, 232
PAPNET, 308
parsimony, *see* phylogenetics
partially directed acyclic graph, *see* PDAG
Pathfinder, 322
pattern recognition, 60
pattern-based learning, 72
PCA, *see* principal component analysis
PDAG, 35, 38, 39
PDM, 162, 168
global versus local, 165
illustration of, 163, 164
PDP++, 479
Pearl's message-passing algorithm, *see* Bayesian networks
peeling algorithm, *see* likelihood method in phylogenetics
penalty term, 14, 42, 53
penicillin resistance, 147
periodic respiration, 436
permutation test, 231
pharmacodynamics, 351, 352, 359, 360
pharmacokinetics, 351, 352, 360–362, 364
PHASE program, 200
PHYLIP, 122, 202
phylogenetic networks, 148, 151
phylogenetic tree
branch lengths, 85
consensus tree, 129, 135, 202
equivalence classes, 113, 114
interpreted as a Bayesian network, 111
mammalian, inferred from RNA genes, 203
of HIV and SIV strains, 87
outgroup, 84, 201, 202
rooted, 84, 85, 140
topology, 84
unrooted, 84, 86, 140
phylogenetics, 83
distance method, 90
failure of, 98
information loss, 100
likelihood method, *see* likelihood method in phylogenetics
parsimony method, 100, 171
failure of, 103
illustration of, 101, 102

long branch attraction, 104
phylogeny, *see* phylogenetics
physiologically-based models, 356
PK/PD models, 352, 365, 367, 368
PKBugs, 367, 477
PLATO, 156, 168
illustration of, 157
polymorphic sites, 152, 156
positive false discovery rate (pFDR), 233
posterior probability, 11
prediction, 391, 398
information for, 398
preprocessing, 77, 391–395
AR model, 393–395
Bayesian, 392–395
lattice filter, 393–395
stochastic model, 392, 393
principal component analysis, 234
principal component analysis (PCA), 77, 379
prior probability, 11
conjugate prior, 11
probabilistic divergence method, *see* PDM
probabilistic graphical models, *see* Bayesian networks
Probabilistic Networks Library, 483
probability
conditional, 3
joint, 3
marginal, 3
posterior, *see* posterior probability
prior, *see* prior probability
probability model, 66
prokaryotes, 192
Promedas, 320
promoter, 257, 258
protein, 212
degradation, 257, 259, 269
dimerization, 257–259
FYN binding, 289
sequences, 138
synthesis, 212
purines, 87, 105, 198
pyrimidines, 87, 105, 198

quantiles, 282, 284
quartet puzzling, *see* likelihood method in phylogenetics
Quick Medical Reference model, 319

R, 476
randomization test, 154
rate heterogeneity, *see* nucleotide substitutions
rate matrix, *see* nucleotide substitutions
Rauch-Tung-Streibel smoother, 276
receiver operator characteristics curve, *see* ROC curve
recombination, 147, 148
in *Neisseria*, 184
in HIV, 150
influence on phylogenetic inference, 149
simulation of, 168, 181
synthetic benchmark study, 167, 169, 170
RECPARS, 170, 182
reference design, 226
regression, 64
function, 64
linear, 64
logistic, *see* logistic regression
polynomial, 64
regularization term, *see* penalty term
REML, 226
reverse engineering, 239, 270, 283
reversibility condition, *see* nucleotide substitutions
reversible jump MCMC, *see* Markov chain Monte Carlo
ribonucleic acid, *see* RNA
RNA, 191
compensatory substitutions, 196
covariation, 195
mismatch (MM) base-pairs, 193, 198
mRNA, 212, 257, 258
mRNA degradation, 257, 259, 269
rRNA, 140, 141, 191
secondary structure, 193, 194
helices, 193, 194, 204
loops, 194, 204
secondary structure prediction, 193
comparative methods, 193
minimum free energy methods, 193
sequence alignment, 192, 195

stacking interactions, 194
tertiary structure, 193
tRNA, 191
Watson-Crick base-pairs, 193
ROC curve, 256, 261, 285–288, 414, 416
RR Intervals, 437
RTS smoother, *see* Rauch-Tung-Streibel smoother

S-Plus, 475
Streptococcus, 147
See5, 484
segmentation, 331
image, 333
sensitivity, 254, 285
sensor fusion, 391, 393, 396, 400, 413, 416
predictions, 413
spatio-temporal, 400, 413, 416
separator relations, *see* DAG, *see* DAG
simian immunodeficiency virus, *see* SIV
singular value decomposition (SVD), 234
SIV, 86
sleep EEG, 435
SNNS, 479
sparse candidate algorithm, 248, 270
specificity, 254, 285
Spiegelhalter–Lauritzen–MacKay approximation, 303
splicing, 212
split decomposition, 148
standard error of difference (SED), 230
state-space models, 272
controllability, 277
extended identifiability, 279
identifiability, 278
observability, 278
stability, 277
Statistica, 479
statistics
Bayesian, *see* Bayesian statistics
classical or frequentist, 5, 6, 127
comparison: frequentist versus Bayesian, 10, 12
step-down method, 232
stochastic model, 360, 364, 366
structural EM algorithm, *see* EM algorithm
structured variational approximation, 422
Stuttgart Neural Network Simulator, 478

T cell, *see* T lymphocytes
T lymphocytes, 289
t-test, 230
test set, 75
Tetrad, 480
ThinksPro, 479
Tiberius, 479
top-hat filter, *see* image analysis
TOPAL, 159, 168
dependence on the window size, 161
DSS statistic, 159
illustration of, 160
transcription, 212, 257–259
transcription factor, 257, 258
transition-transversion ratio, 108
transitions, *see* nucleotide substitutions
translation, 212, 257–259
transversions, *see* nucleotide substitutions
Treat, 452–470
tree metric, *see* metric
tree-based models
CART algorithm, 323, 327
class-probability trees, 323
classification trees, 323
cost-complexity pruning, 324
option trees, 326
surrogate split, 325
tree smoothing, 326
tree-type models
Bayesian tree induction, *see* Bayesian statistics, tree induction
missing data, *see* missing data, tree-type models
triangle inequality, 97

unweighted pair group method using arithmetic averages, *see* clustering, UPGMA
UPGMA, *see* clustering

v-structure, *see* DAG
validation set, 75
variable subset selection, 77, 375

variance-stabilizing transformation, 219
variational methods, 291, 320, 330, 332
  model-free mean-field update
    equations, 442
  cost function, 425
  framework, 420
Venn diagram, 3
VIBES, 484
Viterbi algorithm, *see* hidden Markov
    models

Watson-Crick base-pairs, *see* RNA
WebWeaver, 480
Welch-statistic, 230
WinBUGS, 363, 367, 368, 476

X-ray crystallography, 193
XOR regulation, 244

yeast cell cycle, 247

Printed in the United Kingdom
by Lightning Source UK Ltd.
109803UKS00005BC/15

9 781852 337780